Hip Arthroplasty

Minimally Invasive Techniques and Computer Navigation

Hip Arthroplasty

Minimally Invasive Techniques and Computer Navigation

LAWRENCE D. DORR, MD

Director, Dorr Arthritis Institute

Centinela Freeman Health System

Inglewood, California

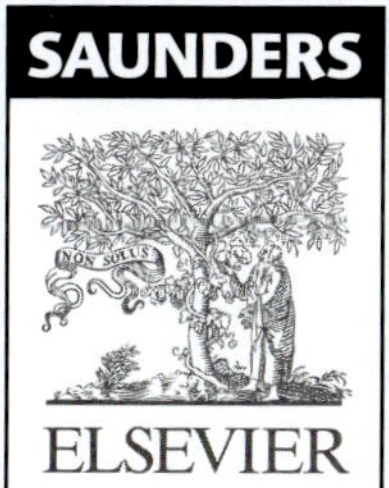

SAUNDERS

ELSEVIER

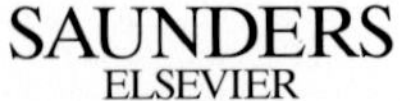

SAUNDERS
ELSEVIER

1600 John F. Kennedy Blvd.
Ste 1800
Philadelphia, PA 19103-2899

HIP ARTHROPLASTY: MINIMALLY INVASIVE TECHNIQUES AND
COMPUTER NAVIGATION

ISBN-13: 9781416022978
ISBN-10: 1-4160-2297-X

Copyright © 2006, Elsevier Inc.

Notice

Knowledge and best practice in this field are constantly changing. As new research and experience broaden our knowledge, changes in practice, treatment and drug therapy may become necessary or appropriate. Readers are advised to check the most current information provided (i) on procedures featured or (ii) by the manufacturer of each product to be administered, to verify the recommended dose or formula, the method and duration of administration, and contraindications. It is the responsibility of the practitioner, relying on their own experience and knowledge of the patient, to make diagnoses, to determine dosages and the best treatment for each individual patient, and to take all appropriate safety precautions. To the fullest extent of the law, neither the Publisher nor the Authors assume any liability for any injury and/or damage to persons or property arising out or related to any use of the material contained in this book.

The Publisher

Library of Congress Cataloging-in-Publication Data

Dorr, Lawrence D.
   Hip arthroplasty : minimally invasive techniques and computer navigation / Lawrence D. Dorr.—1st ed.
     p. cm.
   ISBN 1-4160-2297-X
   1. Total hip replacement. 2. Hip joint—Endoscopic surgery. 3. Computer-assisted orthopedic surgery. I. Title.
   RD549.D67 2006
   617.5′810592—dc22
                                   2005050438

ISBN-13: 9781416022978
ISBN-10: 1-4160-2297-X

Acquisitions Editor: Elyse O'Grady
Developmental Editor: Heather Krehling
Publishing Services Manager: Tina Rebane
Senior Project Manager: Amy Norwitz
Design Direction: Ellen Zanolle

Printed in China

Last digit is the print number: 9 8 7 6 5 4 3 2 1

To the best partner any doctor ever had,
Marilyn A. Dorr.

CONTRIBUTORS

Clive Duncan, MD
Professor and Head
Department of Orthopaedics
Faculty of Medicine
University of British Columbia
Vancouver, British Columbia
Canada
Video: *"Anterior Approach for Total Hip Replacement"*

Charles A. Engh Sr., MD
Medical Director
Joint Replacement Program
Inova Mt. Vernon Hospital
Medical Director
Anderson Orthopaedic Clinic
Alexandria, Virginia
Video: *"Simple Techniques for Revision Total Hip Replacement"*

Richard "Dickey" Jones, MD
Professor of Orthopedic Surgery
University of Texas Southwestern Medical Center
Chief of Orthopedic Surgery
Veterans Administration Medical Center
Orthopedic Surgeon
St. Paul University Hospital
Dallas, Texas
Chapter 9: *Anterolateral Approach for Mini-incision Total Hip Replacement*
Video: *"Anterolateral Approach for Total Hip Replacement"*

Wayne Paprosky, MD
Associate Professor of Orthopaedic Surgery
Rush University Medical College
Chicago, Illinois
Staff Orthopaedic Surgeon
Department of Adult Joint Reconstruction
Central Dupage Hospital
Winfield, Illinois
Video: *"Simple Techniques for Revision Total Hip Replacement"*

Andrew G. Yun, MD
Centinela Freeman Health System
Inglewood, California
Chapter 8: *The Anterior Mini-incision Intermuscular Approach: A Single Incision*

PREFACE

I have learned through my career that there are four stages in the maturation of a surgeon's practice of medicine. Whether a surgeon will progress through all four stages will probably affect his or her enjoyment of and fulfillment in his or her career. Many surgeons become stuck in the second stage, feeling defeated, because they do not recognize the natural progression through these stages. Some surgeons understand these stages early in their careers, while others do not. For some, it seems that the understanding of the fourth stage, which is to give back to the profession, occurs very early, and for these surgeons, a lifetime of contribution to the orthopedic and lay communities will provide substantial recognition and fulfillment.

The first stage of a career is the *thrill of victory*. This begins for most when they are accepted to medical school, and their tremendous boost in self-esteem builds as they endure the years of study. Most physicians share a sense of being a member of a team, or at least a member of a group who has suffered together in the medical training environment. Success in medical school, internship, and residency promotes in many medical students a feeling of victory because these years of study are so difficult, so important, and so rewarding. In the medical training environment the student feels as though everything that he or she will do will be worthwhile, helpful to others, and important. The thrill of seeing a patient be healed from a disease, undergo a successful operation, or overcome the mental and physical adversity of disease creates a sense of triumph for every medical student and the expectation that this is what he or she can accomplish with every patient treated. Certainly every physician enters his or her practice with a high expectation of promise for doing good and doing well.

The second stage of the medical career is the *agony of defeat*. It comes at a different time for each physician, but it usually occurs sooner rather than later after the physician has assumed total responsibility for patients and their care. Treatments do not work, operations fail, and patients do not like their results. The first time this occurs the physician may think it an aberration, but once a few failures have accumulated, the physician realizes that his or her expectations when beginning practice may not come to pass. In fact, the physician/surgeon may have more failures within the first 2 years of practice than he or she expected in a lifetime. How many times during training does a student see a patient transferred from another institution with a complication that causes the student to say, "I would never do something like that!" Yet sometimes within the first 2 years of practice, that physician's patient experiences a complication very similar to one that the student thought would never occur in one of his or her patients.

The most critical issue in the practice of the young physician is whether he or she is able to overcome the sense of failure that occurs during the second stage of the *agony of defeat*. If the physician cannot overcome this agony and comes to live with a fear of failure for every treatment, he or she begins to be like an athlete who plays not to lose, instead of to win. The enjoyment of practice is clouded by anxiety, and decision making is compromised by a fear of failure. For the physician who overcomes this *agony of defeat* and recognizes that it is a natural condition of being human, the chance for a promising career continues. Every leader in medicine has experienced dramatic failures in both research and clinical practice and yet has been able to recognize this as a phenomenon over which he or she has no control and has been able to go beyond these failures. It is absolutely critical that every young physician understand that this second stage of medicine occurs and that he or she must learn to adapt to it.

The third career stage is *There is a God, but it is not me.* It is the recognition of this fact that helps the physician overcome the sense of failure that occurs from the *agony of defeat.* This is the stage in which one recognizes one's limitations. One realizes that he or she must acknowledge that many of the results clearly occur with the help of God, that the ideas of others are sometimes better, and that others have contributed to one's knowledge and skills. There are complications that occur at the hand of the surgeon, and there are complications that occur at the hand of God. One complication that seems to occur at the hand of God is a sciatic nerve palsy. There is almost never a good explanation for why this occurred. Usually the surgery was conducted in the same manner as always and there were no untoward complications during the surgery, and yet at the completion of the surgery the patient has a sciatic nerve injury. Some instances could have an explanation, but most do not. This is a devastating complication for a patient and for a physician, yet there is little that the physician could have done to change this outcome. The surgeon must overcome his or her profound disappointment and depression after this outcome, particularly so that the complication can be treated in a positive and productive manner. On the other hand, there are many instances in which there has been a positive outcome of a surgery or treatment when there is no explanation as to why it was positive. Clearly, the hand of God resulted in the patient's doing better than expected. Every physician has seen an example of this, and I continue to marvel at the ability of the human body to adapt to injury. When the physician/surgeon is willing to accept that some of the good and bad events that occur are out of his or her control, the remainder of the surgeon's career should be full of enjoyment and fulfillment.

The fourth stage of medicine is *give back better than you took.* After acknowledging the previous three stages, it is rewarding to contribute to the orthopedic and lay communities, realizing that helping many with one deed or act is greater than each individual act of care. There are so many ways that physicians/surgeons can give back to their profession and their communities. Even teaching one resident is a tremendous repayment to the profession. I founded an organization called Operation Walk, which operates on economically disadvantaged people, both

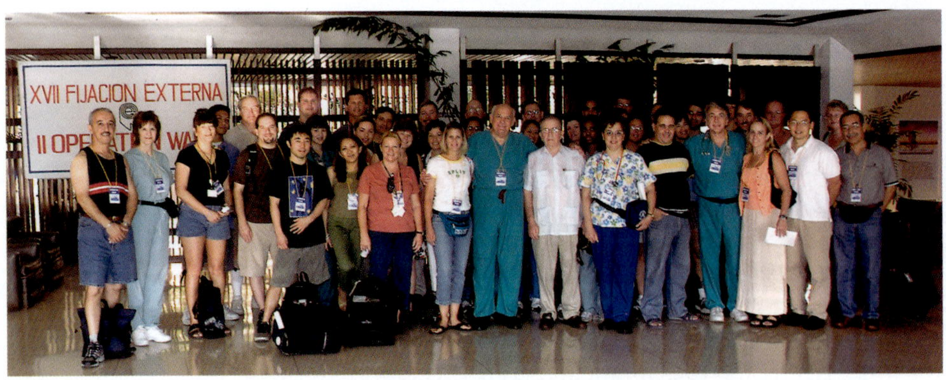

Operation Walk team on a mission to Cuba.

in the United States and in Third World countries. This has been tremendously satisfying for me and every health care professional who has participated in these trips.

This book is one of the final ways in which I can give back to my profession, and it is for that reason that I have written it.

Lawrence D. Dorr, MD

AKNOWLEDGMENTS

I would like to acknowledge all that I have learned from the Fellows with whom I have had the privilege of working and whom I have trained. I thank them for what they have taught me and for the thrill that they have given me as I watch them mature through the four stages of medicine.

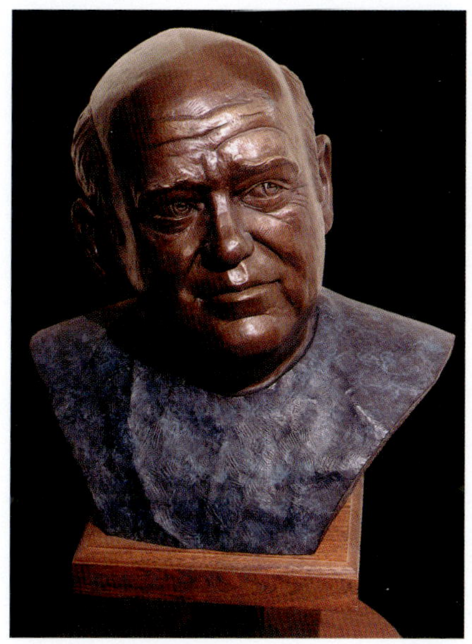

A present from the Fellows to Dr. Dorr in the year 2003.

Michael Absatz
David Apel
Rodney Barnhardt
David Bindelglass
Richard Boirado
Ronald Carn
Jonathan Cohen
Christopher Cox
Rolf Drinhaus
David Forgarty
Juan Frisancho
Lugi Galloni
Ramin Ganjianpour
Martin Hall
Arthur Harris
Michael Harris

Kevin Heaton
Yutaka Inaba
Alan Inglis Jr.
Brian Johnson
Thomas Kane
Joon-Soon Kang
George Kantor
Robert Klapper
David Kull
John Kumar
Kris Lewonowski
William Long
Donald Longjohn
Michael Lucero
Audley Mackel
Byung Woo Min

Lock Ochsner
William Overdyke
Jeffrey Passick
Kurt Possai
Steve Sanders
John Serocki
Cambize Shahrdar
Samuel Tawakkol
John Tozzi
Pacharapol Udomkiat
Zhinian Wan
Alan Wolf
Ye-Yeon Won
Steve Young
Robert Zann
James Zmolek

VIDEO CONTENTS

The following chapters have companion video clips on DVD-ROM.

CONTENTS

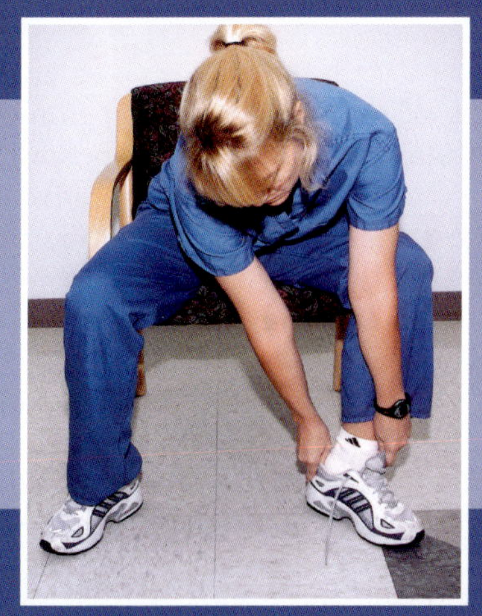

The New Process of Total Hip Replacement

The revolution in the care of the patient undergoing total hip replacement in the first decade of the 21st century has been more the improvement of the art of medical care than scientific improvement in joint implantation and operative technique. The new focus on patient care reflects a different type of incision and resulting operative injury and also important changes in anesthesia, pain management, and recovery. Even if a more standard-length incision is selected, a patient undergoing total hip replacement today has more positive expectations for the operation, enjoys the experience of the operation, recovers better than was previously possible, leaves the hospital sooner, and has the option of returning to work sooner. In this chapter, I outline the methods that will optimize the outcome from total hip replacement. These are categorized as preoperative care and education, intraoperative anesthesia and recovery room techniques, the pain management program, and postoperative rehabilitation and recovery techniques. Specifics of bilateral total hip replacement are also discussed.

PREOPERATIVE PATIENT CARE AND EDUCATION

Most people are intimidated by a visit to a doctor's office because they will have to discuss personal issues and may have to disrobe partially, and they dread learning that they need to have an operation. The initial communication of the surgeon's office with the patient is critical in establishing the patient's confidence in both the surgeon's skill and the care the patient will receive. The best methods of instilling confidence are friendly communication and thorough education. Patient education should include as much information regarding the operation as the patient desires; the patient should be informed about preoperative and operative procedures and the expected outcome.

Once the patient has made an appointment to see the surgeon, he or she should receive information that may relieve the anxiety created by visiting a doctor. The ideal form of communication is a video introducing the patient to the people that he or she will be meeting at the office visit and also perhaps some of the hospital personnel. The patient also will gain confidence by viewing the testimonials of other patients. One of the videos we use is included in the DVD-ROM provided with this book (*see "Patient Testimonials"*).

The preoperative class is one of the best techniques available to educate patients and their families because it provides information on what will happen to them and significantly eases the "fear of the unknown" that patients experience in entering a hospital. The preoperative class should be conducted by a person who is personable, confident, and knowedgeable. It includes information on all aspects of their care, ranging from preoperative logistics to the expectations of the hospital stay and the program of recovery. The preoperative class allows patients to meet some of the physical therapists and nurses with whom they will have contact in the hospital. Through a video, they can meet the anesthesiologist and learn about the type of anesthesia they will receive. The patients can be shown and be allowed to handle the implants. The class provides a forum in which they can ask all of the many questions they have, many of which arise after their initial visit with the doctor. This significantly decreases the burden on the surgeon of providing these answers during office time or in telephone calls. The outline of the preoperative class we use is shown in Table 1–1.

INTRAOPERATIVE ANESTHESIA AND RECOVERY ROOM TECHNIQUES

An important aspect of the patient care program is anesthesia care during surgery and in the recovery room. The goal of anesthesia care is to reduce anxiety and keep the patient safe and comfortable throughout the hospital stay. The anesthesiologist must reassure patients that he or she will stay with them throughout the surgery, monitoring and observing them from the initiation of anesthesia until they are safely awake and in the recovery room. After surgery, the anesthesiologist remains involved in pain control to help speed recovery.

Successful anesthesia for hip replacement has to meet the challenges of rapid ambulation and discharge, if not on the same day, then within 48 hours. The anesthesiologist should (1) address pain control before surgery begins, (2) prophylactically treat nausea and vomiting, and (3) use anesthesia techniques that favor regional anesthesia over the use of general anesthesia with parenteral narcotics.

Our anesthesiologist meets the patient in the preoperative area. By this time, the anesthesia plan has been established and initial reservations, concerns, and questions about different types of anesthesia have been resolved and answered. Our premedication includes oral oxycodone (OxyContin), 10 mg; celecoxib (Celebrex), 400 mg; acetaminophen (Tylenol), 500 mg; and lansoprazole (Prevacid), 30 mg. This combination addresses pain relief and anti-inflammatory response by combining a potent narcotic and a cyclooxygenase (COX)-2 and COX-3 inhibitor. Prevacid, 30 mg, is given orally for gastric mucosa protection, and midazolam (Versed), 1 to 2 mg, is given intravenously for sedation. In the preoperative area, all patients are placed in the seated position and an epidural catheter is placed and tested for efficacy.

Table 1–1
Preoperative Class

The general principle of the preoperative class is to educate patients before surgery to make their recovery easier. The preoperative class is intended to take the "mystery" out of the surgical and hospital experience. Patients are informed of everything from what to bring to the hospital to how their leg will feel during the different phases of recovery. They are taught exercises, how to use walking devices such as crutches and canes, and how to use adaptive equipment to help with showering and dressing. Patients are encouraged to use these devices in class to become comfortable with their use before surgery.

We have found that it is easier for patients and their families to learn in a classroom setting with other patients undergoing the same type of procedures. Patients and family are encouraged to ask questions and interact with the staff.

In Preoperative Class, We Cover

Prehospitalization procedures, including blood donation, clearance by Internal Medicine physician, signing of consents, and time of arrival at hospital on day of surgery date

Preoperative skin cleansing and care

Complete explanation of basic joint replacement surgery: visualization of hip model; hands-on joint replacement components to examine weight, texture, and fit to bone

Preoperative medication planning: when to stop anti-inflammatory drugs and aspirin-containing medications; explanation of what over-the-counter medications and alternative medications to avoid

Hospital admission procedure: where to report for surgery; who will greet you and help prepare you for your operation; what time to report to the hospital

Limb identification for ensuring correct surgery on day of operation

Approximate time the surgery will take; where your family can wait comfortably for you during your operation

Anesthesia: what type is used; reduction of side effects with epidural anesthesia

Postoperative feelings in the leg, and how your leg will feel at different times during recovery

Timing and correct methods for icing and elevating your leg after surgery

Bowel protocol to avoid constipation both before and after surgery

Foods to incorporate into your diet for the benefit of healing and blood rejuvenation

Wound care

Follow-up phone calls and appointments, and when you will be expected to return to the clinic

---

The advantages of epidural versus general anesthetic for total hip and total knee arthroplasties can be summarized in three categories.

1. Decreased intraoperative bleeding (blood loss is less using a regional technique than with general anesthesia, in spite of maintaining a similar mean arterial blood pressure)

2. Decreased deep venous thrombosis and pulmonary embolism (by increasing blood flow to lower extremities, decreasing platelet reactivity, and attenuating the postoperative increase in factor VIII and von Willebrand's factor)

3. Decreased nausea, vomiting, and recovery room time

Although long-term morbidity and mortality statistics are similar for total hip and total knee replacements with general anesthesia versus regional anesthesia, the immediate postoperative recovery represents a clear handicap for patients treated with inhalation anesthesia and intravenous narcotic (increased nausea and vomiting, which delay recovery, and greater problems with pain control). Sickness and lethargy have a negative impact on early ambulation and discharge. Increasing nausea and vomiting, in particular, should be addressed and aggressively treated. A regimen that includes pro-phylactic metoclopramide (Reglan) and ondansetron (Zofran), granisetron (Kytril), or dolasetron (Anzemet) every 4 hours is advised for the first 24 hours.

The Operating Room

In the operating room, an arterial line is started for safe monitoring and control of hypotension (in the case of a bilateral knee procedure, a Swan-Ganz catheter also is started for pulmonary artery blood pressure monitoring).

The epidural catheter is activated with a combination of lidocaine (Xylocaine) 2%, for a total of 80 mg, and ropivacaine (Naropin) 1%, 80 mg (this amount is sufficient for most patients). The combination of these two amides produces a relatively fast-setting block in 10 to 20 minutes that provides ideal conditions for hip and knee surgeries and has a median duration of 2 to 3 hours.

A continuous infusion of propofol (Diprivan), 5 to 10 mg/kg/hour, is initiated. This amount renders most patients unresponsive in 3 to 5 minutes. The airway is managed with either an oral airway or a laryngeal mask; both very well tolerated with a continuous infusion of propofol. This infusion should stop approximately 10 minutes before the end of the procedure. Most patients will be responsive by the time they are moved from the operating room table.

Pain Control

Pain control begins before surgery with oral medications and continues during surgery with an intra-articular injection given by the surgeon. This injection contains ropivacaine, 100 mg, methylprednisolone (Depo-Medrol), 40 mg, and morphine sulfate, 4 mg, administered with 60 mL of saline for volume.

Hip patients have their epidural catheter removed after surgery. Their pain is managed with only oral anti-inflammatory agents and oral narcotics. We use Celebrex, 400 mg orally daily, with hydrocodone and acetaminophen (Norco or Vicodin) or propoxyphene and acetaminophen (Darvon or Darvocet), depending on age and tolerance. For patients older than 80 years of age, acetaminophen (Tylenol) is often the only oral medication given. We do not use a patient-controlled analgesia (PCA) pump, epidural narcotics, or intramuscular or intravenous push narcotics.

The success of this anesthesia and pain management protocol requires that the recovery room nurses, floor nurses, and physician assistants be educated and comfortable in caring for patients who have epidural or femoral nerve catheters. The use of only oral pain medications for the treatment of pain and the program of rapid mobilization and discharge require a culture change on the part of nurses and therapists. It is critically important that they be educated in the advantages of this program, or their cooperation may be insufficient to allow success.

PAIN MANAGEMENT TECHNIQUES

The heart and soul of the new process of total hip replacement is the change in pain management techniques. There is a choice of epidural, spinal, or general anesthesia, and, appropriately administered, any of these three can be used effectively with the new process of total hip replacement. We prefer epidural anesthesia for the reasons previously listed. However, no matter which mode of anesthesia is chosen, the pain management program must be adhered to strictly to allow the patient to be rapidly mobilized and discharged from the hospital and to enjoy the experience of the operation. The pain management program is directed toward preventing the onset of pain sensitization, as prevention is far easier to accomplish than controlling pain that has overcome the patient. Enough knowledge is available about the pathways of the origin and distribution of pain that particular medications can be used to prevent both central and peripheral sensitization. This pain management can be

accomplished without the use of intravenous or epidural narcotics. This change virtually eliminates the occurrence of nausea, emesis, dizziness with ambulation, and postoperative lethargy and depression.

A new world opens up for the surgeon, nurses, and therapists caring for the patient when this pain management protocol is used. Patients get some sleep at night, are not sick, and have a positive attitude toward therapy and discharge from the hospital. Nurses do not spend the majority of their time dealing with the patient's nausea, dizziness, and general feeling of sickness. Therapists are not prevented from mobilizing the patient because of the same symptoms. The surgeon can conduct rounds during which the patient expresses gratitude for the experience and the care, rather than rounds that are filled with complaints and queries about multiple adverse symptoms. The pain management protocol is described next, and an outline of our pain management program is given in Table 1–2.

Pain Protocol

The pain protocol is multimodal, involving use of more than two analgesic agents with different modes of action. We believe that it is easier to prevent pain and inflammation at the central and peripheral levels than it is to reduce it once it is established. For central modulation, we use oral opiates, epidural anesthesia, and COX-2 inhibitors. Locally, we use the "cocktail injection," which consists of 100 mg of ropivacaine, 4 mg of morphine, 40 mg of Depo-Medrol, and 60 mL of saline for volume.

Once tissue is damaged, noxious stimuli initiate a response from peripheral sensory neurons to release neurotransmitters in the dorsal horn neurons of the spinal cord. Acute pain is produced when these neurotransmitters relay the sensory information to the thalamus. If inflammation is treated appropriately, normal hypersensitivity will resolve without causing major biochemical changes. If inflammation persists, an alteration in receptors occurs, causing an increased sensitization of peripheral sensory neurons where the COX-2 isoenzyme is induced in dorsal horn neurons and the thalamus, ventral midbrain, and pons.

Before surgery, we use three medications to prevent postoperative pain. OxyContin (10 mg) is an opioid that mimics the actions of endogenous opioid peptides in the central nervous system. When the medication activates the mu opioid receptors, excitatory pathway transmission of acetylcholine, serotonin, and substance P (a neuropeptide active in neurons that mediate pain sensation) is inhibited. Celebrex (400 mg) is used to decrease inflammation and pain by selectively inhibiting the COX-2 isoenzyme and prostaglandin production. If a patient is unable to take Celebrex because of a sulfa allergy, we give acetaminophen (Tylenol,

Table 1–2
Arthritis Institute Total Hip Arthroplasty Pain Protocol

Note: Patients do NOT need to stop Celebrex before surgery

Preoperative (Morning of Surgery)

1. OxyContin, 10 mg PO
2. Celebrex, 400 mg PO (if allergic to sulfa, then no NSAIDs)
3. Tylenol 500 mg PO
4. Prevacid, 30 mg PO
5. If allergic to sulfa drugs, Lembril 1000 mg

Recovery Room

1. For bilateral hips, keep epidural catheter capped until transferred to floor
2. For primary hips, pull epidural catheter in operating room
3. ASA 600 mg per rectum
4. Toradol, 30 mg IV × 1 dose as need for mild to moderate pain (15 mg IV if older than 65 years)
5. OxyIR, 5 mg PO as needed for severe pain
6. Ice applied to operated hip

Floor Program

1. If younger than 65 years, Norco, 10 mg, 1 tablet PO, alternating with Tylenol ES, 500 mg PO every 4 hours from 6 PM to 6 AM × 2 days
2. If older than 65 years, Darvon, 65 mg, 1 tablet PO, alternating with Tylenol ES, 500 mg PO every 4 hours from 6 PM to 6 AM × 2 days
3. Celebrex, 200 mg PO twice daily, starting postoperative day 1, or Lembril, 500 mg PO twice daily

4. Vicodin, 5 mg/500 mg, 1 to 2 tablets PO every 3 hours as needed for pain
5. Norco, 10 mg/325 mg 1 to 2 tablets PO every 3 hours as needed for pain
6. Darvocet N-100 1 tablet PO every 4 hours as needed for pain (if older than 65 years)
7. Ancef (cefazolin), 1 g IVPB every 8 hours × 24 hours
8. Anzemet, 12.5 mg IV every 6 hr × 24 hours
9. If reflux disease, Zofran, 4 mg IV every 6 hours x 24 hours (instead of Anzemet)
10. Reglan, 10 mg IV IVP every 8 hours x 48 hours
11. Enteric-coated acetylsalicylic acid (ECASA), 325 mg, 1 tablet PO twice a day
12. MOM, 30 mL every 8 hours
13. Colace, 100 mg PO twice a day
14. Dulcolax suppository per rectum daily as needed for constipation
15. Prevacid, 30 mg PO twice a day
16. Dietary for food preferences
17. Regular diet
18. Cream of wheat for breakfast daily to avoid need for iron tablets

Discharge

1. Celebrex, 200 mg PO twice a day x 21 days (total of 3 weeks), or Lembril, 500 mg PO twice a day
2. ECASA, 325 mg, 1 tablet PO twice a day (for 30 days after surgery)
3. Prevacid, 30 mg twice a day (while on ECASA)
4. Pain medications (whatever patient was on while in hospital)

---

500 mg) and Lembril (1000 mg). Tylenol affects the COX-3 receptors and elevates a patient's pain threshold. To prevent stomach irritation from these three pain relievers, we give one dose of the proton pump inhibitor Prevacid (30 mg).

During the operation, we use medications to produce a local response. An epidural infusion of ropivacaine is used, accompanied by propofol. A cocktail of ropivacaine (100 mg), morphine (4 mg), Depo-Medrol (40 mg), and 60 mL of saline for volume is injected into the joint to prevent peripheral sensitization. The cocktail is injected into the capsule, muscle, and subcutaneous tissue to prevent peripheral sensitization. The corticosteroid prevents local inflammation, and morphine stimulates the mu receptors.

In the recovery room, if the patient is having pain, we give ketorolac (Toradol), 15 to 30 mg intravenously, depending on the age and creatinine level of the patient. Toradol is a COX-2 inhibitor that prevents the formation of prostaglandins and decreases inflammation. For moderate to severe pain, we also give a fast-acting opioid, oxycodone (OxyIR), 5 mg orally, to activate the mu opioid receptors.

Once the patient is transferred to the orthopedic floor, we continue COX-2 inhibition by giving Celebrex, 400 mg twice a day, beginning on postoperative day 1. If the patient is sulfa allergic, we substitute Tylenol, 500 to 1000 mg four times daily (maximum dose, 4000 mg/day), or Limbrel, 1000 mg twice a day. For the first two nights, a combination of an oral opioid and Tylenol is given every 4 hours from 6 PM to 6 AM. Patients younger than 65 years of age alternate Norco and Tylenol, 500 mg, every 4 hours, and those older than 65 years of age alternate Darvon, 65 mg, and Tylenol, 500 mg, every 4 hours. During the rest of the hospitalization, patients take either Norco, Vicodin, Darvocet, or Tylenol as needed for pain, depending on tolerability.

Through our research, we have found that this protocol prevents the onset of pain for most of patients, as well as the nausea, dizziness, and vomiting associated with intravenous narcotics. Our patients are able to ambulate on the day of surgery, with pain grades of 1 to 3 on a scale of 10, and leave the hospital within 48 to 72 hours (Tables 1–3 to 1–5). We have a same-day discharge program available for those who wish it.

PHYSICAL THERAPY TECHNIQUE FOR RAPID DISCHARGE

Many years ago, the typical patient undergoing joint replacement surgery was at least 70 years of age. Today, younger patients are being diagnosed with arthritis and searching for ways to resume a pain-free, active lifestyle. With advancements in surgical technology and better implants, these patients can undergo joint replacement surgery much earlier and experience improved longevity of their joint. This group of patients is physically stronger and motivated to get back to a normal life as soon as possible. Therefore, the Arthritis Institute physical therapy staff has created the Minimally Invasive Surgery (MIS) program to meet these demands.

The patient is initiated into the program by attending an extended preoperative teaching class. Patients and family members will meet the physical therapist (PT) and occupational therapist (OT). Techniques for early mobilization (getting in and out of bed, getting out of a chair) and progressive ambulation (using crutches or a cane) while maintaining hip precautions, and education in a home exercise/walking program are provided by the PT. Techniques for using adaptive equipment to complete activities of daily living (bathing, dressing) are demonstrated by the OT. This training session allows the patient and family members to ask questions, alleviate any concerns, and practice with ambulatory devices and adaptive equipment.

Table 1–3
Summary of Pain Score and Analgesia Requirements

	Mini-incision 2002 Group	Mini-incision 2004 Group	P Value
Pain during Hospital Stay*			
Day of surgery	3.0 ± 0.9	0.9 ± 0.9	P < .01
Day 1 after surgery	3.0 ± 0.9	2.0 ± 1.0	P < .01
Day 2	3.6 ± 1.0	2.5 ± 1.1	P < .01
Day 3	2.9 ± 1.1	1.6 ± 0.8	P < .01
Day of discharge	2.4 ± 1.0	1.7 ± 0.7	P < .01
Pain after Discharge†			
6 wk after surgery	40.9 ± 4.6	43.7 ± 1.0	P < .01
3 mo	43.6 ± 0.6	43.9 ± 0.6	N.S.
Analgesia Requirements (Tablets/Person)			
Opioid–Analgesic Combinations			
Day of surgery	0.8 ± 0.7	0.3 ± 0.6	P < .01
Day 1 after surgery	4.1 ± 2.2	1.9 ± 1.7	P < .01
Day 2	4.4 ± 2.2	2.7 ± 2.0	P < .01
Day 3	3.4 ± 2.6	2.1 ± 1.5	N.S.
Nonopioid Analgesia			
Day of surgery	0.3 ± 0.5	0.6 ± 0.6	P < .01
Day 1 after surgery	0.5 ± 0.8	0.6 ± 0.7	N.S.
Day 2	0.7 ± 1.2	1.2 ± 1.0	P < .01
Day 3	0.2 ± 0.6	1.3 ± 0.8	P < .01

*The self-assessment pain score (0–10) was used for the evaluation of pain during the hospital stay.
†The pain component of the Harris Hip Score (10–44) was used for the evaluation of pain at 6 weeks or 3 months.
N.S., not significant.

Table 1–4
Summary of Functional Data

	Mini-incision 2002 Group	Mini-incision 2004 Group	P Value
Length of hospital stay (hr)	95.5 ± 24.8	73.1 ± 17.4	$P < .01$
Transfer to a rehabilitation unit	2 (2%)	0 (0%)	
Assistive Device Use			
At discharge			$P < .01$
Cane	22/86 (26%)	50/86 (58%)	
Single crutch	8 (9%)	17 (20%)	
Double crutches	49 (57%)	15 (17%)	
Walker	7 (8%)	4 (5%)	
At 6 wk after surgery			$P < .05$
No device	54/86 (62%)	67/86 (78%)	
Cane	22 (26%)	12 (14%)	
Single crutch	5 (6%)	1 (1%)	
Double crutches	4 (5%)	6 (7%)	
Walker	1 (1%)	0 (0%)	
At 3 mo after surgery			N.S.
No device	86/86 (100%)	84/86 (98%)	
Cane	0 (0%)	2 (2%)	
Muscle Strength*			
At 6 wk after surgery			
Straight leg raising	4.3 ± 0.7	4.7 ± 0.5	$P < .01$
Straight leg abduction	4.5 ± 0.6	4.8 ± 0.4	$P < .01$
At 3 mo			
Straight leg raising	4.9 ± 0.3	5.0 ± 0.2	N.S.
Straight leg abduction	4.9 ± 0.3	5.0 ± 0.2	N.S.

*Manual Muscle Testing (0–5) was used for the evaluation of muscle strength at 6 weeks and 3 months.
N.S., not significant.

Table 1–5
Numbers of Patients by Length of Hospital Stay

Lengths of Hospital Stay (hr)	Numbers of Patients	
	Mini-incision 2002 Group	Mini-incision 2004 Group
0–12	0	3 (4%)
13–24	0	0
25–48	3 (4%)	11 (13%)
49–72	29 (34%)	57 (66%)
73–96	33 (38%)	15 (17%)
97+	21 (24%)	0

Postoperative Rehabilitation

Early mobilization is crucial to avoid postoperative side effects and complications. Physical therapy begins on the day of surgery and includes instruction in bed mobility, transfers, and gait/stairs and a review of the home exercise/walking program. The PT will see the patient twice a day to help in the rapid progression of their mobility. At the time of discharge, the PT assists the patient with the car transfer. The OT sees the patient once a day for bathing and dressing and instruction in the use of the adaptive equipment. The OT educates the patient in bathroom mobility safety, including a commode transfer and transfer in and out of a tub or shower.

The anticipated discharge may be influenced by the patient's physiologic response to anesthesia, medications, and pain control. For example, the patient may experience prolonged numbness and impaired motor control from epidural analgesia. When this happens, therapy is initiated once these symptoms resolve (usually within a couple of hours). Patients may also experience orthostatic hypotension or nausea from the anesthesia, epidural, or narcotics. Therefore, the PT must check with nursing to ensure administration of medication and monitoring of the patient's blood pressure with positional changes.

The primary focus with physical and occupational therapy is to maximize function and independence while ensuring patient safety on discharge. The patient and family members must verbalize and integrate the safety precautions before release from hospital. Because of thorough preoperative education and extensive training sessions, the length of stay for patients undergoing same-day discharge has been significantly reduced. Patients can be discharged as soon as the day of surgery and no later than 48 hours after surgery.

The typical patient undergoing MIS is younger than 65 years of age. The patient must have family or a caregiver who will be available to assist him or her after discharge. Both the patient and family must be motivated for early discharge to ensure an optimal and safe outcome.

Patients need to be familiar with ambulating with assistive devices before discharge from the hospital. For patients who are discharged on the day of surgery, this education must be provided in the preoperative class, and the patients must work with the assistive devices in the class to ensure safety and confidence. Eighty percent of patients can go home with a cane or a single crutch. A few go home with a walker, and the rest go home with two crutches. Some go home with two crutches because they do not feel safe walking out of doors initially with a cane; they can advance to a cane as soon as they feel comfortable doing so. Patients do go home fully weight bearing on the operative leg. If both legs have been operated on, patients still can walk because they are fully weight bearing on both legs.

There are two therapy programs for the postoperative patient, a walking program and a stretchng program. We do not refer the patient to outpatient physical therapy, and for most patients we do not have a home therapist. With the new process of hip replacement, patients feel so much better and are so much more confident that they can be discharged home and do not require very much supervised therapy. Our use of the hospital Rehabilitation Department after acute care on the hospital floor shrank from 40% in 2000 to 1% in 2004. These data reflect the increased confidence and strength of the patients undergoing surgery with the new anesthesia and pain management program, as well as the use of smaller incisions.

Our walking program is the most important postoperative therapy. We encourage patients to set a goal of walking 1 mile and to do so within 2 weeks. This can initially be done with crutches, and when the patients feel strong with crutches they can advance to a cane and then dispense with assistive devices. This weaning of assistive devices is left to the discretion of the patients, who will make the correct choice because they want to be safe. Patients are instructed in the heel–toe gait pattern, which is of great importance for the restoration of normal muscle function (Fig. 1–1). The heel–toe

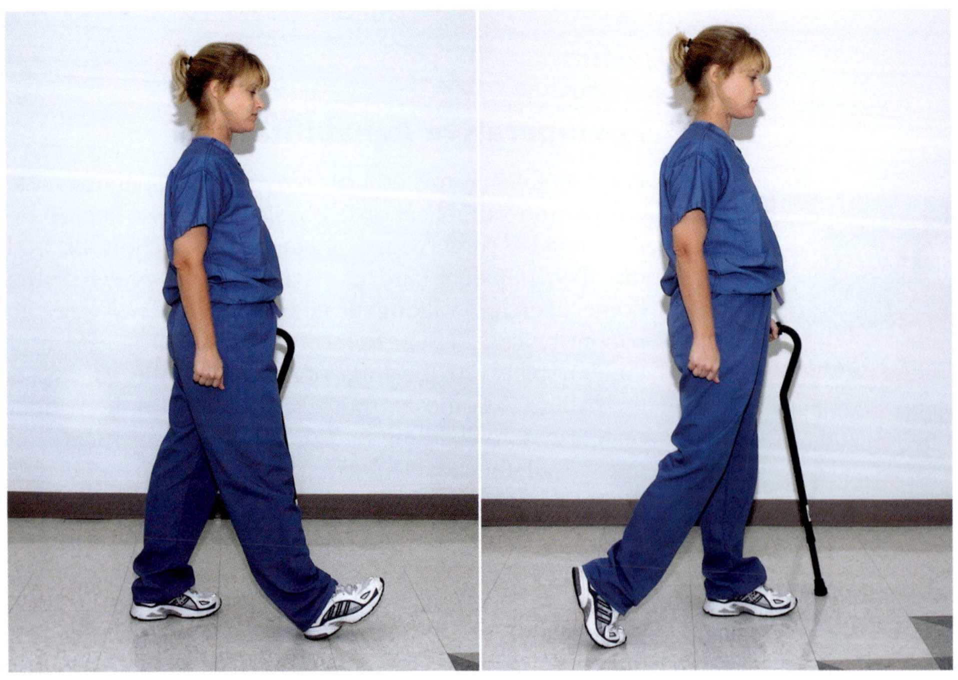

A   B

Figure 1–1 **A,** *The physical therapist demonstrates the heel–toe gait with the cane in the hand opposite the operative hip. This figure illustrates the heel strike.* **B,** *This figure demonstrates the toe-off. Training in the use of the heel–toe gait eliminates the preoperative pattern of a flat-footed gait seen in almost all arthritic patients who require surgery.*

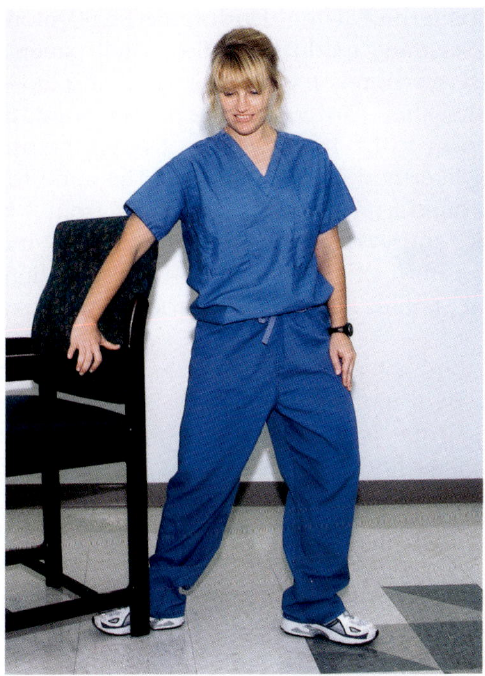

Figure 1–2　*The physical therapist demonstrates the adductor stretch exercise. The foot is fixed against an object and the trunk and hip are internally rotated against this resistance to stretch the adductors.*

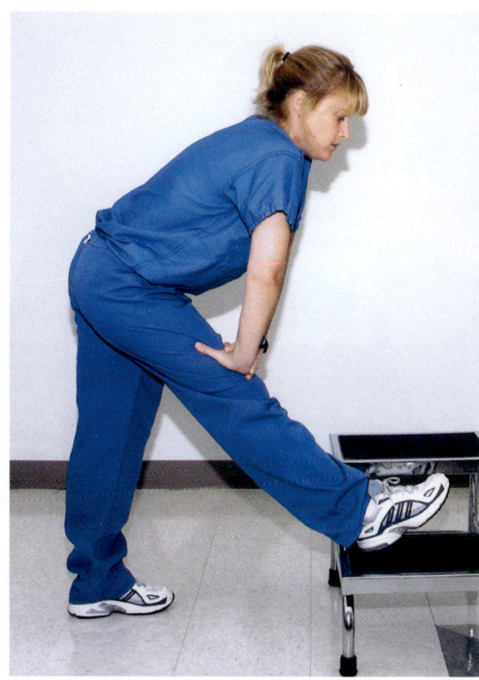

Figure 1–3　*The physical therapist demonstrates the hamstring stretch. The foot is placed on an elevated stool or chair and the trunk is leaned over the hip. The more the hamstring stretches, the farther the trunk can lean.*

pattern is the normal gait pattern, and it retrains the muscles from the stiff-legged arthritic gait pattern. The muscles of the hip have a normal phasic firing pattern that is disrupted with arthritis.[1] We have demonstrated this in gait studies. Our current gait studies with patients with the posterior mini-incision show that these patients function at approximately 80% of normal for stride characteristics by 6 to 12 weeks after surgery (see Table 1–3). Electromyographic tests do not show normal phasic firing of the muscles at 6 to 12 weeks after surgery, but test results return to normal by at least 1 year after surgery.[1] The only muscle with a normal dynamic EMG at 6 weeks is the gluteus maximus.

The second therapy program we use consists of stretching exercises. We want the patient to emphasize strengthening the gluteus medius and abductor complex of muscles. Abduction exercises are taught for this purpose; beyond this, no other specific exercises are critical. Stretching exercises are of great benefit for the patient because they will increase the comfort of the hip and its functional range of motion. The arthritic hip in particular has tightness in the adductors and the hamstrings. Figure 1–2 shows the exercises used to stretch the adductors, and Figure 1–3 shows the exercises for the hamstrings. These can be begun immediately after surgery. The anterior compartment muscles should also be stretched (and the gastrocnemius strengthened); this is done with toe raises (Fig. 1–4). The Achilles tendon, gastrocnemius, and hamstring can also be further stretched by an exercise in which the patient leans

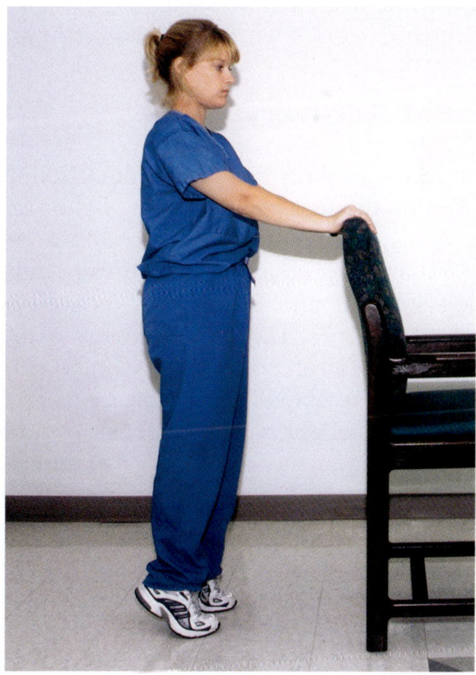

Figure 1–4　*The physical therapist demonstrates toe raises. Toe raises help in strengthening the gastrocnemius muscle and stretching the anterior compartment muscles.*

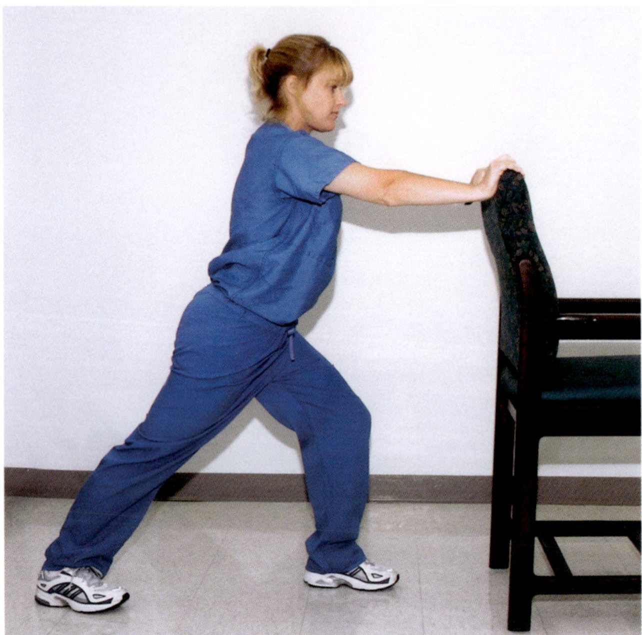

Figure 1–5 *The physical therapist demonstrates the stretch for the gastrocnemius and Achilles tendon. This is most commonly done by leaning into a wall so that there is a pulling sensation across the back of the leg, particularly across the back of the knee and along the calf. As the muscle stretches, the angle of lean into the wall can be gradually increased.*

forward with the leg extended (Fig. 1–5). These are the postoperative exercises we recommend for patients.

Pattern of Recovery

The pattern of healing can be summarized in three phases. During the first phase, which lasts 6 weeks, the patient regains energy and confidence in the body and the hip. Walking is a critical activity during this time to regain leg strength and confidence, as well as build endurance for energy. The loss of energy is much less with the avoidance of postoperative intravenous narcotics. With the use of oral pain medications, in dosages no greater than necessary, the patient's metabolism is not so lethargic and the recovery of energy is faster. Still, it takes 6 weeks before the patient is able to go all day without some rest or without having to retire early in the evening.

The second phase lasts from 6 weeks to 3 months. By 3 months, the patient has good stamina, and traveling is easy. For patients who want to return to golf, they certainly can be playing by 3 months if they use a cart. I tell people who want to play golf that when they can walk 5 miles, they can walk the golf course. This of course will differ by individuals but is a good measuring index. People who like to play golf can go to the golf course and chip and putt 1 week after surgery. It is a good activity to get them out of the house and use their legs, and to feel like they are returning to a more normal pattern of living. During the first 3 months, the patient's stamina gradually builds. I tell patients when they first go home to use the "2-hour plan," which means that they can go anywhere they want, but they should plan to be home within 2 hours because they will feel like they need some rest. This time for activities can build from 2 hours to 3 hours, from 3 hours to 4 hours, and so forth, according to the individual patient's return of stamina. By 3 months patients have sufficient stamina to be easily productive for an entire day.

The third phase lasts from 3 to 6 postoperative months. By 6 months, the patient has a good return of strength in the leg and can participate in more vigorous activities. Sports such as skiing, hiking in the mountains, and lifting and carrying objects can all be reasonably done at 6 months. There is a clear distinction in the coordination of the leg at 6 months compared with 3 months. Even after 6 months, continuing to 1 year postoperatively, the patient will observe a subtle increase in strength, so that at 1 year the leg is clearly stronger than it was even at 6 months. Still, at 6 months the leg has sufficient strength that vigorous activities can be done safely and enjoyed.

Recovery from hip replacement is much easier than that from knee replacement. Perhaps this is because the hip is a ball and socket joint; perhaps it is because it is a deeper joint and pain secondary to swelling of the joint is not so prevalent; or perhaps it is because the struggle to regain flexibility in the knee is more painful. Regardless of the reason, patients with hip replacement can be more active and are more comfortable much sooner than patients with knee replacement. This increased comfort level also allows patients to be more athletically active, more productive in work, and weaned off assistive devices sooner.

Although it has always been true that patients with hip replacement heal more easily than those with knee replacement, the accelerated postoperative recovery for patients undergoing the new process of total hip replacement still has been dramatic. Clearly, the patient's metabolism is not compromised as much with the current anesthesia and pain management techniques, and the patient feels better, sleeps better, and heals better because the mental aspect of the experience is so much more positive. Please view the testimonials of patients who have experienced this new process of total hip replacement to get a full understanding of its benefits for patients (*see "Patient Testimonials"*).

Chapter 11 is a detailed autobiographical history of the healing pattern after total hip replacement. This information will be helpful to the physician in truly understanding what the patient experiences in the first weeks and months after the operation.

Dislocation Precautions

Dislocation has been a complication feared by surgeons and patients throughout the history of total hip replacement. Even worse than the physical compromise and pain that occur with a dislocation is the mental stress it creates for the patient.[2] The patient is constantly fearful of dislocating with any level of activity and therefore avoids going out in public. It is critical to perform an operation that will prevent dislocation, and if the patient does experience dislocation, it is also critical that it be correctly treated.

With current surgical techniques such as the posterior mini-incision, which leaves most of the hip capsule intact, the hip is more stable after surgery. Perhaps the greatest help in avoiding dislocation is the use of the computer, which ensures that impingement is avoided with the hip replacement. Almost all dislocations occur because of instability due to impingement.

The strict dislocation precautions that were previously necessary with posterior hip replacements are no longer required. We now allow patients to sit on regular chairs (Fig. 1–6). To get into and out of the chair, the patient sits on the edge of the chair with a straight leg and, when seated, just slides to the back of the chair. To stand, the leg is drawn back under the trunk as the patient rises from the chair (Fig. 1–7). Patients can cross their legs (Fig. 1–8), although this will cause some pull in the back of the hip for 1 to 2 months after surgery, and they need to be reassured that this is not dangerous and that the activity depends on their comfort.

Patients can bend down between their knees if they always keep the hip in an externally rotated position (Fig. 1–9). They can bend over to pick up objects if they put the operative leg behind them (Fig. 1–10). We do recommend that patients use a raised toilet seat. A raised toilet seat provides great comfort for the patient

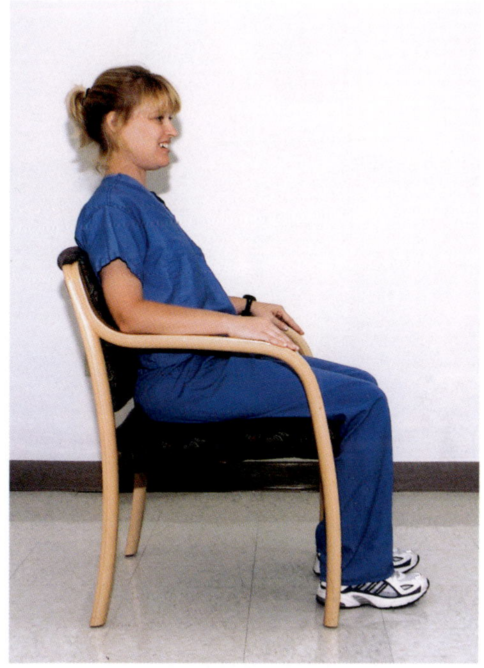

Figure 1–6　*The physical therapist demonstrates sitting in a regular chair in a normal fashion. This is acceptable immediately after surgery even with a posterior incision.*

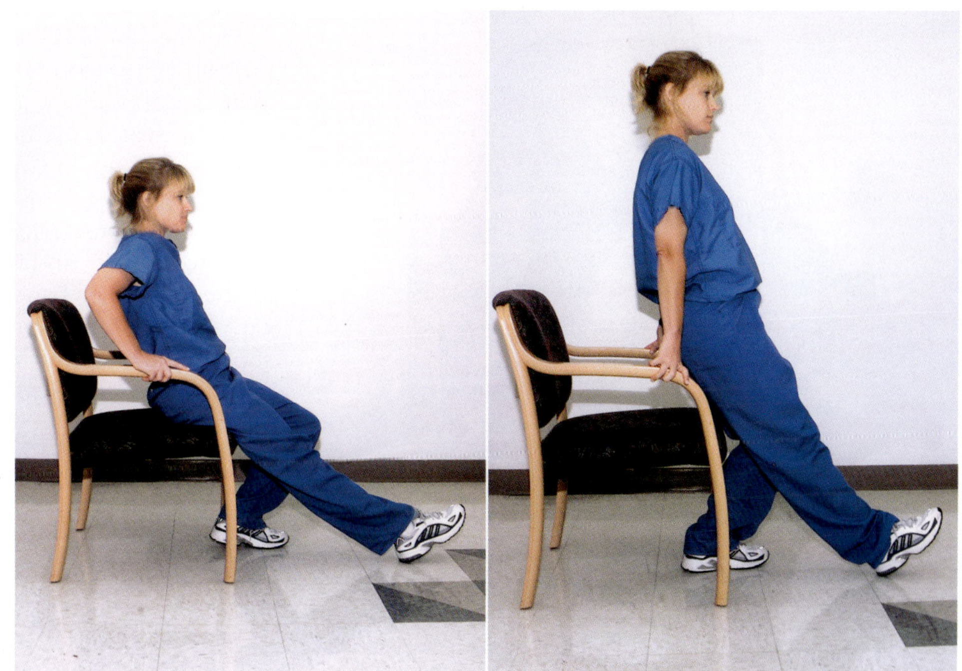

Figure 1–7　**A,** *In the early postoperative period it is safest to get out of the chair by simply sliding to the front of the chair and pushing off with the nonoperative leg with the operative leg extended. The operative leg does not need to be extended as straight as is shown here unless it is more comfortable for the patient.* **B,** *As the patient stands, the leg that was straight is drawn back under the patient to allow him or her to stand with balance and proceed with walking.*

A　　　　　　　　　　　　　　　B

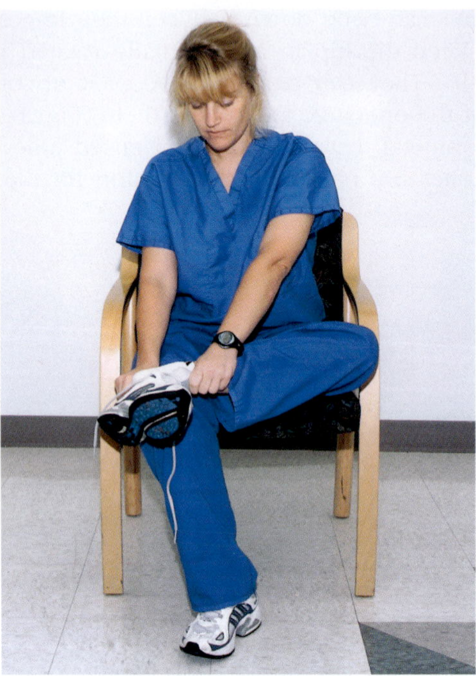

Figure 1–8   *The operative leg can be crossed over the non-operative leg immediately after surgery to allow placement of shoes and stockings. This maneuver causes a pulling sensation in the back of the hip, and it may have to be gradually attained.*

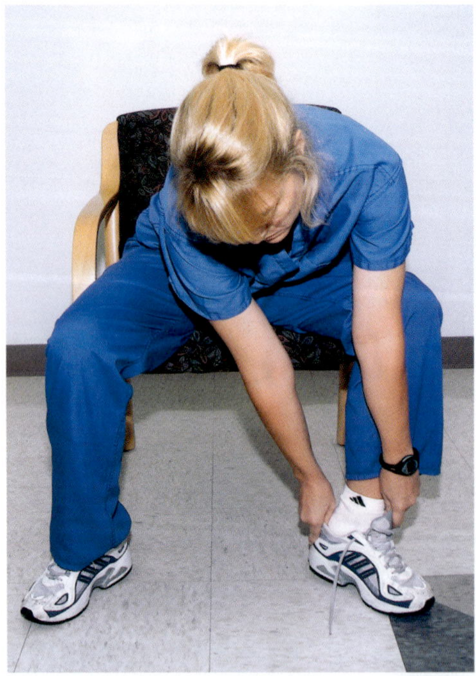

Figure 1–9   *After surgery, the patient may immediately lean down to the foot to put on shoes and stockings. This maneuver should always be done inside the knee of the operative leg, as shown.*

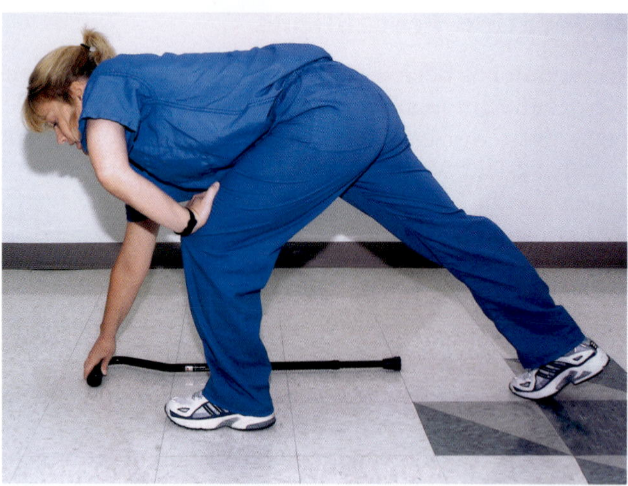

Figure 1–10   *Immediately after surgery, the safest and most comfortable way to lean forward and pick up an object on the floor is to extend the operative leg. If bilateral hip replacements have been performed, in this way the patient can use one of the operative hips for support.*

for about 1 month. The posterior capsule is sore, and sitting on and getting off a low toilet can be painful. Using a raised toilet seat is much more comfortable.

Patients are allowed to turn on their side to sleep in bed. It is painful to turn to the operative side, but they certainly can sleep on the nonoperative hip. Using a pillow between the legs provides comfort for the first 2 to 3 weeks. Some patients elect to use the pillow for a long time, and some patients wish to discard it as soon as possible. It can be discarded when the patient does not feel any pulling in the back of the hip when lying on the side. The pulling in the back of the hip is capsular pain.

Driving is safe when the leg has enough coordination to work the brake and accelerator safely. That, not the ability to get in and out of the car or to sit in the seat, is the main limitation in terms of driving. Getting the leg in and out of the car is difficult for several weeks for all patients and as long as 3 to 6 months for some patients. This is simply because the leg is weakened, and it may be necessary for the patient to use his or her hands to help lift it in and out of the car. In the initial postoperative period, the patient should enter the car by sitting sideways in the car seat and then swinging both legs into the car (Fig. 1–11).

BILATERAL TOTAL HIP REPLACEMENT

Indications

A bilateral total hip replacement is indicated for any patient whose x-ray resembles Figure 1–12 (severe bilateral arthritis) and, in particular, who has contractures in

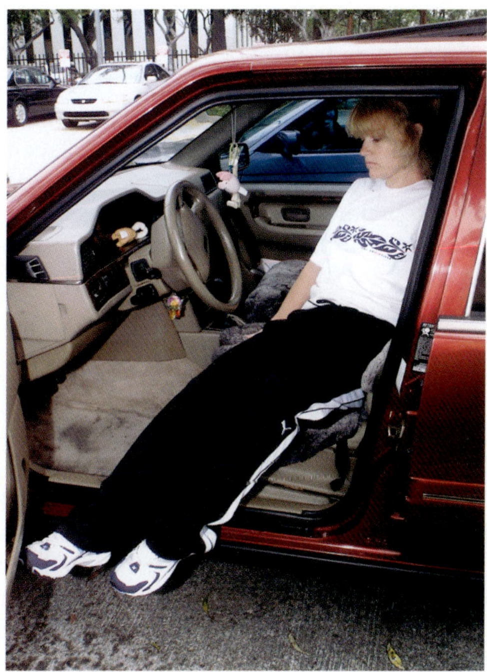

Figure 1–11　*Entering and exiting the car are done most comfortably by facing the door of the car and swinging the legs in for entrance and out for exit. For the first month after surgery, it may be necessary to help the operative leg by sliding it across the floor of the car to the edge of the door or by lifting it with the hands.*

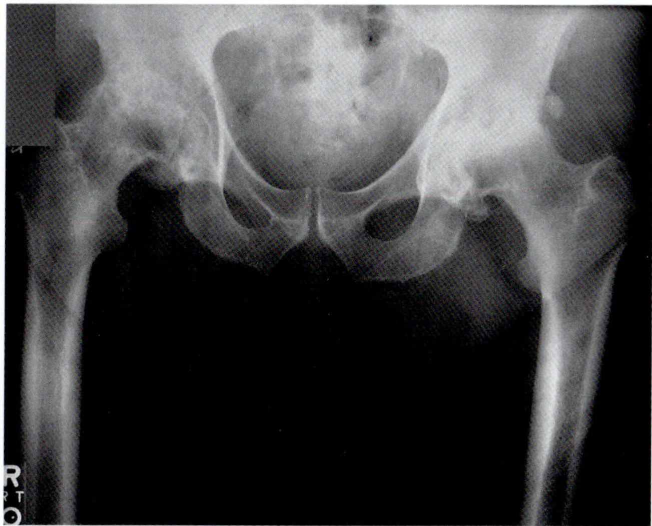

Figure 1–12　*Pelvic x-ray of patient with severe arthritis in both hips. With this much destruction of the hips, the patient has significant stiffness. Bilateral destruction of the hips combined with severe stiffness is the primary reason for bilateral hip replacements.*

rotation of the hip. If the surgeon is capable of performing a single hip replacement within 1 hour, a bilateral hip replacement can be done. The total operating room time should be 3 hours, with each hip operation lasting 1 hour. In our experience, patients tolerate this amount of surgery without any extra complications. We have had no deaths, no increased incidence of venous thrombosis or pulmonary embolism, and no increase in the mechanical complications of hip replacement.

Bilateral total hip replacement has the most benefit for patients who have severe contractures of the hip because it allows them to obtain optimal flexibility. If operation on the second hip is delayed for several weeks or months, the first hip replacement will not be as flexible as it could be. This is because the hips "sympathize with each other": if one hip is stiff, the other will have more stiffness than would be expected after the operation.

A second great benefit of bilateral total hip replacement is that the patient has to endure the anxiety of the operation only once. The patient fears anesthesia and always knows that there is a slight possibility of death with an operation. Therefore, any patient would like to minimize the number of operations he or she must have. For the patient, bilateral hip replacement provides the advantage of one anesthesia, one operation, and one recovery. Because of the single recovery period, it also is a very good operation for patients who need to

be economically productive. A single recovery period obviously reduces the amount of time patients will miss from their employment.

Technique

For many years, we did every bilateral total hip replacement with a Swan-Ganz catheter to monitor cardiopulmonary pressures. We used the same criteria for termination of the second hip procedure that we use for total knee replacement.[1] If the pulmonary vascular resistance was 200 dynes·sec·cm^{-5} or more after the first operation, we would cancel the second hip procedure. This has never happened with either a cemented or a cementless hip replacement. Furthermore, the only possible fat embolism complication of which I am aware during those years was a temporal artery thrombosis. Because we have had no fat embolism complications with either a cemented or a cementless bilateral total hip replacement, we no longer use the Swan-Ganz catheter. There are no fat embolism complications with these bilateral hip replacement procedures because the top of the femoral canal is so open that there is a wide outlet for the fat when it is pressurized in the intramedullary canal. A second reason for the lack of fat emboli is that we do the operations with the patient in the lateral position. There is a 30- to 40-minute gap between the operations, with the closure of the first hip and the change in position of the patient, with subsequent preparation of the skin and draping. If there were any adverse complications from fat embolism, they would be observed during that period. This delay also gives a much greater period of time for any fat that was released into the bloodstream to be metabolized than occurs with bilateral knee replacements. With bilateral knee replacements, the second knee operation is begun while the first knee surgery is being closed.

Postoperative Care

The hospitalization of patients with bilateral hip replacement is 1 to 2 days longer than for a single hip replacement. Such patients require longer to recover their energy level and endurance. However, in our experience, by 3 months after surgery, patients with bilateral hip replacement are equivalent in activity to patients with a single hip replacement. We allow patients to be fully weight bearing after surgery, and therefore patients on whom both hips have been operated can ambulate without assistive devices as soon as they are safe in transfers and ambulation, confident, and strong enough to do so. The postoperative rehabilitation for these patients does not differ from that in patients with a single hip replacement, in that walking and stretching are the primary rehabilitation activities.

Patients with bilateral hip replacement go home on the third or fourth day after surgery and are fully functional for activities of daily living. They are strong enough to go outdoors and begin walking on their return home. This is true whether the patient received a cementless or a cemented stem. The patient most likely will go home on two crutches but commonly by the end of the first week is on a single cane outdoors and perhaps using no assistive device in the house.

The first 4 to 6 weeks after bilateral hip replacement necessitate some compromises by the patient. It is difficult for them to sleep on their sides because they have wounds in both the right and left hips. It is more difficult for them to put on shoes and stockings because the hip capsule is sore in both hips. Their postoperative limitation in driving an automobile is the same as in a patient who has had a right hip replacement, in that the right leg needs to be strong and coordinated enough that braking and accelerating can be done safely; this can take from 2 to 4 weeks after surgery.

Pain Management

The patient who has bilateral total hip replacement should be treated before surgery, in the hospital, and after surgery with the same medications as in the single hip replacement. The primary difference for pain management in the hospital is that the epidural catheter is left in for 24 hours to provide pain relief in both hips during the patient's first night in the hospital. This provides sufficient pain relief that the patient can then take only oral medication and be comfortable. The remainder of the medications used are the same as discussed in the section on pain management for the primary hip replacement. In our experience, patients with bilateral hip replacements do not take more pain medication at home than patients with single hip replacements. These patients can also return to work in the same time frame as those with a single hip replacement. We have not discharged patients with bilateral hip replacements on the same day as surgery.

References

1. Long WT, Dorr LD, Healy B, Perry J: Functional recovery of non-cemented total hip arthroplasty. Clin Orthop 288:73-77, 1993.
2. Dorr LD; Wan Z: Causes of and treatment protocol for instability of total hip replacement. Clin Orthop 355:144-151, 1998.

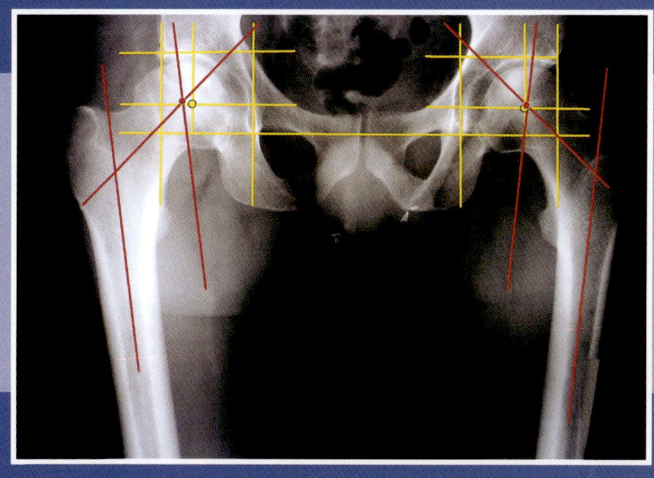

Chapter 2

Biomechanical Reconstruction, Fixation, and Articulation Surfaces

BIOMECHANICAL RECONSTRUCTION

One goal of a successful total hip arthroplasty is to reestablish correct biomechanics for the hip joint. Correct biomechanics are established by reconstructing the hip so that the muscles have a normal resting tension length that will allow them to function in a normal phasic pattern with strength. One of the most overlooked aspects of hip replacement, one that is vital to its successful function, is muscle function. Muscle function must be optimal for the hip to be comfortable and for the patient to have endurance. In my experience, one of the most common causes of a painful hip after primary hip replacement is weakness of the muscle around the hip. If a patient does not have good strength against resistance with the sidelying abduction test (Fig. 2–1), the abductor construct (gluteus medius and upper gluteus maximus) is too weak to allow the hip to function comfortably; most likely the muscles will be fatigued within one block of walking, and the patient will have pain around the hip with any activity equivalent to that time or distance.

Chapter 7 discusses computer navigation to optimize biomechanical reconstruction intraoperatively. This section describes the traditional technical maneuvers necessary to obtain good biomechanical reconstruction.

Requirements of Biomechanical Reconstruction: Soft Tissue Balance of the Hip

Hip Length, Offset, Avoidance of Impingement

The three most important factors for correct biomechanical reconstruction of the hip are hip length, offset, and avoidance of impingement. *Hip length* can be estimated, but not accurately measured, from an x-ray by the position of the lesser trochanters (Fig. 2–2). *Offset* can be estimated by the distance between the ischium and the lesser trochanter. It is difficult to determine the absolute leg length and offset because of rotation of the pelvis and femur. The numerical value of the offset can be estimated by the measurements illustrated in Figure 2–2.

The reward for correct reconstruction of the hip is not simply adequate muscle function, but also *avoidance of impingement*. There are no good consequences of impingement. Impingement is the most common reason for dislocation and for accelerated wear; it can cause increased loosening; and it causes pain. With correct hip length and offset, and with a combined anteversion of 35 degrees combined with as large a femoral head as can be used, the risk for impingement is essentially eliminated.

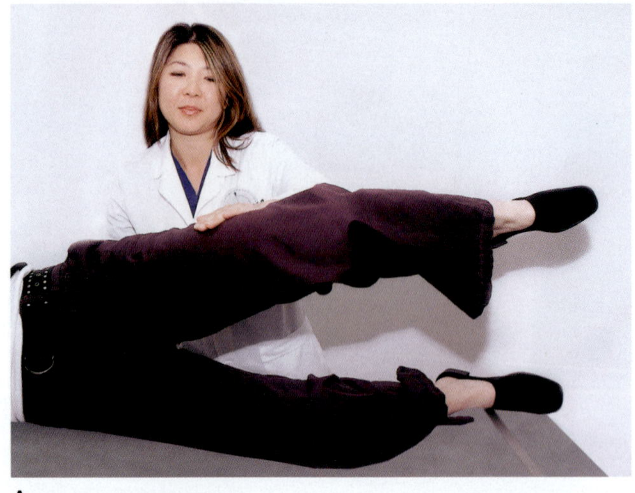

A

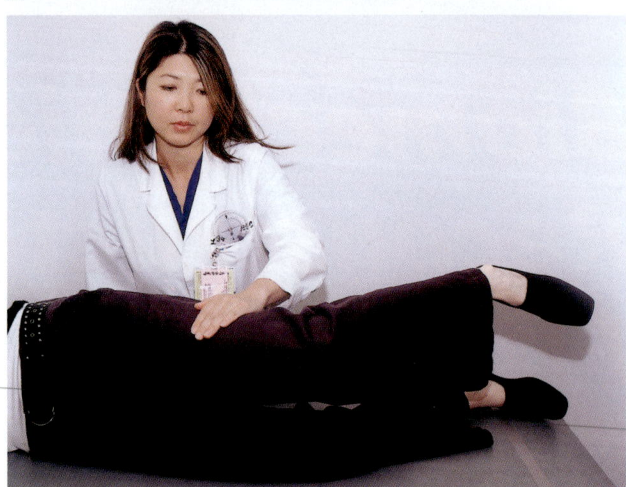

B

Figure 2–1   **A,** *The sidelying abduction test. The knee should be somewhat bent, or the iliotibial band can substitute for the gluteus medius. The assistant pushes against the leg with the patient trying to resist. If the leg cannot be moved, the abductor complex (gluteus medius and upper gluteus maximus) is strong.* **B,** *The assistant was able to push the leg down and break the resistance. In this case, leg strength is graded fair or less.*

Restrictions to achieving correct biomechanics when reconstructing the hip are primarily anatomic. For instance, what position of the cup in the bone is best to provide stability and no impingement? Chapter 5, which deals with acetabular position, and Chapter 7, on computer navigation, provide the answers to this question. An ideal example to consider is a dysplastic acetabulum, which requires placement of the cup more medially and superiorly. This cup position, however, might allow impingement of the femur against the pelvis; hence, dysplastic hips require trochanteric osteotomy to prevent impingement more frequently than other hips. Where should the femoral neck cut be placed to provide correct leg length and offset? The discussion of femoral preparation in Chapter 6 answers this

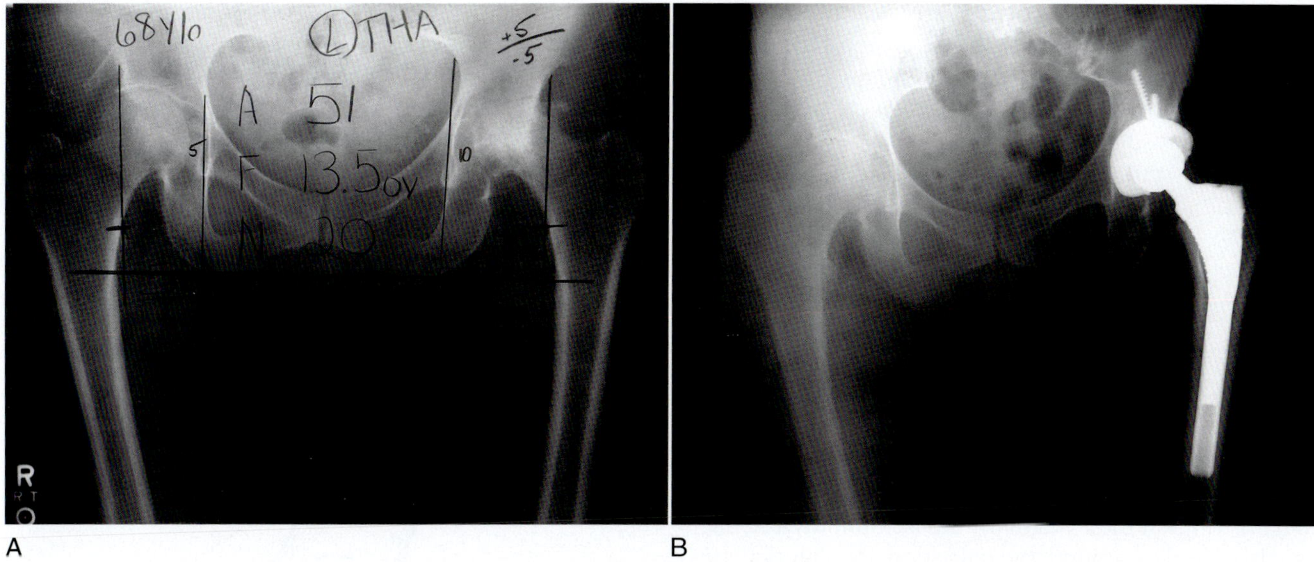

A B

Figure 2–2 **A,** *Preoperative x-ray of 68-year-old patient for left total hip replacement. Placement of a transischial line allows measurement from the lesser trochanter to the transischial line. Lines drawn through the tear drop and through the junction of the lesser trochanter with the femoral neck allow measurement of offset and the change that should be made at surgery. The numbers above the left hip indicate that the hip needs 5 mm more leg length and 5 mm less offset. The number 10 in the left acetabulum means that the medialization, as measured on the computer, will most likely be approximately 10 mm. The other numbers represent preoperative planning. It is anticipated that a 51-mm acetabular cup will be used, that a 13.5 femoral stem will be used, and that the neck cut should be 20 mm superior to the lesser trochanter, which would normally be 15 mm below the periphery of the head. **B,** The postoperative x-ray of the reconstruction shows that the offset and leg length have been restored. The cup was medialized to Köhler's line.*

question. Previous trauma to the femur, a dysplastic femur, or congenital defects such as slipped capital femoral epiphysis (which results in retroversion of the femur) can compromise the femoral component position. When the femoral geometry is abnormal, anteversion of the femoral component may be difficult to obtain and to determine visually (it is for this reason that modular femoral components are popular in these types of femurs). With computer navigation, however, the surgeon can first determine the femoral anteversion and then adjust the cup anteversion to provide a combined anteversion of 35 degrees.

Release of Static and Dynamic Contractures Around the Hip

A second consideration associated with soft tissue balance of the hip is release of static and dynamic contractures around the hip, which provides significant and immediate benefits for the patient and accelerates postoperative rehabilitation. Benefits include a decrease in knee pain, elimination of groin pain, increased hip range of motion, and, perhaps most important for both the patient and surgeon, reduction of functional leg-length difference. A functional long leg occurs when, despite correct hip length and offset, contractures around the hip and a resultant pelvic obliquity make the patient feel that the operative leg is 1 or 2 inches too long. The most common cause is tightness of the gluteus medius muscle

in a hip that was short and had a decreased offset and is corrected to the normal length and offset. Even in a leg that has undergone proper soft tissue balancing, the gluteus medius muscle requires time to adapt to its correct length; failure to perform soft tissue balancing, however, accentuates this abductor stretch. The surgeon must warn patients with the aforementioned characteristics that the operative leg will feel long after surgery, and that the condition can persist for many months until the tissues accommodate to the arthroplasty.

Soft tissue balance of the hip requires release of muscles. There are few negative consequences for the patient with muscle release, except when the iliopsoas tendon is completely released from the lesser trochanter. This can cause weakness when ascending stairs and lifting the leg to enter and exit a car.

The surgeon can anticipate the need for soft tissue release around the hip when a patient has contractures of the hip greater than 20 degrees in abduction and external rotation. Soft tissue release also will be necessary if, radiographically, the hip demonstrates shortening from collapse of the femoral head, particularly if accompanied by superolateral migration and osteophytosis. During surgery, tightness of the hip through the range of motion with the components in place indicates the necessity for soft tissue release. The surgeon's inability to bring the hip to full extension, abduct the hip beyond 20 degrees, and bend the knee beyond 90 to 100 degrees (in the absence of knee arthritis or previous total knee arthroplasty) are indications of soft tissue imbalance. The test for full extension is the ability to extend the leg 10 degrees beyond a line between the anterior superior spine and the patella. A tight tensor fascia muscle results in a positive Ober-Yount sign, with the thigh not settling easily against the other leg.

First, the surgeon must ascertain that the tightness is not due to leg lengthening. We use the position of the lesser trochanter relative to the ischium to determine leg lengthening. On a radiograph, a line is drawn across the bottom of the ischia, and the relationship of that line to the lesser trochanters is used to determine the hip length. During surgery, an accurate assessment can be made by palpating the ischium and observing the position of the lesser trochanter (Fig. 2–3; see Fig. 3–49), although it is important not to mistake the tendons of the hamstrings at their origin for the ischium itself. Offset can also be determined by palpating the interval between the greater trochanter and the pelvis during range of motion, as previously described (see Fig. 3–50).

If the hip is very tight in abduction and external rotation, or if there is tightness in the thigh as it lies against the other leg (positive Ober-Yount sign), release of the tensor fascia is necessary. This is done by grasping the tensor fascia with two Kocher clamps. The vastus lateralis fascia should be retracted down with one hand while the assistant lifts the tensor fascia anteriorly (Fig. 2–4). Division with an electrocautery device includes the muscle fibers so that the muscle and fascia will give. The tensor fascia can be divided completely to the rectus femoris muscle, resulting in improved abduction and external rotation of the hip.

If the tensor fascia has been divided and the knee will not flex beyond 90 to 100 degrees, division of the

rectus muscle is necessary. The rectus muscle can be brought into direct view by lifting the cut edges of the tensor fascia and placing opposite retraction on the vastus lateralis. The rectus muscle is then grasped and pulled toward the wound and divided as necessary to allow the knee to flex fully without resistance (Fig. 2–5). With release of the tensor fascia muscle, iliotibial band

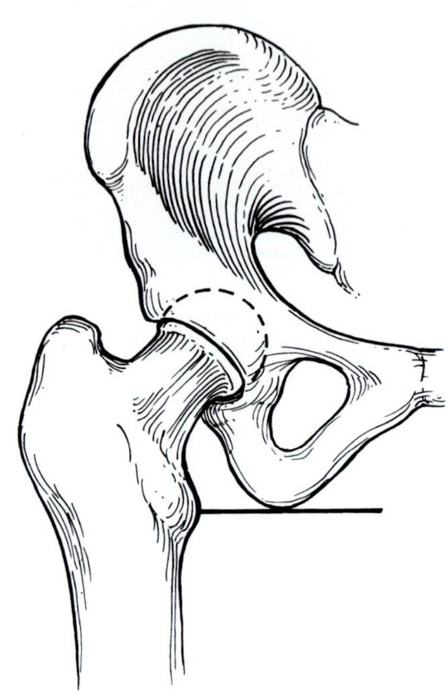

Figure 2–3 *The tip of the lesser trochanter is at the level of the tip of the ischium. If the lesser trochanter is below the ischium, the leg will be too long. In some hips, the lesser trochanter will be above the tip of the ischium; this must be determined from the preoperative x-ray.*

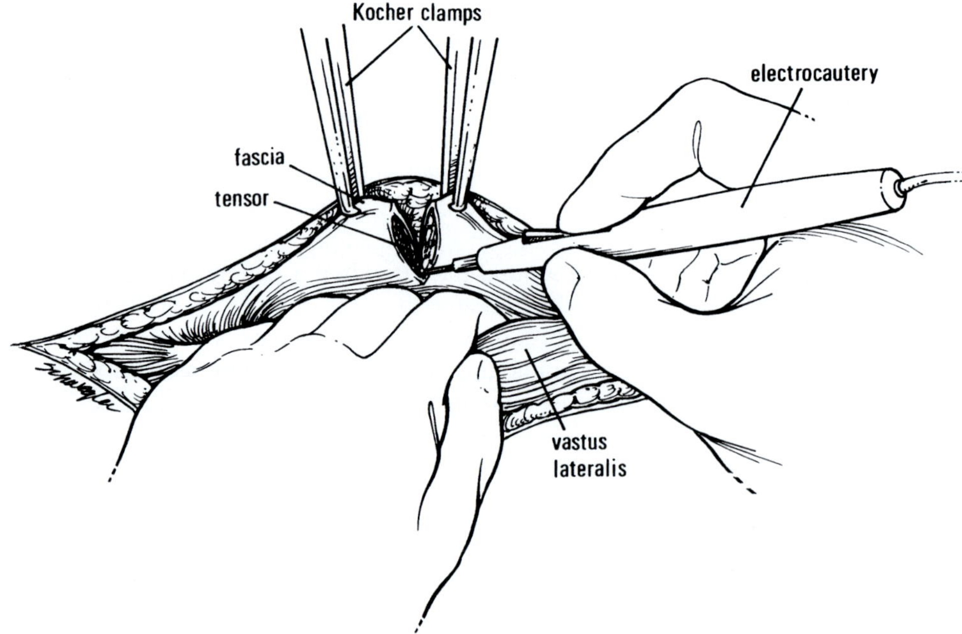

Figure 2–4 *The surgeon retracts the vastus lateralis with his left hand, while the assistant holds the tensor fascia with two Kocher clamps. The fascia and muscle of the tensor are divided by the electrocautery.*

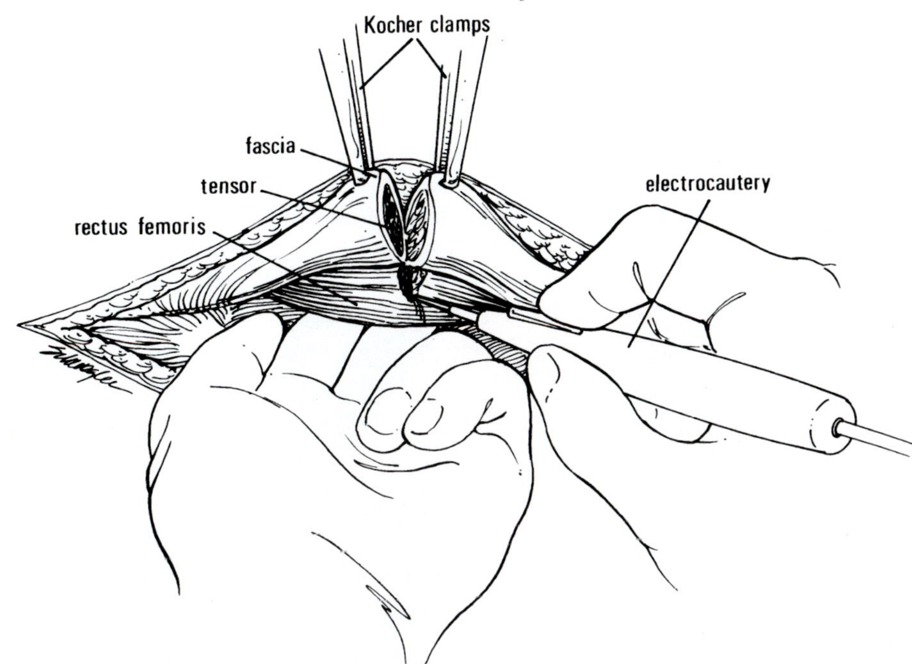

Figure 2–5 The surgeon uses the index and middle fingers of his left hand to grasp the rectus femoris muscle belly and pull it toward the wound. While holding the muscle belly, the electrocautery is used to divide it partially or fully as necessary to allow flexion of the knee. The surgeon's fingers protect the femoral nerve, which runs just medial to the muscle belly. The assistant continues to elevate the tensor with the Kocher clamps.

(which inserts at Gerdy's tubercle), and rectus tendon, postoperative knee pain is significantly reduced.

If the hip does not extend beyond neutral (i.e., a line from the anterior iliac spine to the patella), the surgeon must palpate the iliopsoas tendon. This tendon likely will be very tight, crossing the anterior acetabulum like a "banjo string." The iliopsoas tendon must be recessed or completely released until it is elastic while it is palpated in extension and as it crosses the anterior acetabulum. Leaving the iliopsoas tendon tight can cause groin pain after surgery from irritation of the tendon as it crosses the anterior acetabulum. The anterior capsule also may be very tight, preventing extension of the hip. This static structure must be released by excision or incision (step cuts) sufficiently to allow the hip to extend 10 degrees

Technique of Biomechanical Reconstruction

With a hip replacement, ideally the center of rotation of the acetabulum is restored, the hip length and offset are restored, the largest head size possible is used, and a combined anteversion of 30 to 40 degrees of the femoral and acetabular components is achieved. If all of these goals are achieved, the hip replacement will function well for a long time. The margin of error for any of these individual components of the reconstruction is 1 cm, and for the combined anteversion it is 35 ± 5 degrees. That means that if the hip length (measured from the center of the head to the lesser trochanter) is 1 cm too long, the offset as well as the center of rotation of the cup must be correct, or the hip

will be uncomfortable for the patient. Clearly, any individual component of the reconstruction can deviate by 1 cm, but if more than one component deviates by 1 cm, the patient will be uncomfortable. If the combined anteversion is not at least 30 degrees or is greater than 45 degrees, the risk for hip instability significantly increases.

The center of rotation of the cup is restored by properly preparing the acetabulum and placing the acetabular component correctly. This is described in detail in Chapter 5, Posterior Mini-incision: Acetabular Preparation and Implantation. The process can be summarized as shown in Figure 2–6. When the acetabulum is correctly prepared, reaming is done by removing all floor osteophytes, removing the acetabular ridge, and stopping at the cortical bone of the cotyloid notch. When the cup is correctly implanted, its metal edge does not overlie the cortical bone of the cotyloid notch by more than 2 to 3 mm, the anteroinferior edge of the cup is 5 mm below the peak of the pubic tubercle, the anterosuperior edge of the cup is below the osseous edge of the acetabulum, and the posterosuperior metal edge of the cup may be exposed for 5 mm; the posteroinferior edge of the cup is below the osseous edge of the ischium. The center of rotation of the hip will be most closely reproduced in this position. The anterior wall of the acetabulum is not a good guide because it has four variable structures[1]; nor is the acetabular anatomy itself a good guide, because the normal inclination of the acetabulum is greater than 50 degrees, and 20% of acetabula are retroverted (see Chapter 7).

The hip length is best restored by matching the characteristics of the implant to the bony anatomy of the femur using the preoperative template. When computer navigation is not used, preoperative templating is critical because implants differ by their offsets and their neck shaft angles. An implant with a neck shaft angle of 125 to 130 degrees is the easiest to use to reconstruct femoral mechanics. The APR stem (Zimmer, Warsaw, Ind.) has a neck shaft angle of 130 degrees. With that neck shaft angle, I can adapt it to almost any hip. With a neck shaft angle of 135 degrees or more it is more difficult to balance the hip length and offset. By using a template on the x-ray (Fig. 2–7), one can judge the fill of the implant in the femur. This allows one to estimate the size of the implant to be used. The level of the neck cut of the osseous femoral neck can be determined. This level of neck cut will restore the hip length and offset if the center of rotation of the acetabulum is reestablished. If it is judged from preoperative templating of the acetabulum that the acetabular component will need to be placed superiorly or excessively medially, the femoral neck will need to be adjusted to allow the hip length and offset to be restored as nearly correctly as possible (Fig. 2–8). Without computer naviga-

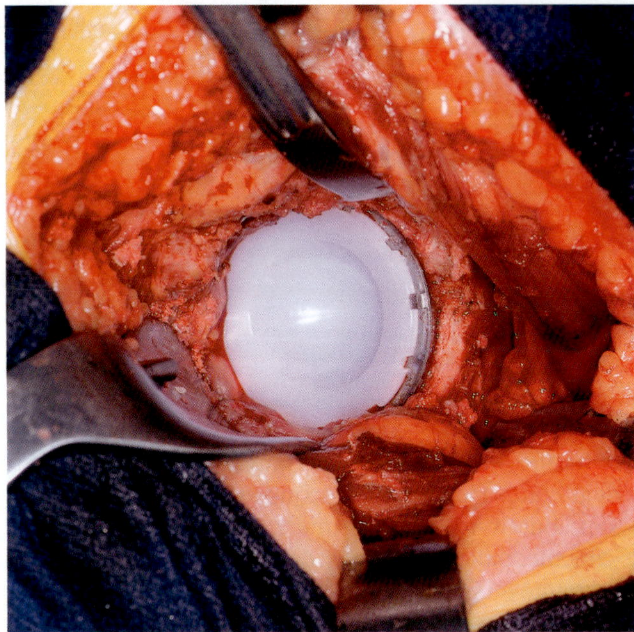

Figure 2–6 *An acetabular cup in the correct position. The retractor in the center top is the snake retractor. The retractor in the left margin is the retractor that rests on the ischium. A long incision was used and a Charnley retractor placed. The anterosuperior edge of the cup (just under the snake retractor) is flush with the acetabular bone. The posterosuperior cup is not covered by bone for approximately 5 mm. The medial cup (against the #7 retractor) is flush with the edge of the cortical bone, as demonstrated by the fact that it is just adjacent to the retractor. Anteriorly but not well visualized, the anteroinferior cup is 5 mm below the pubic tubercle. The anterior edge of the cup should not stand proud of anterior bone, or it can cause irritation of the iliopsoas tendon.*

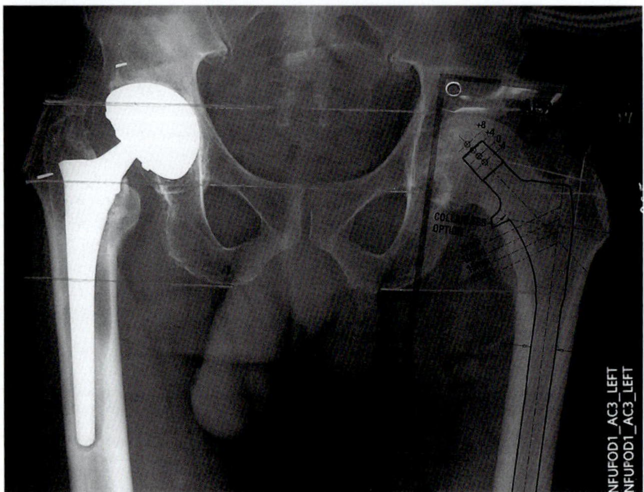

Figure 2–7 *A template is placed onto the x-ray of the left hip so that the center of the femoral head approximates the zero head length. The cut should be 10 mm above the lesser trochanter. There would be complete fill of the stem and the bone. This x-ray also illustrates the principle that the hip needs to be reconstructed correctly regardless of the situation of the opposite hip. Clearly, the opposite hip is shortened from a loose femoral stem, and that hip will need revision. The left hip still must be correctly reconstructed.*

Figure 2–8 **A,** *This patient has a long valgus femoral neck in the right hip. It will be necessary to leave a long femoral neck cut to get the correct offset and leg length. Furthermore, it is known from the left hip that the cup will need to be medialized because of the dysplasia, which can require even more neck length. These considerations must be recognized during preoperative planning.* **B,** *The postoperative x-ray has a long length of retained femoral neck, so a plus 8-mm femoral head was needed to provide the correct length and offset. As expected, the cup was slightly superior and medial because of the dysplasia.* **C,** *These hips are the opposite of those seen in* **A.** *They have a short varus neck, and either a very short neck cut will be required or a short head length will be needed, depending on which is better for the offset.* **D,** *In this patient a short head length was used to allow restoration of the hip length and offset, which are well reconstructed. There was no impingement with this patient because the cup anteversion, which was known from the computer, was adjusted to the femoral position.* **E,** *In this situation the hip is quite short compared with the opposite side, and care must be taken to size and position the acetabulum correctly so that the femoral neck cut does not need to be long to produce the correct leg length. The opposite hip is an APR stem and cup that has been in place for 15 years with no evidence of osteolysis or significant wear.* **F,** *The right hip was reconstructed so that the offset and hip length are similar to those of the left hip. The cup was positioned at the correct level with the inferior edge of the cup at the inferior edge of the tear drop. The cortical bone in zone 2 behind the acetabulum can also be visualized on the preoperative x-ray.*

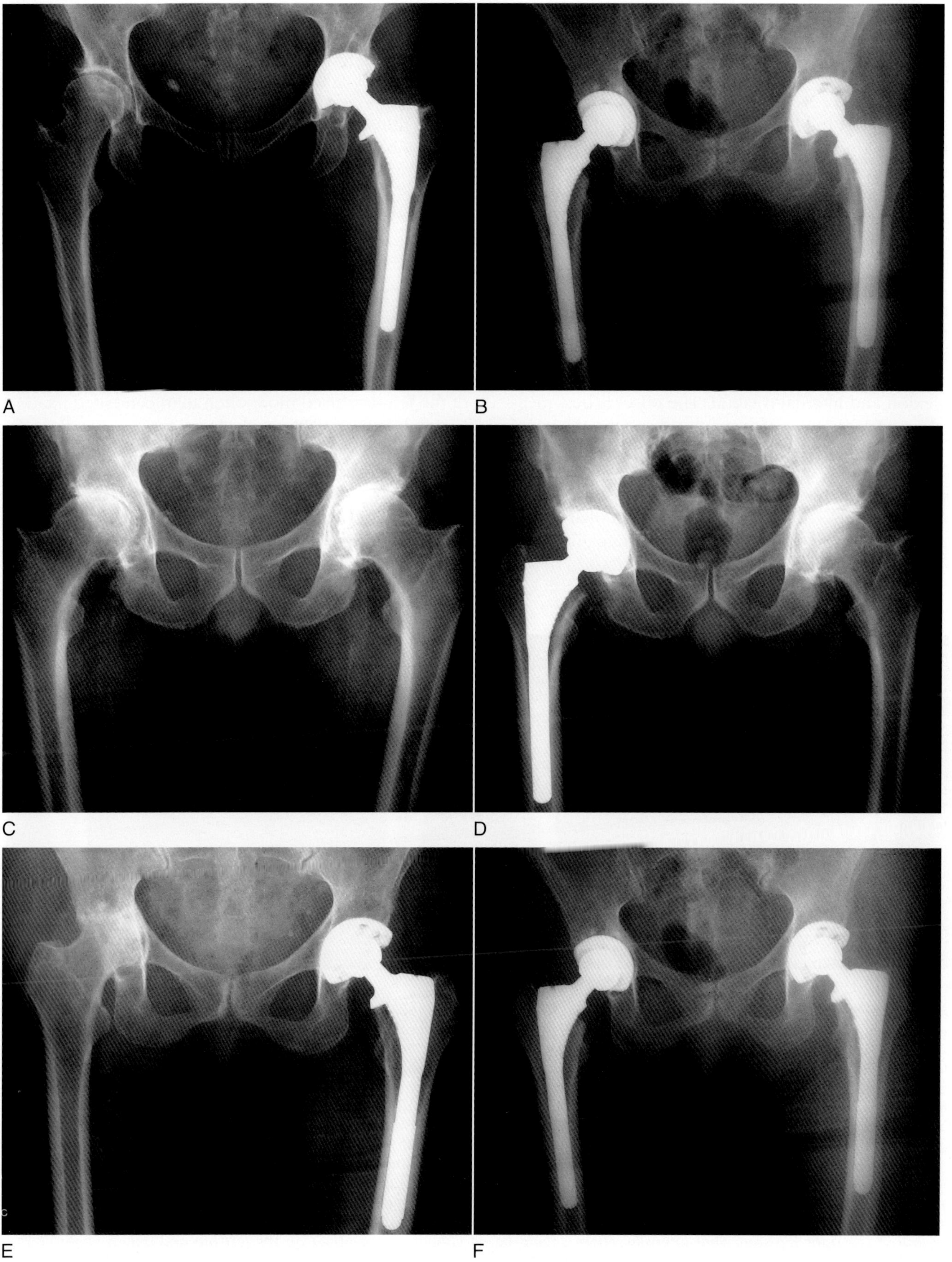

Legend on opposite page

tion, preoperative templating is necessary to judge sizes of implants, positions of implants, and the necessity for any intraoperative adjustments to perform the operation successfully (*see "Templating for Total Hip Arthroplasty"*).

The offset of the hip is critical because it permits the correct positioning of the femur relative to the pelvis. If the femur is not positioned correctly relative to the pelvis, impingement of the femoral bone against the pelvic bone can occur during range of motion of the hip. This is painful and can result in hip dislocation. The femur must clear the pelvis throughout the range of motion after hip replacement. I judge this by using 1 fingerbreadth clearance of the greater trochanter in extension and external rotation; of the lesser trochanter and the ischium in full extension and external rotation; and of the trochanter and femoral neck in 90 degrees of flexion and internal rotation. The offset is best measured on an x-ray by measuring the change in the center of rotation of the hip (Fig. 2–9), because offset is affected so much by rotation, unlike the round femoral head. It is incorrect to use the measurement of offset from the center of the stem in the intramedullary canal, as it is a measure of the offset of the implant and is

determined by the manufactured offset of that stem; it does not indicate that the femur will be offset correctly from the pelvis.

The use of as large a head as possible for the size of the osseous acetabulum and the femoral component lowers the risk of impingement and improves joint range of motion. Also, it decreases the dead space of the hip. Hence, it reduces the amount of capsular thickening that will occur with healing, which speeds capsular healing and increases the patient's comfort. Large head sizes are available with all articulating surfaces in current use.

FIXATION

Femoral Stem Fixation

In contemporary hip replacement, cementless fixation of the femur is used more often than cemented fixation. Certainly, in patients with Dorr type A or B bone, cementless fixation can be performed easily, with the expectation that the patient's comfort will be the same as with cemented fixation. Only older patients with Dorr type C bone (Fig. 2–10) may be less comfortable with cementless than with cemented fixation, because bone

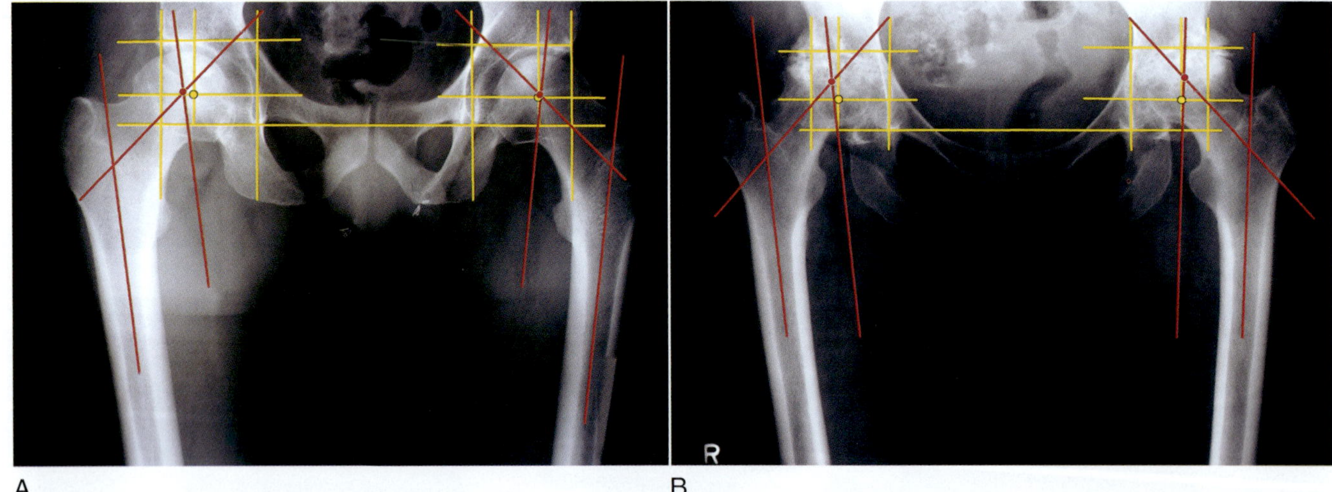

A   B

Figure 2–9 ***A,*** *The left hip in this patient is normal; the center of rotation of the acetabulum is shown by the yellow dot, and the center of rotation of the femur by the red dot. The center of rotation of the femur is determined by drawing a line that bisects the intramedullary canal of the femur and by drawing a parallel line that goes through the junction of the femoral head and neck. The acetabular center of rotation is determined by drawing a perpendicular line to the line that connects the tear drops. The perpendicular line goes through the tear drop, and then a parallel line is drawn through the edge of the acetabulum. Two thirds of the distance from the tear drop line to the edge of the acetabulum is the distance of the center of the acetabulum. A third line is drawn parallel to the tear drop line from this point. Two thirds of the distance caudad along this line marks the point of the acetabular center of rotation. The right hip of this patient has avascular necrosis and a change in the position of the femur, so that the femoral center of head has moved laterally. The lines are drawn by the same rules. The femoral center of rotation is drawn in the same fashion, and it can be seen that the femoral center of head has moved laterally and a bit superiorly. This distance can be measured on an actual x-ray and will give the change necessary for offset and leg length.* ***B,*** *Hips with much greater destruction than seen in* ***A*** *on the right hip. In these hips, the femoral center of rotation has moved superiorly and in the right hip somewhat laterally. There should be no change in the offset on the left hip and only a slight change in the offset on the right hip. The center of rotation has to be brought caudad, however, and this causes the leg length change. This can be measured on an actual x-ray.*

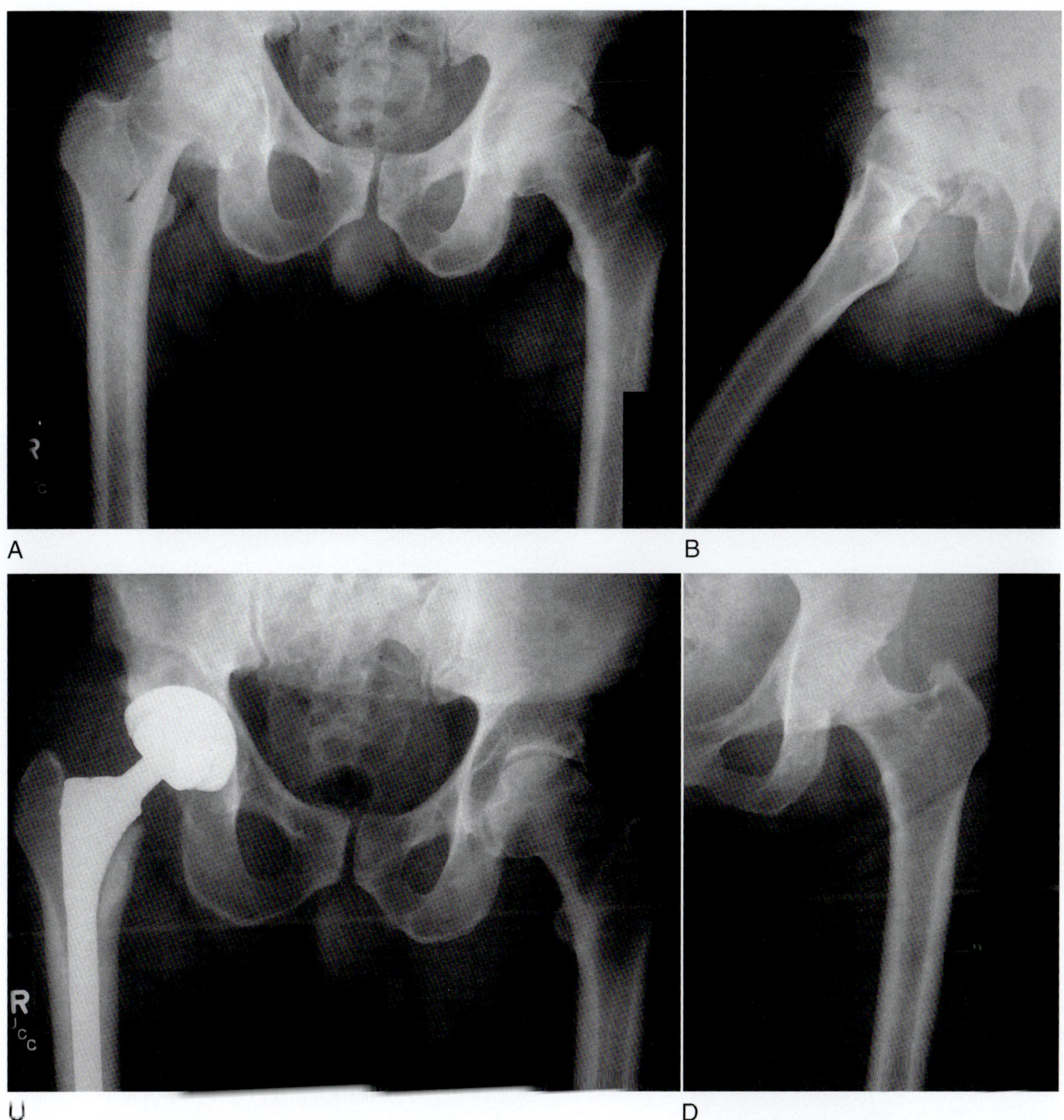

Figure 2–10   **A,** *In Dorr type A bone, there are thick cortices and a thin intramedullary canal.* **B,** *Lateral x-ray with type A bone again shows thick cortices, and sometimes the femoral canal is even thinner on the lateral x-ray than the anteroposterior (AP) x-ray, although this is not the case in this patient. There is no erosion of the posterior fin of the posterior cortex in type A bone.* **C,** *Postoperative radiograph of the patient in* **A.** *The femoral stem always fits superbly in type A bone.* **D,** *Dorr Type B bone still has thick cortices on the AP x-ray, but irregularity of the endosteal surface is usually visible, which is indicative of osteoblastic activity in this bone.*

Illustration continued on following page

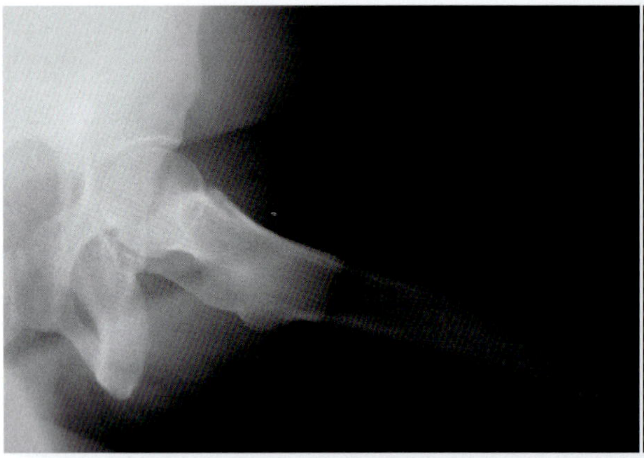

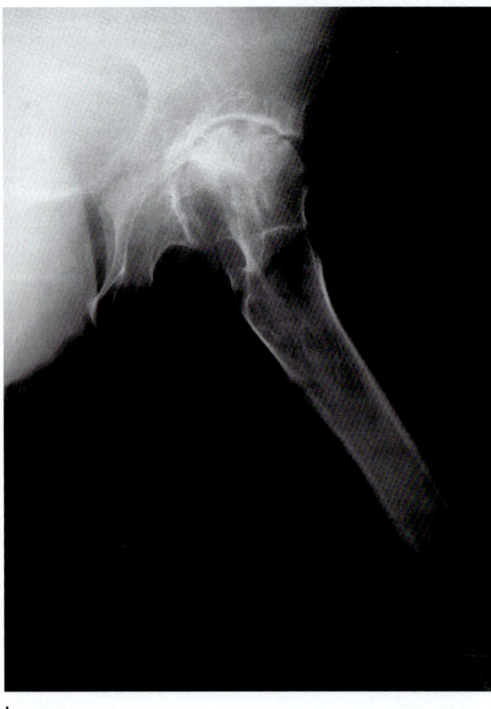

Figure 2–10, cont'd   **E,** *Lateral x-ray of type B bone shows thinning of the cortices and erosion of the thick fin of the posterior cortex; in type B bone the posterior fin is often absent, which widens the intramedullary canal on the lateral x-ray.* **F,** *Postoperative x-ray of a different patient than in* **D.** *This patient also has type B bone, and the AP x-ray shows good cortices and a good fit of the stem.* **G,** *Lateral x-ray of same patient shows equal thicknesses of the anterior and posterior cortices in type B bone. Again, there is always an excellent fit of the stem in type B bone.* **H,** *Dorr Type C bone has thinning of the cortices, although medial and lateral cortices remain evident.* **I,** *Lateral x-ray of type C bone often has no distinct cortices and, as seen here, the cortices are always thinned and blurred. This means that the intramedullary canal on the lateral x-ray is wide; it is always wider than on the AP x-ray. For this reason, in type C bone we often pack slurry obtained from the acetabulum into the canal to provide better contact of the stem to bone in the lateral x-ray (AP plane).*

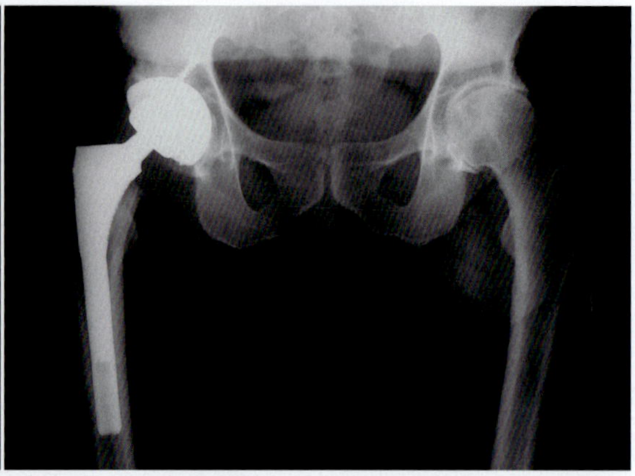

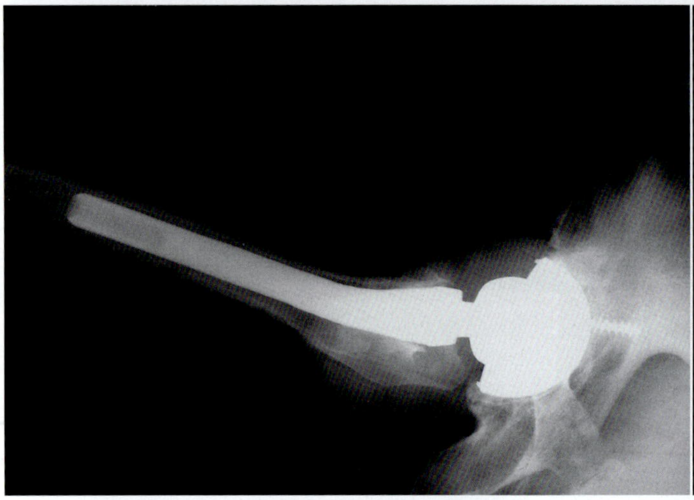

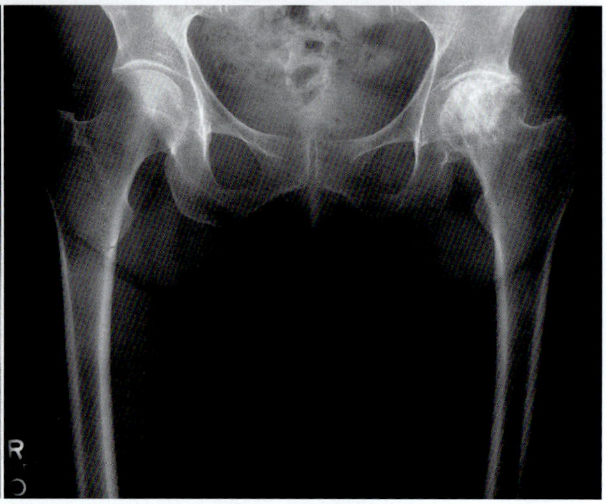

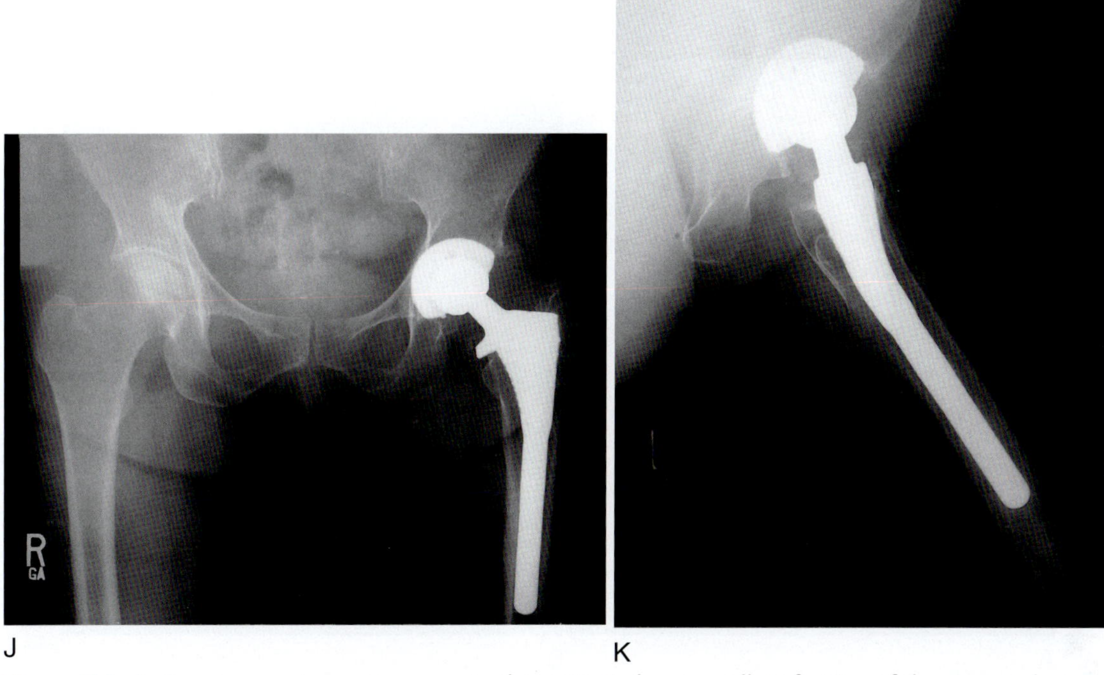

Figure 2–10, cont'd *J, One-year postoperative x-ray in this patient shows excellent fixation of the stem and cup, with no radiolucent lines and excellent biomechanical reconstruction of the hip. There is proximal osteopenia of the femur, and distal and medial there is significant thickening of the cortex, which means that there is fixation and load transfer into the bone occurring here. The thickening of this bone can cause thigh pain for patients until the remodeling is complete, which usually takes 18 months. K, Lateral x-ray of same patient again shows significant osteopenia proximally, which always occurs in type C bone with any noncemented stem. Distally, there is thickening of bone around the tip of the stem and a lucency in zone 4 at the tip of the stem. This stem had room to move in this lateral x-ray, and it did have some motion. However, the endosteal bone is healing to the metal of the grit-blasted stem. Packing cancellous chips from the acetabular reamings facilitates endosteal bone healing.*

remodeling, which is slower in older patients, is needed to allow adaptation of the bone to the stem (see Fig. 2–10H–K). However, cementless stems can perform well in this bone type. The Zweymüller stem (Alloclassic; Zimmer) has not been reported to perform differently in type C bone than in other bone types. I perform almost exclusively cementless fixation with the APR stem. The AML stem produces higher stress shielding in type C bone but equivalent fixation to nonosteoporotic bone. All stems result in increased stress shielding in type C bone because of the reduced rate of metabolism of this bone. I perform cemented fixation in older patients if I believe they will experience greater comfort with that type of fixation; this is true in probably 2 or 3 of every 100 patients on whose hips I operate.

I have used the APR stem, the Natural hip stem, and the Zweymüller stem. These stems represent three different geometric types, and success with all three has been reported in the literature.[2-4] Our most recent data with the APR stem show that with this stem, when combined with the APR cup (now called the Converge cup), there is no loosening of the stem or the cup at 10 years,

and the only reoperations have been for infection or dislocation.

The best cementless stems provide fixation in both the metaphysis and the diaphysis, and there are several surface types that have given durable bony fixation to the metal. The proximal metaphyseal fixation using a porous coating seems to be better than proximal fixation obtained with a grit-blasted surface. In the diaphysis, grit-blasted surfaces have provided very stable fixation. The APR stem has a grit-blasted diaphyseal stem, as does the Natural hip. The Zweymüller Alloclassic stem is grit blasted throughout its surface. The AML stem has provided long-term durable results and is fully porous coated. The Mallory-Head stem has a plasma spray coating in the metaphyseal portion and grit blasting in the diaphysis. Several surgeons have reported that once they observed bone ingrowth in the femur, they have not seen it deteriorate for up to 20 years (Fig. 2–11).

Chapter 6 describes the techniques for both cementless and cemented fixation of the femur, but cementless fixation should be used in almost all patients.

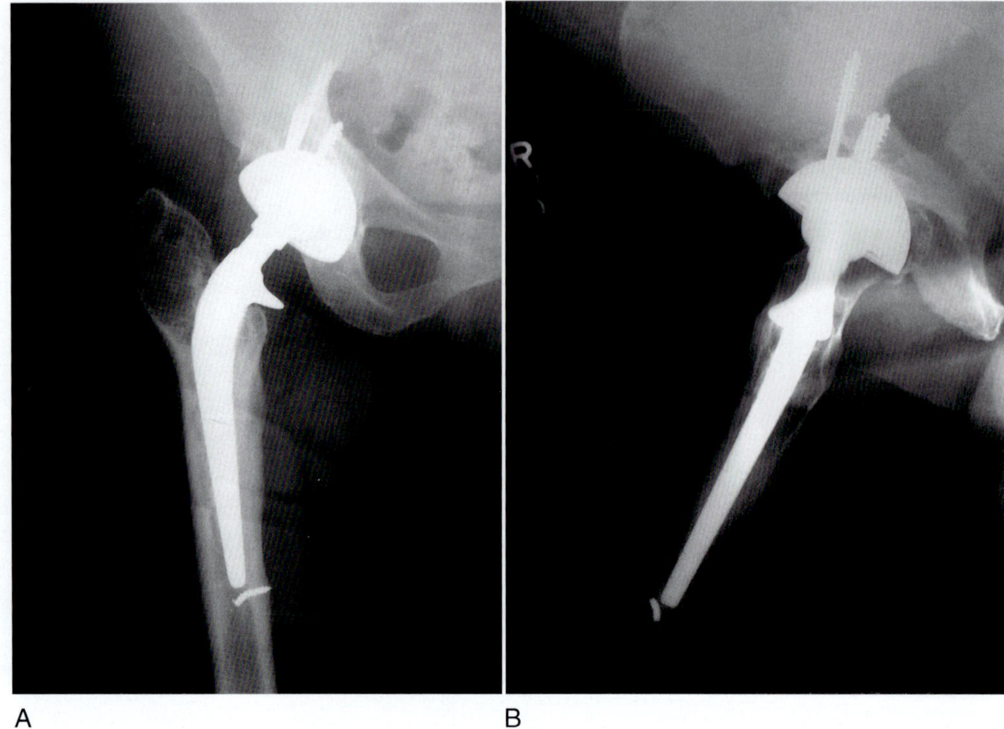

A   B

Figure 2–11   **A,** *Anteroposterior x-ray of a 21-year-old cementless hip replacement. There is remodeling of the bone around the femoral component, with endosteal bone healed immediately adjacent to the stem. There are no radiolucent lines around the cup and there is no significant osteolysis, even though there is some gross wear.* **B,** *Lateral x-ray of the same hip replacement as in part* **A.** *The endosteal bone in zones 3 and 5 immediately adjacent to the stem are clearly evident, as is the bone adjacent to the porous coating in the proximal portion of the stem. There is no lucency or osteolysis evident in the acetabulum except at the peripheral edges of the acetabulum superiorly and inferiorly.*

Cup Fixation

Cementless fixation of the acetabular component has been the dominant practice since 1990. The best cementless shells are those that have the most flexibility. Initially, the thin titanium shells of the Harris-Galante I (Zimmer) and the APR (Zimmer) acetabular components were associated with the best results. There was the least amount of osteolysis around these cups, and because of their thinness there was almost no mechanical loosening. Loosening is more commonly associated with thicker acetabular shells because the acetabular bone is more likely to be stress shielded as the thickness of the metal increases. This stress-shielded acetabular bone becomes thin and weak, which promotes migration of the acetabular component. The thin titanium shells had equivalent fixation records whether or not screws were used to augment the initial fixation. I still implant cups in primary hip replacement chiefly without screw augmentation. However, I do not hesitate to use a screw if there is any question of the quality of the press-fit at surgery.

A new fixation surface called *trabecular metal* has been in use since in the first decade of 2000. This surface mimics the appearance of cancellous bone and

has shown superb bone fixation in animal studies and with implant retrievals (Fig. 2–12). The trabecular metal surface is versatile, which makes it particularly beneficial in revision surgery. It is possible to drill holes through this surface for screw fixation, and it is possible to cement liners into this surface so that it can be used as a modular surface. It is available as a monoblock cup. Surgeons such as Thomas Sculco from the Hospital for Special Surgery in New York City and Arlen Hanssen from the Mayo Clinic in Rochester, Minnesota, have experienced superior results with this cup (personal communication, 2005). The technical use of this cup is described in Chapter 10 on revision surgery.

ARTICULATION SURFACES

Three articulation surfaces are used today, all with the expectation of 30 years of durability. Two of these are hard-on-hard articulations consisting of metal-on-metal and ceramic-on-ceramic. The third is a hard-on-soft articulation consisting of metal against cross-linked polyethylene. I have had extensive experience with the Metasul (Zimmer) metal-on-metal articu-

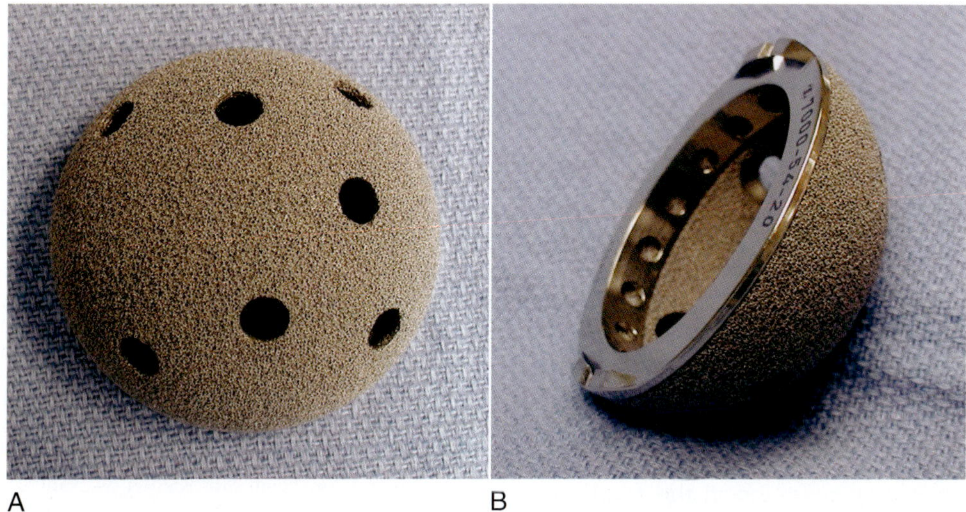

A   B

Figure 2-12   **A,** *Trabecular metal cup. This photograph clearly shows the porous surface that mimics cancellous bone and is very flexible, so that the stiffness of this cup is the best available for approximating the stiffness of cancellous bone.* **B,** *Face of the trabecular metal cup. The thick walls are not detrimental because of the highly flexible coating.*

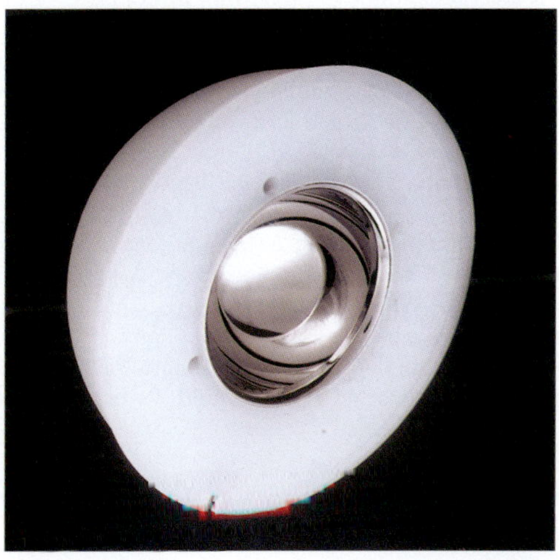

Figure 2-13   *The Metasul insert for the Converge cup. This is a 28-mm articulating surface. The highly polished quality of the surface is evident.*

lation (Fig. 2–13). The cross-linked polyethylene with which I have had experience is Durasul (Zimmer). I have not had experience with the ceramic-on-ceramic articulation, but the results with this have been excellent for surgeons such as James D'Antonio, William Capello, and Benjamin Bierbaum (personal communication, 2005).

Metasul Articulation

Total hip replacements in patients using the Metasul articulation are successful. On our original cohort of 127 hips, we had four revisions (3.2%), one for loosening of the cup and three for dislocation. It is important to verify that all components are well fixed. In many published studies, fixation of either the stem or cup is reported in detail, but not fixation of both, with a failure and reoperation rate of 13% to 56% for the other component. Metasul is associated with fewer cup revisions than most of the cementless total hip replacements commonly used in the 1990s.

New articulation couples such as Metasul were designed in response to osteolysis. Osteolysis was radiographically absent in patients receiving the Metasul articulation. Calcar resorption, which appears as small, focal radiolucent areas immediately beneath the collar of the prosthesis, was seen in 6 of 96 hips. Some surgeons do not include calcar resorption in the definition of osteolysis because it is difficult to determine whether calcar resorption was caused by stress shielding or lysis. We have elected to consider this phenomenon as caused by lysis, for completeness of reporting.

Radiographic views other than the anteroposterior and lateral femur and pelvic oblique views may reveal osteolytic lesions not visible with these plain radiographs. Claus and associates reported that anteroposterior radiographs had a sensitivity of 47% (i.e., a 47% chance of detecting a lesion) and that the iliac oblique view added only 16% sensitivity.[5] Four views (anteroposterior, lateral, iliac, and obturator oblique views) gave 73% sensitivity. Therefore, unobserved osteolysis may have been present.

Focus on articulation surfaces in the next 5 years will help clarify whether changes made in polyethylene preparation in the 1990s, such as increased cross-linking, sterilization in inert gases, and design changes for better congruence, have lessened the need for hard-on-hard couples.

Durasul Articulation

Durasul shows the same qualitative pattern as conventional polyethylene regarding bedding-in (immediate 3-month penetration) and running-in (period of creep, or plastic deformation, of the polyethylene in the first 2 years) leading to a steady state of wear. The steady state seems to be reached after 2 years with Durasul. Our data[6] showed penetration of 0.074 mm in the first postoperative year and penetration of 0.082 mm during the second postoperative year; the rate precipitously dropped to 0.01 mm during the third year and stayed steady with 0.02 mm of penetration in the fourth year and 0.01 mm in the fifth year after surgery. Our mean linear wear at 5 years was 0.03 mm. The mean linear wear has not differed with 28-, 32-, or 38-mm-diameter femoral heads.

The quantitative pattern of wear of Durasul is different after postoperative year 2 from that of conventional polyethylene, which was gamma irradiated in air and packaged in an oxygen-free environment. At year 1, we observed 0.15 mm of total wear for conventional polyethylene versus 0.074 mm total wear for Durasul. At 2 years, the annual penetration was 0.09 mm in conventional liners versus 0.08 mm in Durasul liners. The linear wear rate at 5 years was 0.03 mm for Durasul and 0.065 mm for conventional polyethylene. The wear rate of Durasul has been 45% of that of conventional polyethylene. Comparison of wear between Durasul (0.03 mm/year) and conventional polyethylene in studies by Sychterz and colleagues (0.17 mm/year),[7] Dowd and associates (0.18 mm/year),[8] and Pederson and colleagues (0.14 mm/year)[9] shows an 80% reduction in linear wear for Durasul.

The Durasul data are early results. Time is needed to observe whether the steady-state wear remains steady and well below the osteolysis threshold of 0.1 mm identified in hips on which we operated.

References

1. Maruyama M, Feinberg JR, Capello WN, D'Antonio JA: Morphologic features of the acetabulum and femur: Anteversion angle and implant positioning. Clin Orthop 393:52-65, 2001.
2. Kang JS, Dorr LD, Wan Z: The effect of diaphyseal biologic fixation on clinical results and fixation of the APR-II stem. J Arthroplasty 15:730-735, 2000.
3. Hofmann AA, Feign ME, Klauser W, VanGorp CC, Camargo MP: Cementless primary total hip arthroplasty with a tapered, proximally porous coated titanium prosthesis. J Arthroplasty 15:833-839, 2000.
4. Garcia-Cimbrelo E, Cruz-Pardos A, Madero R, Ortega Andrew M: Total hip arthroplasty with use of the cementless Zweymuller Alloclassic system. J Bone Joint Surg 85A:296-303, 2003.
5. Claus AM, Engh CA Jr, Sychterz CJ, et al: Radiographic definition of pelvis osteolysis following total hip arthroplasty. J Bone Joint Surg 85A:1519-1526, 2003.
6. Dorr LD, Wan Z, Shahrdar C, Sirianni LE, et al: Five year clinical performance and wear of a highly crossed-linked polyethylene acetabular liner. J Bone Joint Surg Am 87:1816–1821, 2005.
7. Sychterz CJ, Engh CA Jr, Shah N, Engh CA Sr: Radiographic evaluation of penetration by the femoral head into the polyethylene liner over time. J Bone Joint Surg 79A:1040-1046, 1997.
8. Dowd JE, Sychterz CJ, Young AM, Engh CA: Characterization of long-term femoral-head penetration rates. Association with and prediction of osteolytes. J Bone Joint Surg 82A:1102-1107, 2000.
9. Pederson DR, Callaghan JJ, Johnston TL, Fetzer GB, Johnston RC: Comparison of femoral head penetration rates between cementless acetabular components with 22-mm and 28-mm heads. J Arthroplasty 16S(1):111-115, 2001.

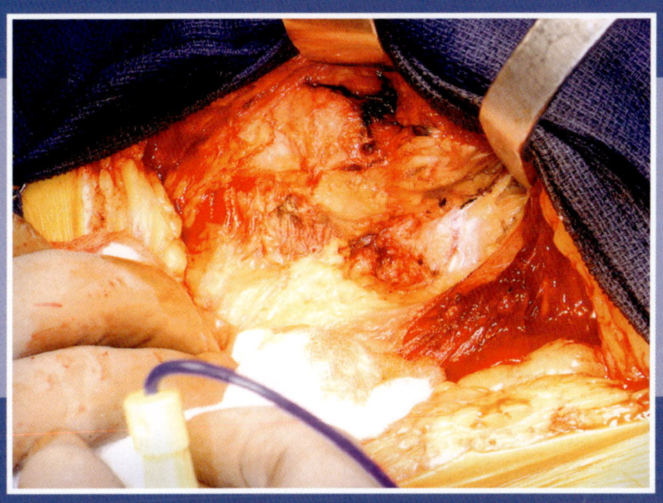

Chapter 3

Standard Posterior Exposure for Total Hip Replacement

EXPOSURE OF THE HIP JOINT

Proper exposure of the hip is the key to successful total hip replacement. A perfectly performed hip replacement controls soft tissue injury, positions the acetabular and femoral components with solid initial fixation to allow immediate weight bearing, and mates the femoral and acetabular components such that there is no impingement of the implants or bone through a wide range of motion. To accomplish these goals, the exposure must allow the surgeon to place the components correctly without significant soft tissue injury.

Most surgeons use the hip exposure they learned during training. Comfort with the hip exposure has a significant bearing on the surgeon's stress level during the operation, and learning a new exposure is associated with a learning curve during which the stress level and risk of surgical errors are higher. Therefore, the surgeon should maximize his or her education about a surgical exposure before applying it.

The first goal for a surgeon learning a new exposure is to gain a clear mental picture of the operation. Then, the achievement of flawless technique requires repeated practice. Most surgeons continue to learn new technical maneuvers throughout their careers. This happens by critically evaluating one's performance and by observing the techniques of other master surgeons and incorporating them into one's repertoire.

In this chapter, I describe the standard posterior exposure for total hip replacement, in the hope that readers will be able to develop their own mental picture of the procedure. Repeatedly viewing the accompanying video, "*Posterior Total Hip Replacement Traditional Incisions,*" will help reinforce the various technical moves necessary to perform the operation skillfully.

STANDARD POSTERIOR EXPOSURE FOR TOTAL HIP REPLACEMENT

The standard posterior approach for the hip is accomplished with the patient in the lateral position on the operating table. The patient should be stabilized securely so that body position will not change during the operation. Secure stabilization of the body also allows the table to be tilted forward or backward to enhance visualization of the acetabulum or femur without changing the body position. Secure stabilization is achieved through supports that fix the pelvis and chest (Fig. 3–1). We use a commercially available support system consisting of four separate supports (SunMedica; Redding, Calif.). The pelvic supports rest against the bones to minimize the chance of tissue damage. The posterior support is placed against the posterior iliac spines of the pelvis with padding between the skin and the post. The anterior pelvic support is placed against the down-side anterior iliac spine and the pubis. Some patients experience postoperative edema of the genitalia from the anterior support, particularly if the operation was longer than 2 hours. However, this edema resolves within 2 weeks and is not painful.

The chest supports are placed at the level of the scapular tips posteriorly and just below the breasts anteriorly, against the xiphoid of the sternum. Again, soft padding is used to protect the skin. The chest supports should be tightened securely, but not so tightly that they interfere with chest expansion for ventilation during the operation. The patient should be aligned on the table in the support system so that the sagittal axis through the chest and pelvis is a straight line. This usually means that the tip of the shoulder, the high point of the ilium, and the trochanter are all on the same line (Fig. 3–2). The hips and knees each should be bent approximately 30 degrees, and padding should be placed along the lower leg to protect the peroneal nerve as it crosses the fibula (Fig. 3–3). With the patient securely stabilized in this position, the surgeon may concentrate on preparation and component placement without worrying about pelvic position.

The skin incision should be centered over the posterior third of the trochanter and extend for 4 fingerbreadths above the tip of the greater trochanter and 4 fingerbreadths below the vastus tubercle (Fig. 3–4). The length of the incision can vary from 6 to 15 inches, depending on the surgeon's preference. The incision through the skin and subcutaneous tissue is done on this curvilinear path. Only the aggressively bleeding vessels in the subcutaneous tissue need to be cauterized; most of the subcutaneous bleeding vessels will clot on their own. Using the coagulation arm of the Bovie electrocautery for incision of the subcutaneous tissue also helps to control bleeding.

The fascia over the gluteus maximus and the tensor fascia are also incised along this same path. After incision of the fascia, the gluteus maximus muscle is split in line with its herringbone pattern. (I do this with a Bovie so that if I come near the nerve of the gluteus maximus, the muscle contracts vigorously, and I can avoid cutting the nerve between the upper and lower heads of the muscle.) The gluteus maximus can also be split with a finger, using gentle pressure to protect the nerve. Once the fascia and gluteus maximus muscle fibers are split, a self-retaining retractor is placed to hold the edges of the fascia and the muscle is separated to allow exposure of the deep structures of the hip (Fig. 3–5).

The deep structures of the hip are visualized, including the greater trochanter, the gluteus medius cephalic, and the fascia of the vastus lateralis muscle on the femur. The fat overlying the external rotators is visible

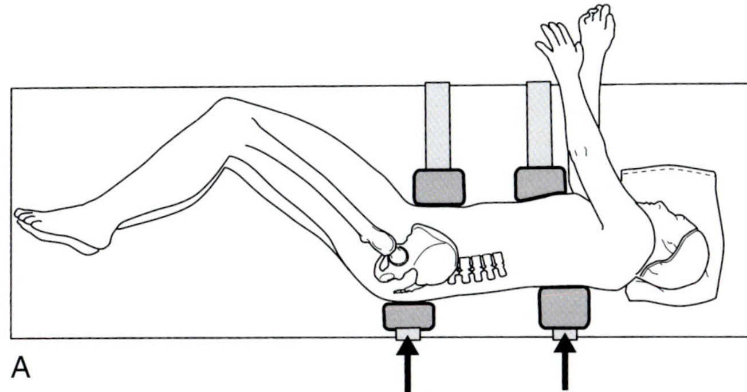

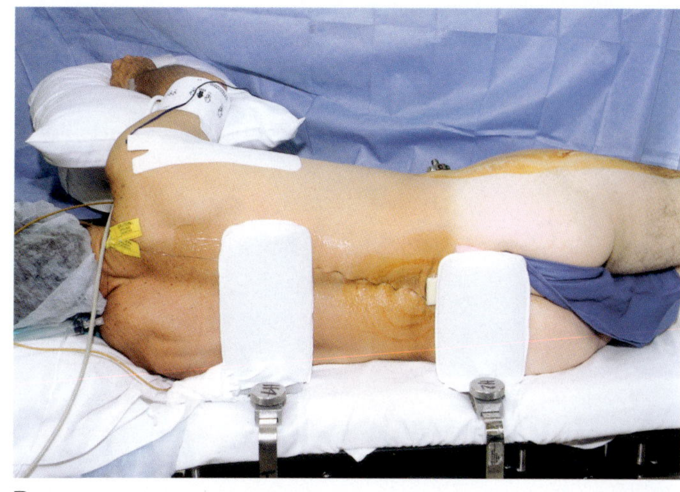

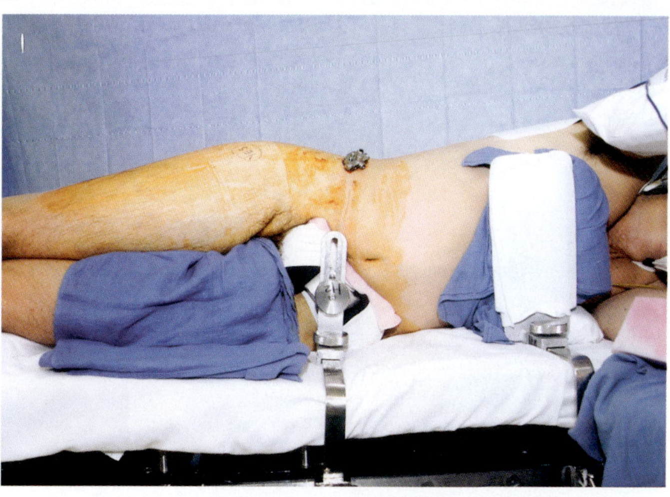

Figure 3–1 **A,** The patient in the lateral position is supported by two chest supports and two pelvic supports. These four supports maintain the patient in a rigid position that stabilizes the pelvis for acetabular placement, as well as allowing the table to be turned to or away from the surgeon without changing the longitudinal axis of the pelvis. **B,** Operating room view of the posterior supports. The posterior pelvic support is placed against the posterior inferior iliac spines, and the posterior chest support is placed at the base of the scapulae. The posterior pelvic support can be elevated to rest higher against the posterior pelvis in patients who are fatter or more muscular, which will prevent the upper buttock from rotating over the support. **C,** Operating room view of the anterior supports. The anterior pelvic support is placed against the down-side anterior superior iliac spine and the pubis, and the anterior chest support is placed just below the breast. Padding is placed between the supports to protect the skin and genitalia with the pelvic support and the breasts with the chest support.

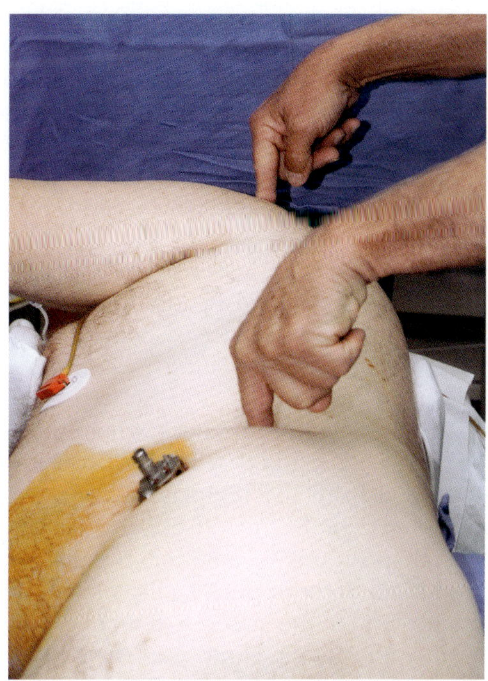

Figure 3–2 The patient's body is properly aligned if the upper finger on the tip of the shoulder and the longer finger on the high point of the iliac crest are aligned with the high point of the hip, which is the greater trochanter. The pelvic base for the computer is attached to the pelvis. When the patient is aligned in this manner, the longitudinal axis of the body is controlled by the supports shown in Figure 3–1.

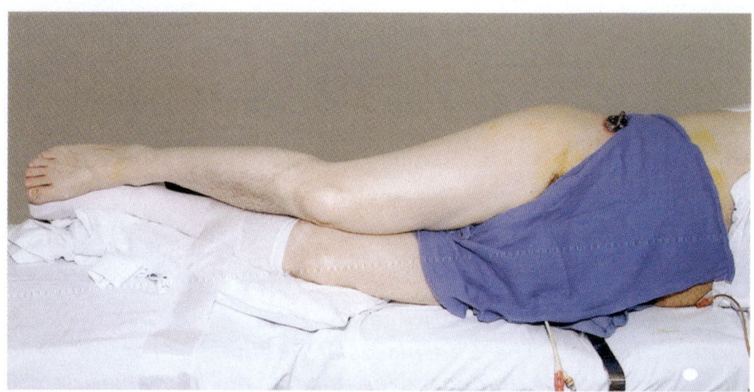

Figure 3–3 The patient's hips and knees should be bent at approximately 30 degrees each. Padding is placed under the lower leg from the knee to the ankle to protect the peroneal nerve. We usually put only a towel between the legs and tape across the lower leg. This allows us to feel the relative positions of the patellae and the soles of the feet to judge leg lengths. A pillow or padding placed between the legs distorts the relative positions of these anatomic structures.

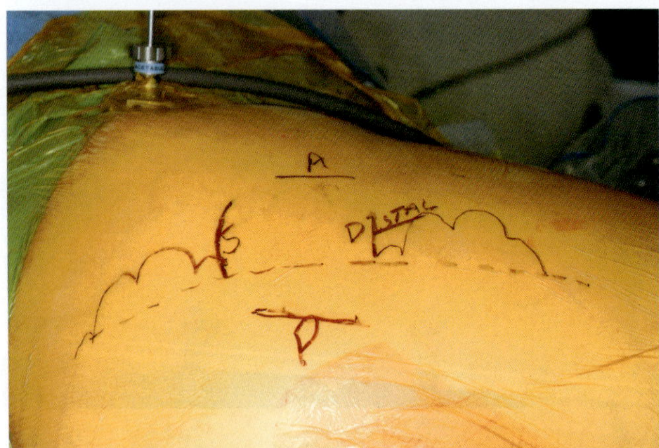

Figure 3–4 *The long skin incision encompasses 4 finger-breadths above the tip of the greater trochanter and 4 below the vastus tubercle.*

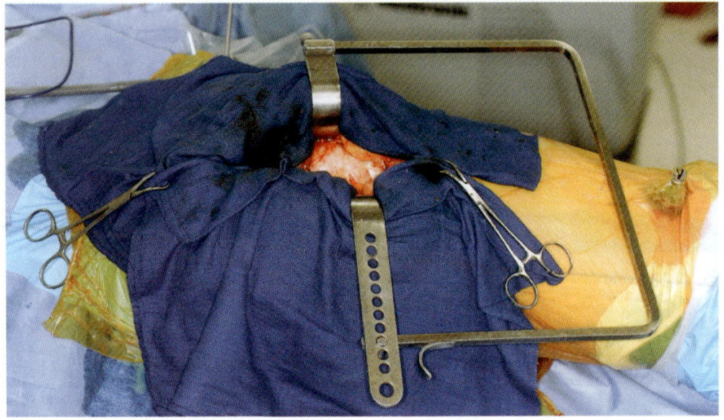

A

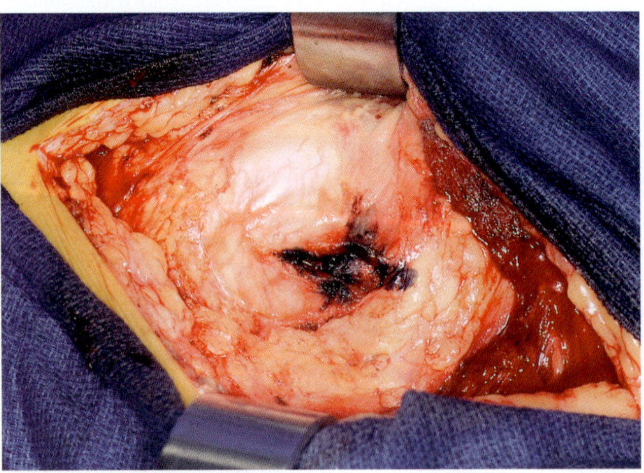

B

Figure 3–5 *A, The Charnley self-retaining retractor separates the anterior and posterior flaps of the long incision and exposes the greater trochanter and posterior structures of the hip. B, Exposure of the hip using the Charnley retractor shows the greater trochanter, marked by a methylene blue "X," and the fat overlying the posterior hip musculature.*

posterior to the trochanter. The hip is internally rotated, which moves the posterior edge of the trochanter anteriorly to give easier access to the external rotators and the posterior capsule, as well as to provide separation between the sciatic nerve lying on the ischium and the posterior aspect of the greater trochanter (Fig. 3–6). The fat is incised off the posterior trochanter using the coagulation arm of the Bovie to expose the external rotators and tendon of the gluteus maximus. A bent Homans retractor is placed under the gluteus medius tendon and on top of and over the piriformis tendon to protect the gluteus medius muscle. This retraction exposes the piriformis and gluteus minimus muscle at the superior edge of the posterior trochanter (Fig. 3–7).

The external rotators from the intertrochanteric ridge (thereby including the quadratus femoris muscle) and the capsule are incised off the femoral neck and onto the superior edge of the acetabulum, which necessitates incision into the gluteus minimus muscle for approximately 3 cm. This creates a flap of external rotators and capsule that can be retracted during the operation and repaired after its completion (Fig. 3–8). The gluteus maximus tendon is incised from its attachment onto the femur (Fig. 3–9). This allows easy retraction of the femur anterior to the acetabulum and also prevents compression of the sciatic nerve, which runs under this tendon, during anterior retraction of the femur. The tendon is repaired during closure.

Dislocation of the hip exposes the entire neck and head of the femur, including the lesser trochanter and the insertion of the iliopsoas tendon (Fig. 3–10). I release one third of the iliopsoas tendon, which is the portion of the tendon that wraps around the superior aspect of the lesser trochanter. This is done to recess the tendon and reduce the risk for groin pain from the abrasion of the tendon across any exposed anterior edge of the metal shell. Recession of the tendon also exposes the lesser trochanter, which can be used as a measuring point.

The distance from the lesser trochanter to the estimated center of the femoral head is measured using a ruler (Fig. 3–11). This distance is compared with that from the preoperative templating to confirm that the magnification of the x-rays was close to the actual size of the bone. The level on the neck where the neck cut should be made is marked with the Bovie; this level was determined from the templating based on reconstruction of hip length and offset. The cut should be oblique, from posterior to anterior, because leaving a somewhat longer anterior neck facilitates the placement of a retractor under the anterior femoral neck during preparation of the femur. Bone wax is placed onto the cut surface of the neck to prevent blood from dripping into the acetabulum during preparation of the acetabulum (Fig. 3–12).

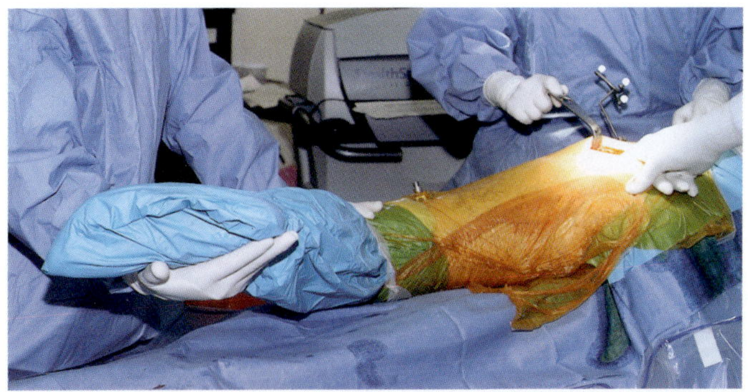

Figure 3–6 **A,** *The leg is internally rotated by applying pressure against the knee and lifting the lower leg, rotating the greater trochanter and its attached musculature away from the sciatic nerve to permit a safer incision through the posterior structures.* **B,** *The trochanter in the externally rotated position shows its approximation to the fat overlying the sciatic nerve and the greater trochanter (GT) and nerve (N).* **C,** *When the leg is internally rotated, the greater trochanter (GT) moves away from the fat containing the sciatic nerve (N). QF, quadratus femoris.*

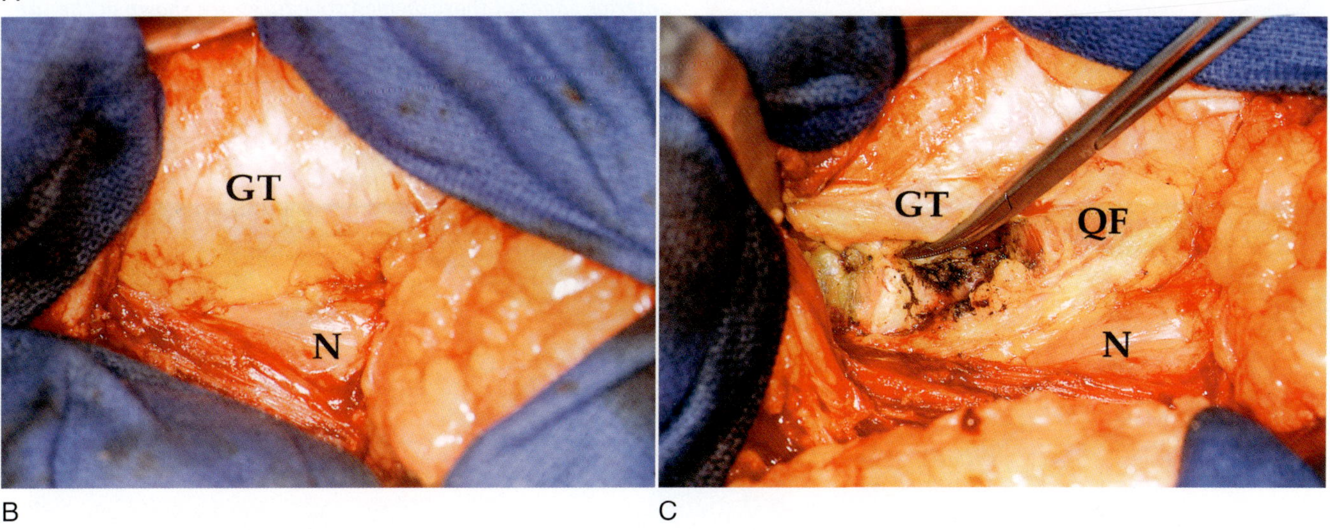

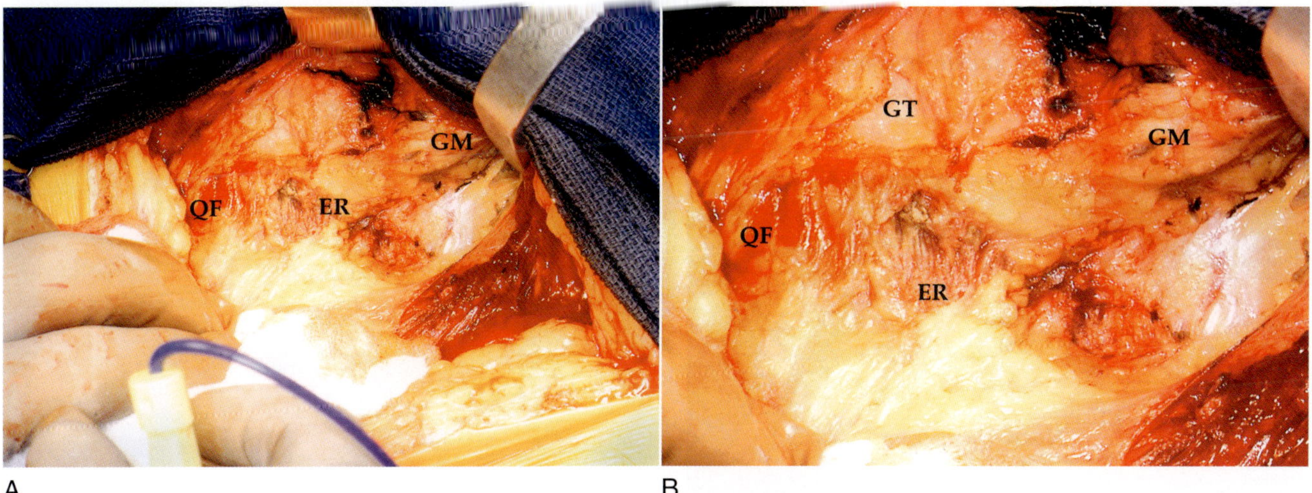

Figure 3–7 **A,** *The deep structures of the long incision. The metal retractor in the upper right is retractor #2, which retracts the tendon of the gluteus medius (GM). The GM muscle lies distal to the retractor and attaches to the greater trochanter (GT). The gluteus minimus muscle is visible below the GM muscle, and distal to that are the external rotators (ER), the last of which is the quadratus femoris (QF).* **B,** *Close-up view of the posterior structures of a left hip with the retractor under the GM tendon, barely visible in the upper right; the gluteus minimus lies below the GM. The ERs are visible below the GT, with the QF the most distal of them.*

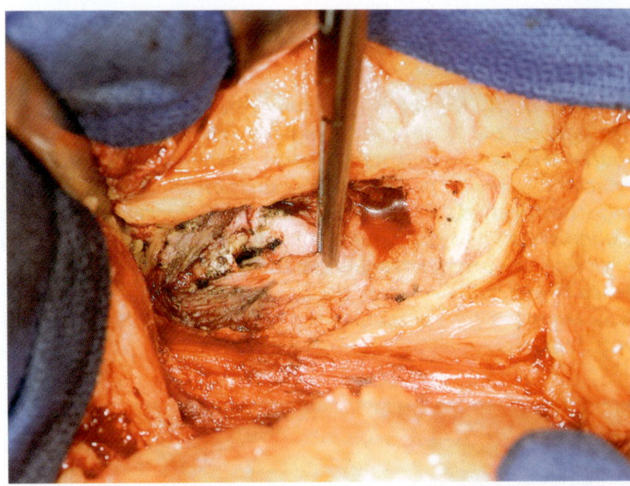

Figure 3–8   *Division of the external rotators and capsule of a right hip allows exposure of the femoral head and neck. The anterior edges of these divided structures are shown at the superior edge of the femoral head, and the posterior edges are held by a Kocher clamp. These edges are repaired by sutures at the conclusion of the reconstruction.*

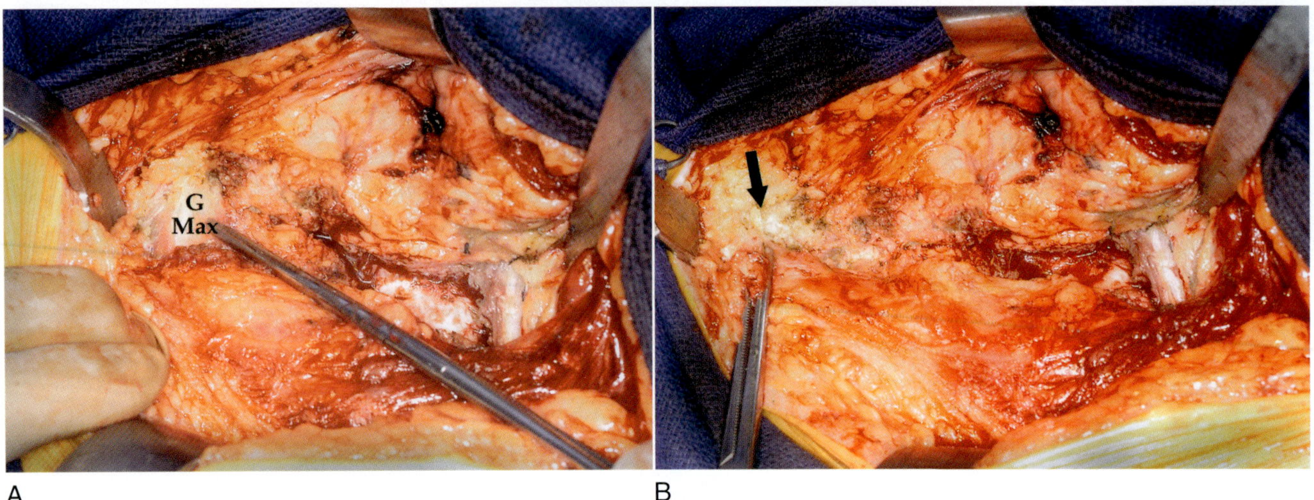

Figure 3–9   *A, In a left hip, the gluteus maximus (G Max) tendon attaches to the femur distal to the quadratus femoris. B, The gluteus maximus tendon is partially or completely incised from its attachment to the femur (arrow) to facilitate retraction of the femur anterior to the acetabulum as well as release tension on the sciatic nerve during femoral retraction. The sciatic nerve runs in the fat just below the gluteus maximus tendon.*

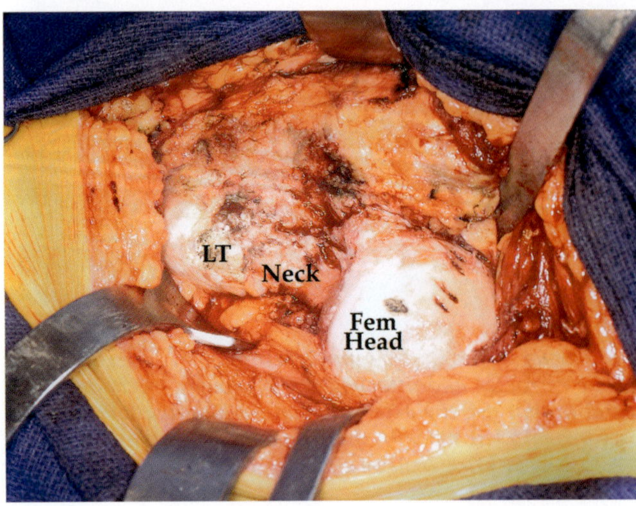

Figure 3–10   *The femoral head has been dislocated from the acetabulum and the entire length of the hip can be seen, including the femoral head, femoral neck, and lesser trochanter, with the insertion of the iliopsoas tendon to the lesser trochanter.*

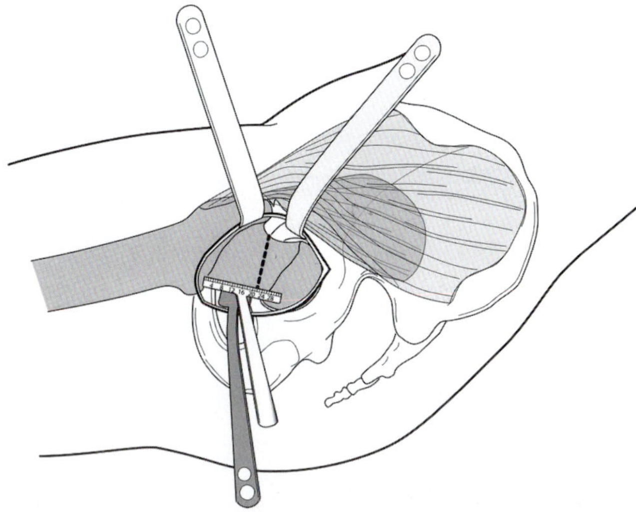

A

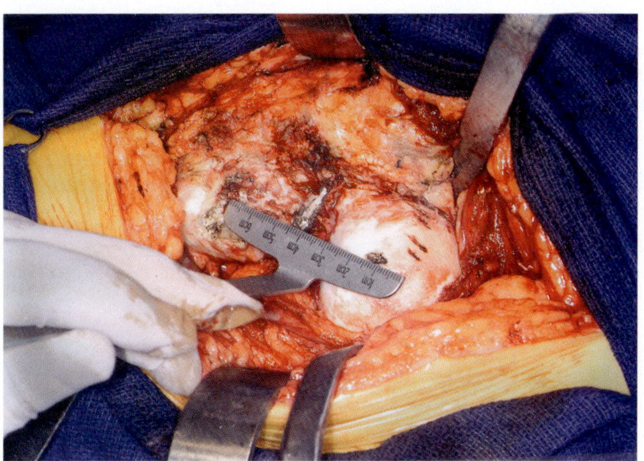

B

Figure 3–11 **A,** *Use of the ruler to measure the length of the hip from the lesser trochanter to the center of the femoral head. The desired neck cut can be marked with a Bovie electrocautery. The neck cut has been determined from preoperative templating and is validated by hip length measurement.* **B,** *Intraoperative view of measurement of hip length from the lesser trochanter to the center of the femoral head. The upper third of the iliopsoas tendon attachment has been removed from the lesser trochanter, and the center of the femoral head has been marked by the Bovie. A Bovie mark is made on the femoral neck at the desired level of the neck cut.*

Acetabular Preparation

A bent Homans retractor (or the retractor from the posterior mini-incision instrument set) is placed between the capsule and the labrum of the acetabulum at the posterosuperior corner of the acetabulum (Fig. 3–13). This can usually be malleted into position so that it does not need to be held by an assistant. The anterosuperior corner of the capsule is excised between the cut level of the femoral neck and the superior acetabulum (see Fig. 3–13B). The labrum is removed from the edge of the acetabulum using a long-handled knife (see

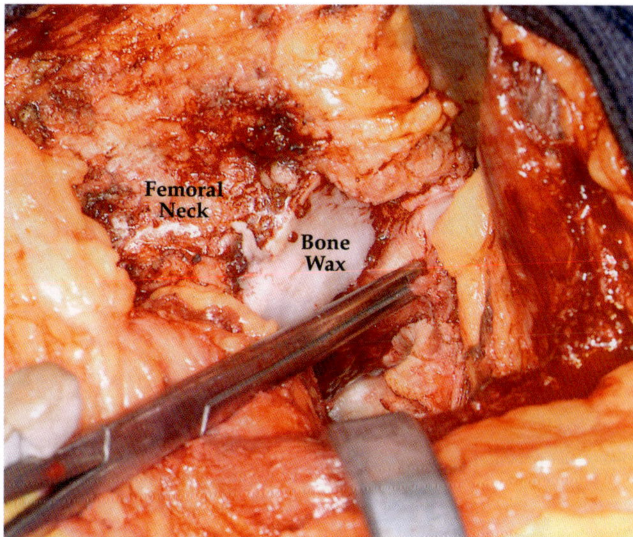

Figure 3–12 *The cut surface of the femoral neck has been covered with bone wax and is marked.*

Fig. 3–15B). The "snake retractor" is placed under the tip of the greater trochanter and onto the ilium, and the tip of this retractor is malleted into the bone (Fig. 3–14). This retractor gives excellent leverage for retracting the femur anterior to the acetabulum, and the trochanteric bone acts as its fulcrum so that it does not damage the gluteus medius muscle (Fig. 3–15). The snake retractor should not be placed against the anterior wall of the acetabulum because it can fracture the anterior wall, as well as put the femoral nerve at risk for a traction injury. I have never had a femoral nerve palsy in my patients when placing the snake retractor on the ilium. If the trochanter needs to be retracted further anteriorly, incise the reflected head of the rectus muscle and the remaining anterior capsule.

The posterior medial capsule of the hip is incised. This capsule runs from the posterior acetabulum to the femur and runs across the medial aspect of the acetabulum (which looks like the inferior aspect of the acetabulum with the patient in the lateral position). It also covers the transverse acetabular ligament (see Fig. 3–15). This capsule is incised across its width to the level of the transverse acetabular ligament; I also incise the transverse acetabular ligament. Incision of this capsule is the final step to allow easy retraction of the femur anterior to the acetabulum. Incision of the capsule also removes any arthritic contraction, which helps to mobilize the hip postoperatively into flexion and rotation (Fig. 3–16).

A Cobra retractor (or the #7 retractor from the mini-incision set) is placed with the tip around the cortical bone of the cotyloid notch, exposing the medial aspect of the acetabulum (Fig. 3–17). If a Cobra is used, a posterior retractor is placed along the posterior acetabulum with the tip just cephalic to the ischium, and the paddle of this retractor sits on the ischium to retract the

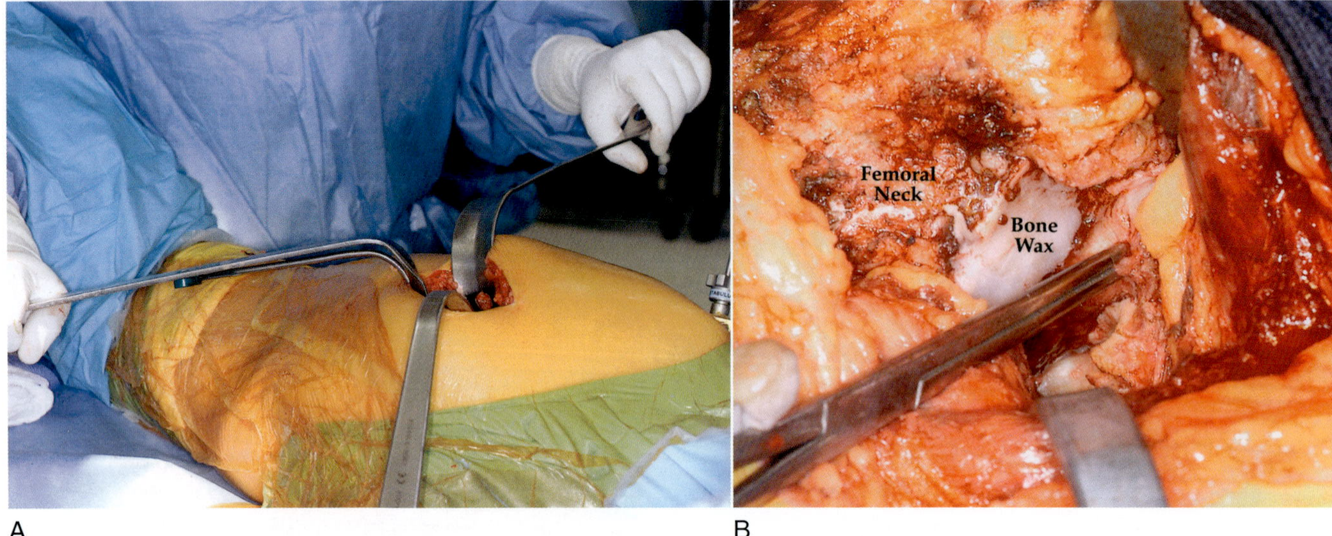

A   B

Figure 3–13   **A,** *Surgical view with a small incision, showing positioning of the #4 retractor in the posterosuperior corner of the acetabulum. The assistant cradles the leg in her right arm and holds the #7 retractor in her right hand. She holds the #5b anterior retractor in her left arm, at the upper side of the wound. The #4 retractor emerges from the posterosuperior corner of the wound; its tip has been malleted into the bone so that it sits in position without having to be held. **B,** The acetabulum is exposed by instrumentation designed specifically for this purpose. The #4 retractor is positioned at the posterosuperior corner of the acetabulum between the posterior flap of the capsule and the labrum (metal retractor at lower center of wound). This protects the posterosuperior capsule and begins exposure of the acetabulum. The Kocher Clamp grasps the anterior superior capsule that is to be excised.*

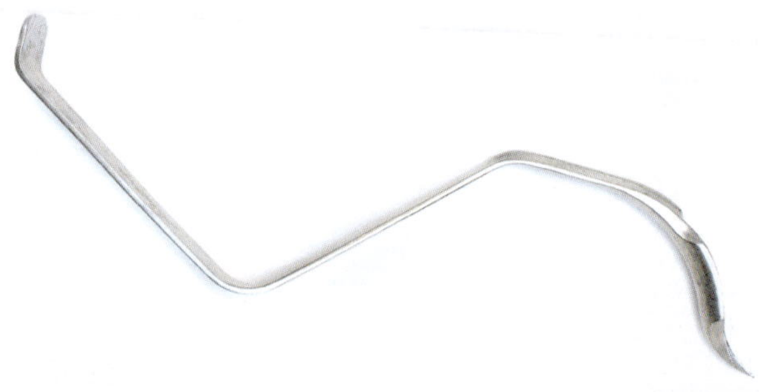

Figure 3–14   *The anterosuperior #5 retractor ("snake retractor") has its tip malleted into the ilium and pulls the greater trochanter anterior to the acetabulum. The anterosuperior corner of the capsule is excised between the cut level of the femoral neck and the superior acetabulum to allow placement of this retractor. Resection of the capsule also helps eliminate flexion contractures of the hip.*

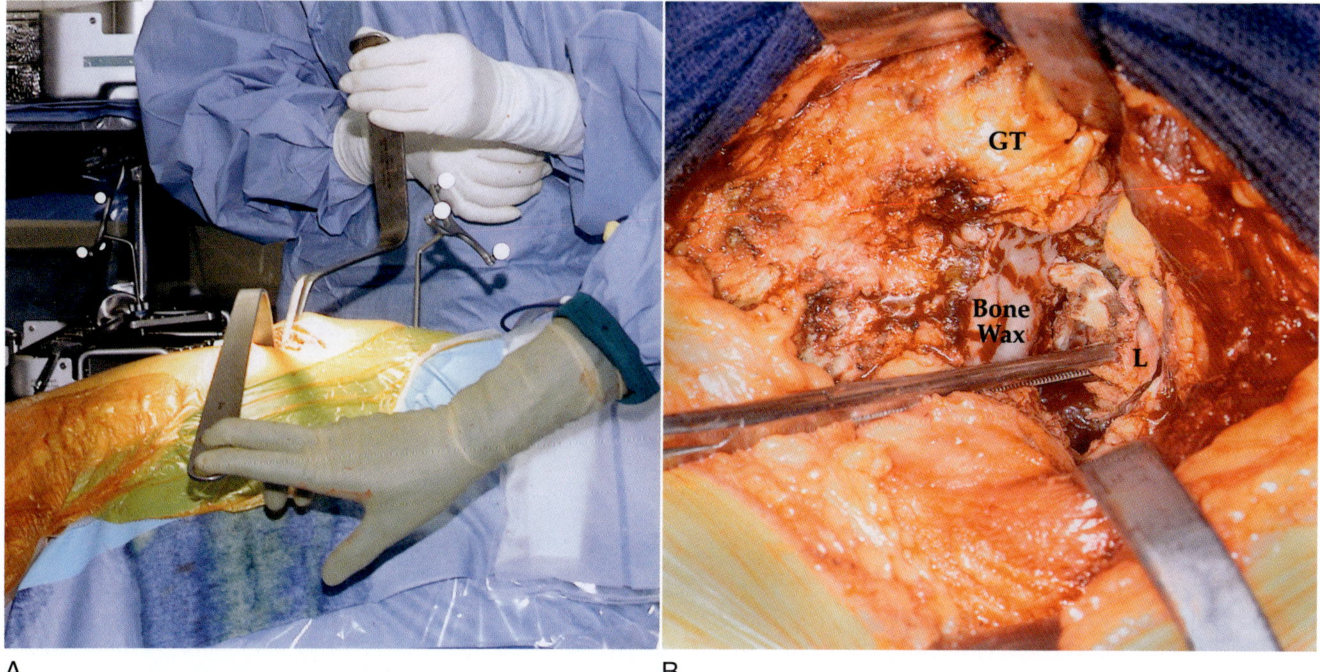

Figure 3–15 **A,** *Long view of the #5 retractor at the upper side of the wound. The #4 retractor is on the lower side of the wound.* **B,** *The #5 retractor anteriorly and the #4 retractor posteriorly give good exposure of the superior acetabulum. The labrum (L) can be excised to expose the bony rim of the acetabulum. GT, greater trochanter.*

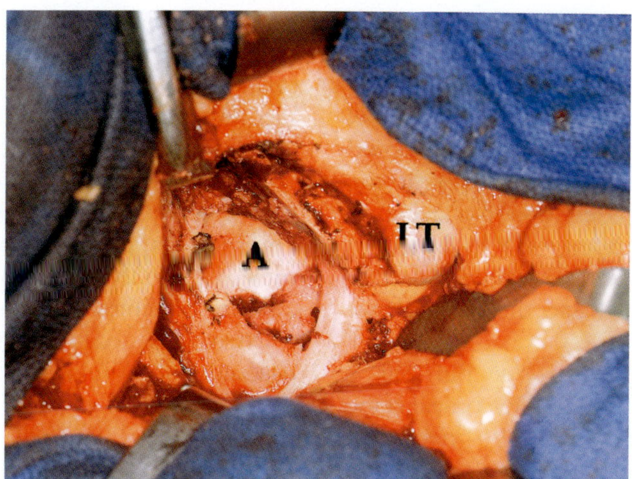

Figure 3–16 *The #6 retractor is positioned between the medial-inferior capsule (seen intact across the right side of the acetabulum [A]) and the external oblique muscle with its tip at the level of the transverse acetabular ligament. This retractor protects the medial circumflex artery and vein from being cut while the medial inferior capsule (which includes the ischiofemoral ligament) is incised vertically through the transverse acetabular ligament. LT, lesser trochanter.*

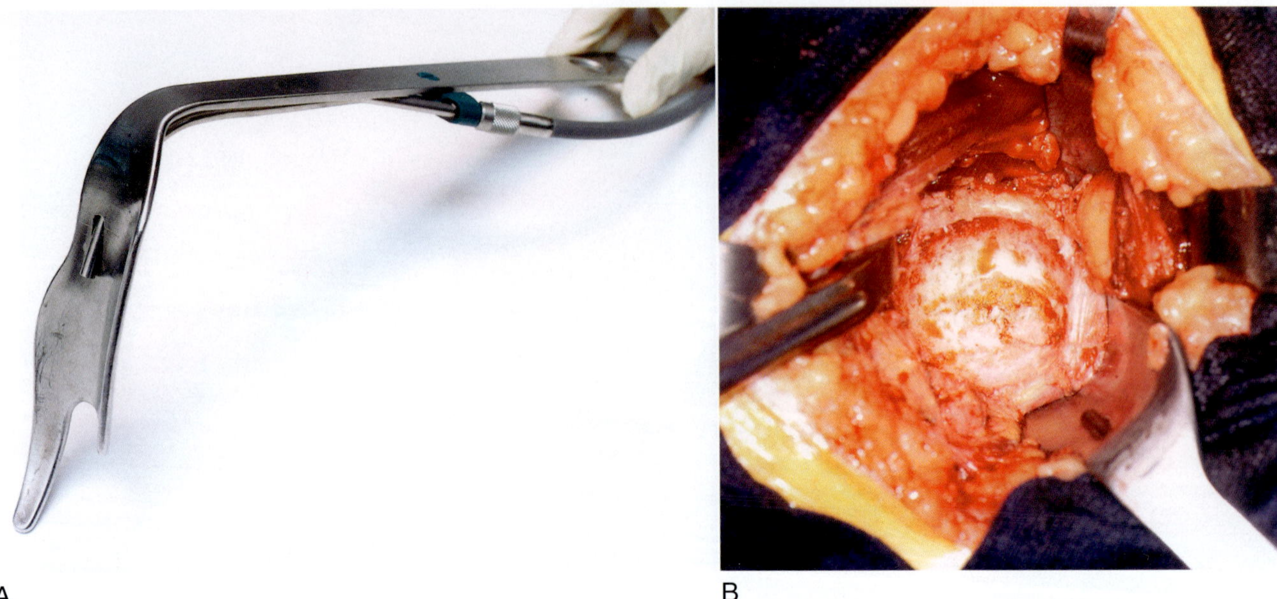

A

B

Figure 3-17 *A, The #7 retractor is shown with its fiberoptic light source attachment. The tip of the retractor is placed against the cortical bone of the cotyloid notch and the paddle sits on the ischium. The light source helps illuminate the acetabulum during its preparation. B, The attached fiberoptic light source is shown illuminating the acetabulum. The snake retractor is seen at the upper anterior corner of the acetabulum with its tip in the ilium. The #4 retractor is visible at lower right. There is complete visualization of the acetabulum.*

posterior capsule and protect the sciatic nerve (Fig. 3–18). The leg is laid on the table with the hip and knee flexed so that the remaining femoral neck is rotated away from the anterior wall of the acetabulum. Sometimes the best position is with the leg flat on the table, and sometimes it is with the foot on a Mayo stand and the leg slightly internally rotated (Fig. 3–19). If the gluteus medius muscle overlaps the superior acetabulum enough to occlude visualization, or is in danger of injury with reaming, it should be retracted cephalad by the placement of a Charnley pin into the ilium above the superior acetabular rim.

The hip is prepared for reaming. The pulvinar is excised from the cotyloid notch so that the cortical bone of the cotyloid notch is visible, which is necessary because this bone is the medial end point for reaming (Fig. 3–20). The first reamer chosen should be of a size that barely touches the anterior and posterior walls of the acetabulum, and the direction of the reamer should be in anteversion of the acetabulum, but at a steep angle (nearly transverse) to allow removal of the acetabular ridge (Fig. 3–21). This reamer will remove the bone to the level of the cortical bone of the cotyloid notch. The next reamer should make just enough contact with the anterior and posterior walls that it prepares the bone for peripheral contact of the cup but does not weaken the walls. This reamer is directed cephalad to begin to form a hemisphere with the superior surface of the acetabulum. A third reamer is usually needed to contact the entire periphery of the acetabulum, and this is

also directed cephalad into the direction of anteversion desired to complete the formation of a hemisphere. The size of the osseous acetabulum is also determined by this last reamer (Fig. 3–22). Reaming should result in a bleeding bed of cancellous bone (Fig. 3–23). In some cases, there is cortical bone in the cotyloid notch, and most of the superior surface of the acetabulum is bleeding cortical bone. All cartilage should be removed. Osteophytes may need to be removed, but this is most commonly done after the trial is placed so that the amount of removal necessary can be visualized.

Next, the trial cup is placed into the prepared osseous bed. Trial cups have holes through which the bone can be visualized to ensure complete contact of metal to bone (Fig. 3–24). The trial cup should fit snugly enough that it needs to be malleted into position. If it can simply be placed into position, the acetabulum has been reamed too large for the cup, and the next larger-size trial cup must be used. If the trial cup is not fully seated in its position after malleting, the acetabulum needs to be reamed again to achieve a complete fit. When the trial cup is fully seated into the bone, the acetabular position must be determined. Commonly, anterosuperior and anterior wall osteophytes are present and must be removed so that they do not cause impingement during flexion (Fig. 3–25). If posterosuperior and posterior wall osteophytes also are present, they need to be removed to prevent impingement during extension (Fig. 3–26).

Text continued on page 42

Figure 3–18 **A,** The tip of this posterior retractor used with the long incision is placed superior to the ischium, with the paddle sitting on the ischium. This retractor is used to retract the posterior capsule and protect the sciatic nerve if a Cobra retractor is placed around the edge of the cotyloid notch. **B,** The posterior retractor in place. The retractor is somewhat obscured in this view (outlined by arrows), *but its position is well illustrated as it retracts the posterior capsule and protects the sciatic nerve.*

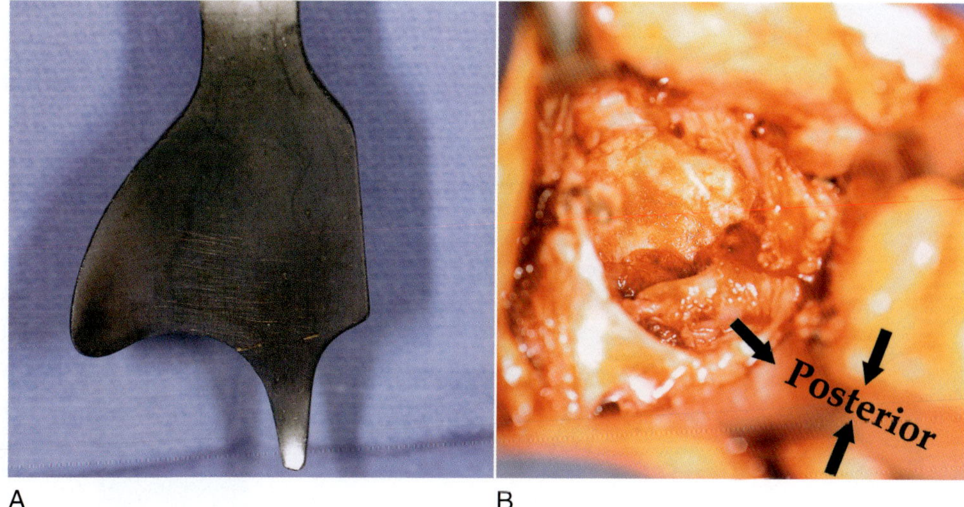

A   B

Figure 3–19 View of the operating table with the patient's foot on the Mayo stand, which slightly internally rotates the leg. This position can help clear the femoral neck from the anterior edge of the acetabulum, but sometimes the femoral neck is best cleared with the leg laying flat on the table. The #5 and #4 retractors are in place in the acetabulum.

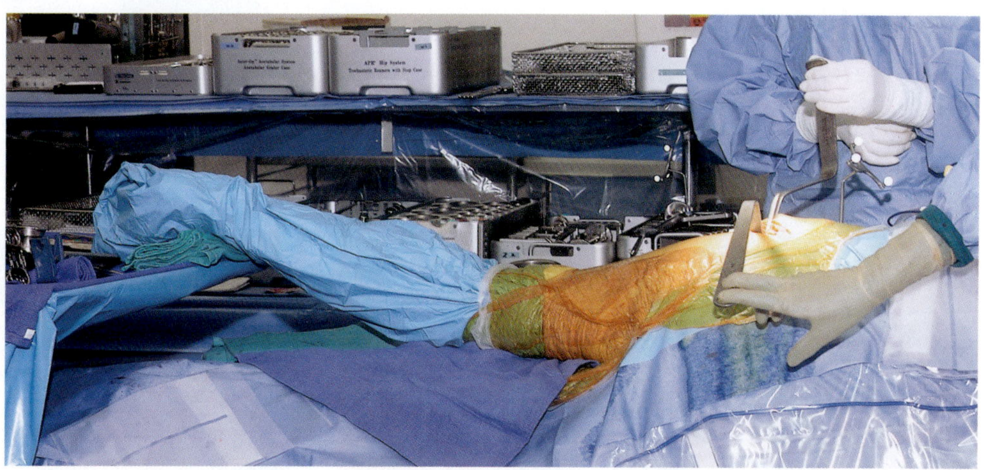

Figure 3–20 The cortical bone of the cotyloid notch has been exposed by removal of an osteophyte, and the pulvinar has been removed using the Bovie. A thin film of blood covers the cortical bone. The #7 retractor is seen in the lower right at the base of the cotyloid notch. The #4 retractor is in the lower left, and the #5 retractor is in the upper right. An additional retractor is placed superior to the acetabulum to provide increased exposure for the photograph.

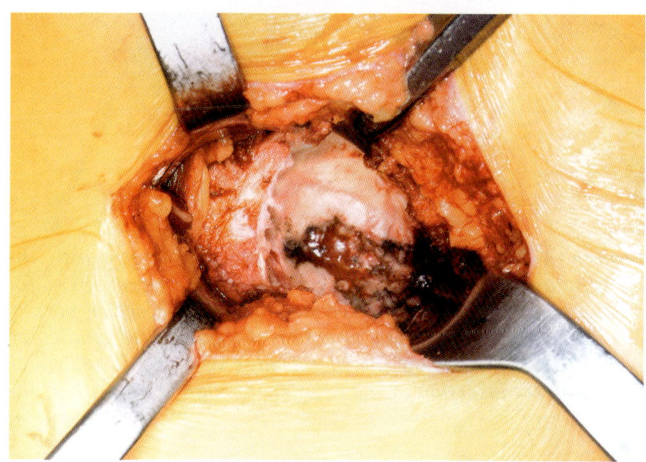

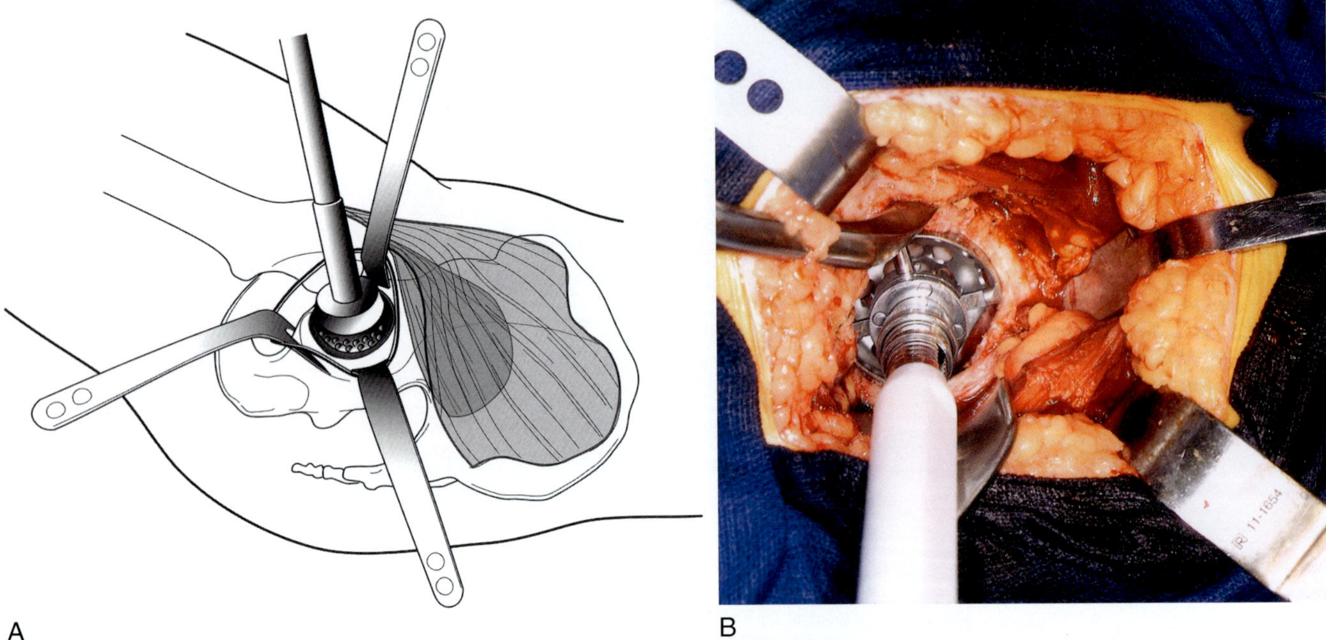

A

B

Figure 3–21 **A,** *Transverse placement of the reamer into the acetabulum to remove the acetabular ridge and ream to the level of the cortical bone of the cotyloid notch.* **B,** *Intraoperative view of the reamer placed directly into the acetabulum for removal of the acetabular ridge. This is a half-reamer, which gives better visualization of the acetabular walls during reaming.*

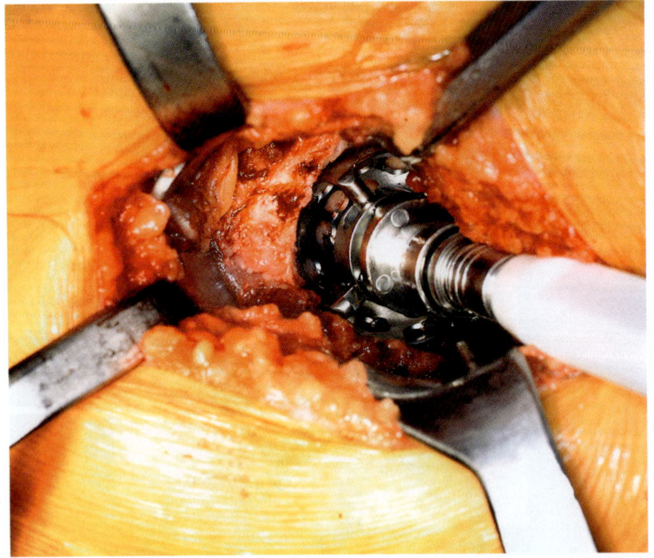

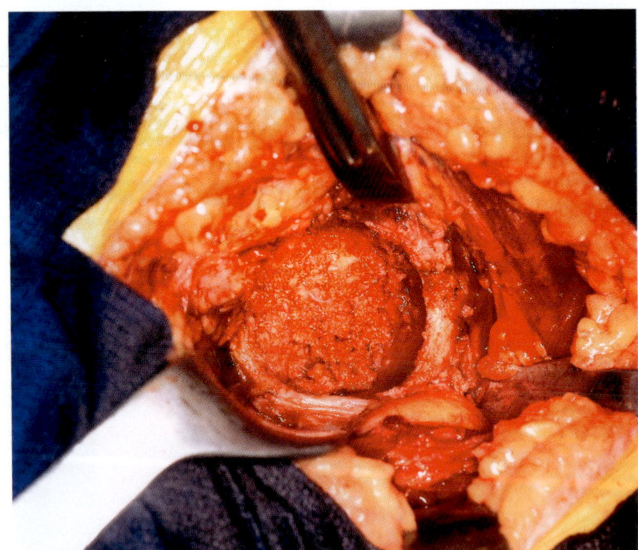

Figure 3–22 *The last reamer is placed directly into the acetabulum along its axis to form the final hemisphere for placement of the cup. This reamer touches the entire periphery of the acetabulum. The direction of the reamer is indicated by the handle crossing the distal edge of the wound, which allows direct insertion of the reamer through the mouth of the acetabulum.*

Figure 3–23 *The bleeding cancellous bone of the acetabulum provides an excellent bony bed for fixation of a porous-coated cup.*

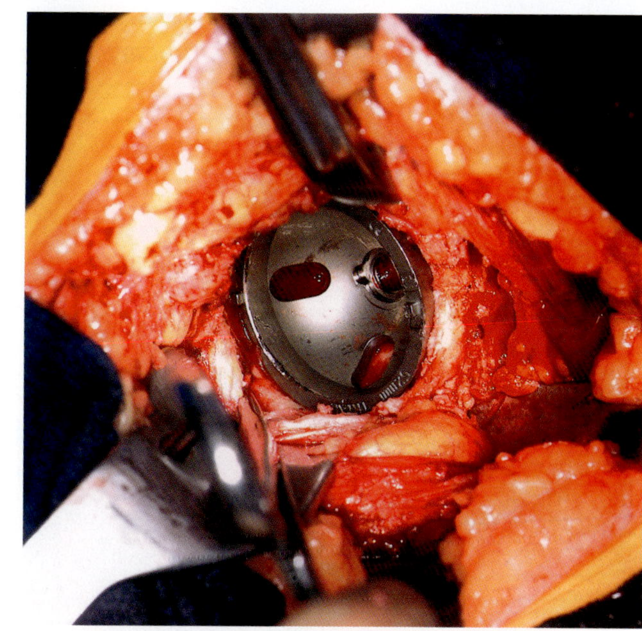

Figure 3-24 *A trial cup placed into the acetabulum. The holes in the trial allow visualization of the contact of the metal shell to the acetabular bone. The periphery of the metal shell is in direct contact with the periphery of the entire acetabulum.*

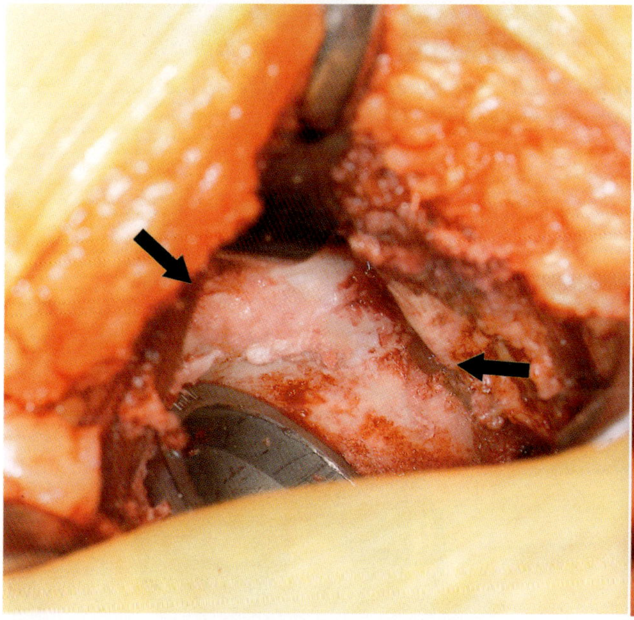

A

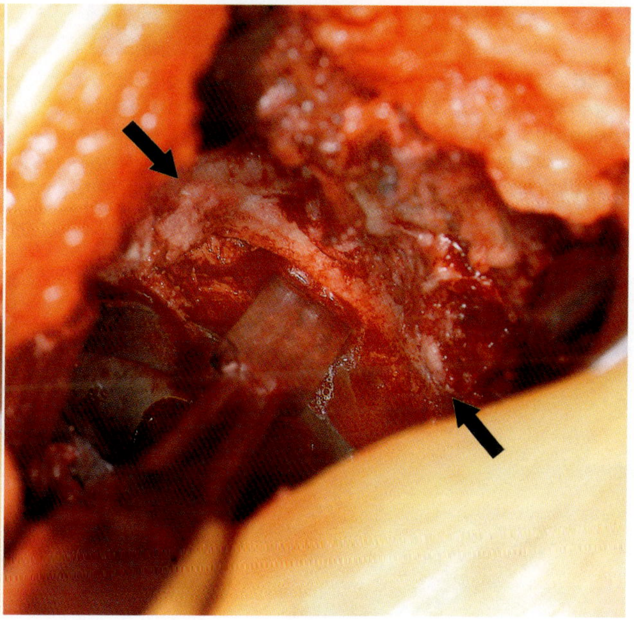

B

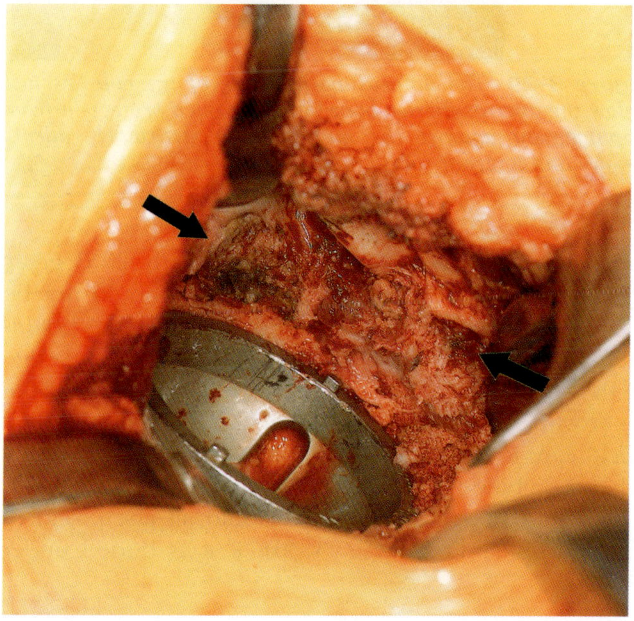

C

Figure 3-25 **A,** *A large anterior osteophyte (arrows) protrudes above the anterior edge of the metal shell when it is in its correct position.* **B,** *An osteotome is used to fracture the osteophyte (arrows) above the anterior edge of the metal shell.* **C,** *The osteophyte has been removed (arrows) in such a way that the anterior capsule remains in place.*

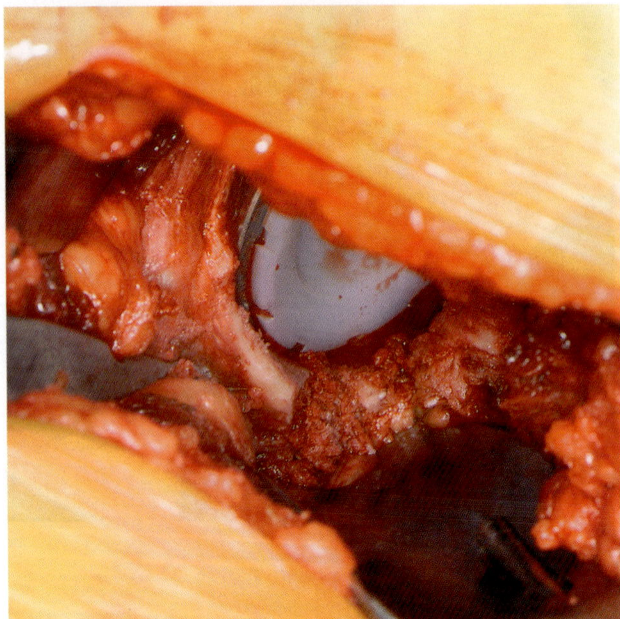

Figure 3–26 *A posterior osteophyte protrudes above the posterior metal edge of the cup from the posterosuperior corner, continuing distally on top of the ischium. The osteophyte has already been removed where it overlaid the transverse acetabular ligament. The #7 retractor is seen at bottom.*

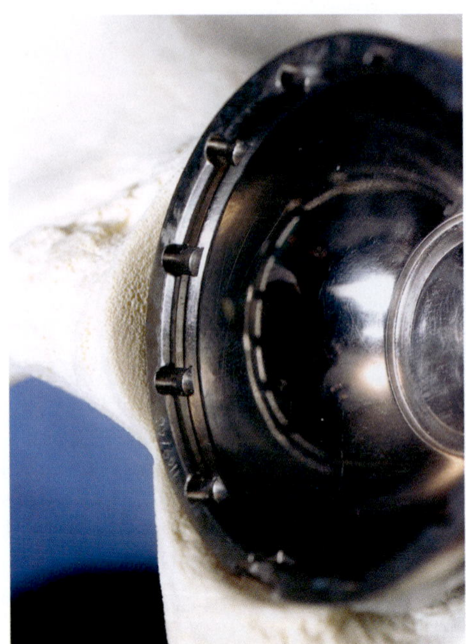

Figure 3–28 *The anteroinferior edge of the cup sits 5 mm below the pubic tubercle.*

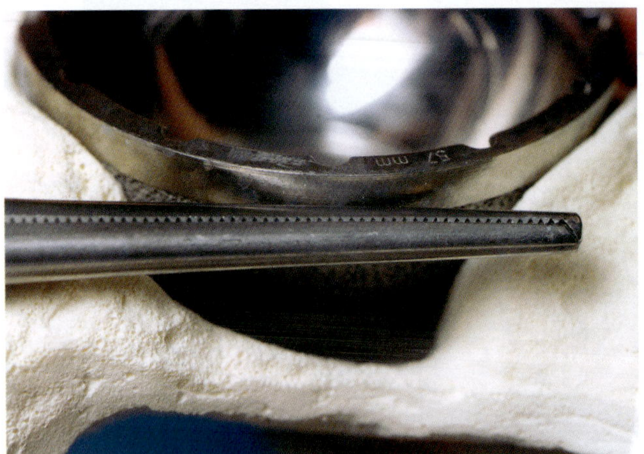

Figure 3–27 *A Kocher clamp imitating the position of the transverse acetabular ligament. The metal edge of the shell is shown in its correct position relative to the pubis, ischium, and transverse acetabular ligament.*

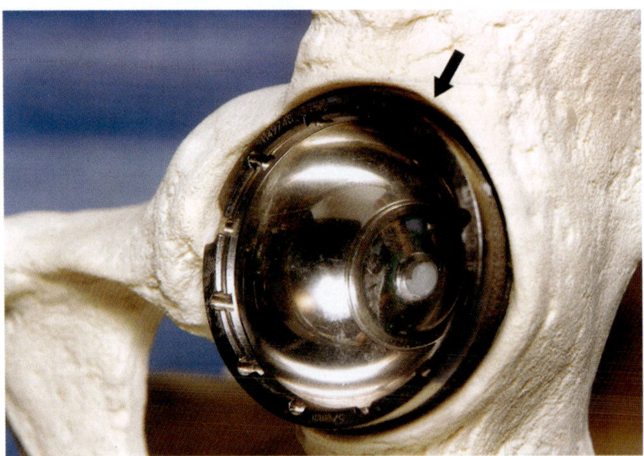

Figure 3–29 *The anterosuperior edge of the cup lies just below the anterosuperior bone (arrow), which protects it from impingement against the metal neck, particularly during flexion and internal rotation.*

The position for the acetabular cup can now be determined. The medial edge of the cup should not overhang the edge of cortical bone of the cotyloid notch (the tear drop) by more than 5 mm, which can be verified by placing an index finger or tonsil clamp against the bone and feeling for the transverse ligament or the cortical bone of the notch (Fig. 3–27). The anterior edge of the cup should be 5 mm below the pubic tubercle (Fig. 3–28). This gives a good approximation of the correct anteversion for the acetabulum and usually means that the acetabular cup is in nearly 20 degrees of anteversion. The anterior bony wall should not be used to judge alignment of the cup because of its potentially variable geometry.[1] The anterosuperior metal edge of the cup should sit just below bone (Fig. 3–29). If the anterosuperior edge of the cup is left proud, the metal neck can impinge against it with flexion, especially when combined with internal rotation. The posterosuperior metal edge of the cup should sit just proud to the acetabular bone (Fig. 3–30); if it is buried under

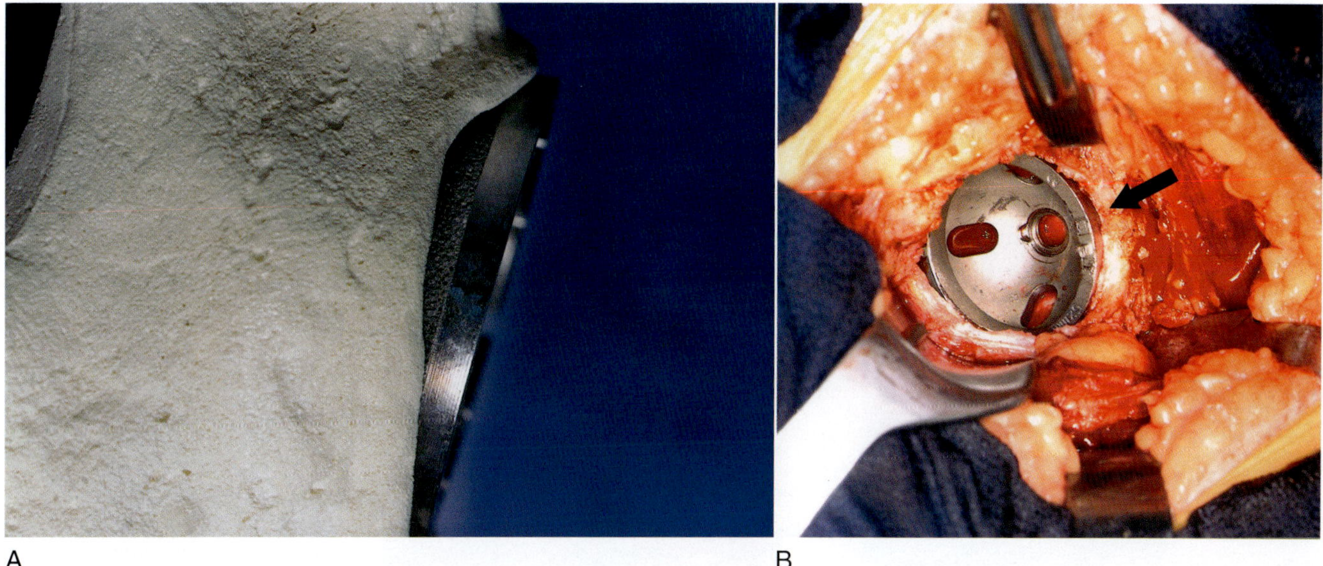

A   B

Figure 3–30 **A,** *The posterosuperior edge of the metal shell stands proud of the bone. This should almost always be the case because the osseous acetabulum has an average inclination of 55 to 60 degrees. Therefore, if the posterosuperior corner of the metal shell is buried under bone, the cup is too vertical.* **B,** *Intraoperative view shows the posterosuperior edge of the trial shell standing proud of the posterosuperior bone* (arrow).

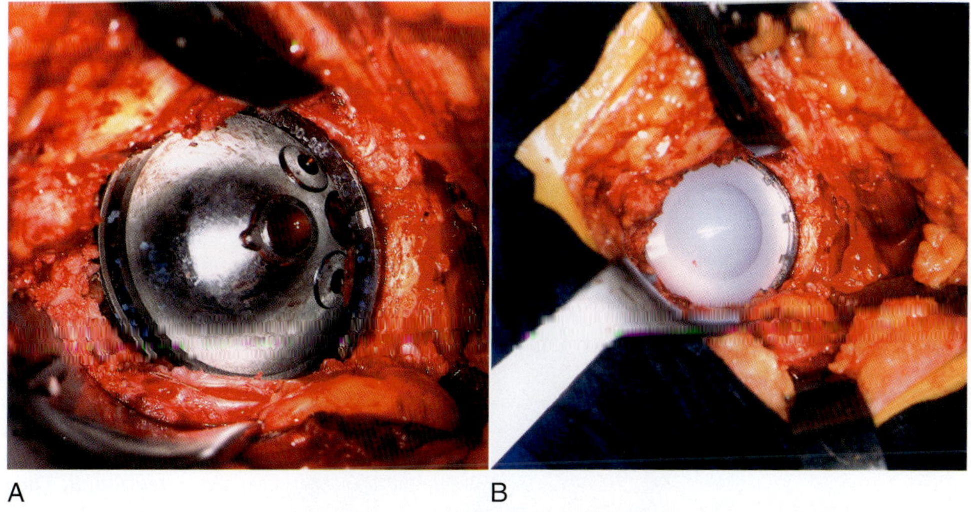

A   B

Figure 3–31 **A,** *The metal shell correctly positioned in the osseous acetabulum. The screw holes should be placed posterosuperiorly because this is the safest position for screws. The posterosuperior edge of the metal cup stands above the posterosuperior bone, and the anterosuperior bone lies below the anterosuperior edge of the cup. The anteroinferior edge of the cup lies below the pubic tubercle, and the posteroinferior edge is below the ischium. The medial-inferior edge of the cup is in line with the edge of the cortical bone of the cotyloid notch.* **B,** *The same cup with the insert in place. The thickness of the insert does not affect the principles of cup placement. The plastic liner is easy to insert because the edge of the cup is free of soft tissue.*

bone, the inclination of the cup is too steep (greater than 40 to 45 degrees). The posteroinferior metal edge of the cup should never project above the ischium; if it does, the cup is either too anteverted or too lateral. Figure 3–31 shows visual and palpable anatomic landmarks demonstrating the cup position.

Finally, the trial cup should be tested for stability by hitting of its edge with a sharp blow with the heel of the hand or by tapping with the mallet; if the cup tilts easily, it is not fixed securely and a screw is needed (Fig. 3–32). Sometimes the trial cup exhibits slight motion that would not be present with the permanent cup if the real cup is 1 mm bigger than the trial; also, the permanent cup gets some frictional fit from its porous coating. The second test for cup stability consists of pulling on the handle used to insert the trial cup; if the trial cup cannot be lifted out of the bone, the press-fit is secure (Fig. 3–33). The trial cup is

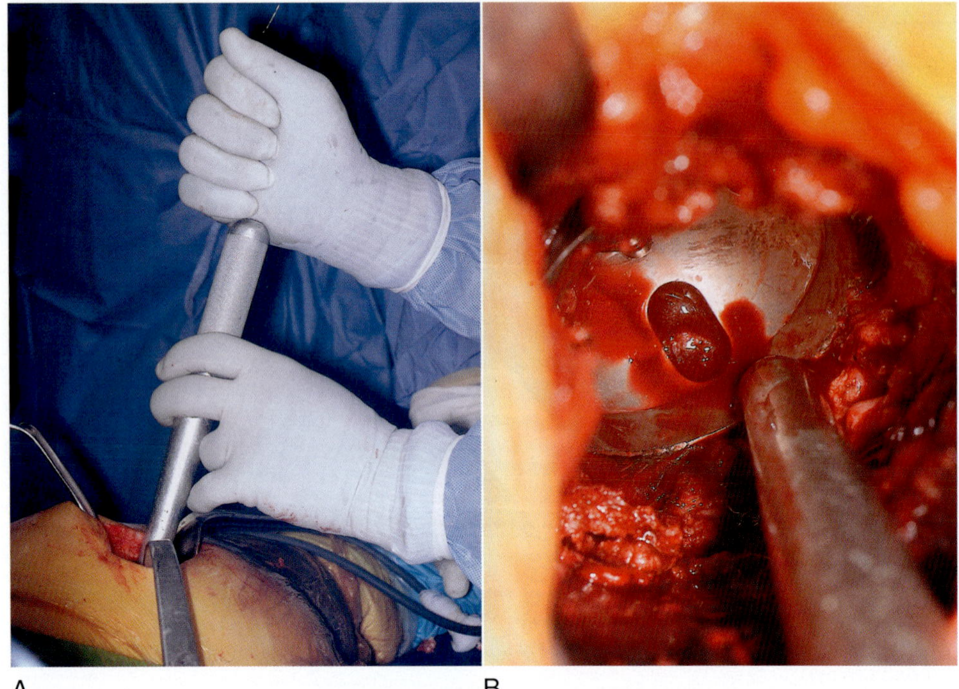

A   B

Figure 3–32 **A,** *A long bone tamp is placed against the edge of the cup and is struck with the heel of the hand to check for cup movement.* **B,** *The bone tamp against the edge of the trial.*

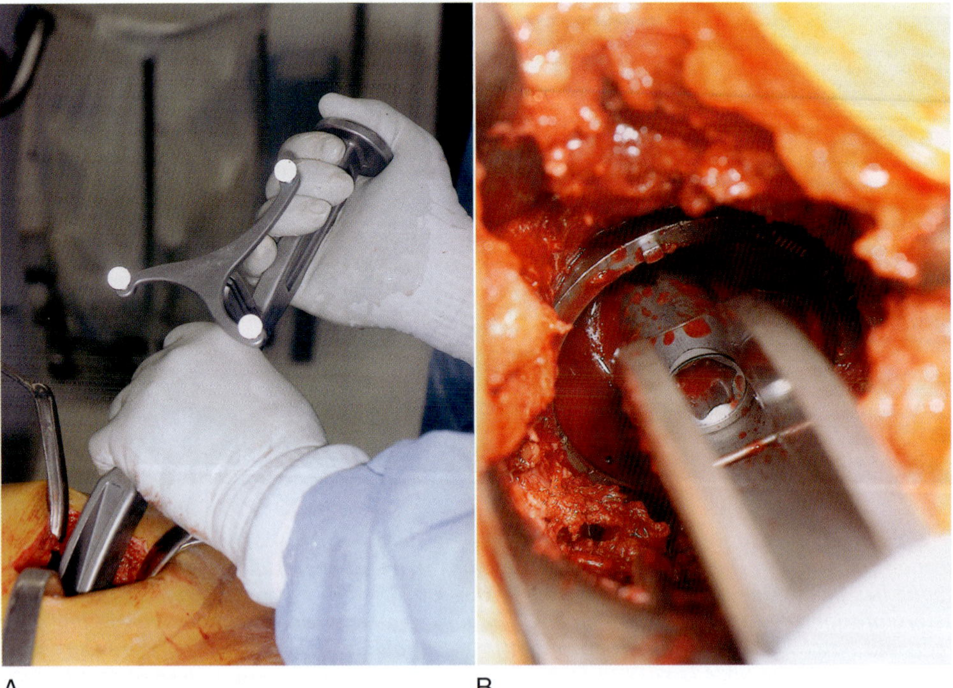

A   B

Figure 3–33 **A,** *Both hands are used to pull on the cup holder. Enough force should be used to pull out a loose cup easily. This cup holder has three light-emitting diodes for computer registration.* **B,** *The cup holder is being pulled, but the trial cup remains stable in the acetabulum. If the trial cup is stable, then certainly the cup, which has a rough surface, will have a secure press-fit that will not need screws.*

removed by hitting it on the edge vigorously with a tool and mallet to tilt the cup so that it can be gripped with a Kocher clamp in one of its holes and rotated out of the bone (Fig. 3–34).

The actual acetabular component is implanted by placing it into the position determined to be correct with the trial cup. It should need to be malleted into position (*see "Posterior Total Hip Replacement Traditional Incision"*).

If the trial cup can simply be placed into the acetabulum without any malleting or can be easily moved once placed, it is too small and a larger size must be used (*see "Posterior Total Hip Replacement Traditional Incision"*).

Fixing a loose cup with screws is unsatisfactory because of the difficulty in keeping the cup in correct inclination and anteversion during application of screws, and the tenuous fixation of cup to bone.

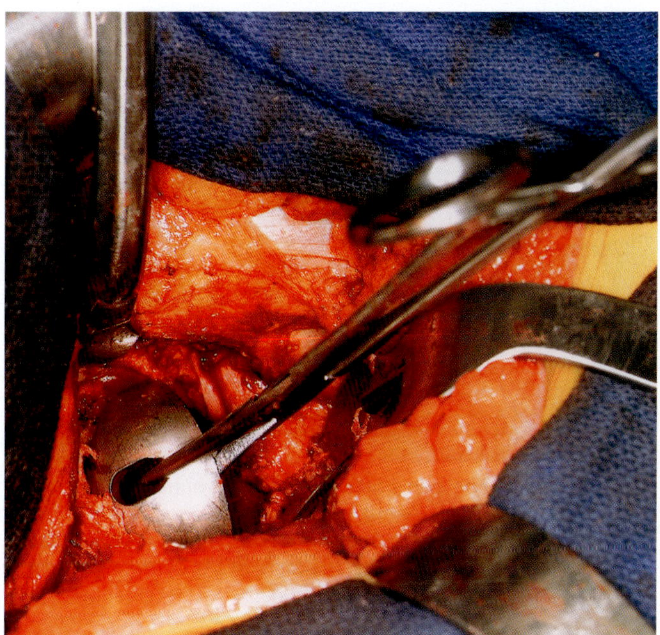

Figure 3–34 *The trial cup is gripped with a Kocher clamp to rotate it and lift it out of the acetabulum.*

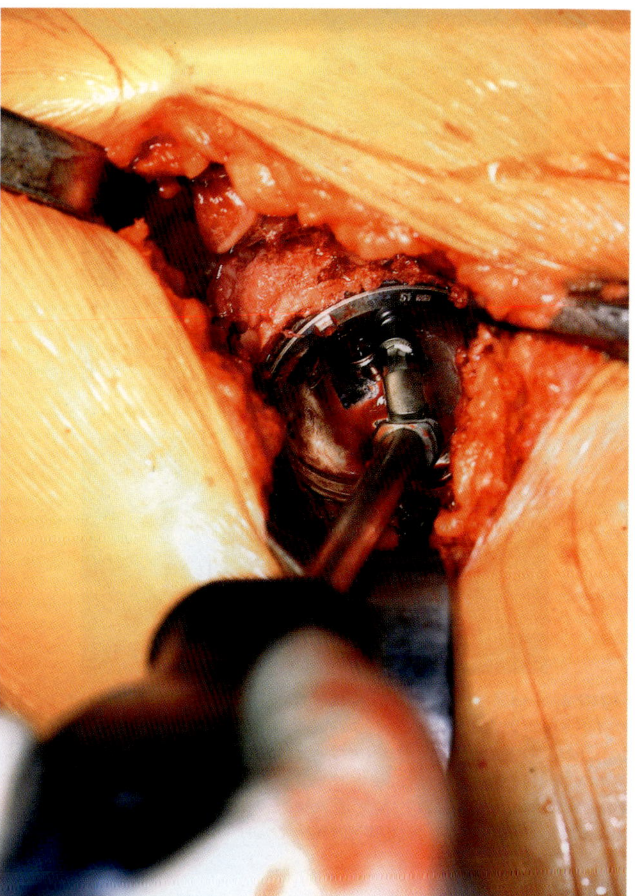

Figure 3–35 *A 6.5-mm screw is placed into the acetabulum using a flexible screwdriver to ensure correct angle of insertion.*

When the cup is press-fit into the osseous acetabulum, the same landmarks should be checked as for the trial cup (see earlier). If one or two screws will be used with the cup, the cup should be placed in slightly greater anteversion and slightly flatter (less inclination) than actually desired because the cup can move 5 to 10 degrees during insertion and tightening of screws. This positioning is not necessary if there is a solid press-fit and the screw is being used only for extra fixation. As with the trial cup, the surgeon checks the stability of the cup by attempting to pull it out of the osseous acetabulum once it has been inserted (see Fig. 3–33). When the handle of the cup inserter is removed and the cup's position is determined to be satisfactory, the edge of the cup is again lightly struck with a fist, hand, or tool to ensure that it does not tilt (see Fig. 3–32).

If screws are added, the hole is drilled with a 4.5-mm drill, which should be advanced through the inner table to obtain secure purchase for the screw. Drilling must be done slowly and carefully so that the drill does not plunge into the pelvis. The length of the screw can be measured by the amount of blood on the drill or with a measuring guide. The hole should be tapped for a 6.5-mm titanium screw, and the screw is then tightened into the cup (Fig. 3–35). If tightening the screw causes the cup to move excessively, the edge of the cup should be held with a tool to prevent motion while the screw is tightened (Fig. 3–36). A second screw is needed only if the cup moves with the insertion of the first screw.

At this time, a trial insert can be placed into the cup, or, if the surgeon is satisfied with the position and

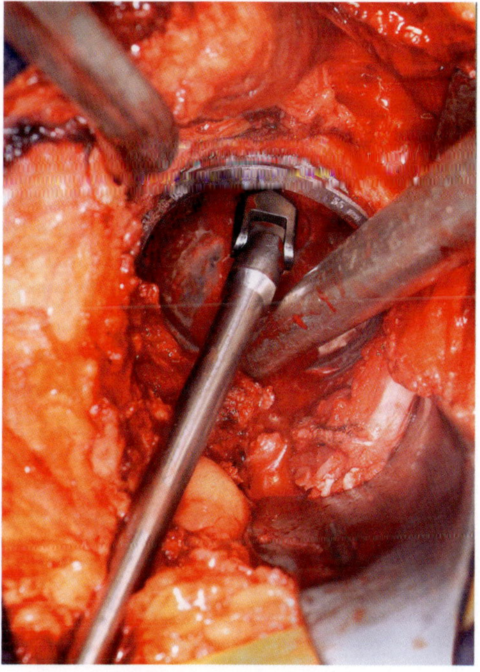

Figure 3–36 *If tightening of the screw results in rotation of the cup into an unwanted position, a long tool is used to push against the edge of the cup to prevent this rotation.*

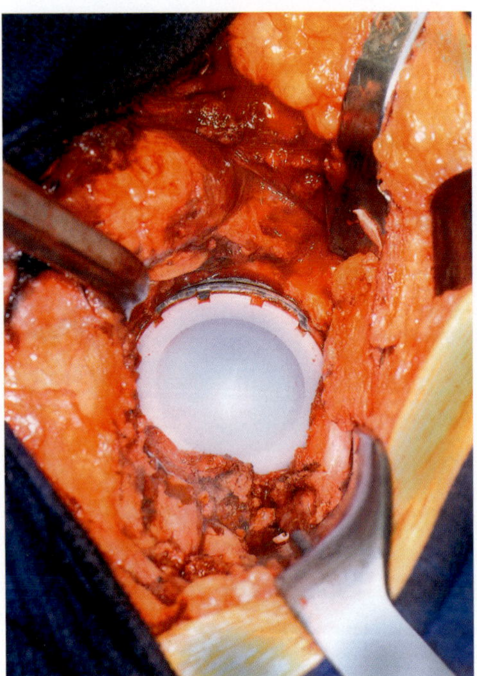

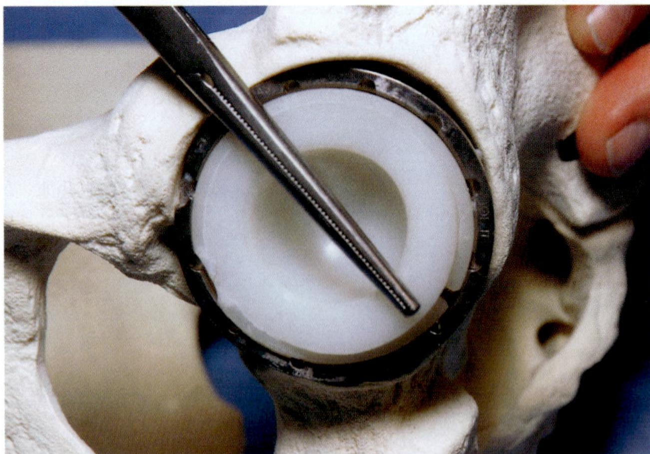

Figure 3–38 *The cup placed in this sawbones represents a left hip. The Kocher clamp points to the apex of the plastic hood, which is at 4 o'clock. The hood in this position lessens the risk for impingement, particularly in the common hip position of flexion and external rotation.*

Figure 3–37 *I insert the plastic liner after fixation of the metal shell is complete. Because I seldom use screws, this does not limit my options for changing the position of the cup by tapping it on the edge, even with the plastic insert in place, to change the anteversion if needed. If screws are used, it is safer to use a trial insert rather than the final insert.*

stability of the cup, the real insert can be placed (Fig. 3–37). The insert is simply locked into the fixed cup.

Whether a hood is used is also at the discretion of the surgeon. In my experience, computerized modeling has shown that a hood should not be used when the cup position is at least 25 degrees of anteversion because the hood can cause impingement in extension. If the anteversion of the cup is suspected to be 20 degrees or less, the hood can give additional mechanical support for the coverage of the head during flexion and internal rotation. Because the hood primarily gives mechanical protection during flexion and internal rotation, it should be placed with the apex at 4 o'clock in the left hip and 8 o'clock in the right hip (Fig. 3–38) These positions give maximum coverage of the head when the joint position poses the greatest risk for posterior dislocation. Once the insert has been implanted, the acetabular portion of the operation is complete. If the real insert has been placed, a gauze sponge should be placed into the insert to protect it from being scratched during preparation of the femur (Fig. 3–39).

FEMORAL PREPARATION

Before the leg is brought into position for preparation of the femur, all acetabular retractors must be removed to prevent tissue damage. The leg is then brought into

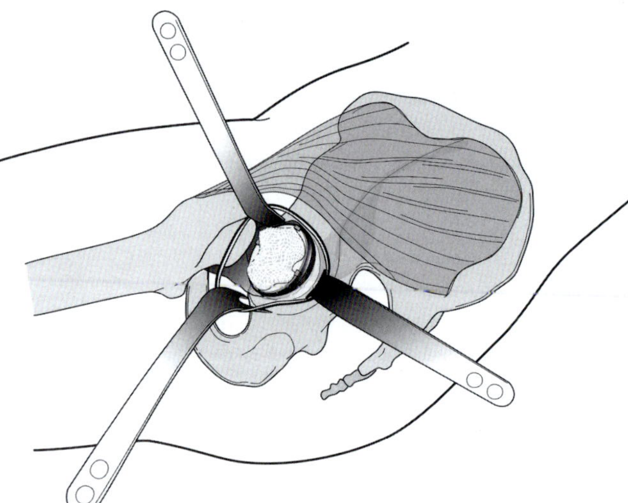

Figure 3–39 *A gauze sponge is placed into the acetabulum. If the real acetabular liner has been placed into the metal shell, this is particularly important to protect the liner during preparation of the femur.*

a position of flexion and internal rotation with the tibia at 90 degrees to the femur (Fig. 3–40). This position exposes the proximal cut end of the femur into the wound. A "jaws" retractor (#8 retractor—see Fig. 3–41A) is placed under the anterior aspect of the femoral neck to help lift the femur into the wound for easier access (Fig. 3–41). A curved retractor can be used to protect the gluteus medius muscle so it is not damaged with reaming and broaching (see Fig. 3–41). A retractor (#3 from the mini-incision set) is placed at the level of the lesser trochanter to protect the posterior wound edge and tissues from injury during femoral preparation (see

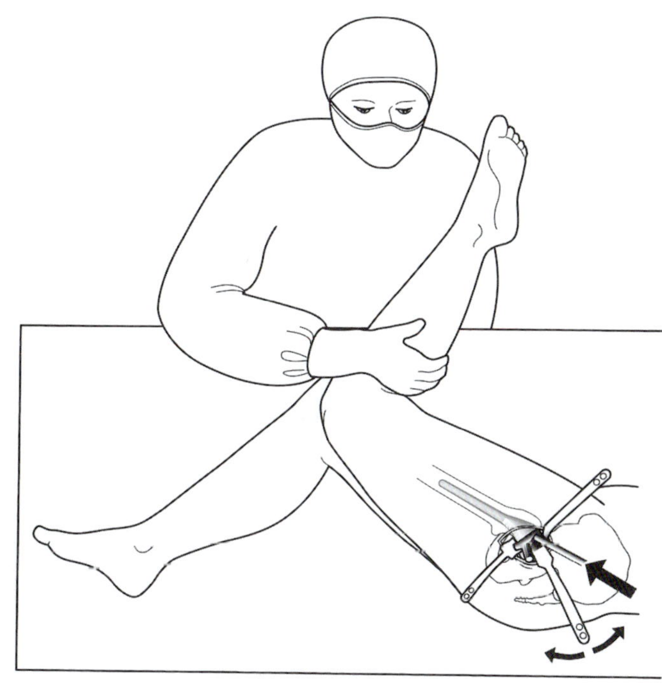

Figure 3–40 The operative leg rests on the lower leg in flexion and approximately 60 degrees of internal rotation. This is the best position for placement of the retractors before the leg is moved over the side of the table into 90 degrees of internal rotation.

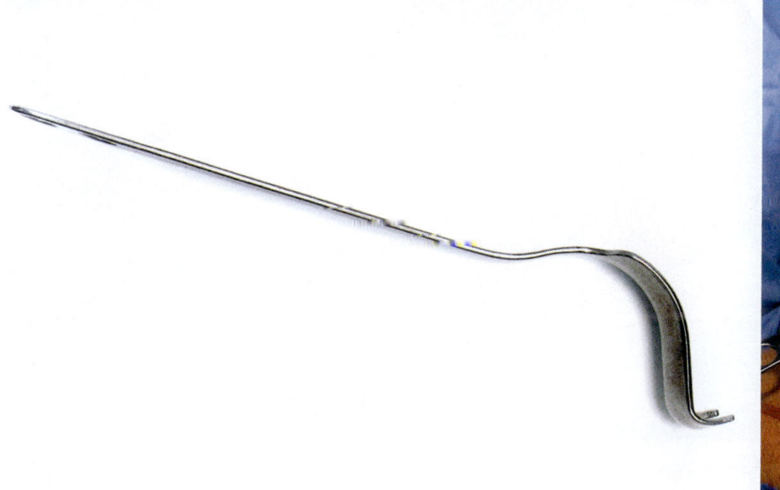

A

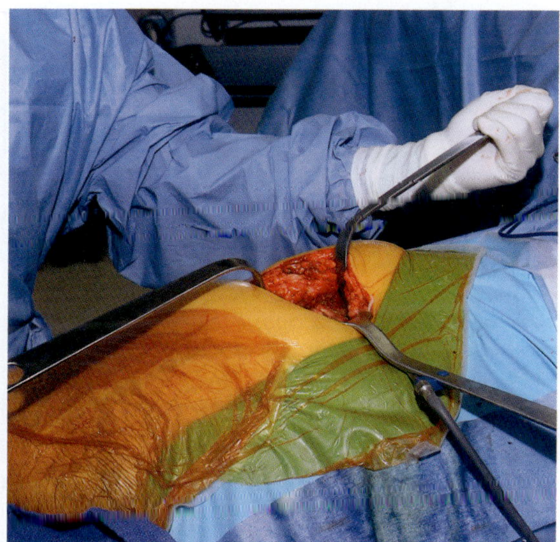

B

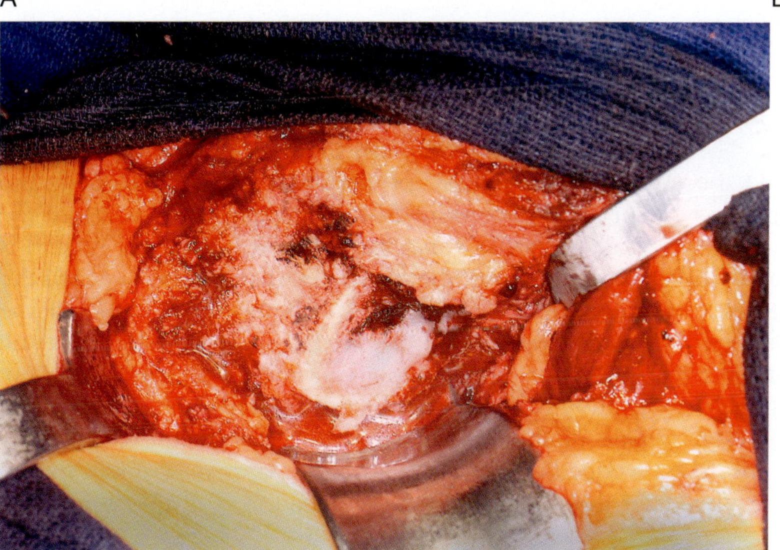

C

Figure 3–41 A, The #8 retractor ("jaws") has a radius of curvature that allows retraction of the posterior flap of the wound without excessive tension on skin and soft tissues. B, The #8 retractor is seen at lower right, with an attached fiberoptic light source. The retractor depresses the posterior edge of the wound to expose the cut edge of the femoral neck. Retractor #9 is held in the assistant's left hand. Retractor #4, around the medial neck, is visible in the lower left of the wound. C, The #9 retractor is seen on the right side of the wound, protecting the gluteus medius tendon. The #3 retractor on the left side of the wound, against the lesser trochanter, protects the posterior tissues and sciatic nerve.

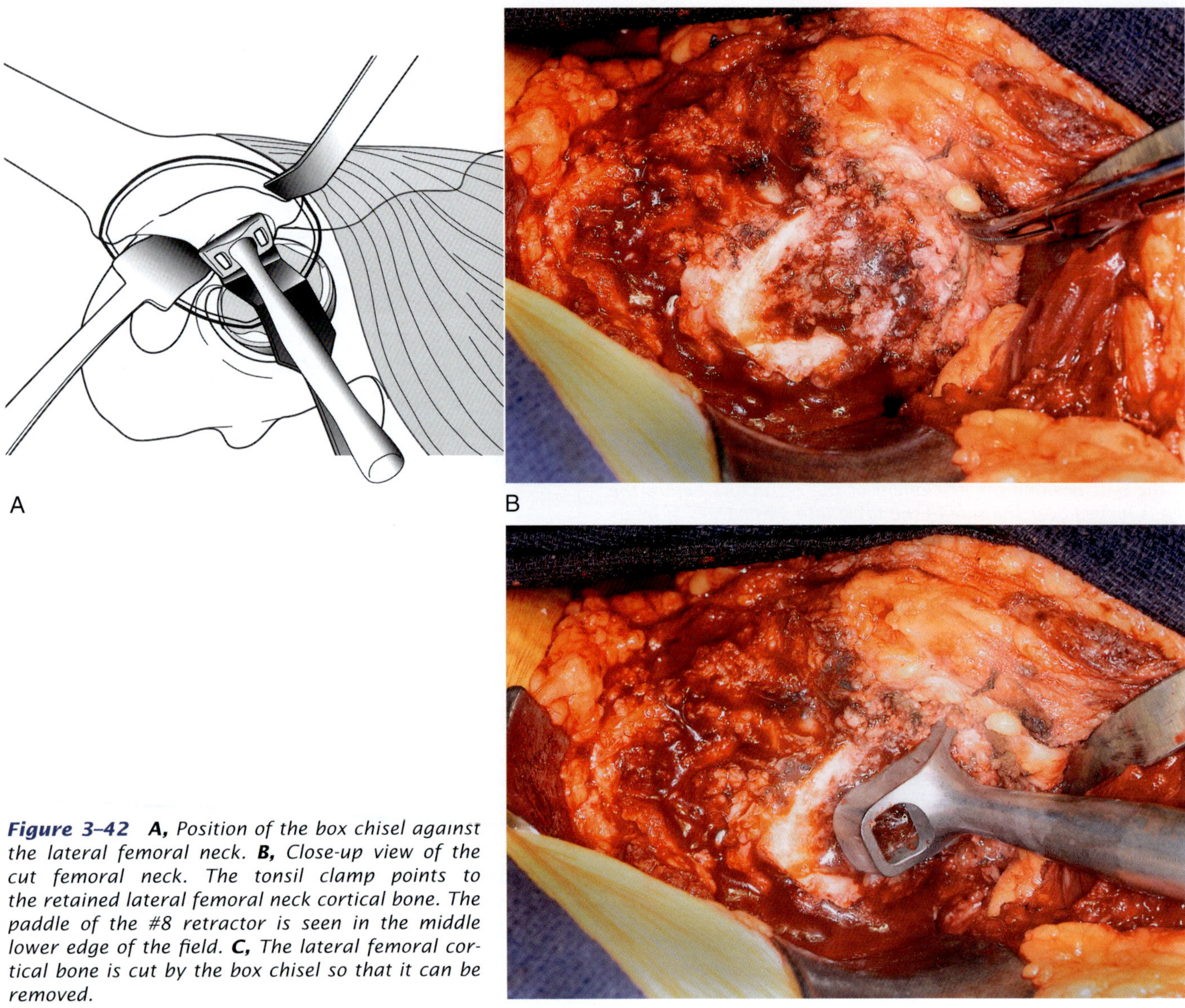

A

B

C

Figure 3–42 A, *Position of the box chisel against the lateral femoral neck.* **B,** *Close-up view of the cut femoral neck. The tonsil clamp points to the retained lateral femoral neck cortical bone. The paddle of the #8 retractor is seen in the middle lower edge of the field.* **C,** *The lateral femoral cortical bone is cut by the box chisel so that it can be removed.*

Fig. 3–41). Any soft tissue that overlies the remaining lateral neck should be excised. The remaining lateral neck is removed with a box chisel (Fig. 3–42), which gives a view of the entire cut femoral neck from the bed of the trochanter to the medial femoral neck. The length of the remaining femoral neck should be checked with a ruler to ensure that it matches the preoperative template (Fig. 3–43).

A burr can be used to open the femoral canal for insertion of the reamers and broaches (Fig. 3–44). Once the canal has been established, reaming is done sequentially until the reamer grips endosteal bone over a distance of approximately 5 cm, the length of contact necessary to ensure a good fit of the prosthesis (Fig. 3–45). The trochanter bed needs to be reamed to ensure that the implant is optimally lateralized. Once the

femoral canal size is established by the reamer, the appropriate broaches are used to prepare the femoral canal for implantation of the stem.

For a description of the use of the broaches for different-shaped stems, see Chapter 6 on femoral preparation. Regardless of the type of broach used, the surgeon can ensure that the broach (and therefore the stem) is not in varus if the lateral side of the broach is under the tip of the greater trochanter; this is called the *anti-varus sign* (Fig. 3–46). If the medial side of the broach lies against the medial neck, the stem can still be in varus in the diaphyseal canal (Fig. 3–47). The stem portion of the broach is not in varus only if the lateral side of the proximal broach is as lateral as possible, wedged against the bed of the trochanter under the tip of the greater trochanter. Regardless of the stem used,

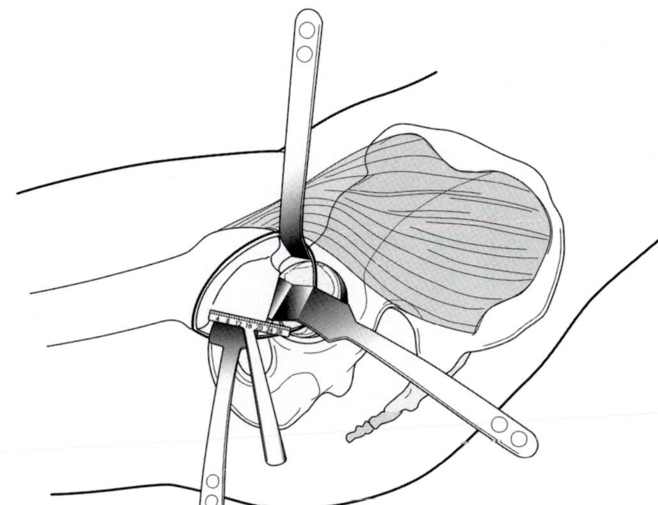

Figure 3–43 *Use of the ruler to confirm the cut level of the femoral neck. Using preoperative templates, the cut level has been determined as correct for restoration of hip length and offset in the prosthesis.*

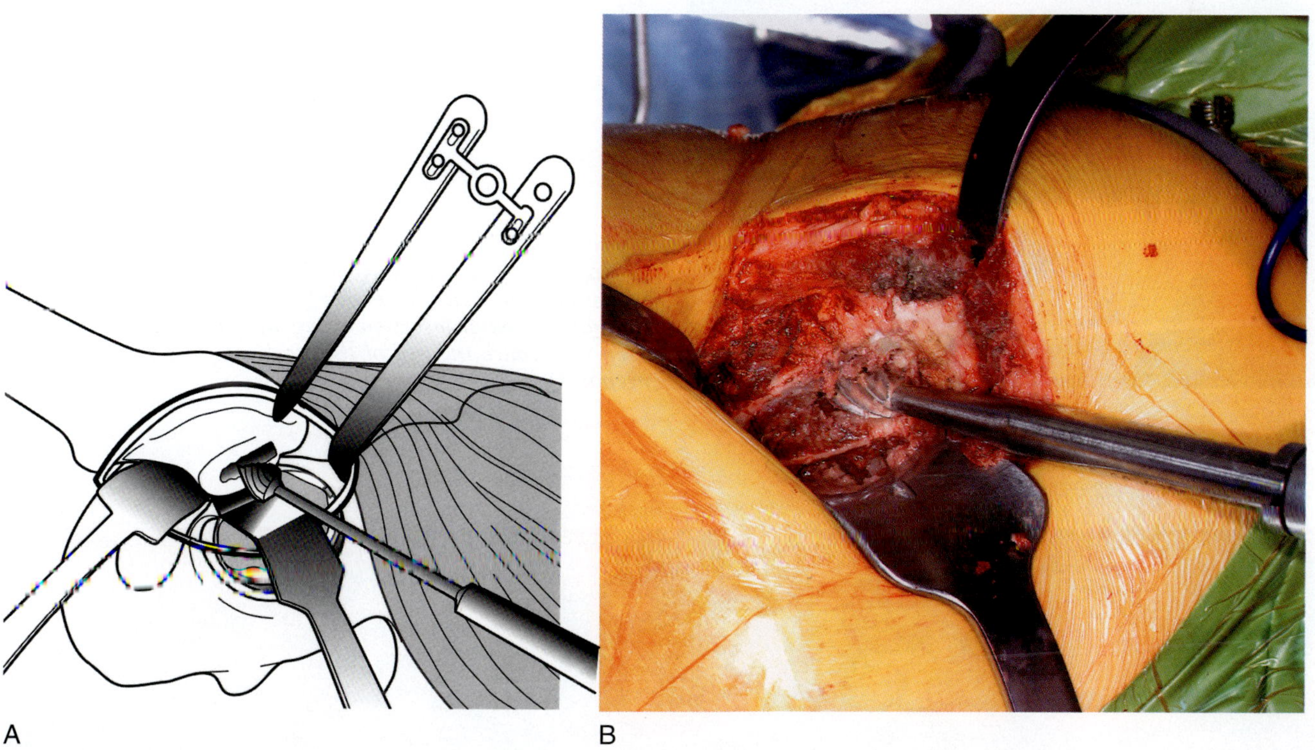

A

B

Figure 3–44 **A,** *Use of the burr to open the femoral canal for preparation with a reamer or broach.* **B,** *Correct placement of the burr to open the femoral canal.*

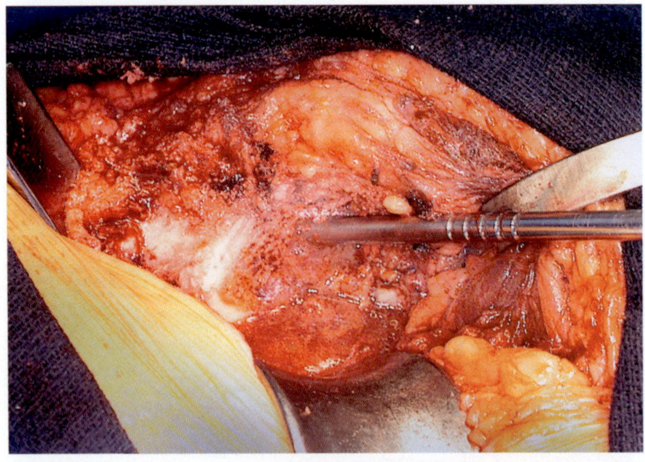

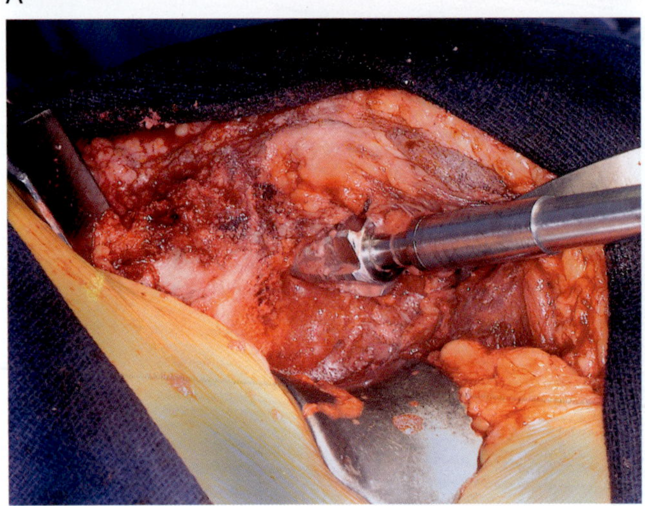

Figure 3–45 **A,** *Placement of a reamer through the hole made by the burr. This hole must be placed lateral and posterior in the femoral neck; it is incorrect to try to open the femoral canal through a medial insertion point.* **B,** *A trochanteric reamer is used to prepare the bed of the trochanters to facilitate broach preparation of the femoral bone.*

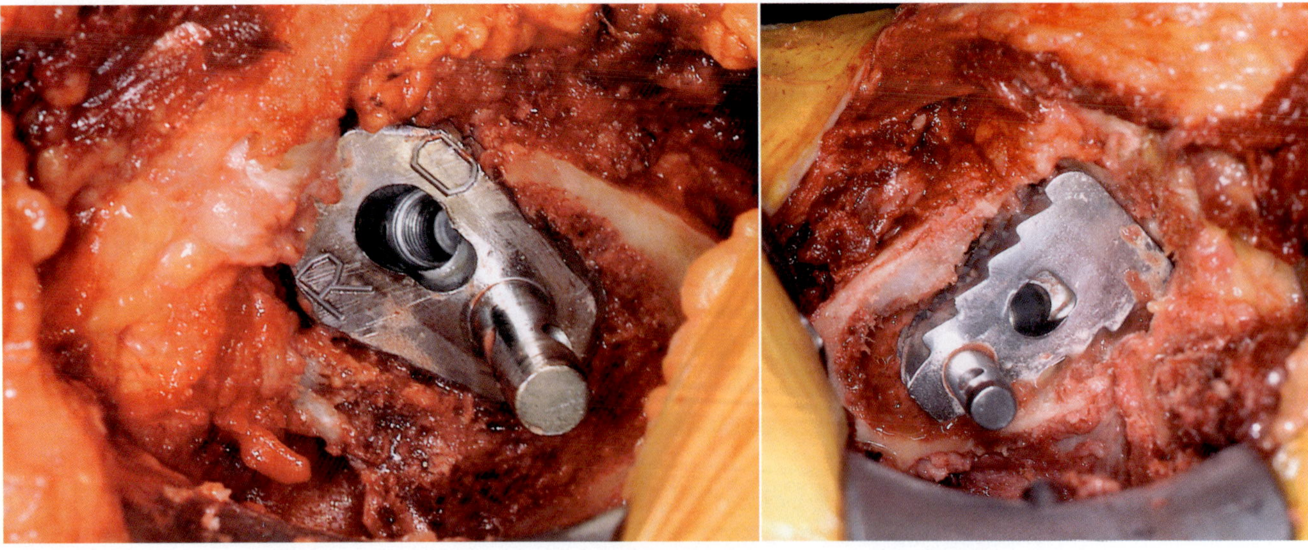

Figure 3–46 **A,** *The tip of the greater trochanter overlying the lateral edge of a broach (this is the Natural hip broach).* **B,** *The lateral side of this APR broach is clearly in the bed of the greater trochanter, and the medial side of the broach is not touching the medial cortical bone. This lateral broach position is called the* anti-varus *sign.*

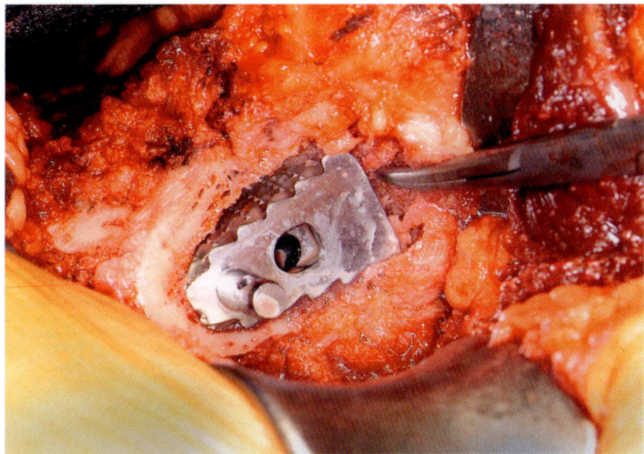

Figure 3–47 *The medial side of the broach touches the medial cortical bone, but the lateral side of the broach is not in the cancellous bed of the trochanter and not under the tip of the greater trochanter, which is just above the tip of the tonsil clamp. This broach position means that the stem is in varus and that the diaphyseal fit of the stem is too small.*

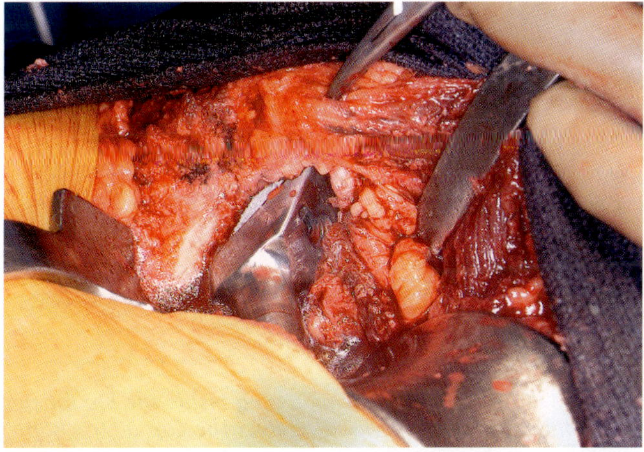

Figure 3–48 *The posterior side of the metal stem is aligned parallel to the posterior cortex of the femoral neck. This position of the stem in the femur practically ensures that the femur will not fracture, which could occur with an attempt to antevert the stem beyond the anteversion of the femoral bone.*

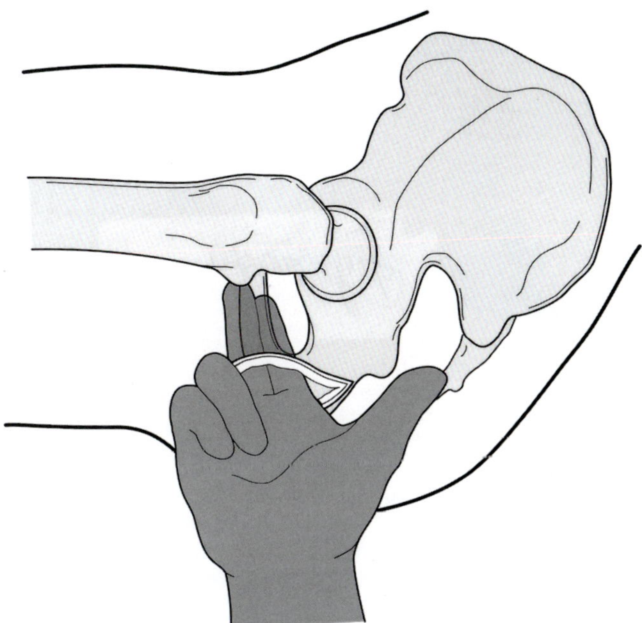

Figure 3–49 *The surgeon's finger palpates the tip of the lesser trochanter and then the tip of the ischium to relate the position of the lesser trochanter to the ischium.*

the broach and stem should be aligned with the posterior cortical bone of the femoral neck; this will be the anteversion of the stem that the femur will accept without fracturing (Fig. 3–48). How much of the proximal femur is filled by the broach depends on the stem selected.

With the broach in place, a trial neck and head are placed and the hip is reduced and taken through range of motion. Hip length and offset should be balanced (see next section). Hip length can be judged by comparing the level of the lesser trochanter with the ischium (Fig. 3–49), and offset is satisfactory if the trochanter is 1 fingerbreadth from the pelvis in extension and exter-

nal rotation, and in flexion and internal rotation (Fig. 3–50). The metal neck should be palpated to ensure that it does not impinge against the metal edge of the cup (Fig. 3–51).

When the correct balance of hip length and offset is obtained, the broach can be removed. The stem is inserted to the same level as the broach. The stem is simply malleted into the femoral "envelope" that has been developed for the implantation (Fig. 3–52). The trial head is placed on the femoral stem and a trial reduction and range of motion accomplished. The permanent femoral head is then placed, after which the hip can be closed. The femoral head size used should be as large as possible to reduce the dead space in the hip after closure. This will accelerate capsular healing and provide better stability and comfort.

The capsule and external rotators are closed using three sutures to reattach the posterior flap to the cut edge of the capsule and gluteus minimus (Fig. 3–53). The sutures are placed with the leg slightly internally rotated and the foot on a Mayo stand (Fig. 3–54). When all three sutures have been placed, the leg is laid flat on the table, which effectively externally rotates it, and the sutures are tied. This gives complete coverage of the metal neck and head and eliminates any dead space between the head and capsule because the capsule and external rotators are closed adjacent to the metal femoral head and neck and secured to the gluteus minimus (Fig. 3–55). It also provides tension to the gluteus minimus, which contracts against the femoral head and helps hold it in place. For these reasons, I

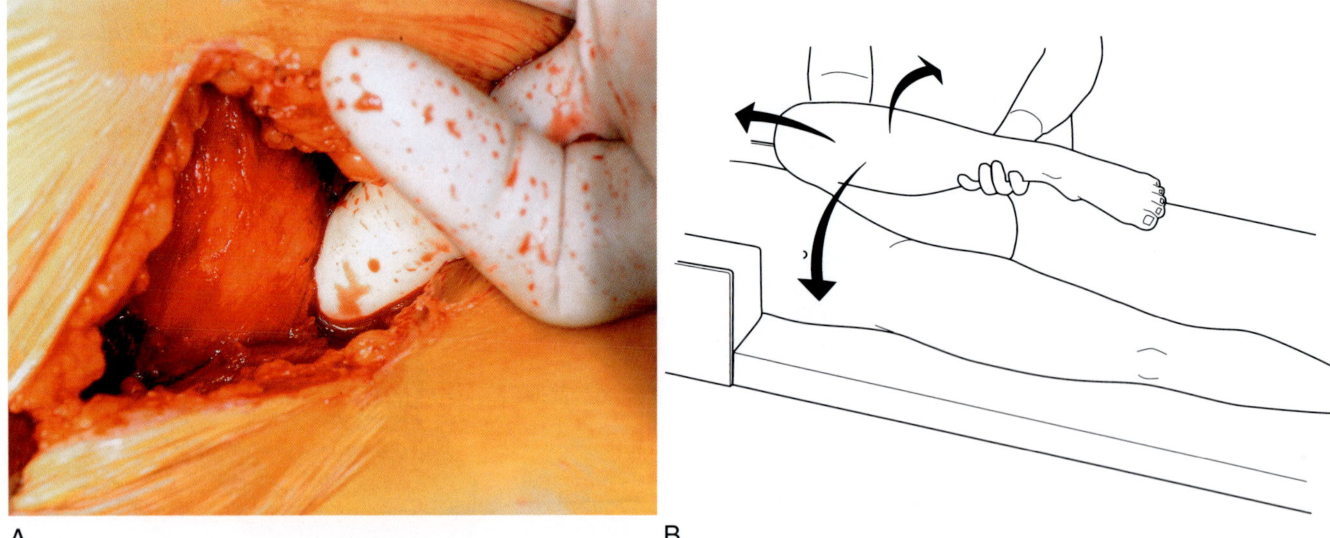

A

B

Figure 3–50 **A,** The surgeon's finger is placed between the greater trochanter and the pelvis to ensure that there is no contact between these structures throughout the range of motion of the hip. **B,** With the left hand, the surgeon places the hip through its entire range of motion, while a finger of the right hand palpates the relationships of the greater trochanter to the pelvis and the metal neck to the edge of the cup. This test detects impingement of the bone or the metal neck.

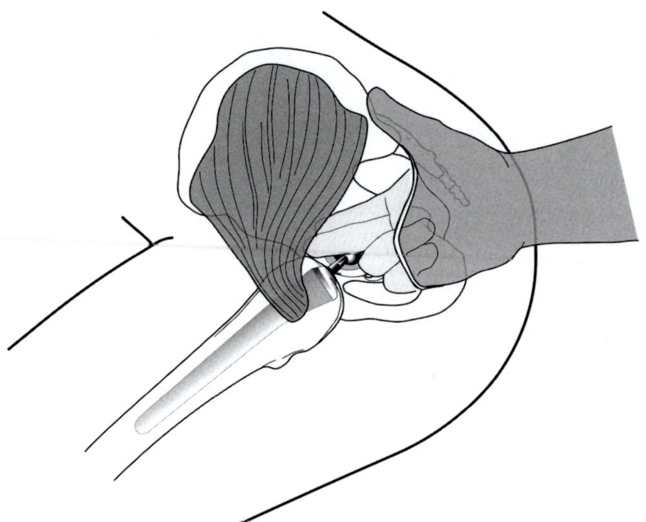

Figure 3–51 Technique for palpating inside the hip for possible impingement of the neck against the cup or trochanter against the pelvis.

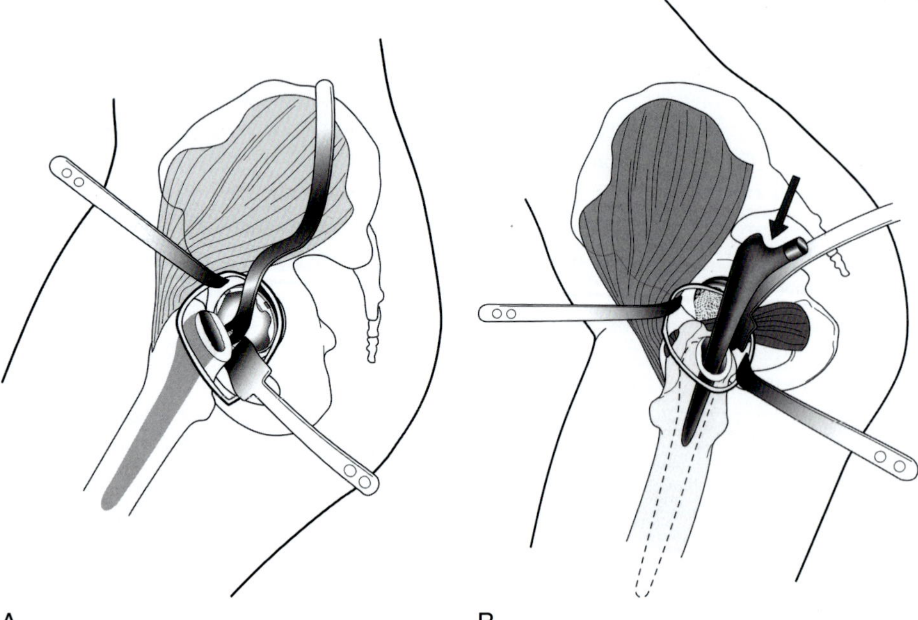

A

B

Figure 3–52 **A,** The envelope inside the femoral bone created by the broach for insertion of the stem. **B,** Technique for inserting the stem into the envelope. Insertion of the stem into the envelope created by the broach essentially eliminates the possibility of femoral fracture.

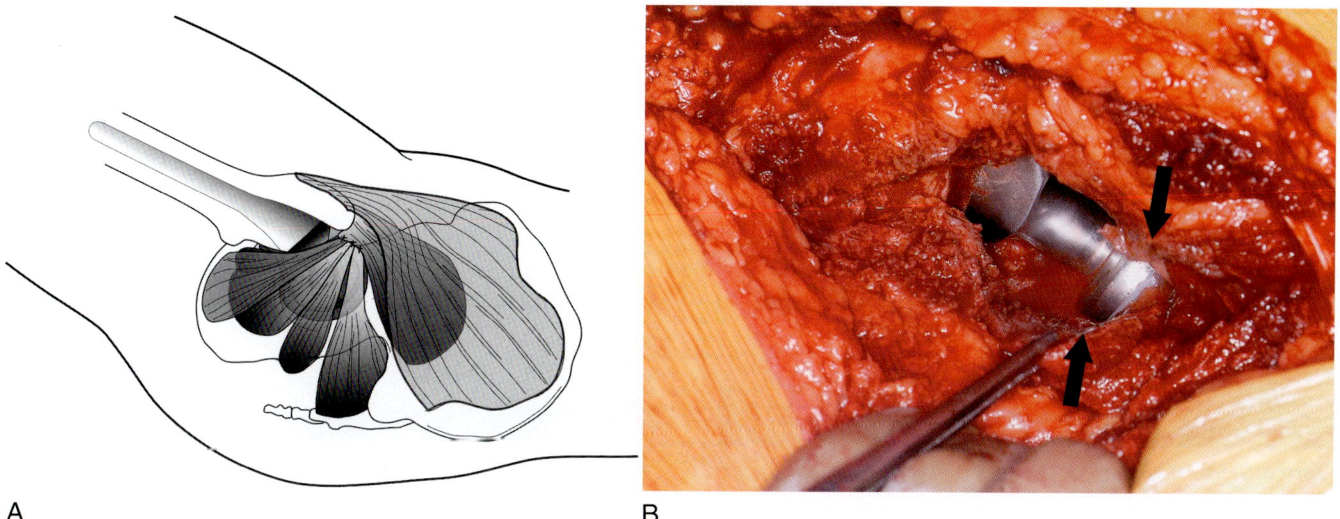

A   B

Figure 3-53 **A,** *The posterior flap has been closed to the anterior flap (see Fig. 3–8). Closing the flap eliminates dead space in the posterior hip.* **B,** *The two edges of the flap are visible (arrows), with the metal neck and head of the hip replacement reduced into the acetabulum. The Kocher clamp holds the posterior flap, which will be brought into apposition to the anterior flap for suture closure.*

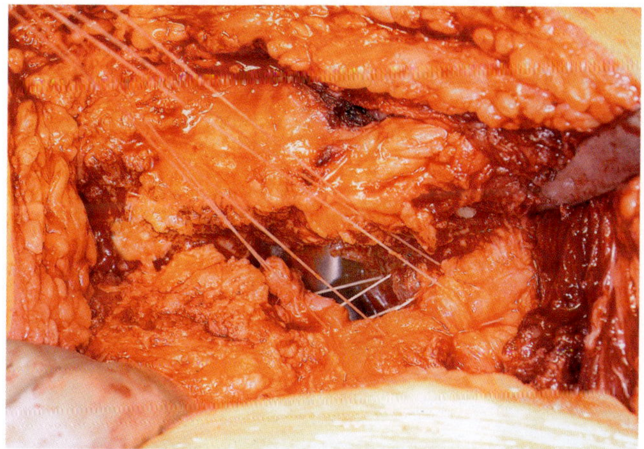

Figure 3-54 *Sutures through the anterior and posterior flaps have been placed with the hip in internal rotation. The foot is usually placed on a Mayo stand. The #2 retractor is seen to the right, retracting the gluteus medius muscle. Once the sutures are placed, the leg is laid on the table to eliminate internal rotation, the #2 retractor is removed to eliminate tension on the edges of the closure, and the sutures are tied to repair the posterior capsule/external rotator flap.*

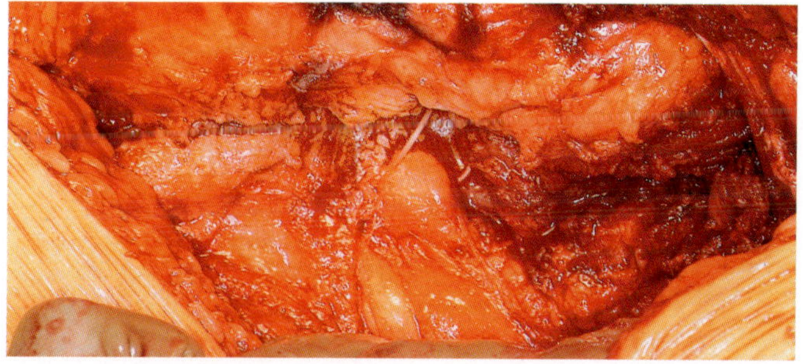

Figure 3-55 *The hip has once again been internally rotated to show the closure for this photograph. The entire posterior hip is closed, with anatomic closure of the posterior flap eliminating any dead space. The gluteus medius muscle is on the right, and at the top middle of the wound the methylene blue mark on the greater trochanter shows the orientation of the greater trochanter to the closure.*

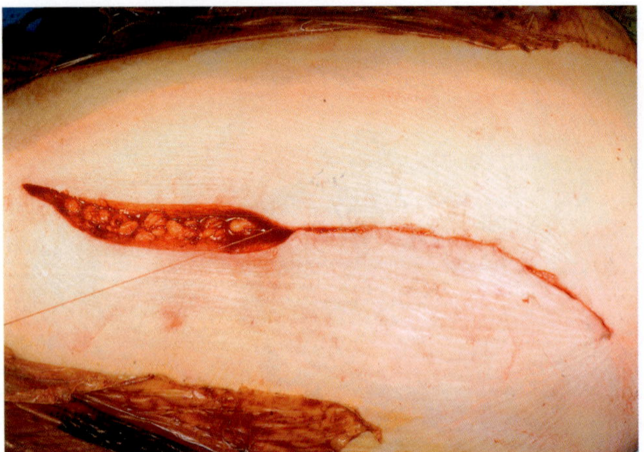

Figure 3–56   *The skin is closed with a subcuticular suture.*

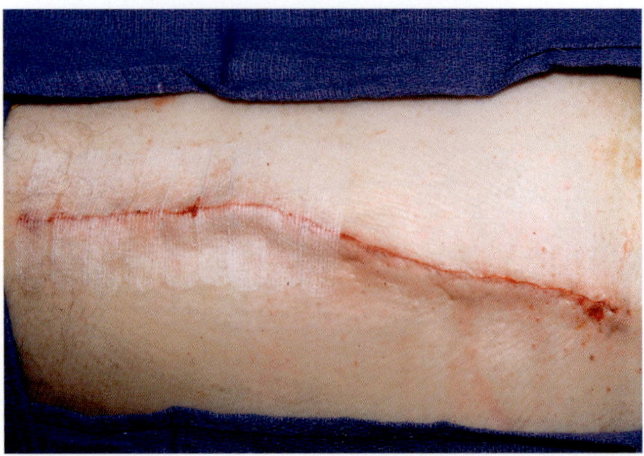

Figure 3–57   *The wound is closed with a subcuticular suture, and Steri-Strip tapes are placed over the closure.*

prefer this closure technique to drilling holes in the trochanter.

The remainder of the closure is done in sequence, with the fascia closed with interrupted sutures of 1.0 Vicryl, the subcutaneous tissue closed with 2.0 Vicryl, and the skin closed with a subcuticular suture (Fig. 3–56). I recommend the use of subcuticular sutures (Fig. 3–57) instead of staples because it saves the patient from the inconvenience and discomfort of returning to the hospital for staple removal. The scar with a subcuticular suture is also much more acceptable to the patient.

Reference

1. Maruyama M, Feinberg JR, Capello WN, D'Antonio JA: Morphologic features of the acetabulum and femur: Anteversion angle and implant positioning. Clin Orthop 393:52-65, 2001.

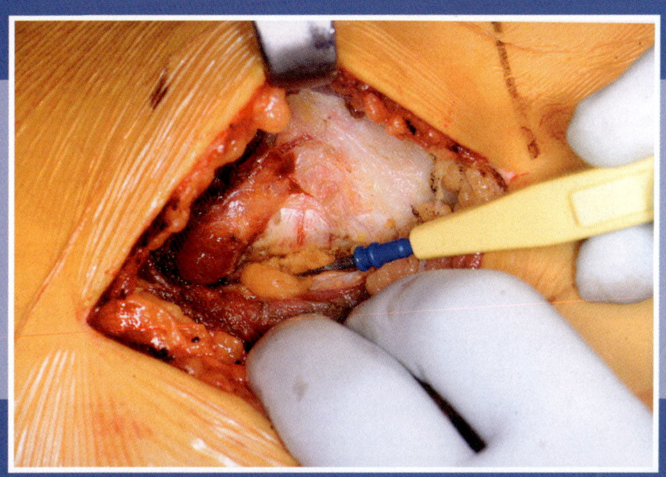

Posterior Mini-incision: Exposure*

*In conjunction with this chapter on the DVD-ROM is the video *"Posterior Minimally Invasive Surgery (MIS) Total Hip Replacement."*

RATIONALE

The primary difference between the posterior mini-incision and the standard posterior incision is the length of the skin cut and muscle incision. With the posterior mini-incision, the muscle incision is significantly shorter, which improves postoperative function. Second, the mini-incision requires only two capsular cuts and no capsular excision, which improves the stability of the components, particularly because the posterosuperior capsular cut is repaired. Avoidance of capsular excision also provides better postoperative comfort. Third, there is no iliotibial band incision. Fourth, there is no gluteus maximus tendon incision; the upper and lower heads of the gluteus maximus are not separated (separation can interfere with the phasic firing of the muscle).

These changes in the exposure of the hip eliminate dead space in the hip joint after closure of the capsule, which in turn promotes more rapid healing of the capsule and stabilization of the joint, with less pain. Reduced tissue injury results in less swelling, a significant cause of postoperative pain. Postoperative muscular strength and stance improve earlier because of the reduced muscular injury, as shown in gait studies we have performed.[1] Finally, the smaller incision provides improved cosmesis, a factor that was important for 100% of respondents to our patient satisfaction questionnaire (see Tables 4–1 and 4–2). Combined with the new process of total hip replacement described in Chapter 1, the posterior mini-incision operation results in reduced hospitalization time, easier rehabilitation, and earlier return to work.

The main disadvantage of the posterior mini-incision is decreased visualization of the anatomy, with a concomitant increase in stress for the surgeon performing the operation and an increased chance for errors. Proper instrumentation is a key factor in increasing the anatomic visualization and the surgeon's comfort with the operation. The addition of computer-assisted navigation (see Chapter 7) for the procedure completely resolves this disadvantage of the smaller incision. With appropriate instrumentation and image guidance, the risk of cup malposition and femoral fracture is eliminated.

Perhaps the most compelling reason to become proficient with the mini-incision operation is that patients want this exposure. Our patient satisfaction ques-

Table 4–1
Patient Satisfaction Questionnaire: Patients Undergoing the Mini-incision Procedure for Total Hip Arthroplasty

	Preoperative (%)			Postoperative (%)		
	Yes	No Difference	No	Yes	No Difference	No
Question: *Do you feel that a patient who has had a small hip incision (2–4 inches) is more likely to have the following than one who has had a traditional incision (10–12 inches)?*						
A shorter time in surgery	82.5	7.2	1.3	91.0	8.0	1.0
Fewer days in the hospital	83.5	8.2	8.2	64.0	28.0	8.0
Less muscle tissue cut in surgery	87.6	12.4	0	100	0	0
Less pain in the first days after surgery	88.7	11.3	0	87.0	4.0	9.0
Quicker healing after surgery	87.6	12.4	0	100	0	0
The ability to walk without pain sooner after surgery	91.8	8.2	0	94.0	6.0	0
A better cosmetic appearance of scar	100	0	0	100	0	0
A feeling the body is less violated	92.8	7.2	0	99.0	1.0	0
The ability to be independent in daily activities sooner	97.9	2.1	0	93.0	7.0	0
Less limp in the affected leg during recovery period	94.8	5.2	0	91.0	9.0	0
More confidence in success of the surgery	80.4	19.6	0	94.0	6.0	0
A more positive attitude toward the surgery	90.7	9.3	0	99.0	1.0	0
Better overall satisfaction with the *results* of surgery	87.6	12.4	0	96.0	4.0	0
Better overall satisfaction with the results of the *recovery* from surgery	86.6	13.4	0	95.0	5.0	0

These percentages represent answers from patients (N = 100) who had their total hip arthroplasty through a mini-incision. The survey was conducted before surgery and at 6 weeks after surgery.

Table 4–2
Patient Satisfaction Questionnaire: All Patients Undergoing Total Hip Arthroplasty

	Preoperative (%)			Postoperative (%)		
	Yes	No Difference	No	Yes	No Difference	No
Question: *Do you feel that a patient who has had a small hip incision (2–4 inches) is more likely to have the following than one who has had a traditional incision (10–12 inches)?*						
A shorter time in surgery	86.1	5.7	8.2	92	6.3	0.8
Fewer days in the hospital	86.9	6.6	6.6	71.4	22.2	6.3
Less muscle tissue cut in surgery	90.2	9.8	0	100	0	0
Less pain in the first days after surgery	86.9	13.1	0	89.7	3.2	7.1
Quicker healing after surgery	86.1	13.9	0	100	0	0
The ability to walk without pain sooner after surgery	93.4	6.6	0	95.2	4.8	0
A better cosmetic appearance of scar	100	0	0	100	0	0
A feeling the body is less violated	94.3	5.7	0	99.2	0.8	0
The ability to be independent in daily activities sooner	98.4	1.6	0	94.4	5.6	0
Less limp in the affected leg during recovery period	95.9	4.1	0	92.9	7.1	0
More confidence in success of the surgery	84.4	15.6	0	95.2	4.8	0
A more positive attitude toward the surgery	92.6	7.4	0	99.2	0.8	0
Better overall satisfaction with the *results* of surgery	90.2	9.8	0	96.8	3.2	0
Better overall satisfaction with the results of the *recovery* from surgery	89.3	10.7	0	96.0	4.0	0

These percentages represent answers from all patients undergoing total hip arthroplasty (mini-incisions and standard incisions; N = 125). The survey was conducted before surgery and at 6 weeks after surgery.

tionnaire clearly shows that most patients favor this approach to hip surgery. The questionnaire in Table 4–1 gives answers from 100 patients who received the mini-incision; Table 4–2 represents answers from those 100 patients plus 25 patients who had a long incision. Patients completed the questionnaire before surgery and 6 weeks after surgery; unanimity is defined as assent to a question by 99% to 100% of patients. In Table 4–1, factors with unanimously favorable answers for the posterior mini-incision on the postoperative questionnaire were less muscle cut (100%), quicker healing (100%), better cosmesis (100%), less violation of the patient's body (99%), and a more positive attitude toward the surgery (100%). For these same factors in Table 4–2, note that at the time of the postoperative questionnaire, virtually all 25 patients with a long incision favored the mini-incision.

These responses clearly demonstrate that the posterior mini-incision results in a patient's better attitude toward the overall results and an improved recovery. The psychological aspect of medicine—the art of medicine—is just as important as its physiologic aspect. The surgeon who can develop the competence to perform the posterior mini-incision with predictable and reproducible results should do so.

Interestingly, the factors associated with responses showing a postoperative decrease in the percentage of mini-incision patients favoring the mini-incision were those pertaining to physical response to the operation. Fewer patients postoperatively felt that the mini-incision would result in fewer postoperative days in the hospital (preop 87% versus postop 71% in Table 4–2); there was almost no increased impression that there was less pain in the first days after surgery with the smaller incision (preop 87% versus postop 90%); there was a decrease in the impression that the patient could become independent in daily activities sooner with a smaller incision (preop 98% versus postop 94%); and there was a decreased impression that there was less limp during the recovery period (preop 96% versus postop 93%). Surgeons, however, often concentrate more on the purely physical response to their work, to the detriment of the overall patient response. In some studies, this clearly has led them to grade surgical results by factors that are of less importance to the patient. For the patient, if the operation can be performed just as safely, the mini-incision is overwhelmingly favored.

The surgeon should learn the technique of the posterior mini-incision operation by gradually decreasing the size of the incision used, while familiarizing himself or herself with the new instrumentation to ameliorate the decreasing field of vision. By the time the operation is performed through an 8- to 10-cm incision, the surgeon is comfortable with the reduced field of vision and understands the instrumentation. Training at an organized course or studying technique videos, or both, is recommended. This book and the accompanying videos allow the surgeon to study the techniques repeatedly and develop a mental picture of the stepwise progression and pattern of the operation technique, the necessary precondition for operating on patients. Finally, performing the initial operation with a surgeon experienced in the procedure lessens the stress for the learning surgeon.

INSTRUMENTATION

The posterior mini-incision operation requires the use of specialized tools, including retractors, reamers, and implant holders, to protect against excessive soft tissue tension. The retractors in particular have long handles to provide retraction with a minimum of soft tissue tension, to keep the assistants' hands and bodies clear of the wound and the operating surgeon, and to allow an assistant to hold multiple retractors, which minimizes the number of assistants needed.

The retractors used for exposure of the posterior hip and the femoral head during osteotomy of the femoral neck, with the rulers used to measure the neck cut, are shown in Figure 4–1. The acetabular retractors are shown in Figure 4–2, and their numbers correspond with the order of their use at surgery. Perhaps the most important of these is the unique retractor for the posterior capsule (#7 retractor), which has a long tip to engage the cortical bone of the cotyloid notch (just below the transverse acetabular ligament) and a paddle that sits on the ischial bone to protect the sciatic nerve during retraction of the posterior capsule (Fig. 4–3). This retractor is attached to a fiberoptic light source to illuminate the acetabulum. The so-called snake retractor (#5 retractor), used to displace the femoral bone anterior to the acetabulum, was designed by Dr. Chit Ranawat (Lennox-Hill Hospital, New York, N.Y.; Fig. 4–4). This retractor has a point that engages on the anterior ilium, just lateral to the anterior inferior iliac spine, to give secure fixation. It also has a radius of curvature that gives great leverage for retracting the femur anteriorly without damaging the bone. A second choice for anterior retraction of the femur is the curved, two-pronged retractor (#5b retractor) that can be placed against the anterior wall of the acetabulum (see Fig. 4–2). Which retractor is used is largely a matter of the surgeon's preference, although the advantages of not placing a retractor against the anterior wall of the acetabulum include protecting the wall from breakage and protecting the femoral nerve

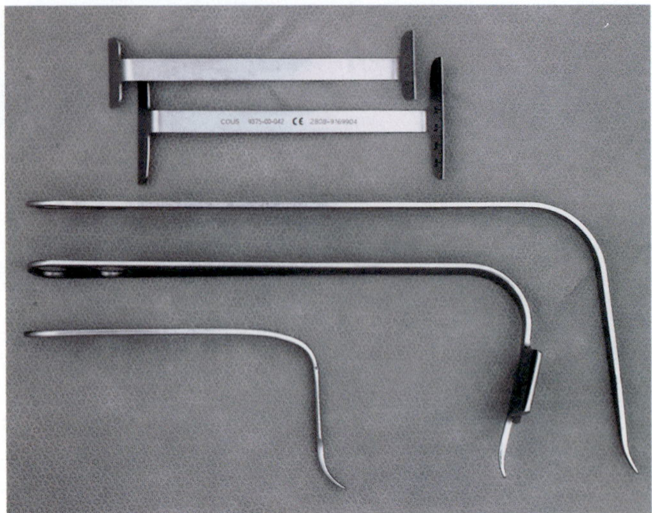

Figure 4–1 *The rulers at top measure 40 mm and 70 mm. Below the rulers, in order from top to bottom, are the #2 retractor, which retracts the gluteus medius tendon away from the piriformis and gluteus minimus; the #3 retractor, which retracts the quadratus muscle and protects the sciatic nerve during osteotomy of the femoral neck; and the #1 retractor.*

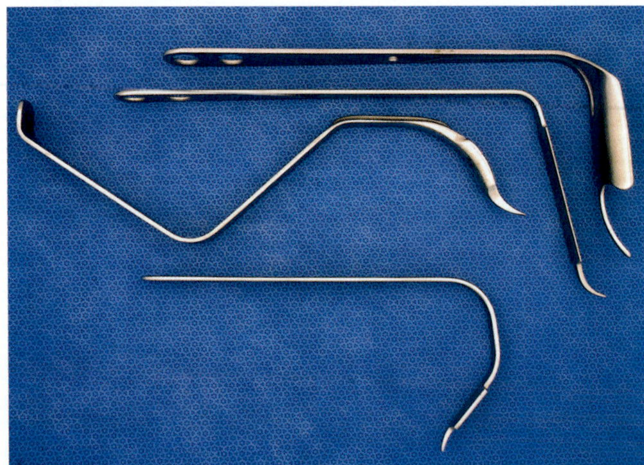

Figure 4–2 *The acetabular retractors are shown in order from bottom to top. The #4 retractor retracts the posterior superior capsule with its point malleted into bone; the #5 retractor retracts the greater trochanter to expose the anterior edge of the acetabulum, also with its point malleted into bone; the #6 retractor is placed between the medial capsule and the external oblique muscle to protect the medial circumflex artery and vein while the medial capsule is incised to the transverse acetabular ligament; the #7 retractor is the posterior medial retractor; the tip of the retractor is hooked against the cortical bone of the cotyloid notch, and the paddle sits on the ischium, with the blade retracting the posterior and medial capsule and protecting the sciatic nerve. There are left and right #7 retractors.*

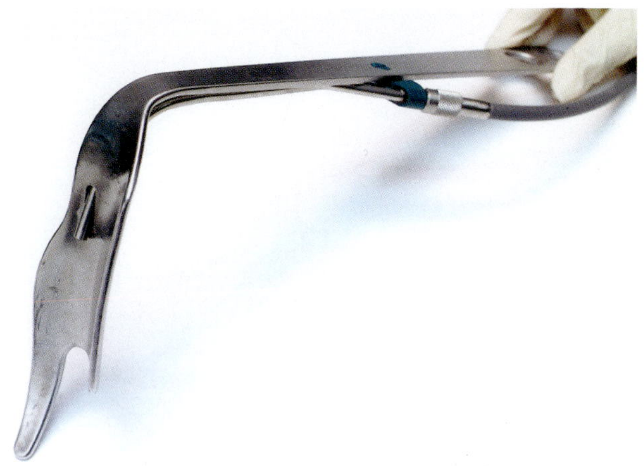

Figure 4–3 *The #7 retractor has a hook for the edge of the cotyloid notch, a paddle that sits on the ischium, and a blade to retract the posterior medial capsule and protect the sciatic nerve. A light source is attached to this retractor to aid visualization during acetabular preparation.*

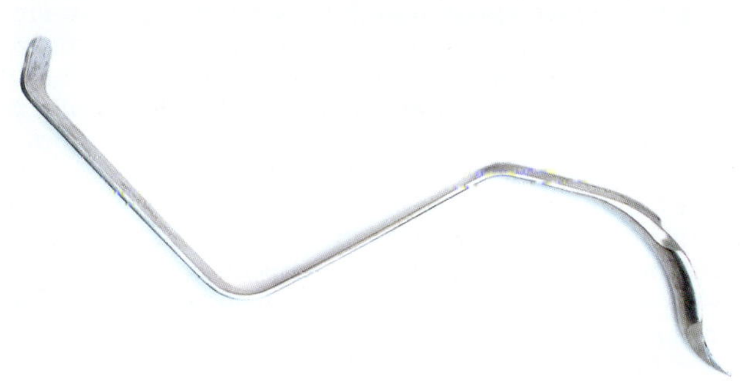

Figure 4–4 *The #5a retractor is nicknamed the "snake." The point is malleted into the ilium just above the anterosuperior border of the acetabulum and gives excellent leverage in retracting the greater trochanter anterior to the acetabulum. The force of retraction is taken against the greater trochanter, which protects the anterior skin.*

from tension. In some patients, one retractor may work better than the other. The posterosuperior retractor (#4 retractor) has a point that can be pounded into the bone to stabilize it as it retracts the posterosuperior capsule and small external rotators.

The femoral retractors are also designed to maximize exposure of the cut surface of the femoral neck without applying excessive retraction force (Fig. 4–5). The radius of curvature and long handle of the "jaws" retractor (#8 retractor) were designed to elevate the cut surface of the femoral neck into the wound by retracting the posterosuperior flap of the wound. This retractor also is attached to a light source to illuminate the distal cut end of the femur. A thinner #8 retractor is favored by some surgeons for retraction of the poste-

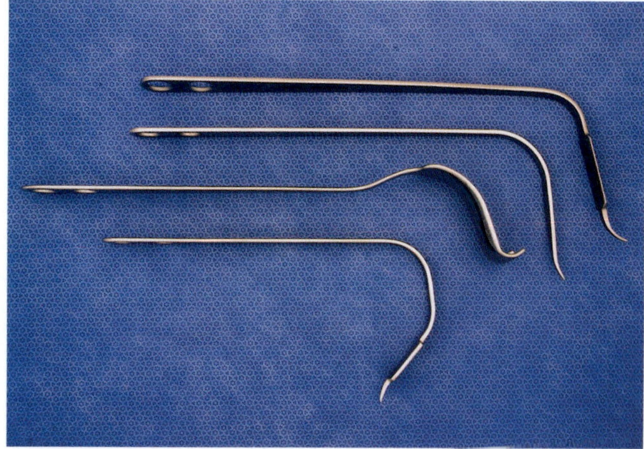

Figure 4–5 *The #4, #8, #9, and #10 retractors (bottom to top) are shown. The #4 retractor retracts the quadratus femoris from the medial bone of the cut femoral neck; the #8 retractor retracts the posterior flap of skin and gluteus maximus from the cut surface of the femoral neck; and the #9 retractor is used to retract the gluteus medius and the anterior skin and fat in most patients. In some patients, the #9 retractor retracts the anterior skin and fat over the greater trochanter, and the #10 retractor is used to retract the gluteus medius tendon and muscle.*

rior flap (Fig. 4–6). The #4 retractor, which also was used for posterosuperior retraction over the acetabulum, is placed on the medial femoral neck under the quadratus femoris muscle to protect this muscle and expose the medial cortex of the neck (see Fig. 4–6 B and C). Anterior skin and gluteal muscle overhanging the greater trochanter are retracted with the trochanteric retractors (#9 and #10 retractors), which can be joined by a linking tool. The #9 retractor is for the gluteus maximus and skin, whereas the #10 retractor is for the gluteus medius muscle (see Fig. 4–6). The choice of which of the two retractors to use, or the use of both, depends on the thickness of skin and fat and position of the gluteus medius and maximus muscles.

TECHNIQUE

Patient Positioning

The patient is placed in the lateral position supported by pelvic and chest supports (Fig. 4–7), as described for the standard incision (see Chapter 3). The incision runs proximally from 2 cm proximal to the tip of the greater trochanter to the vastus lateralis ridge of the femur distally (Fig. 4–8). Visibility of the femur for conventional total hip replacement is enhanced when the incision is made just cephalic to the tip of the greater trochanter to the vastus tubercle because the cut distal surface is easily accessed. An incision proximal to the tip of the greater trochanter is better for surface replacement because it allows better access to the femoral head. The

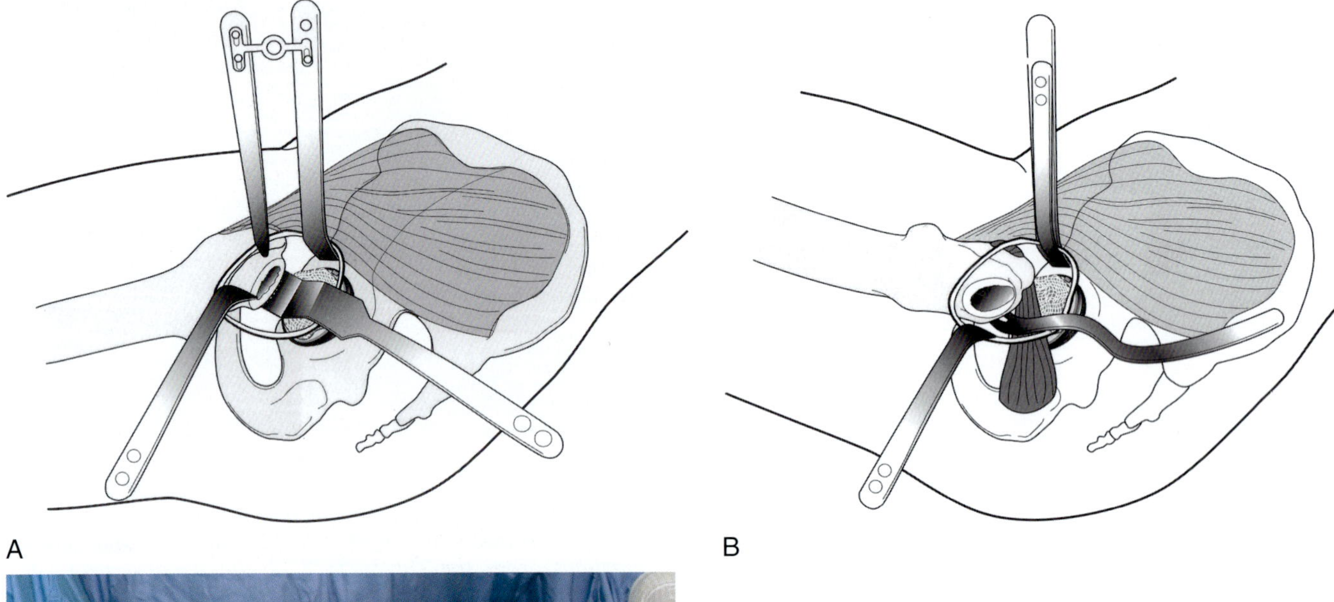

A

B

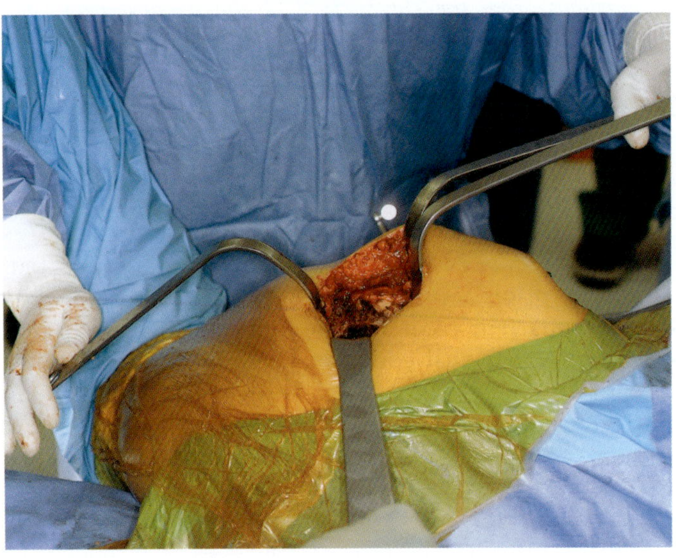

C

Figure 4–6 ***A,*** *The #8 retractor has a radius of curvature and a long handle that allow retraction of the posterior flap of skin, fat, and gluteus maximus muscle while transmitting minimal force into the soft tissues, yet allowing elevation of the cut femoral neck into the wound for preparation of the femur. This retractor is nicknamed "jaws." The #9 and #10 retractors can be joined by a linkage.* ***B,*** *The #8b retractor, a second form of the #8 retractor, with the #4 retractor positioned on the medial side of the femur and the #9 retractor retracting the gluteus medius muscle. The thinner #8b retractor can be used with thin patients and can be more easily moved out of the way of the tools used for preparation of the femur and insertion of the femoral stem.* ***C,*** *Intraoperative view of the femoral retractors. The thin #8b retractor is seen at lower center; at left, the #4 retractor is around the medial neck and retracting the quadratus femoris, and the #9 and #10 retractors are being held at right.*

incision along the posterior third of the greater trochanter facilitates the visualization of both bones of the hip. The bigger the muscle or the thicker the layer of fat over the greater trochanter, the closer the incision should come to the posterior border of the greater trochanter. In heavier patients, the incision should run directly along the posterior border of the greater trochanter (see Fig. 4–8).

Incision

The average length of the skin incision is 8 to 10 cm, which provides the best visual exposure for the surgeon and assistants. The length of the incision may be changed somewhat according to the height of the patient; very tall patients have a longer trochanter and therefore need a longer skin incision. Because the muscle incision is only 6 cm long, the skin incision could be as short as 5 to 6 cm, but this reduces visibility for the assistants and increases tension on the skin with retraction. Furthermore, the patient does not benefit from 2 or 3 cm less of skin incision; it is the extent of injury to the underlying tissues that counts. What the patient does *not* want is a 10- to 15-inch incision!

The procedure includes only three cuts of the hip muscle and capsule.

First Incision

The first cut is to the gluteus maximus muscle. The fascia over the gluteus maximus is incised for the 8-cm length of the skin incision. The actual incision through the portion of the gluteus maximus overlying the posterior greater trochanter is 6 cm in length (Fig. 4–9).

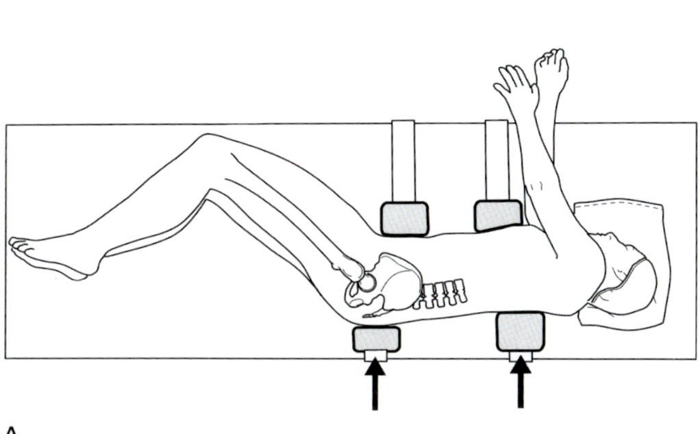

A

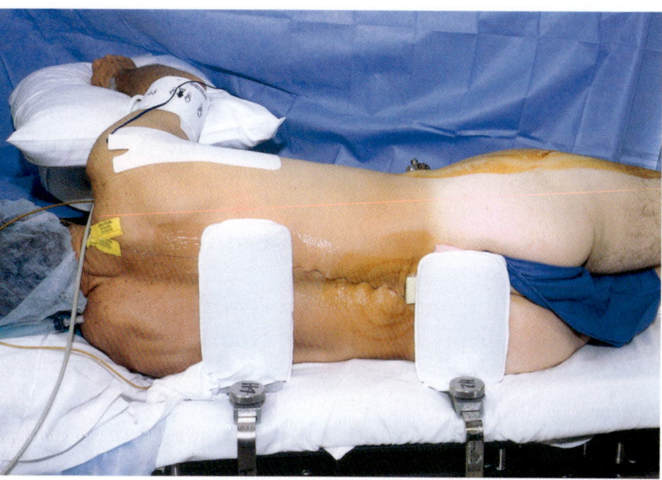

B

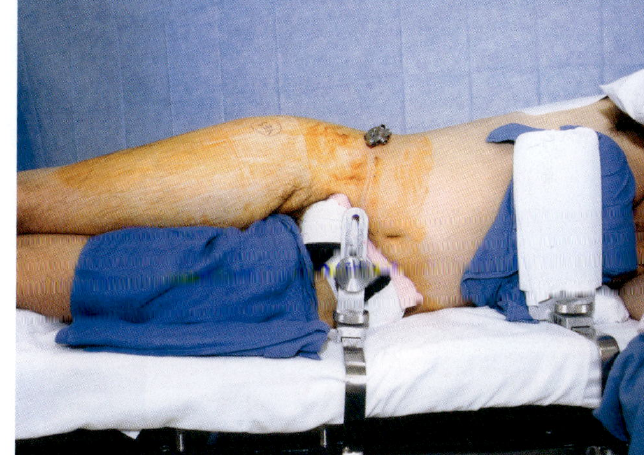

C

Figure 4–7 **A,** The patient is placed in the lateral position and secured with two chest supports and two pelvic supports. The pelvic supports are placed posteriorly against the posterior superior iliac spines and anteriorly against the down-side anterior superior iliac spine and pubis. The chest supports are placed posteriorly against the base of the scapulae and anteriorly at the xiphoid. **B,** The posterior supports rest against the posterior spines of the pelvis and at the distal end of the scapulae. **C,** The anterior supports rest against the chest and the down-side anterior superior iliac spine and pubis.

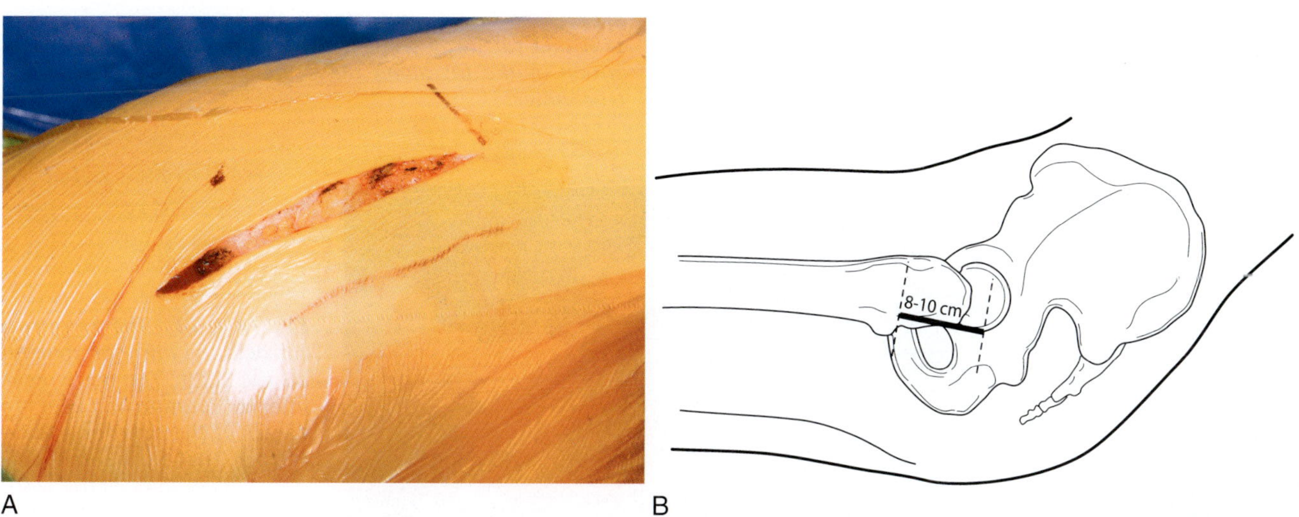

A

B

Figure 4–8 **A,** The incision is made just anterior to the posterior border of the greater trochanter. The dot represents the tip of the greater trochanter, and the transverse line represents the vastus tubercle. **B,** In heavier people, because of the thickness of muscle or fat, the incision is made along the posterior border of the trochanter.

Some surgeons prefer to separate these muscle fibers, but I prefer to cut them. I do not believe the injury to the muscle separated by an incision with the Bovie electrocautery is any greater than that sustained by pulling it apart with retractors. Furthermore, our gait studies indicate that this small incision is of little functional consequence to the gluteus maximus muscle, which regains 100% of its preoperative performance level 6 weeks after surgery.

As soon as the muscle incision is made, the #1 retractor is placed; this is a small, bent Homans retractor that retracts the anterior gluteus maximus muscle to expose the posterior greater trochanter (Fig. 4–10). The leg is internally rotated and kept in the center of the table, lying on top of the lower leg (Fig. 4–11). It is important not to let the knee drop over the side of the table because this puts too much tension on the soft tissue structures in the posterior hip. To prevent bleeding, the fat over the external rotators and the gluteus medius tendon is incised with the Bovie. This exposes the exter-

nal rotators and the gluteus medius tendon (Fig. 4–12). The surgeon's index finger is inserted over the top of the piriformis tendon and moved back and forth to separate the thin fascia between the gluteus medius and gluteus minimus muscles (Fig. 4–13). The gluteus medius muscle is retracted from the gluteus minimus muscle using the #2 retractor.

Second Incision

The second incision of hip tissue separates the small external rotators and the posterior capsule from the

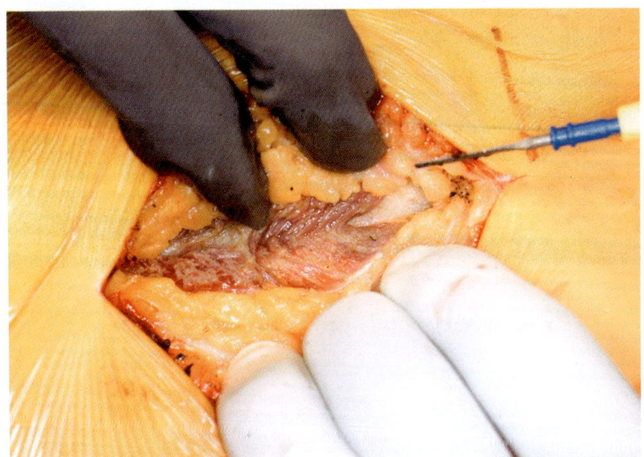

Figure 4–9 *The incision is made through the gluteus maximus muscle along the posterior border of the greater trochanter; the length of this incision, 6 to 7 cm, is less than that of the skin incision.*

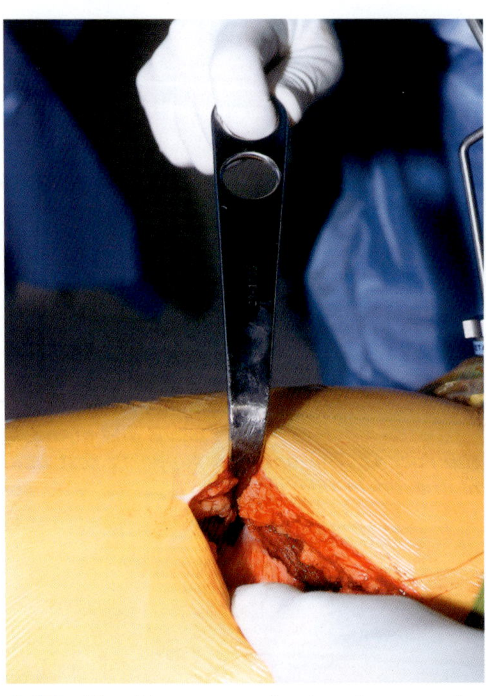

Figure 4–10 *The #1 retractor is placed across the anterior greater trochanter and retracts the anterior gluteus maximus skin and fat away from the trochanter to give good visualization of the fat along the posterior border of the greater trochanter.*

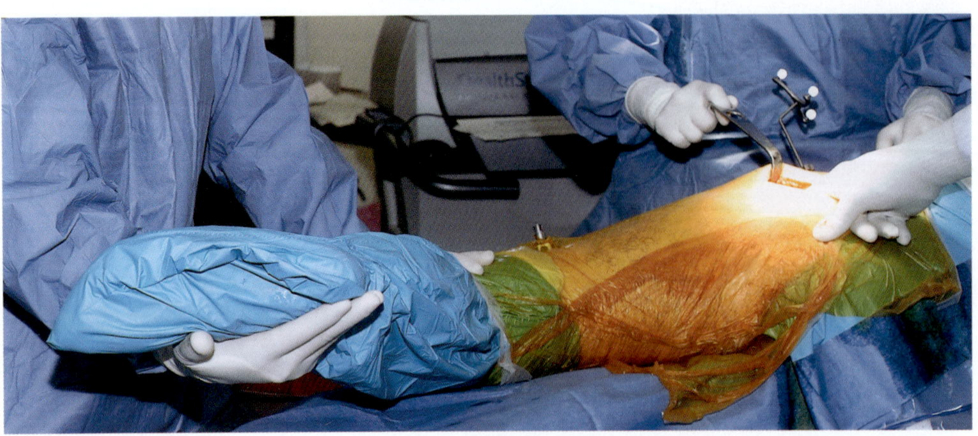

Figure 4–11 *The #1 retractor retracts the anterior structures on the right. The leg is held in internal rotation and kept in the center of the operating table to retract the trochanter anteriorly, which gives better visualization of the posterior hip structures and moves the posterior border of the trochanter away from the sciatic nerve.*

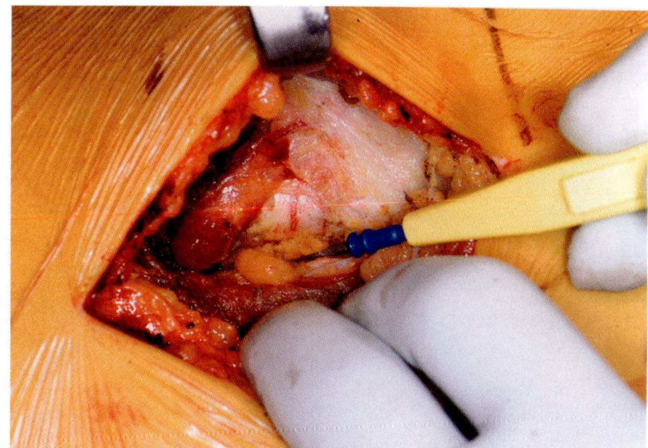

Figure 4–12   *The greater trochanter is seen in the upper right of the wound. The #1 retractor lies over the top of the greater trochanter. The lower gluteus maximus muscle is below the surgeon's fingers. The gluteus medius muscle runs to the greater trochanter. The piriformis tendon is visible below the gluteus medius muscle, and a small vessel runs across it just above the tip of the Bovie electrocautery. The Bovie incises the fat that overlies these structures.*

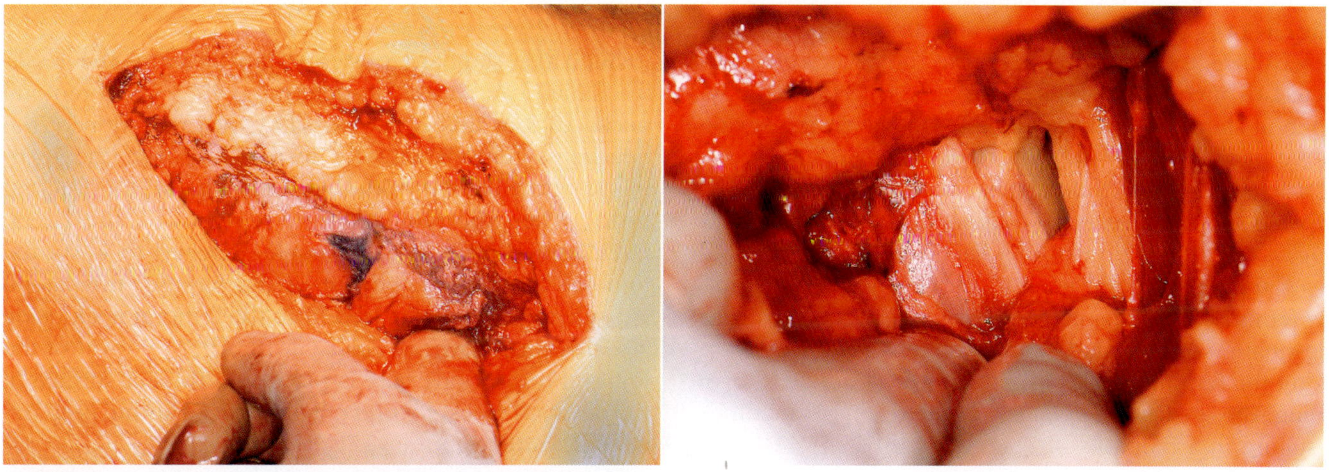

A

B

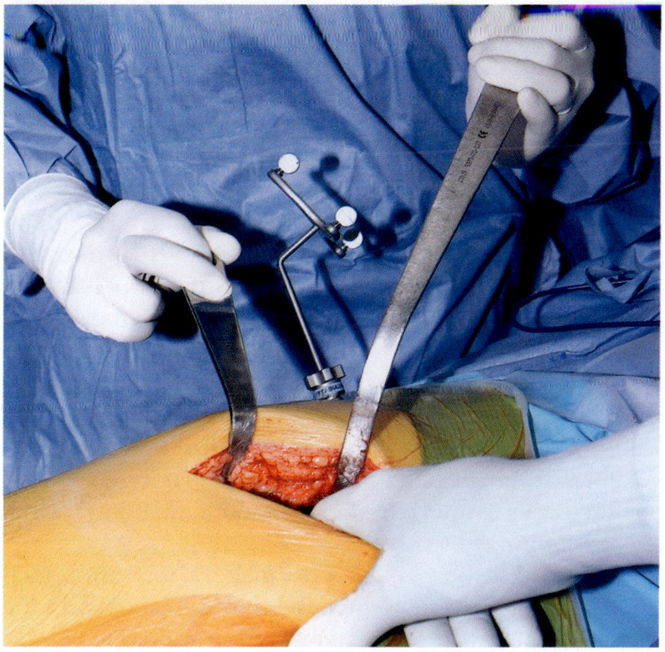

C

Figure 4–13   **A,** *The surgeon's finger opens the interval between the gluteus minimus and gluteus medius muscles by feeling the piriformis tendon and sliding over this tendon and under the gluteus medius tendon.* **B,** *The #2 retractor is placed in the interval between the gluteus medius and gluteus minimus so that its tip is in the gluteus minimus proximal to the piriformis and the blade retracts the gluteus medius tendon, which exposes the piriformis tendon and gluteus minimus muscle and protects the gluteus minimus tendon.* **C,** *The #1 retractor (short handle) and #2 retractor (long handle) are held by an assistant.*

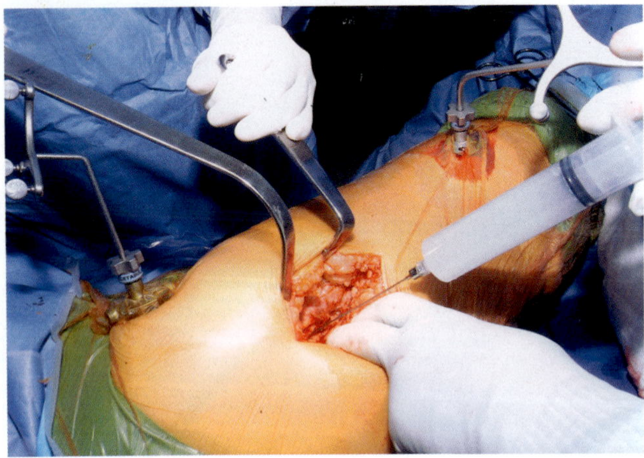

Figure 4–14 *Anesthetic cocktail is injected into the posterior structures of the hip before their incision. The tracker and pelvic base plate for the computer guidance system are visible in the left corner. The #2 retractor is seen in the upper left of the wound, and the #1 retractor in the center right. The femoral base plate and tracker for the computer guidance system are visible at upper right (see Chapter 7).*

greater trochanter. Just before these tissues are cut, they are injected with the cocktail described in Chapter 1 (Fig. 4–14). The timing of the injection is such that it desensitizes the nociceptors before the tissues are subjected to mechanical injury; also, the injection can be done at this time without risk of damage to the sciatic nerve.

The second incision results in a posterior flap of capsule and small external rotators that can be retracted (Fig. 4–15). Retraction of this flap exposes the femoral head and the femoral neck to the level of the quadratus femoris. The capsule can be further incised beneath the quadratus femoris by simply moving the Bovie tip along the femoral neck underneath the quadratus. In so doing the orbicular ligament is also cut, sometimes resulting in a palpable or even audible "snap." The orbicular ligament surrounds the femoral neck about 1 cm below the edge of the femoral head.

The hip is dislocated. This can be done fairly easily by simply rocking the femoral head out of the acetabulum with the leg flexed and internally rotated. I have both cut the femoral neck in situ and dislocated the hip, and have seen no difference in postoperative pain or patient response. It is easier to perform the operation by dislocating the hip, however.

When the hip is dislocated, the #3 retractor is placed around the femoral neck with one edge inserted under the quadratus femoris to retract the muscle away from the femoral neck (Fig. 4–16). Sometimes tightness of the muscle or a small hip prevents the wing of the #3 retractor from sitting between the quadratus and the medial femoral neck, in which case the #4 retractor should be used. The fat between the quadratus muscle and the neck must be excised so that the femoral neck can be cut. The length of the femoral neck cut is measured from the inferior edge of the femoral head and is usually 15 or 20 mm (Fig. 4–17). This level of the cut, which is estimated based on the preoperative x-rays, is that which will recreate hip length and offset for the

patient. Computer navigation enables more accurate determination of the correct neck cut, as described in Chapter 7.

With the standard posterior hip incision, the lesser trochanter can be used to determine the level of femoral neck cut, but this is not possible with retention of the quadratus femoris muscle; instead, we use the technique of measuring from the distal edge of the femoral head. When the femoral head is removed, the lateral neck sometimes still has capsule attached to it. As the femoral head is rotated out of the wound, this lateral capsule needs to be incised from the femoral neck using a scalpel, as shown in Figure 4–18. After removal of the femoral head, bone wax is placed on the cut surface of the femoral neck to prevent bleeding during preparation of the acetabulum (Fig. 4–19).

After removal of the femoral head, the acetabulum can be visualized, and the #4 retractor is placed on the posterosuperior acetabulum between the bone and the posterosuperior capsule/external rotator flap. This also exposes the labrum along the posterosuperior aspect of the acetabulum (Fig. 4–20). The #5 (snake) retractor is inserted anteriorly onto the ilium to retract the femur anteriorly. The anterior capsule is dense, and in some patients it is difficult to insert this retractor without catching a fold of capsule anterior to the retractor, which makes reaming more difficult. If this occurs, the capsule should be incised at its junction with the acetabular bone, and the tip of the retractor placed through this incision to pull the capsule anteriorly with the bone (Fig. 4–21). With the #4 and #5 retractors in place, the labrum of the acetabulum is visualized and can be excised from the edge of the acetabular bone, which better exposes the peripheral osseous anatomy of the acetabulum.

It may also be necessary to make a relaxation incision into the capsule to give the best retraction with the retractor placed against the anterior wall (Fig. 4–22). With this retractor, the leg should be in the same posi-

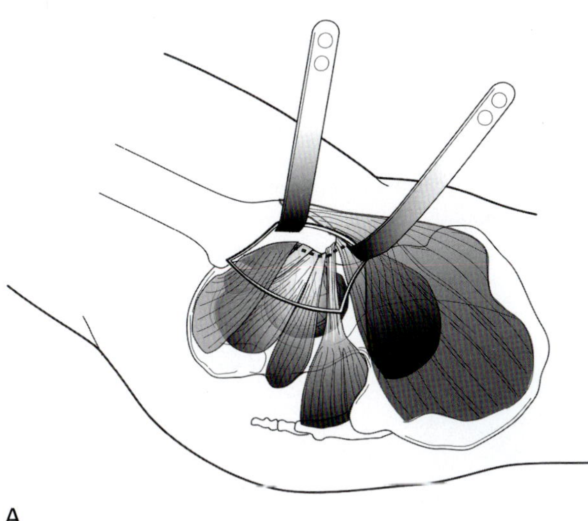

A

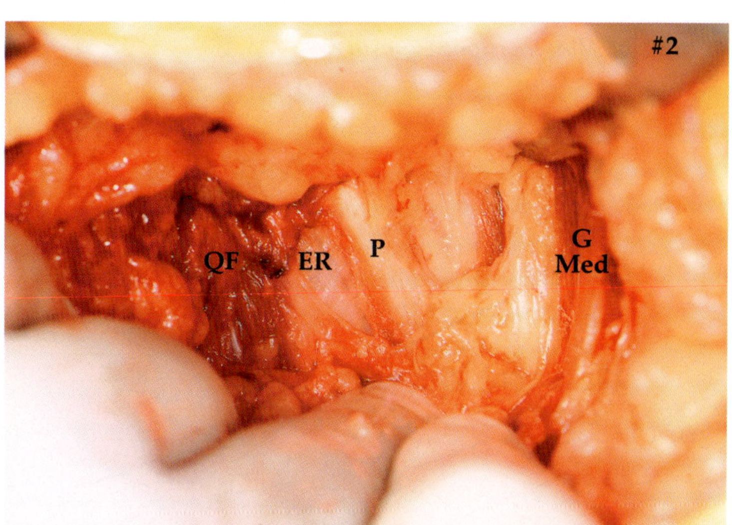

B

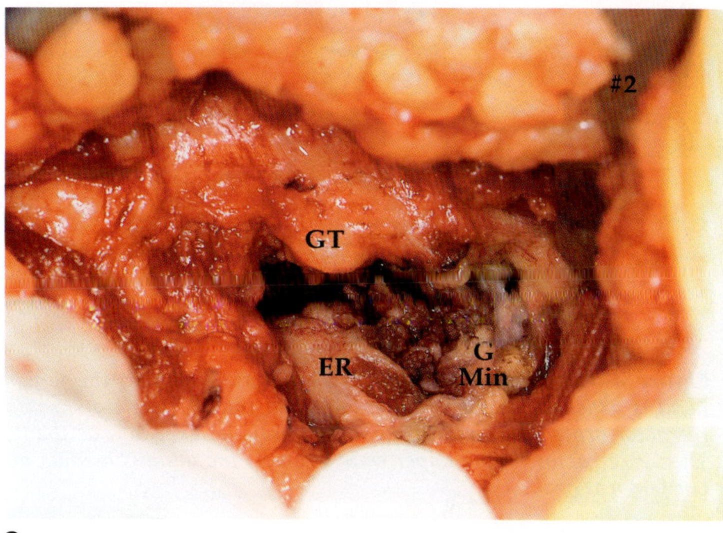

C

Figure 4–15 ***A,*** *The #1 retractor lies over the greater trochanter and the #2 retractor retracts the gluteus medius tendon. The incision line for the posterior structures is outlined, running through the gluteus minimus just above the piriformis and then extending distally through the obturator externus and internus and the inferior and superior gemellus muscles to the border of the quadratus femoris.* ***B,*** *Close-up of the posterior structures that are incised. The fat has been incised off the posterior hip muscles. At the extreme right, just next to the fat at the edge of the figure, the #2 retractor retracts the gluteus medius (G Med) muscle. Next is the gluteus minimus muscle and then the piriformis (P), external rotators (ER), and quadratus femoris muscle (QF).* ***C,*** *The posterior flap created by incision of the capsule and small external rotators. The capsule is under the muscles and not visible. GT, greater trochanter; G Min, gluteus minimus; ER, external rotators.*

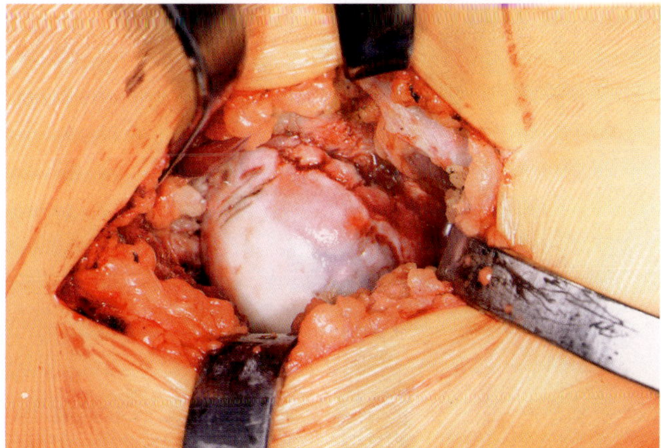

Figure 4–16 *The #4 retractor is placed around the medial neck to protect the sciatic nerve and retract the quadratus femoris muscle during osteotomy of the femoral neck. The #1 and #2 retractors are superior. An accessory retractor exposes the femoral head for this view, but is not usually used.*

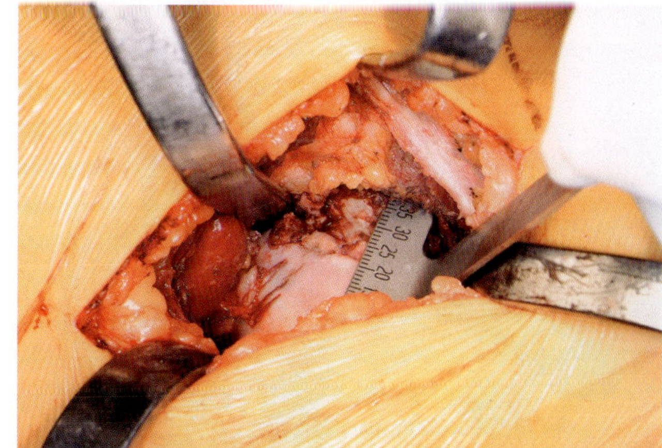

Figure 4–17 *A 40-mm ruler is used to measure from the inferior border of the femoral head along the femoral neck to mark the level of the femoral neck cut. The cut, which is being made between the 25- and 20-mm marks, is 15 to 20 mm long. The distal end of the ruler is against the edge of the quadratus, which is protected by the #4 retractor on the right side of the wound. The #2 retractor protects the gluteus medius muscle superiorly in upper left of the wound. The #1 retractor lies across the trochanter at the top of the wound, and the #3 retractor in the lower left is around the femoral head. The #3 retractor is not usually used, but it provides exposure for this view.*

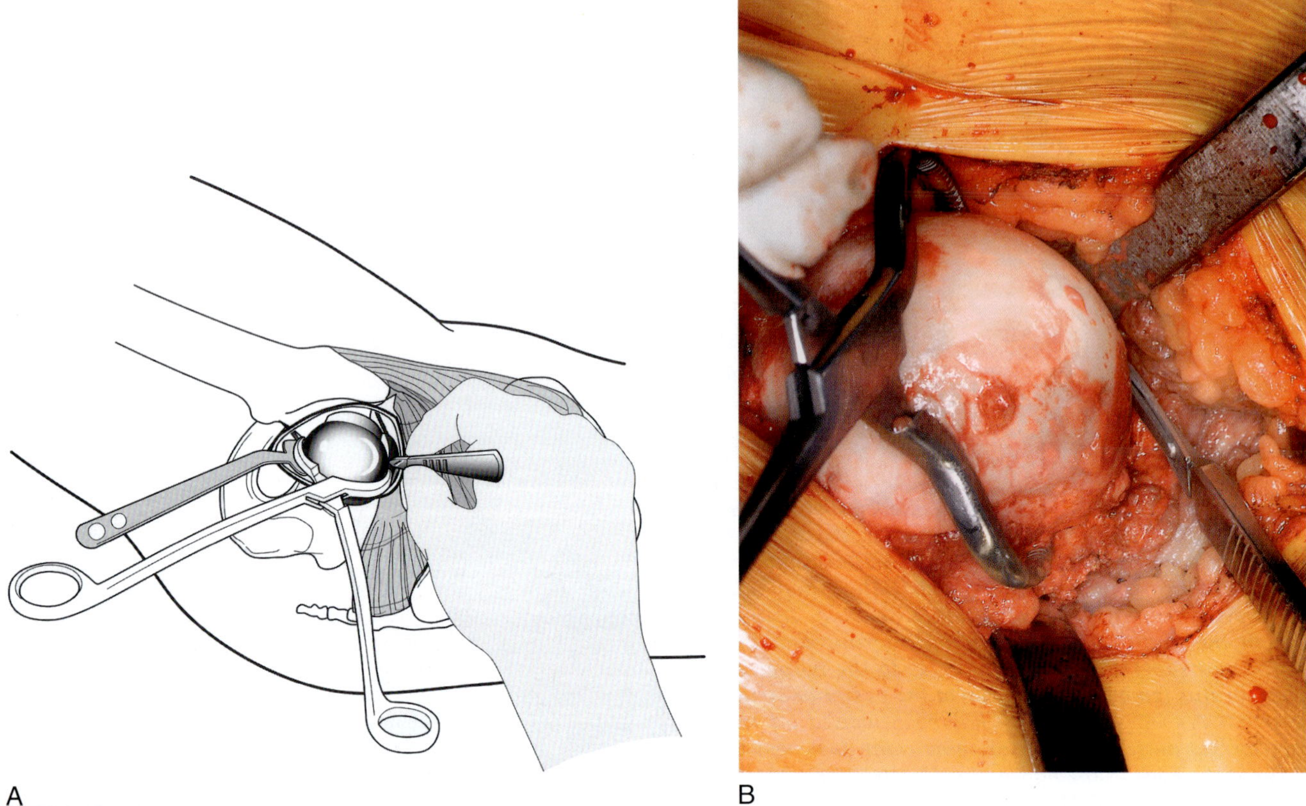

A

B

Figure 4–18 **A,** *Incision of the lateral capsule holding the femoral head and neck during removal of the femoral head. The head is grasped with a Lewin clamp, and the #3 retractor protects the sciatic nerve.* **B,** *On the inside of the wound, the #3 retractor protects the sciatic nerve and provides exposure as the head is rotated out of the wound, grasped with a Lewin clamp. The #2 retractor on the upper right protects the gluteus medius muscle, and the scalpel incises the capsule still attached to the cut femoral neck.*

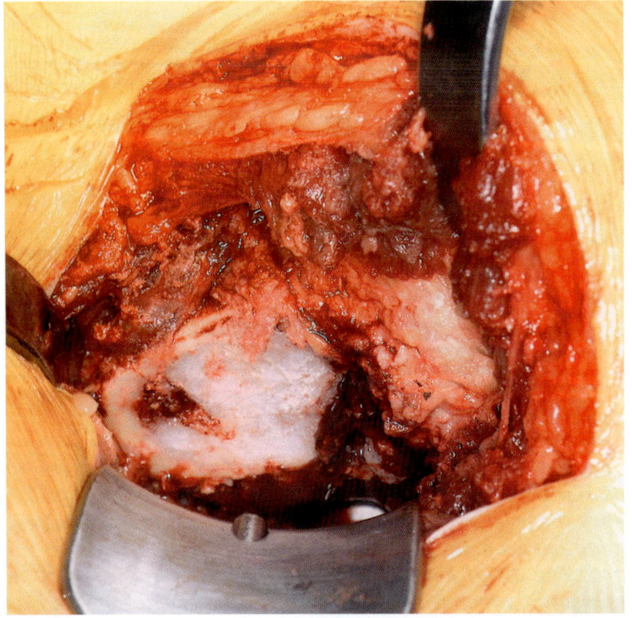

Figure 4–19 *Bone wax has been applied to the cut surface of the femoral neck to prevent bleeding into the acetabulum during preparation of the acetabulum.*

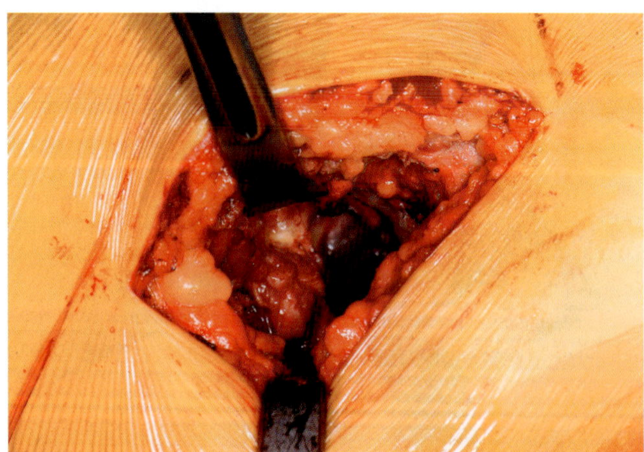

Figure 4–20 *The labrum overhangs the acetabulum in the center of the wound. The #5 (snake) retractor is seen in the upper portion of the wound, and the #4 retractor retracts the posterosuperior capsule at bottom.*

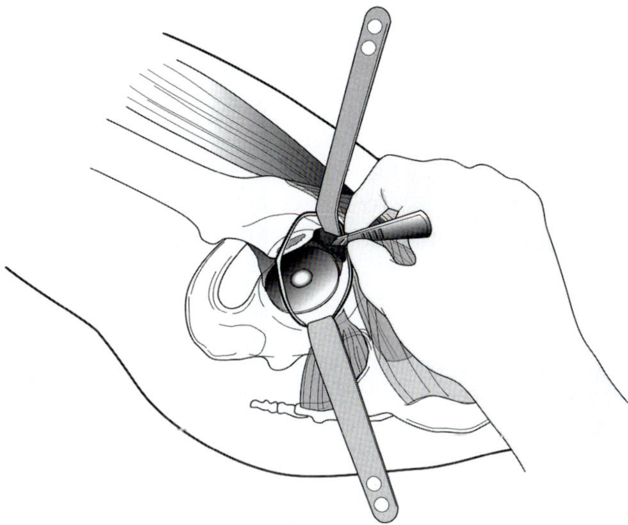

Figure 4–21   *The #5 (snake) retractor retracts the greater trochanter from the anterior edge of the acetabulum. An incision is being made into the anterosuperior capsule, which is necessary if the capsule is too tight to allow the femur to be fully retracted anteriorly. In addition, sometimes there is capsule in front of the #5 retractor that needs to be incised, and the retractor replaced with the capsule behind it so that the capsule does not overhang the acetabulum.*

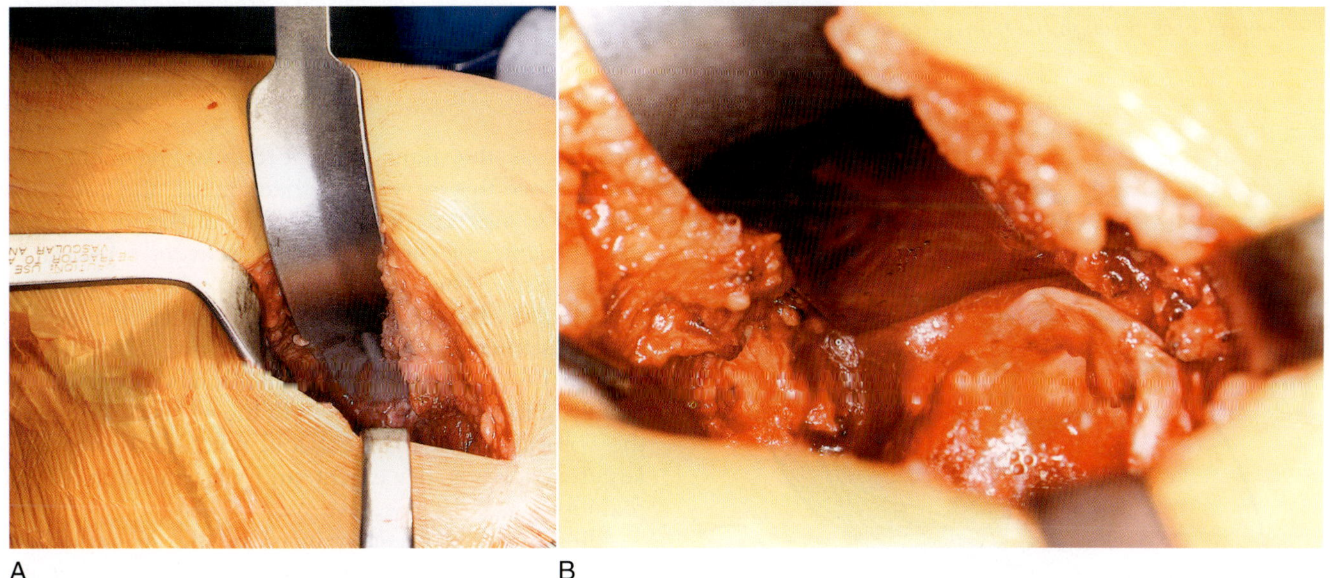

A   B

Figure 4–22   **A,** *The alternative technique for retraction of the femur uses the curved anterior retractor placed against the anterior acetabular wall and hooked on the trochanter to retract anteriorly.* **B,** *The broad, curved anterior retractor holds the greater trochanter at upper left and is placed against the anterior wall of the acetabulum. The labrum is evident on the superior wall of the acetabulum.*

tion on the table as for the snake retractor. The curved radius of this retractor fits against the trochanter to provide easy leverage for anterior retraction of the bone.

Third Incision

The third incision into hip tissue is made through the medial capsule, which includes the posterior ischiofemoral ligament that runs from the posterior acetabulum to the femur. This tissue is exposed by placing the #6 retractor between the capsular/ligamentous tissue and the external oblique muscle (Fig. 4–23). This retractor also protects the medial circumflex artery and vein, which run with the external oblique muscle, preventing them from being cut during division of the capsule. The capsule is divided all the way to the cortical bone of the cotyloid notch, including an

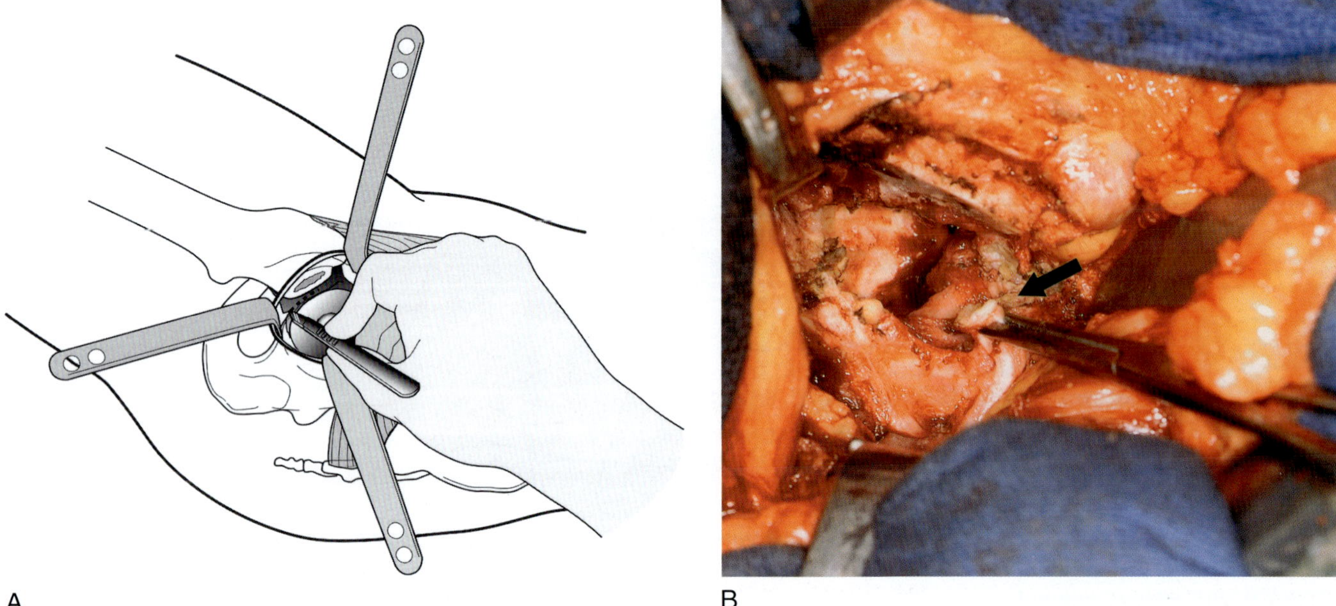

A

B

Figure 4–23 **A,** *The third hip cut. The #5 retractor is on the upper side of the wound; the #4 retractor is at the posterosuperior corner of the acetabulum, under the thumb; and the #6 retractor is placed behind the capsule that runs from the ischium to the anterior femur, and separates this capsule from the external oblique muscle. An incision is made through this capsule to the cotyloid notch of the acetabulum.* **B,** *Intraoperative view of the cut medial capsule. The incision (arrow) runs from the anterior femoral neck through the transverse acetabular ligament. The Kocher clamp holds the cut edge of this capsular incision.*

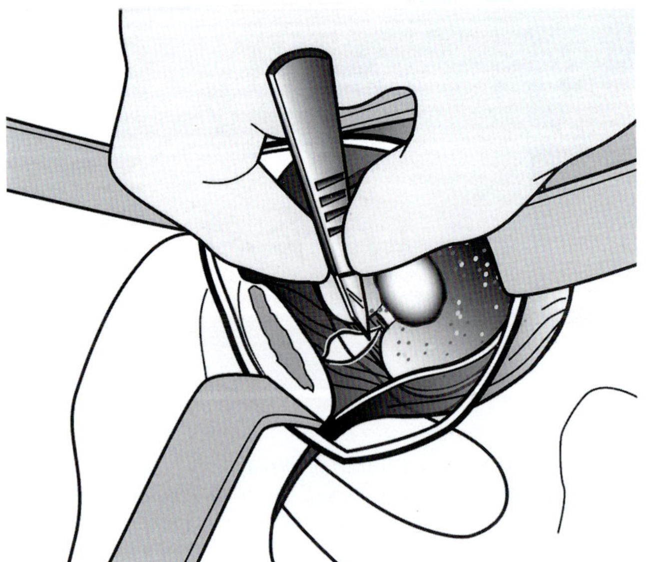

Figure 4–24 *The incision is made through the medial capsule to the base of the acetabulum. The #6 retractor lies adjacent to the cut femoral neck.*

incision of the transverse acetabular ligament (Fig. 4–24). Once this incision has been made, the anesthetic cocktail is injected along the edges of the incision and into the anterior capsule to help prevent sensitization of this tissue. This capsular incision relaxes contracted tissue, allowing the femur to be retracted anteriorly with less force (which helps protect the sciatic nerve), and to be internally rotated and flexed more easily. Finally, it facilitates placement of the #7 retractor against the cortical bone of the cotyloid notch and provides a larger space for placement and manipulation of the reamers.

After the final capsular incision, the #6 retractor is removed and the leg is laid onto the table; the foot also may be placed on a Mayo stand to give slight internal rotation. This relaxes the leg, improving blood flow and helping prevent venous thrombosis (Fig. 4–25). The #7 retractor, which has a light that significantly enhances visualization during preparation of the acetabulum (Fig. 4–26), is placed with its tip against the cortical bone of the cotyloid notch and its paddle sitting on the ischium, which retracts the posteroinferior capsule and protects the sciatic nerve. With the #4, #5, and #7 retractors in position, the acetabular exposure is complete (Fig. 4–27). Preparation and implantation of the acetabulum are described in Chapter 5.

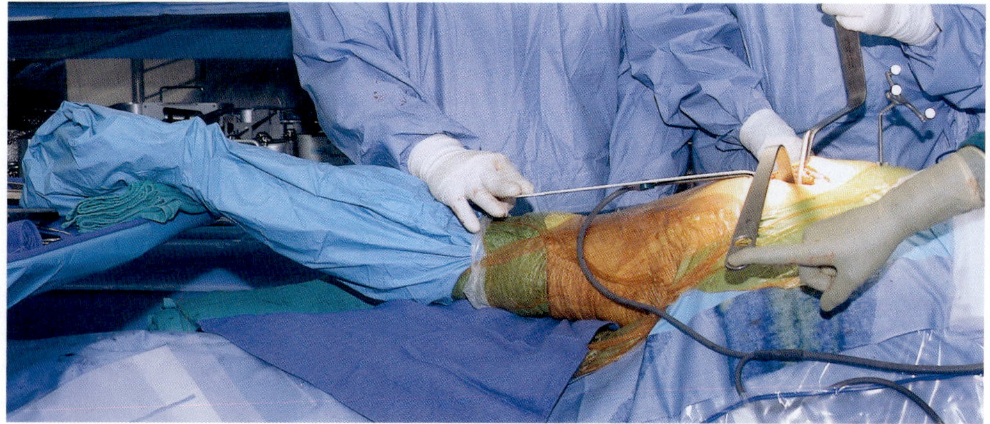

Figure 4–25 *The leg is positioned during preparation of the acetabulum by laying it in the center of the table on top of the lower leg. The femur is usually best retracted anterior to the acetabulum with the foot laid on the edge of the Mayo stand. The three acetabular retractors are seen, with the #5 (snake) retractor being held next to the light-emitting diodes used for the computer guidance system. On the posterior side, the #4 retractor holds the posterosuperior capsule, and retractor #7, the long handle of which is visible along the posterior thigh, retracts the posterior and medial capsule and protects the sciatic nerve.*

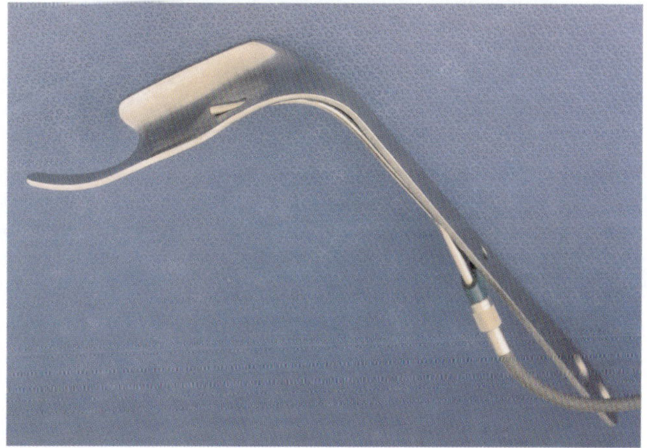

Figure 4–26 *The #7 retractor is attached to a fiberoptic light source. The light is seen at the front of the retractor blade and enhances visualization of the acetabulum during preparation.*

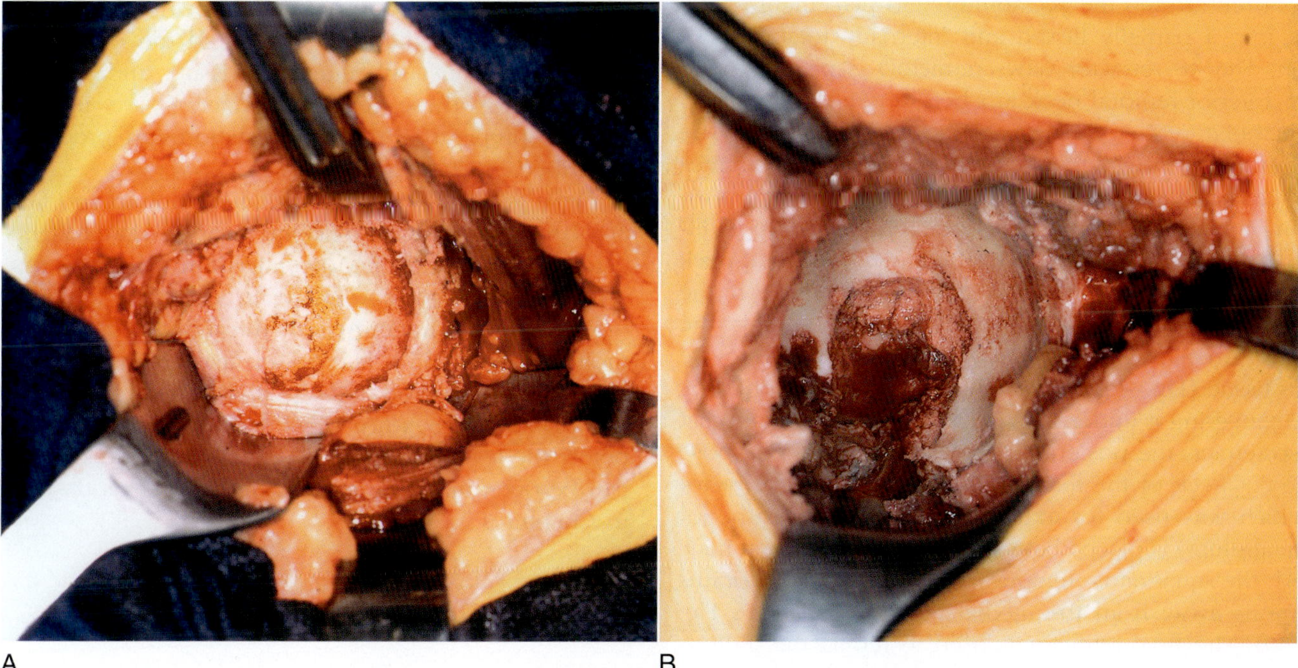

A

B

Figure 4–27 ***A,*** *The acetabulum can be visualized in its entirety, with the #5 retractor in the upper middle portion of the wound and the #4 retractor in the lower right. The efficacy of the #7 retractor, in the lower left, is clear. The tip of the #7 retractor is against the cortical bone of the cotyloid notch, just behind the osteophyte covering the transverse acetabular ligament, and the paddle is seated on the ischium, which retracts the capsule behind it and protects the sciatic nerve.* ***B,*** *In this mini-incision exposure of the acetabulum, the #5 retractor is on the upper left; the #4 retractor in the upper right; and retractor #7 at bottom. The acetabulum is clearly visualized. The osteophyte over the floor of the acetabulum has been removed from the cotyloid notch using the Anspach high-speed burr.*

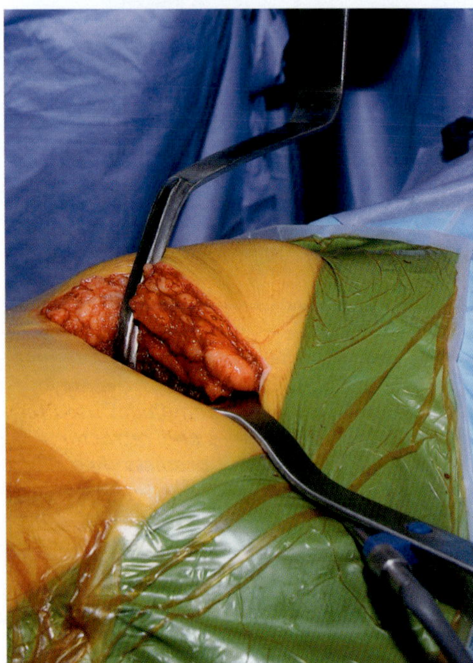

Figure 4–28 *The #8 retractor, with an attached fiberoptic light, is placed under the cut edge of the medial neck while the #5 (snake) retractor is still in place. The snake retractor facilitates palpation and visualization of the femoral neck for placement of the #8 retractor.*

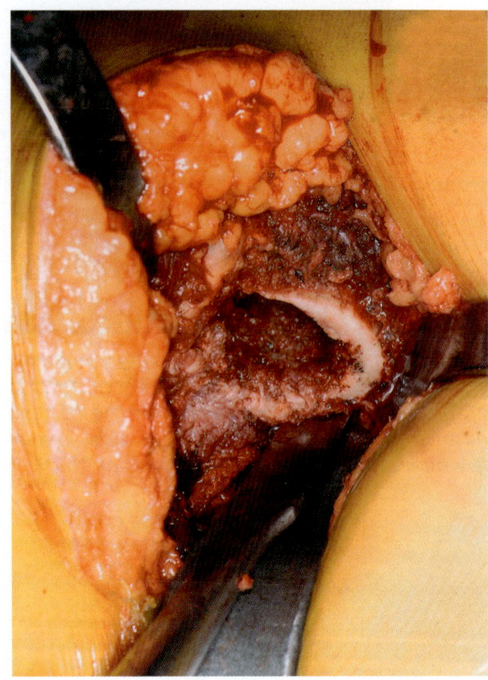

Figure 4–29 *The cut femoral neck is seen in the center of the wound. The #4 retractor next to the medial neck retracts the quadratus femoris. The #9 retractor at upper left retracts the fat and gluteus maximus muscle from the anterior trochanter. An osteotome is being used along the anterior side of the femoral neck to incise a tight anterior capsule from the neck, which will allow the neck to be lifted higher into the wound. The osteotome can also be used to remove osteophytes from the anterior neck.*

FEMORAL EXPOSURE

After completion of the acetabular implantation, femoral exposure begins with removal of the #7 and #4 retractors from around the acetabulum and placement of the leg into a partially flexed and internally rotated position. The #8 retractor (jaws retractor) is placed under the anterior femoral neck just before removal of the #5 acetabular retractor (snake retractor) (Fig. 4–28). The leg is rotated fully into a flexed position with 90 degrees of internal rotation so that the tibia is in a vertical position. If a complete 90 degrees of internal rotation is difficult, the capsule attached to the anterior femoral neck should be incised and, if necessary, elevated off the neck, to release contracted capsule restraining the femur. An osteotome is the most effective tool to elevate this tissue (Fig. 4–29). The #8 retractor is positioned by maneuvering it under the anterior neck at an angle that also retracts the posterior flap of the incision to expose the cut neck of the femur (Fig. 4–30). The #4 retractor (which was used for exposure of the posterosuperior acetabulum) is placed between the medial femoral neck and the quadratus femoris to retract the quadratus femoris away from the medial femoral neck (see Fig. 4–30). The final retractor is used to retract the gluteus medius muscle and any overhanging gluteus maximus muscle, subcutaneous tissue, and skin (Fig. 4–31). If the patient has a thick layer of subcutaneous tissue and skin or a large gluteus maximus muscle, it may be necessary

to use the linked #9 and #10 retractors in order to retract both the gluteus medius muscle and the overhanging gluteus maximus, subcutaneous tissue, and skin (Fig. 4–32). Once these femoral retractors are in place, femoral preparation and implantation can proceed as described in Chapter 6.

Once the implantation of the acetabulum and femur are complete and the femoral head length has been determined, the hip is articulated and placed through a range of motion. The greater trochanter should clear the pelvis by 1 fingerbreadth throughout the range of motion (Fig. 4–33). The lesser trochanter should be aligned with the level of the ischium as determined from the preoperative x-ray (Fig. 4–34); it should not lie below the level of the tip of the ischium. The leg length can be determined by overlaying the legs as described in Chapter 6.

CLOSURE

The wound is closed in a similar fashion to the standard incision. The posterior flap of capsule/small external rotator muscles is repaired to the anterior edge of

Text continued on page 76

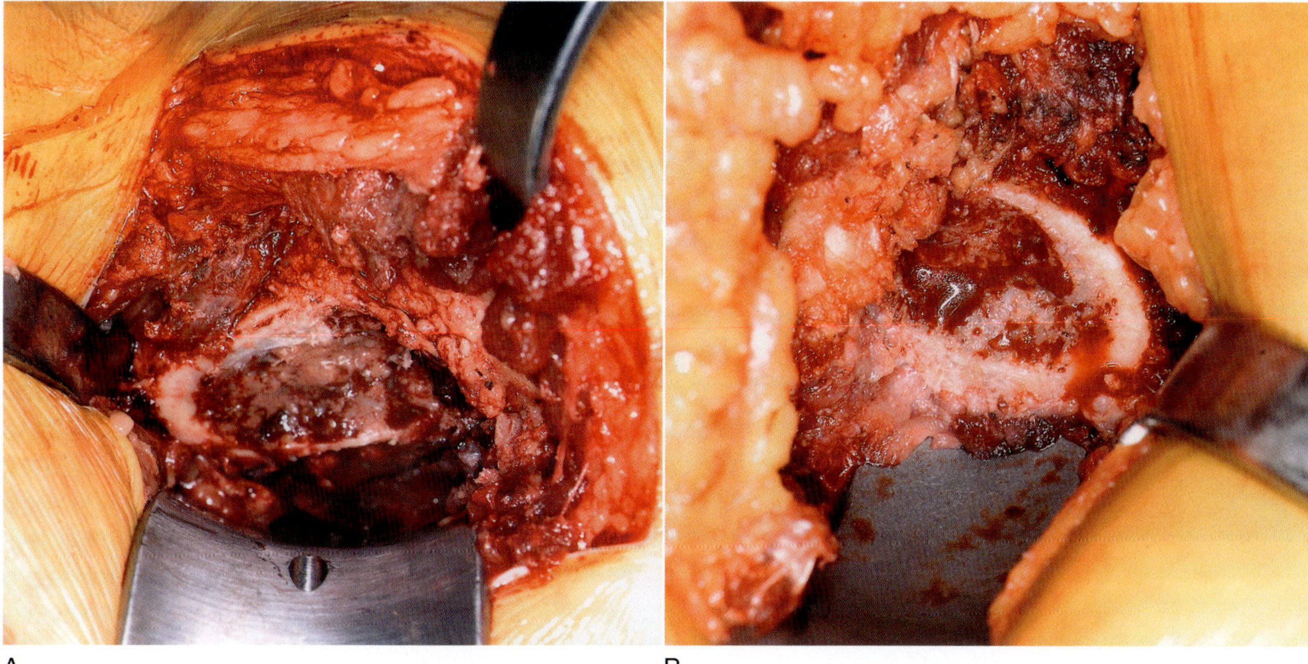

A   B

Figure 4–30 **A,** *The #8a retractor is placed under the anterior surface of the cut femoral neck, retracting the posterior skin and fat flap as well as the posterior gluteus maximus muscle. This retractor is designed to provide leverage to lift the femur into a position in which femoral preparation can easily be done. The #4 retractor is against the medial neck and retracts the quadratus femoris, which overlies the femoral neck. The #9 retractor on the right retracts the gluteus maximus muscle and anterior skin and fat from the top of the greater trochanter.* **B,** *The #8b retractor, which is thinner and has two prongs to lift the femoral neck, is also placed under the anterior femoral neck (see Fig. 4–6B and C). Designed for use in thinner patients, this narrow retractor can be easily moved from side to side to provide more clearance for tools and the femoral stem.*

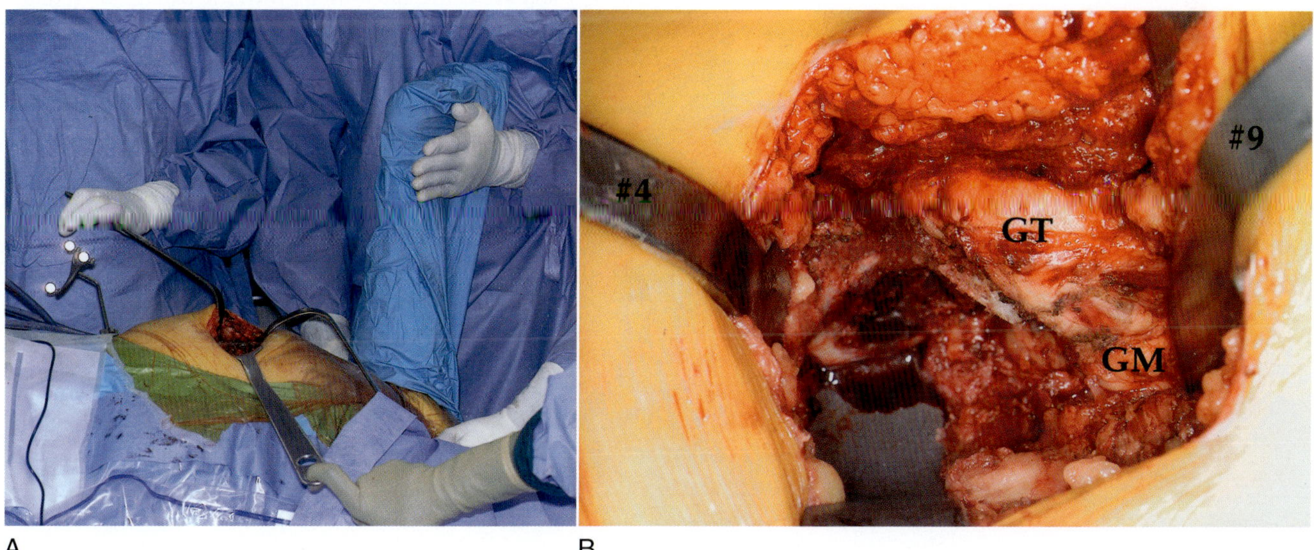

A   B

Figure 4–31 **A,** *The three retractors are in place to expose the femur for femoral preparation. The #8a retractor is seen at lower center. At right, the #4 retractor retracts the quadratus femoris from the medial femoral neck, and at left the #9 retractor retracts the gluteus medius muscle and anterior fat and skin.* **B,** *A close-up view of these retractors in the wound. The #9 and #4 retractors are labeled, and the thin posterior (#8b) retractor is under the anterior neck. GT, greater trochanter; GM, gluteus medius muscle.*

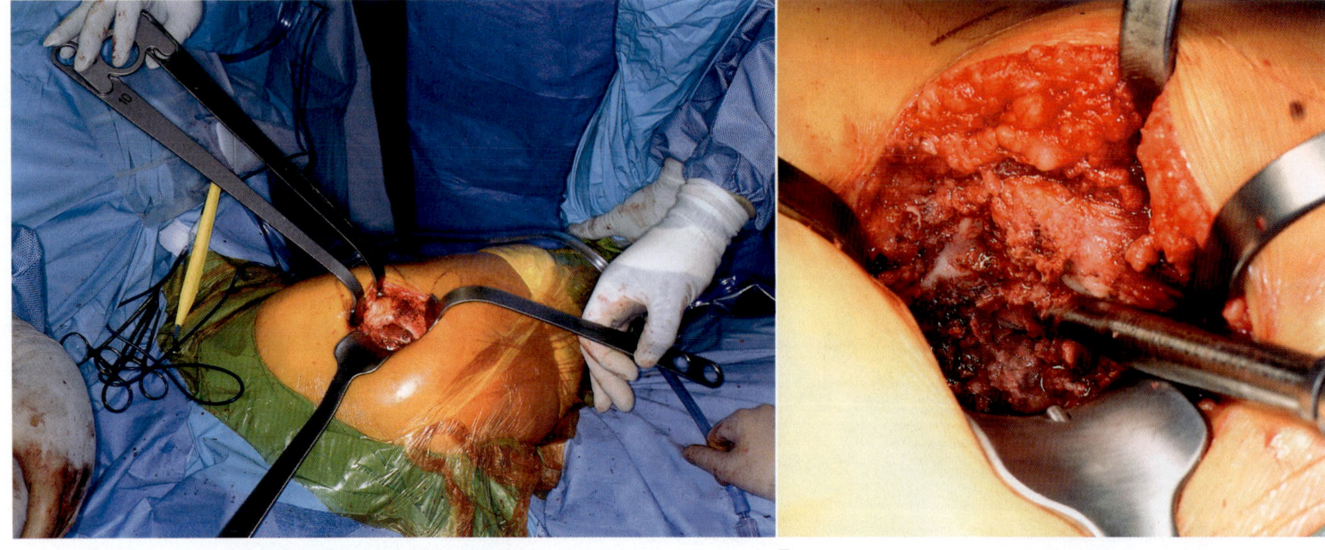

A

B

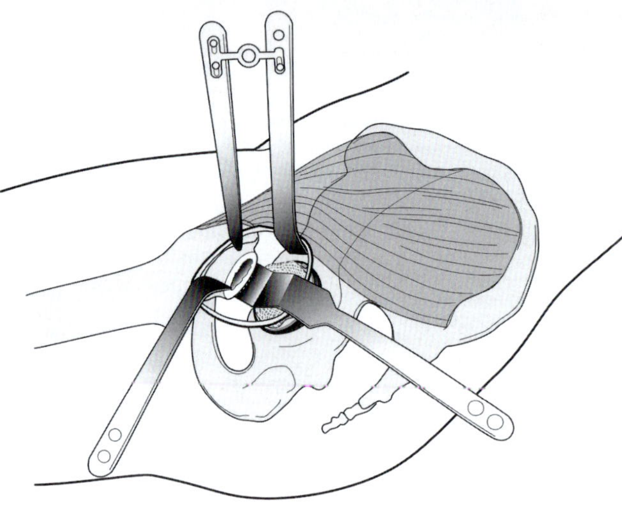

C

Figure 4–32 **A,** *The same retraction as in Figure 4–31, except that the #9 retractor is now on top of the greater trochanter, retracting the skin and fat, the #10 retractor retracts the gluteus medius muscle as well as the skin and fat, and these two retractors are linked at the top so that they can be held easily by the assistant with two fingers in the circular length.* **B,** *Close-up view showing the #9 retractor on the left over the top of the greater trochanter and retractor #10 above the tip of the greater trochanter, retracting the gluteus medius tendon. There is a burr in the femoral canal.* **C,** *Illustration of the #9 retractor over the greater trochanter and the #10 retractor holding the gluteus medius muscle, with the two linked together. The #8 retractor is under the anterior neck, and the #4 retractor retracts the quadratus muscle.*

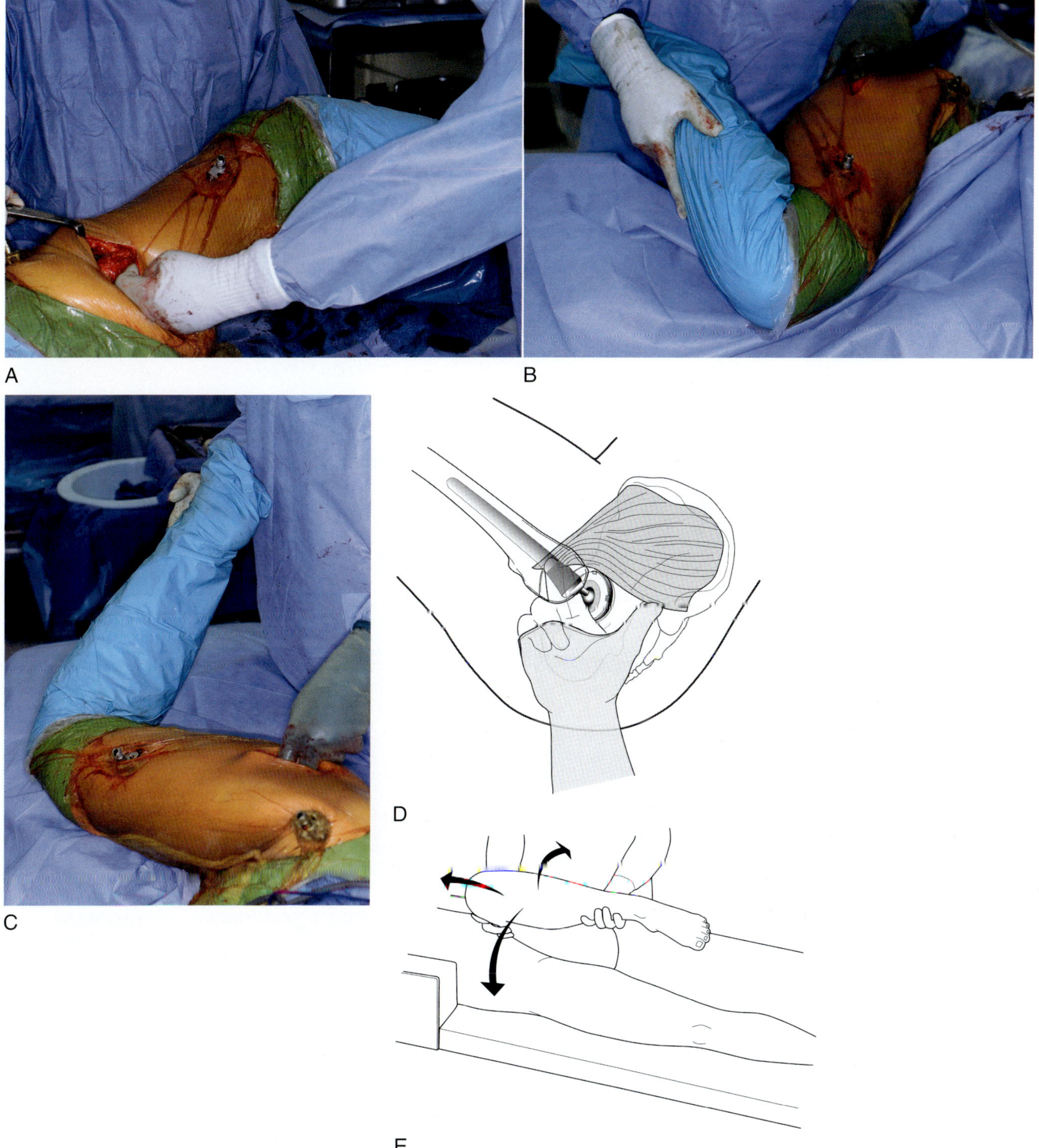

Figure 4–33 **A,** The surgeon's index finger palpates the interval between the greater trochanter and the pelvis as the leg is brought into external rotation and abduction. The femoral base plate for the computer guidance system is attached to the femur. **B,** The greater trochanter is palpated with the leg in adduction and internal rotation to ensure that it does not impinge on the pelvis. **C,** Ranawat's sign is elicited by internally rotating the leg until the femoral head fits symmetrically in the acetabular cup. The degree of internal rotation indicates the combined anteversion of the stem and cup. The pelvic and femoral base plates for the computer guidance system are visible. **D,** Illustration showing the index finger palpating the clearance of the trochanter from the pelvis and the metal neck from the acetabular cup during hip range of motion. **E,** The hip is taken through a complete range of motion, from full extension and external rotation to full flexion and internal rotation, to test stability and impingement.

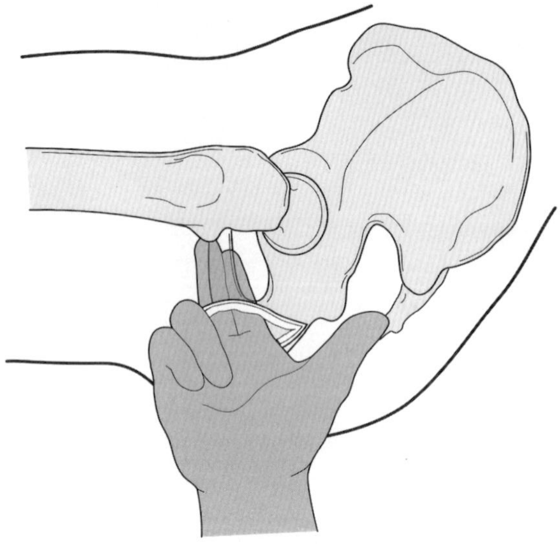

A

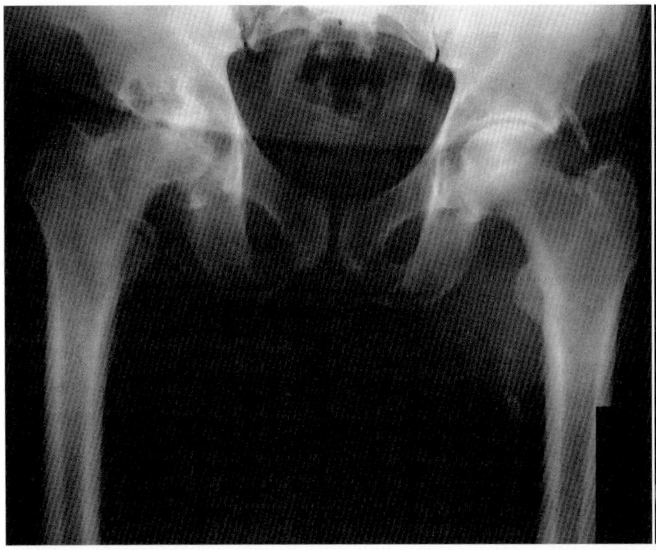

B

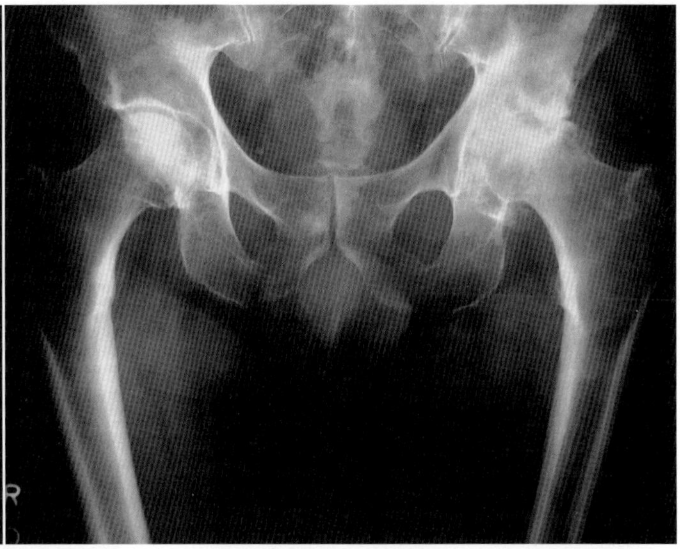

C

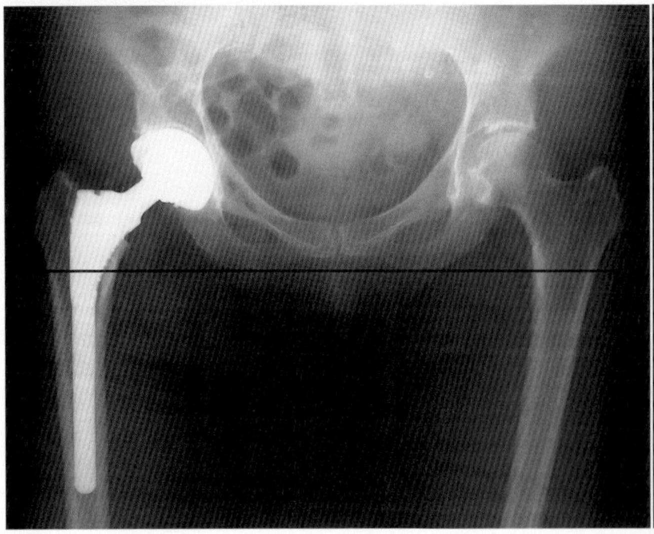

D

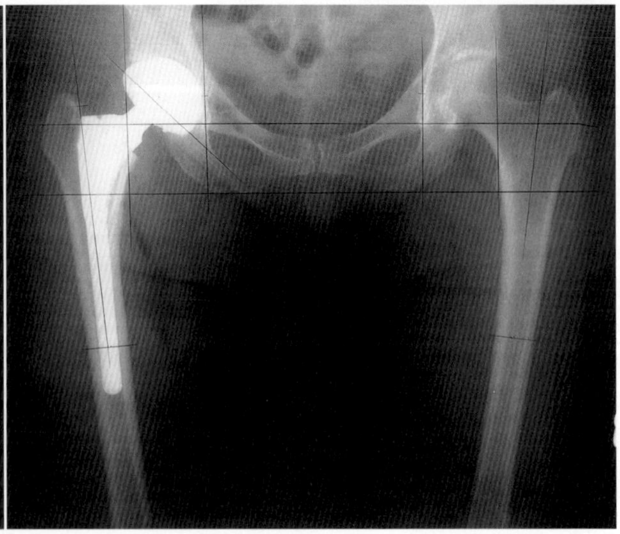

E

Legend on opposite page

Figure 4–34 **A,** *The surgeon's finger palpates the relationship of the lesser trochanter to the ischium; the correct relationship is known from the preoperative x-ray. When the hip is reconstructed, the lesser trochanter should be at the same position as on the opposite side, if that hip is normal. The tip of the lesser trochanter should never be entirely below the tip of the ischium because a long leg will result.* **B,** *A patient with a short femoral neck and the lesser trochanter superior to the tip of the ischium. When the hip replacement is done, the lesser trochanter of the reconstructed side should also be superior to the tip of the ischium by palpation.* **C,** *In a patient with a long femoral neck, the lesser trochanter is at the tip of the ischium and can be palpated in this position intraoperatively. In the reconstructed hip, the lesser trochanter should be at the tip of the ischium, but not below!* **D,** *Postoperative x-ray showing that the hip has been lengthened because the lesser trochanter is distal to that in the normal hip, as demonstrated by the transischial line. We obtain such x-rays in the operating room, and for any hip showing lengthening and unequal offset such as this, we immediately reopen the wound and equalize the leg lengths.* **E,** *The same patient as in* **D,** *after reoperation to place a shorter femoral head and equalize hip length and offset.*

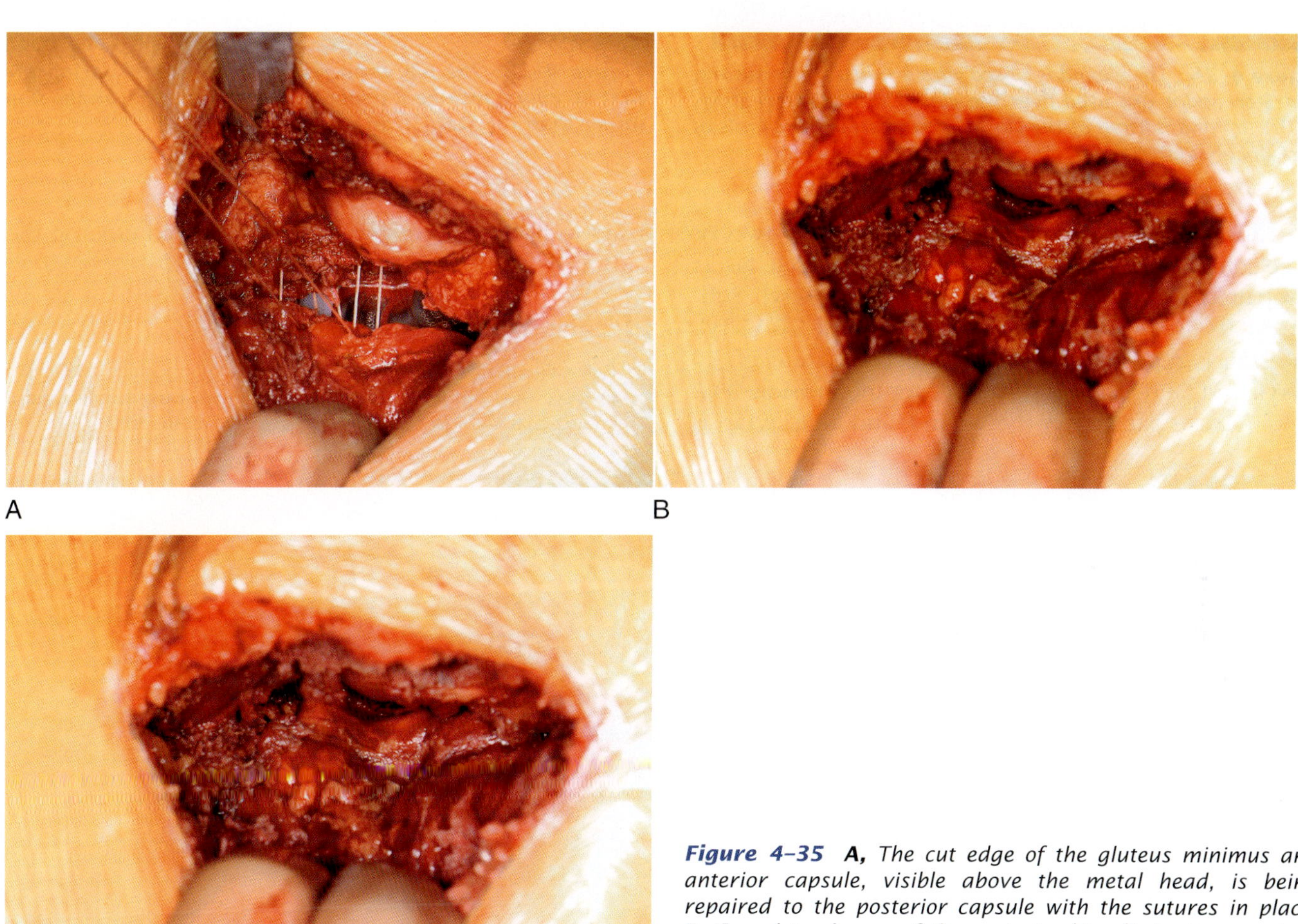

A

B

C

Figure 4–35 **A,** *The cut edge of the gluteus minimus and anterior capsule, visible above the metal head, is being repaired to the posterior capsule with the sutures in place.* **B,** *Complete closure of the posterior hip eliminates any dead space between the capsular repair and the metal femoral head and neck.* **C,** *The flaps are closed, which closes the hip.*

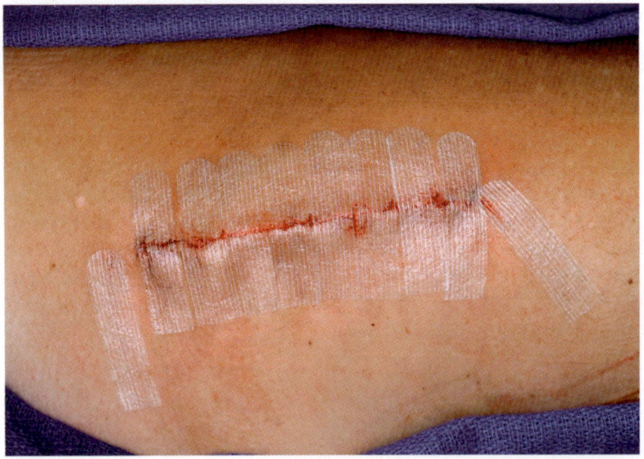

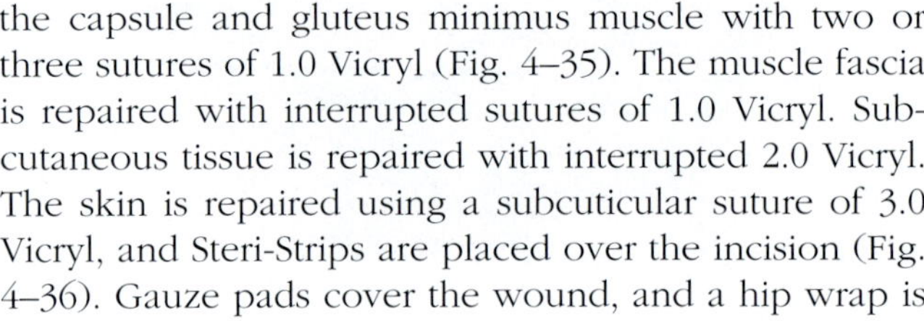

Figure 4–36   *The wound is closed with a subcuticular suture, and Steri-Strips are used over the closed wound. Steri-Strips at the top and bottom of the closed wound secure the ends of the subcuticular suture.*

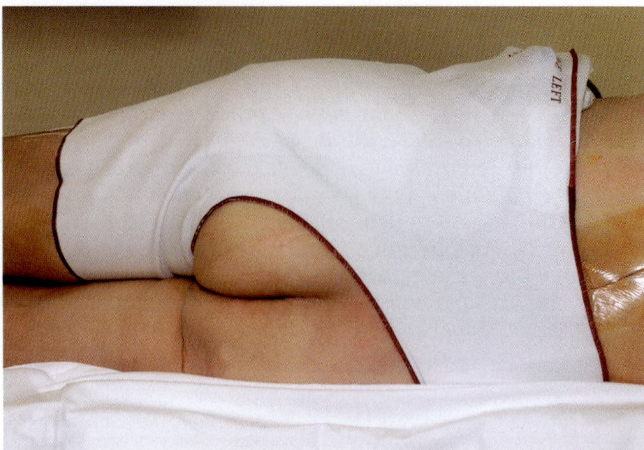

Figure 4–37   *The hip wrap protects the wound during the first 36 hours, making it unnecessary to place tape on the skin (other than the Steri-Strips).*

the capsule and gluteus minimus muscle with two or three sutures of 1.0 Vicryl (Fig. 4–35). The muscle fascia is repaired with interrupted sutures of 1.0 Vicryl. Subcutaneous tissue is repaired with interrupted 2.0 Vicryl. The skin is repaired using a subcuticular suture of 3.0 Vicryl, and Steri-Strips are placed over the incision (Fig. 4–36). Gauze pads cover the wound, and a hip wrap is used to hold the dressing in place to avoid tape on the skin (Fig. 4–37).

Reference

1. Berry DJ, Berger RA, Callaghan JJ, et al: Symposium: Minimally invasive total hip arthroplasty. Development, early results, and a critical analysis. J Bone Joint Surg 85A:2235-2246, 2003.

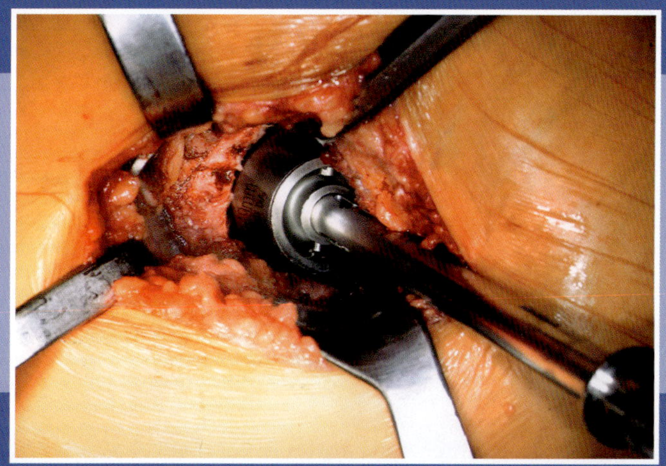

Chapter 5

Posterior Mini-incision: Acetabular Preparation and Implantation*

*In conjunction with this chapter on the DVD-ROM is the video "*Posterior Minimally Invasive Surgery (MIS) Total Hip Replacement.*"

This chapter discusses preparation of the acetabular bone for implantation of a hemispheric cup. It is difficult to use the existing acetabular anatomy for implantation of the acetabular component. First, the osteoarthritic acetabulum has a wide range of geometries. Our data show that the inclination of the native acetabulum can range from 30 to 70 degrees (average, 55 degrees), and the anteversion can range from 15 degrees of retroversion (average, 10 degrees) to 30 degrees of anteversion (average, 12 degrees). Second, the anterior acetabular wall has four different anatomic configurations.[1] Computer-assisted guidance renders most of these difficulties moot (see Chapter 7), but when the acetabulum is being prepared and implanted manually, the technique described in this chapter should be used.

EXPOSURE

With the posterior mini-incision, exposure of the acetabulum is accomplished by three incisions of hip tissue.

First Incision

The first incision is an approximately 6-cm division of the gluteus maximus fibers along the posterior border of the greater trochanter (Fig. 5–1). A small, bent Homans retractor is placed on the greater trochanter to retract the anterior fibers of the gluteus maximus. The surgeon's finger is used to retract the posterior fibers and reveal the posterior structures of the hip (Fig. 5–2).

The external rotators of the hip are exposed by dividing the thin fascial membrane between the gluteus medius and gluteus minimus muscles and placing a long-handled #2 retractor over the piriformis tendon and under the gluteus medius muscle to retract the gluteus medius tendon anteriorly. This exposes the insertion of the gluteus minimus muscle into the trochanter, with the piriformis tendon on top (Fig. 5–3). The surgeon can visualize the posterior hip structures from the gluteus minimus and piriformis cranially to the quadratus femoris muscle caudally (Fig. 5–4).

Second Incision

Before the second incision is made, the tissues are injected with the drug cocktail described in Chapter 1 to avoid injection into the sciatic nerve. This incision is made from the superior border of the quadratus femoris muscle through the piriformis tendon proximally. The incision produces a single flap of tissue that includes the capsule with the small external rotator muscles, including the piriformis (Fig. 5–5). The incision should be made so that the flap is incised from its attachment on the greater trochanter. This maximizes the size of

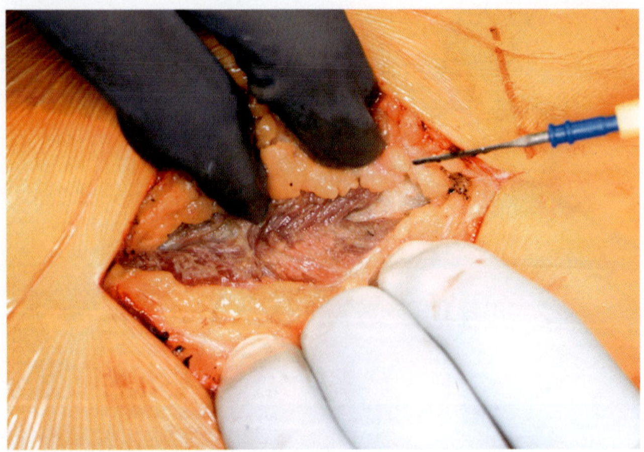

Figure 5–1 *Division of the gluteus maximus fibers along the posterior border of the greater trochanter is the first of three hip tissue cuts with the posterior mini-incision.*

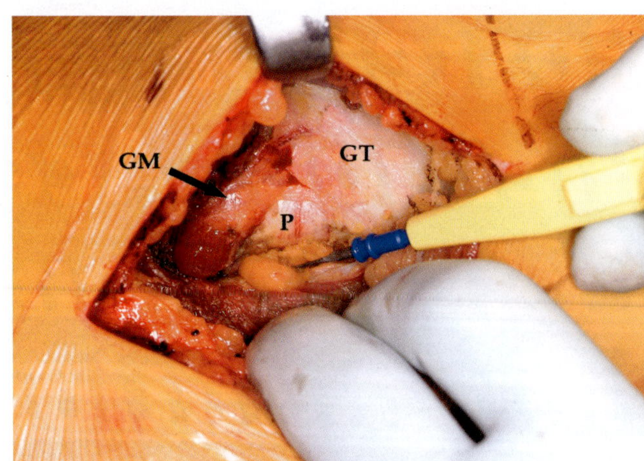

Figure 5–2 *The surgeon's fingers retract the posterior cut edge of the gluteus maximus and the #1 retractor at the top of the finger retracts the anterior cut edge. This retractor is placed over the top of the greater trochanter (GT). The gluteus medius (GM) muscle is attached to the GT, and the piriformis (P) tendon lies under the GM.*

the posterior flap and allows posterior closure of the flap after reconstruction of the hip. Creation of this flap should also include incision of the orbicular ligament, which lies across the femoral neck just distal to the inferior border of the femoral head. This can be done by pushing the Bovie electrocautery tip beneath the quadratus femoris muscle and running it along the bony surface of the femoral neck. Often, the orbicular ligament divides with an audible "snap." Once these tissue structures have been divided, the hip can be easily dislocated.

With the hip dislocated, the #2 retractor remains superior to and provides partial exposure of the femoral head. The #4 retractor is placed around the femoral neck with its distal portion retracting the quadratus femoris muscle to protect it from damage by the saw.

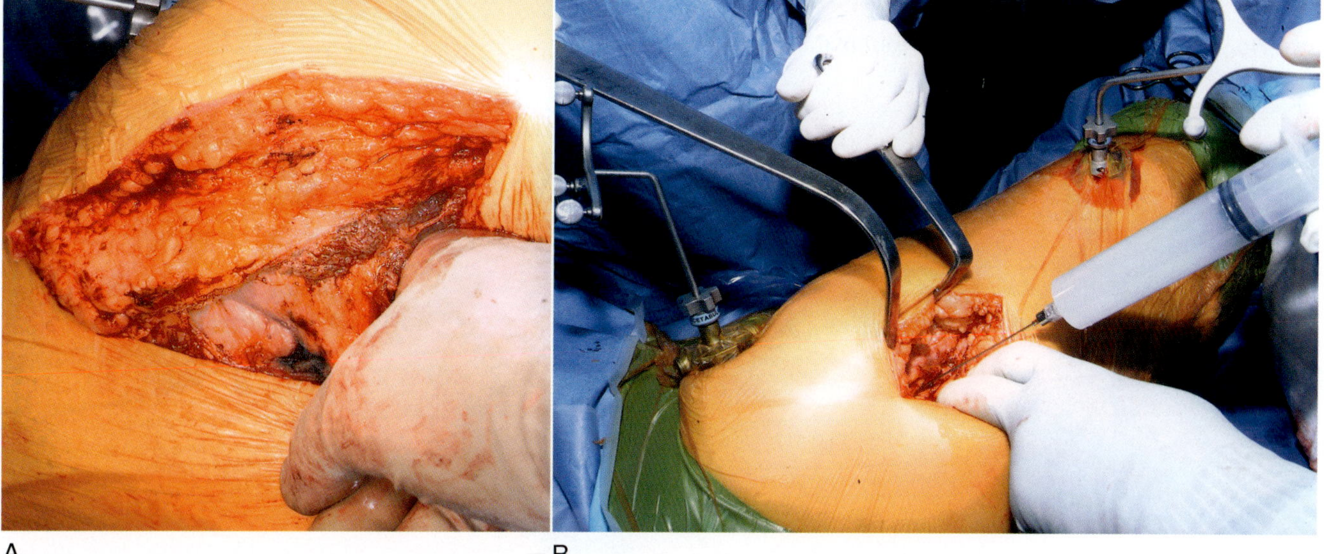

Figure 5–3 **A,** *The surgeon's finger separates the interval between the gluteus medius muscle and the piriformis for placement of the #2 retractor, which will retract the gluteus medius tendon and expose the gluteus minimus and piriformis. The small external rotator muscles are adjacent to the bottom of the surgeon's finger. The cut edge of the gluteus maximus is above the surgeon's finger. This photograph is taken from a long incision so that the maneuver is clearly visible.* **B,** *The #2 retractor is the long-handled retractor on the left edge of the wound adjacent to the computer antenna. The #1 retractor lies over the top of the greater trochanter. The anesthetic cocktail is being injected into the posterior tissues. Even with a small incision, there is excellent visibility of the posterior hip with these two retractors.*

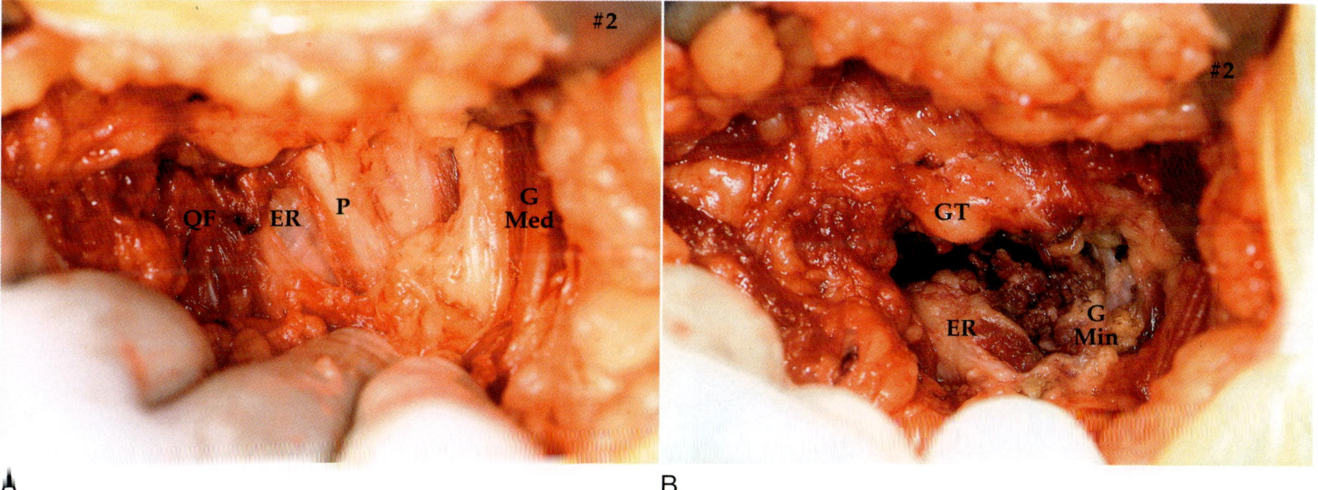

Figure 5–4 **A,** *Close-up view of the posterior hip structures visible with the mini-incision. In the upper right, the #2 retractor retracts the gluteus medius (G Med). The muscle between the piriformis (P) and the gluteus medius is the gluteus minimus. ER, external rotators; QF, quadratus femoris.* **B,** *Same view as in* **A.** *The gluteus minimus (G Min) and external rotators (ER) have been incised. The capsule is not visible under the cut muscles. In the right corner, the #2 retractor retracts the gluteus medius muscle. GT, greater trochanter.*

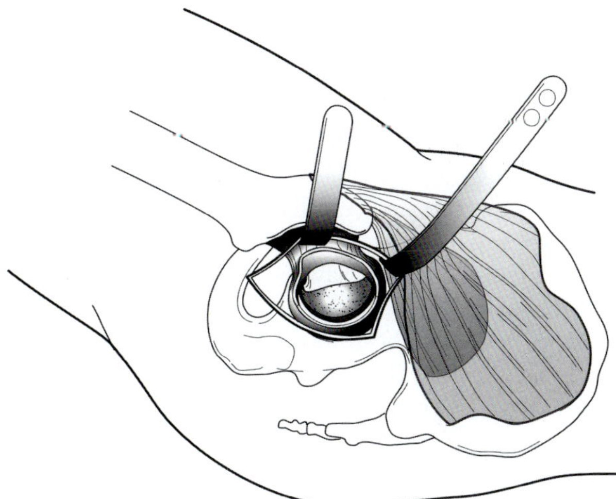

Figure 5–5 *Incision of the capsule is demonstrated; there is no capsular excision. Anterior and posterior flaps are created. The #1 and #2 retractors are in place to allow visualization of the capsule for its incision.*

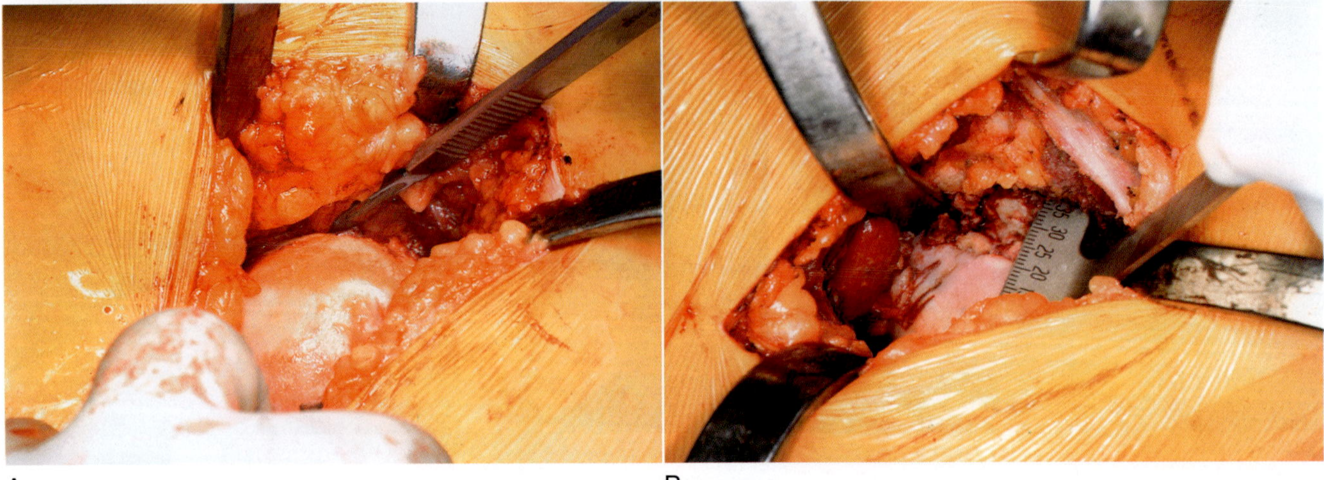

A   B

Figure 5–6 **A,** *The femoral neck is exposed by incising capsular fibers over the neck. The quadratus femoris is visible distal to the scalpel. The #4 retractor is around the medial neck; the #1 retractor, above the scalpel, is on the greater trochanter; and the #2 retractor in the left corner of the wound retracts the tendon of the gluteus medius.* **B,** *The level of the neck cut from the distal end of the femoral head is measured with a ruler. The distal end of the ruler is against the quadratus femoris muscle. The #4 retractor is medial to the femoral neck and the #2 retractor is superior to the femoral neck; the retractor at lower left was used only to improve the exposure for this view.*

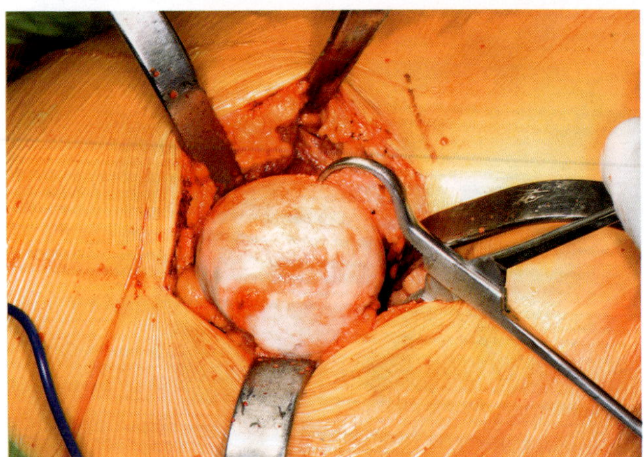

Figure 5–7 *The femoral head is grasped with a Lewin clamp and rotated out of the wound.*

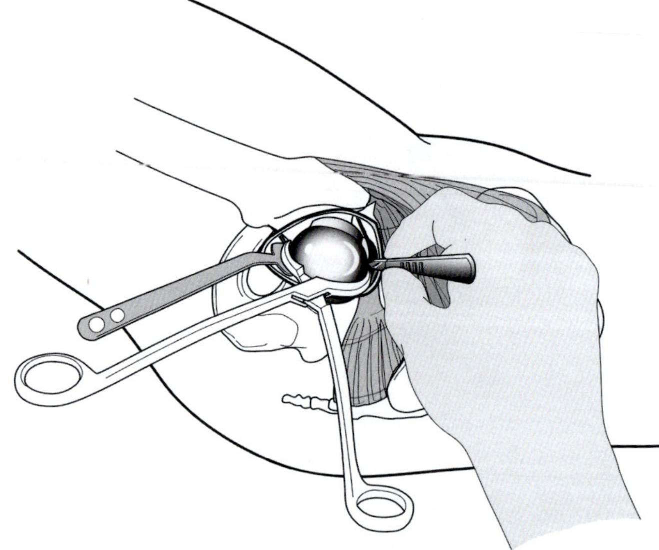

Figure 5–8 *While the femoral head is grasped by the Lewin clamp, a scalpel is used to incise the lateral capsule from the femoral neck to allow removal of the head.*

The femoral neck is exposed distal to the inferior border of the femoral head for the distance necessary to allow it to be cut at the level that will reproduce correct leg length and offset for the patient (Fig. 5–6). This level was determined during preoperative planning (see Chapter 2). The #3 retractor is shifted as needed during cutting of the femoral neck to protect the skin edge from damage by the saw. The saw cut should be angled cranially from posterior to anterior. Making the cut at this oblique angle leaves sufficient length of the anterior neck to allow the #8 ("jaws") retractor to be placed under the neck during apreparation of the femur. The cut femoral head can be removed either by gripping it with a Lewin clamp (Fig. 5–7) or by fixing it with a corkscrew tool and rotating it out of the wound. Often,

some lateral capsule attached to the cut neck must be excised before the head can be removed from the wound (Fig. 5–8). After removal of the femoral head, the #4 retractor is placed between the labrum and capsule at the posterosuperior border of the acetabulum. This instrument retracts the posterior capsule from the posterior bony wall of the acetabulum, exposing it for removal of the labrum.

The #5 ("snake") retractor is placed on the anterior proximal ilium to retract the femur anterior to the acetabulum (retractor #5a, Fig. 5–9). This retractor is inserted through the anterior capsule just lateral to (in front of) the anterior inferior iliac spine. The anterior capsule may be thickened by the arthritic changes, and sometimes there is a fold of capsule between the #5 retractor and the wall of the acetabulum when this retractor is placed (Fig. 5–10). Because this tissue can interfere with reaming, an incision is made in the anterior capsule at its bony junction and the retractor re-placed through the cut to permit the entire anterosuperior capsule to be retracted with the femoral bone, exposing the antero-superior bony wall of the acetabulum (Fig. 5–11). The acetabulum is easily visualized with the #4 retractor placed posteriorly and the #5 retractor anteriorly, and the femur is retracted anterior to the acetabulum. The femur can also be retracted using the #5b retractor (Fig. 5–12). This retractor should be placed against the ante-

rior wall (as opposed to the #5a retractor, which is placed on the ilium); it has a radius of curvature that provides effective retraction of the femur anterior to the acetabulum. The surgeon's preference dictates whether the #5a or #5b retractor is used.

Third Incision

The third incision of hip tissue is through the medial capsule (which appears to be the inferior capsule with the patient in the lateral position). This capsule is exposed by placing the #6 retractor between the capsule and the external oblique muscle to protect against cutting the medial circumflex artery and vein (Fig. 5–13). The incision in the capsule is made through the transverse acetabular ligament to the cortical bone at the edge of the cotyloid notch (the tear drop on an anteroposterior x-ray). Once the incision is complete, the anesthetic cocktail described in Chapter 1 is injected into the cut edges of the medial capsule, into the anterior capsule, and into the gluteus minimus muscle superiorly; the posterior capsule was injected before its incision to prevent injection into or near the sciatic nerve. The cut edges of the gluteus maximus muscle and the subcutaneous tissue are also injected.

The #6 retractor is removed and the leg is changed from the internally rotated and flexed position to either lying flat on the operating table or in slight internal rotation with the foot supported on a Mayo stand (Fig. 5–14). The #6 retractor is removed before the leg position is changed to protect against impingement on the sciatic nerve as the leg is moved. The #7 retractor

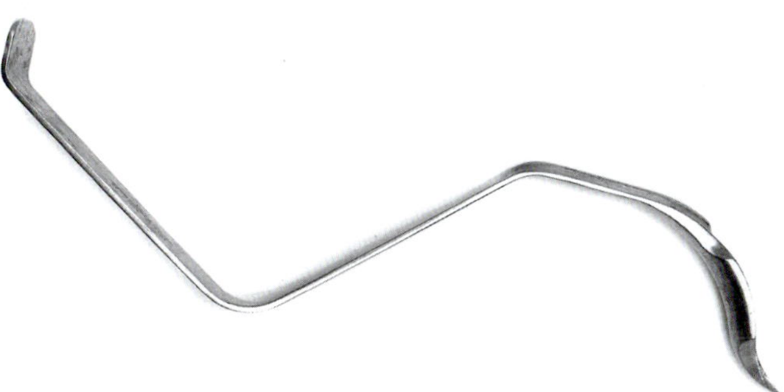

Figure 5–9 *The #5 ("snake") retractor is shaped to retract the greater trochanter anterior to the acetabulum. The point of the retractor is malleted into the ilium.*

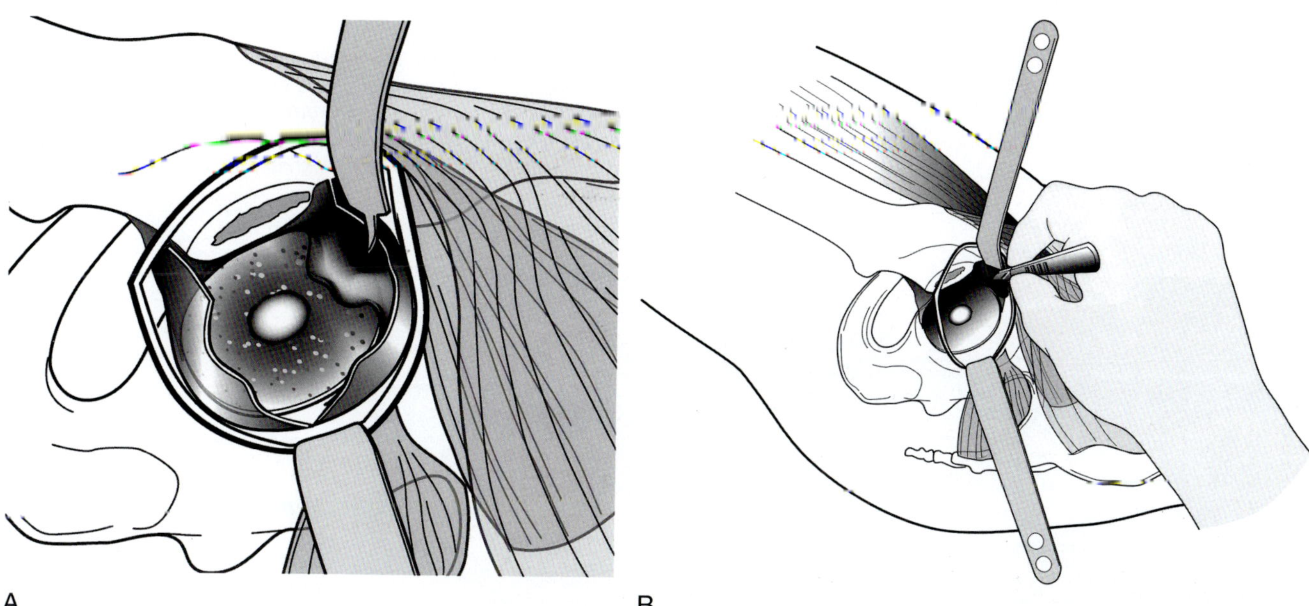

A   B

Figure 5–10 **A,** *With the snake retractor (top) placed into the ilium, a fold of capsule is extruded over the anterosuperior acetabulum and occludes exposure of the entire acetabulum.* **B,** *An incision is made into the overhanging capsule so that the snake retractor can be replaced to retract this capsule out of the acetabulum.*

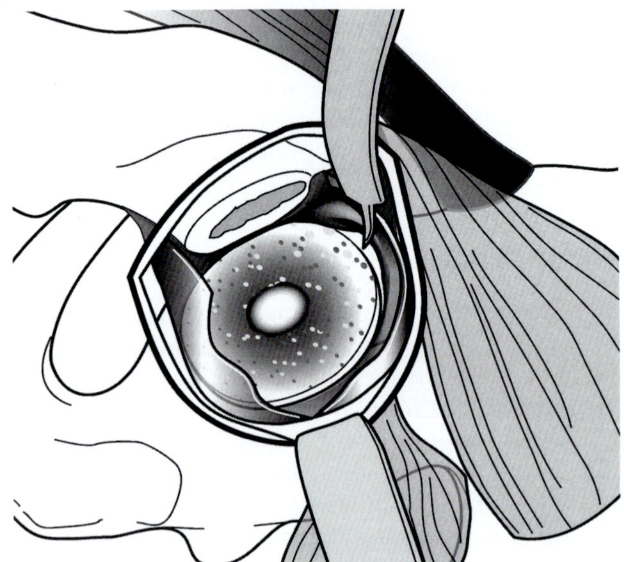

Figure 5–11 The #4 retractor retracts the posterosuperior capsule and the #5 retractor retracts the anterosuperior capsule to expose the superior acetabulum. The #5 retractor is set against the greater trochanter and pulls the femur anterior to the acetabulum.

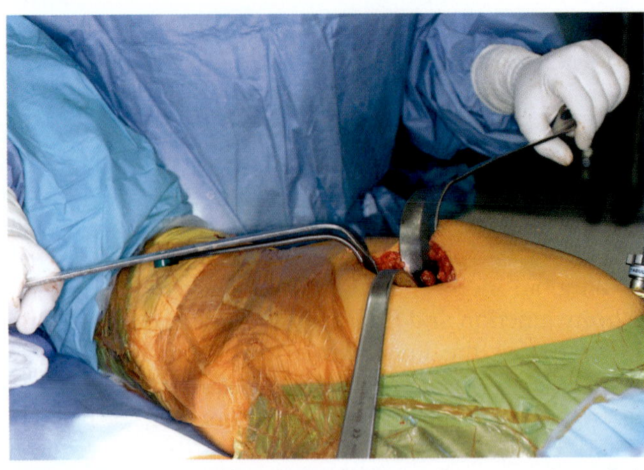

Figure 5–12 Another choice for anterior retraction of the femur and the anterior capsule is the curved #5b retractor. The #5b retractor is on the anterior wound, the #4 retractor is on the posterior (bottom) wound, and the #7 retractor is in the distal wound. The #5b retractor can be placed either on the ilium or against the anterior wall of the acetabulum to retract the femur and the capsule anteriorly. Placing the retractor against the anterior wall of the acetabulum risks fracture of the anterior wall; the tip can perforate the anterior wall and interfere with reaming; and there is an increased risk of femoral nerve irritation.

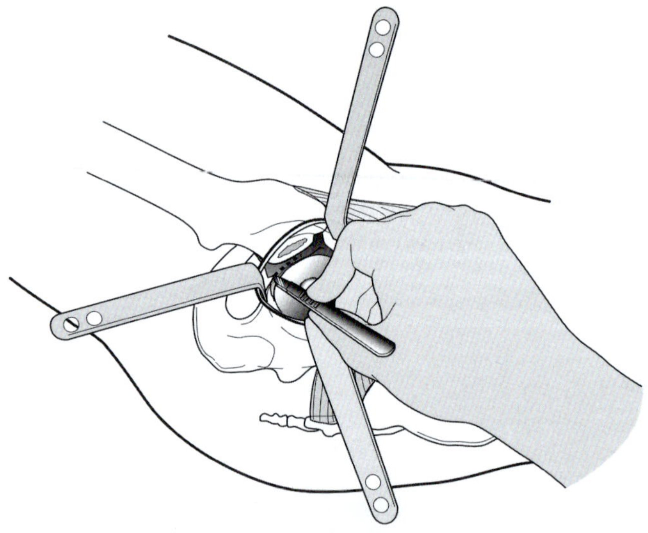

Figure 5–13 The medial capsule is incised. The #6 retractor is behind the medial capsule and retracts the external oblique muscle, through which the medial circumflex artery and vein run. Incision of this capsule allows easy retraction of the femur anterior to the acetabulum without placing tension on the posterior structures, including the sciatic nerve. The #5 retractor is visible superiorly, and the #4 retractor is under the surgeon's thumb.

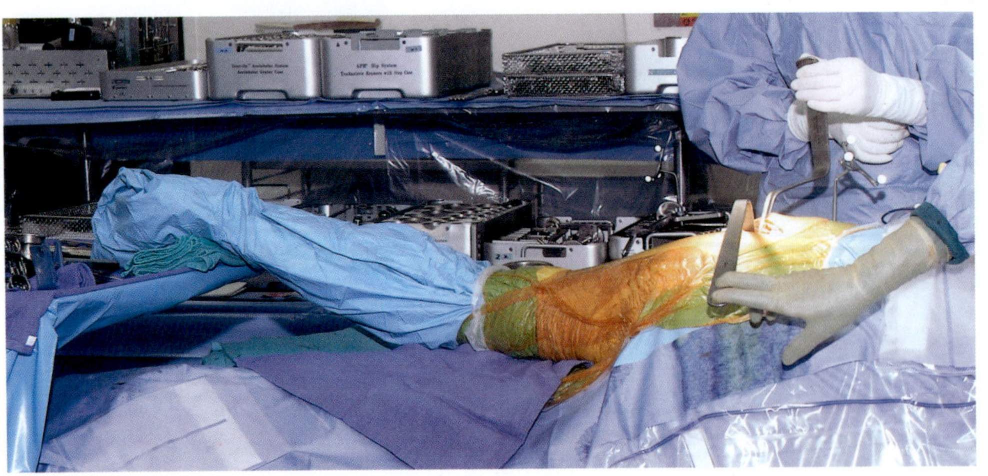

Figure 5–14 The leg is in extension, lying on top of the lower leg with the foot supported on a Mayo stand. This position facilitates retraction of the femur anterior to the acetabulum. The #4 and #5 retractors can be seen exposing the acetabulum.

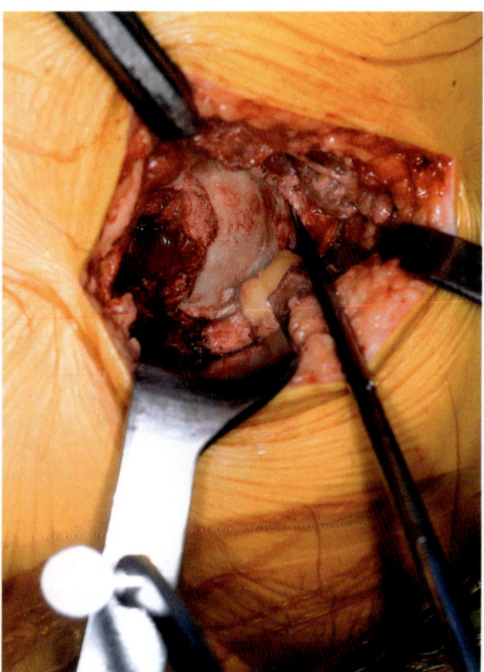

Figure 5–15 *The #7 retractor (bottom of wound) provides excellent exposure of the acetabulum. The tip of the retractor is against the cortical bone of the cotyloid notch and its paddle sits on the ischium, with the capsule and the sciatic nerve behind the paddle. The #4 retractor is in the upper right of the wound, and the #5 retractor is in the upper left. A metal pointer for the computer guidance system touches the acetabulum.*

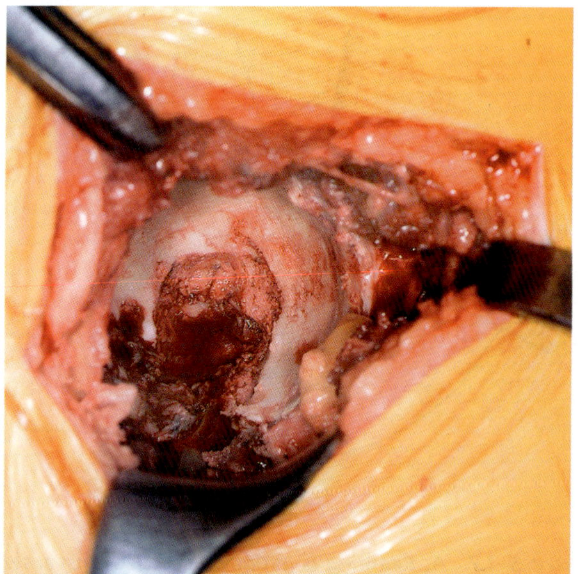

Figure 5–16 *The pulvinar is removed along with an osteophyte over the cortical bone of the cotyloid notch. The #4, #5, and #7 retractors are in position, exposing the entire acetabulum.*

is placed with its tip against the cortical bone of the cotyloid notch and its paddle on the ischium to retract the posterior capsule and protect the sciatic nerve (Fig. 5–15). This retractor is attached to a fiberoptic light source for improved visualization of the acetabulum, and when it is in place the retraction is complete (the #4 retractor is posterosuperior; the #5 retractor is anterosuperior; and the #7 retractor is medial and posterior). The pulvinar is excised from the cotyloid notch to expose the cortical bone of the cotyloid, which will be the limit of reaming for all acetabula except those with congenital dysplasia (Fig. 5–16). Exposure of the cortical bone of the medial wall also allows this bony wall to be registered on the computer, and the surgeon can use this information during reaming to assess when the medial wall has been reached (see Chapter 7).

ACETABULAR PREPARATION AND IMPLANTATION OF THE OSTEOARTHRITIC HIP

Reaming

The acetabulum was sized before surgery by the templating method (see Chapter 2) so that reaming can

proceed more efficiently. Although the size is only an estimate because the measurements on the x-ray can vary somewhat from the actual size, usually it is correct within 2 mm. The scrub technicians prepare the reamers based on the estimated size. Three reamers should be used: the first is 3 mm smaller than the acetabular cup size, the second is 2 mm smaller than the cup size, and the third is 1 mm smaller than the cup size. Use of three successive reamers helps ensure that the acetabulum will be prepared into a hemisphere and not reamed eccentrically.

The first reamer is directed transversely and removes the acetabular ridge. This reamer should be of a size that barely touches the anterior and posterior walls so that it can be directed centrally between those walls without reaming them away (Fig. 5–17).

The second reamer completes the reaming of the medial wall and reams the anteroposterior wall, and it also begins to shape the superior slope of the acetabulum into a hemisphere (Fig. 5–18). If computer guidance is being used, the tracking guide should be attached to this reamer so that the surgeon knows that the reamer has reached the medial wall and is within the peripheral boundaries of the acetabulum to prevent eccentric reaming. If reaming is performed manually, without computer assistance, the use of "half-reamers" allows better visualization of the reamer and acetabulum in the wound (Fig. 5–19). With the mini-incision technique, use of a full reamer limits visibility of the reamer within the bony acetabulum, making it easier to ream eccentrically into either the anterior or posterior

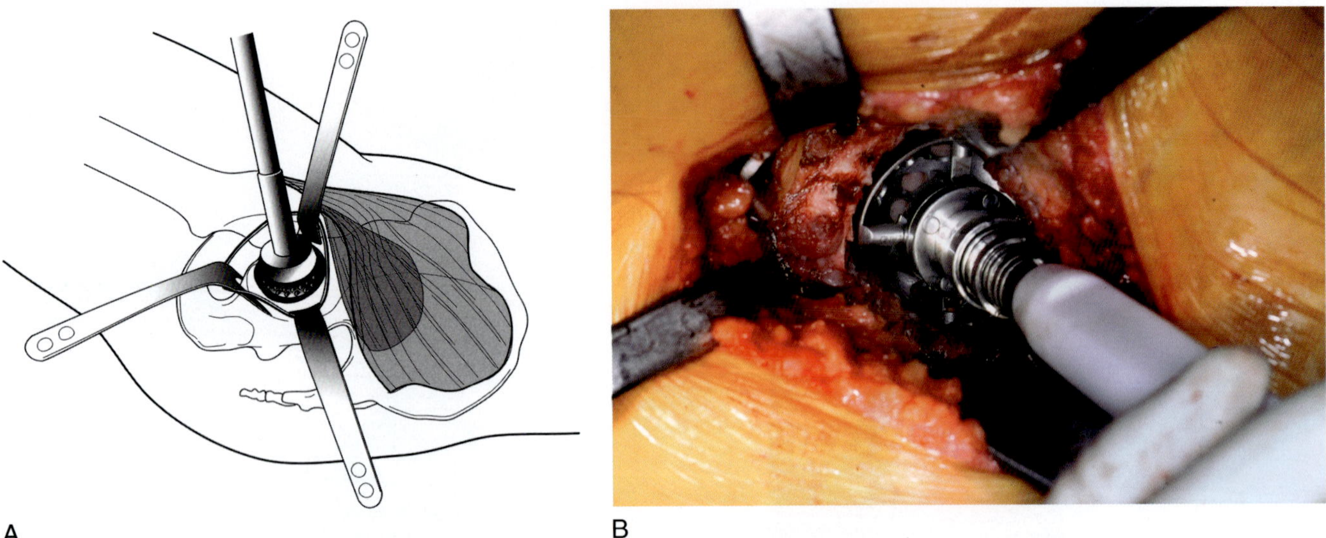

A   B

Figure 5–17 **A,** *Reaming is initially directed transversely into the acetabulum.* **B,** *The reamer is directed transversely into the acetabulum to remove the acetabular ridge and ream to the level of the cortical bone of the cotyloid notch. This reamer is two sizes smaller than the expected size of the acetabular trial.*

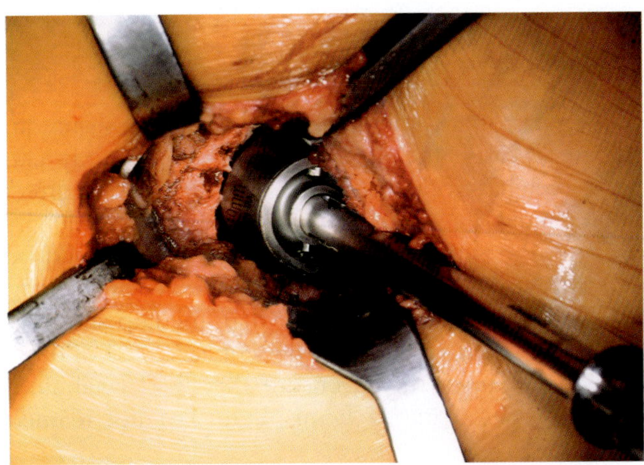

Figure 5–18 *The second reamer is directed obliquely into the acetabulum to avoid exerting excessive pressure against the distal end of the wound with the handle of the reamer. If the reamer were placed directly in line with the acetabulum, additional pressure against the distal end of the wound could cause the superior edge of the reamer to translate superiorly and ream away the superior wall. This reamer contacts the circumferential peripheral wall of the acetabulum and begins to form a hemisphere for the cup.*

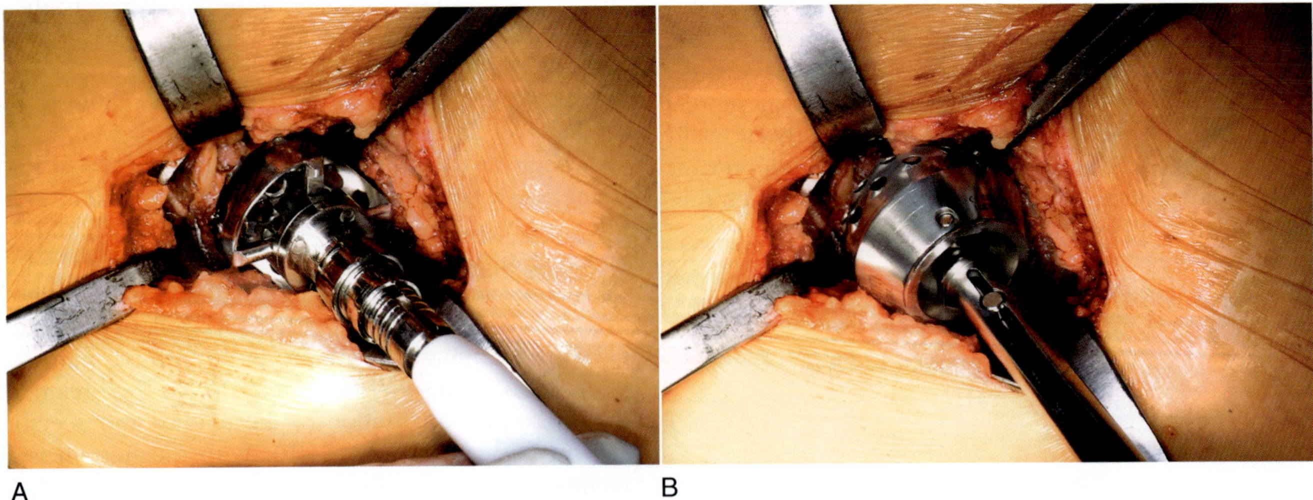

A   B

Figure 5–19 **A,** *The smaller half-reamer is advantageous because of ease of insertion into the wound and the additional visibility it provides.* **B,** *It is more difficult to insert a full reamer into the wound.*

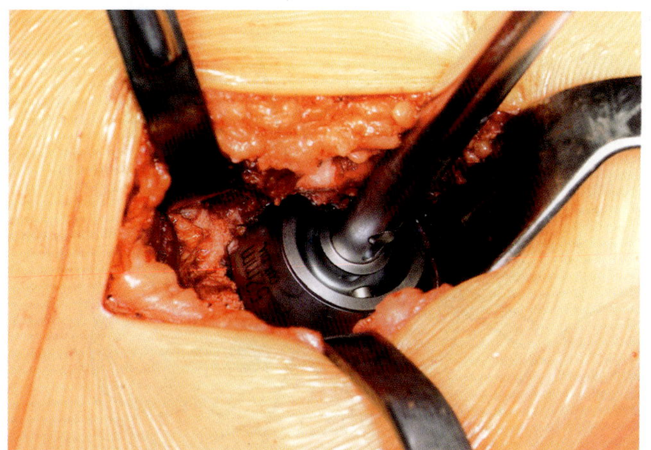

Figure 5–20 *A full reamer blocks part of the view of the acetabular wall anteriorly and inferiorly, so the direction of reaming is not as controlled as with the half-reamer.*

wall (Fig. 5–20). With a standard incision, the full reamer does not obstruct this view.

The third reamer completes the creation of a hemisphere in the bony acetabulum. With a mini-incision this reamer must be angulated, whereas with the traditional incision a straight reamer can be used (Fig. 5–21). A straight reamer abuts against the distal edge of the mini-incision wound, and because it often is levered against the superior wall of the acetabulum, it could actually ream away the superior rim of bone (Fig. 5–22). Furthermore, because of tissue pressures on the handle, it is not possible to keep a straight reamer directed centrally and in correct anteversion.

Insertion of the Trial Cup

I recommend the use of trial cups. Some surgeons prefer to go directly to implantation of the noncemented

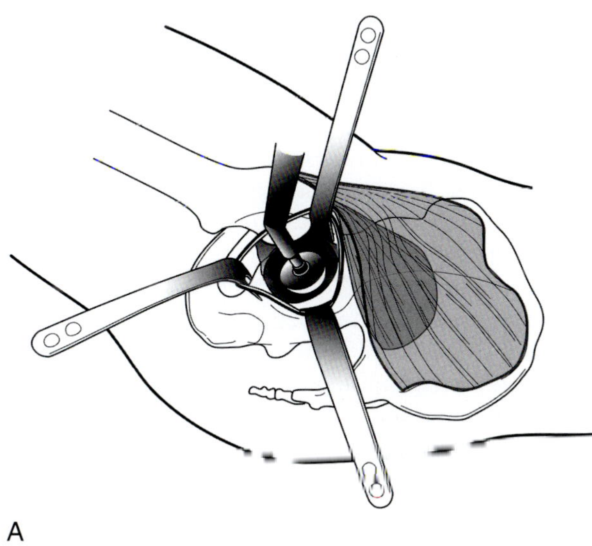

A

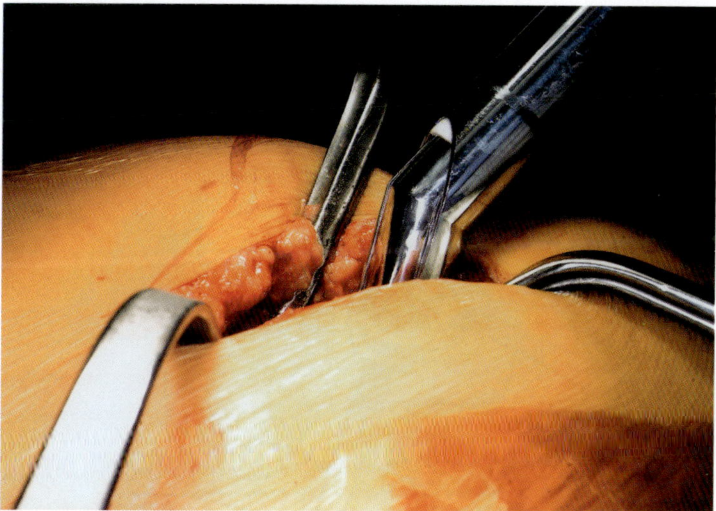

B

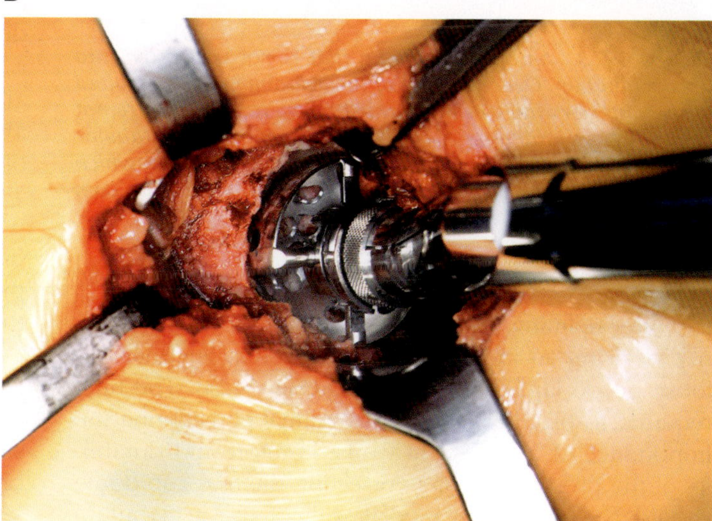

C

Figure 5–21 **A,** *The curved acetabular reamer has the advantage of not impinging against the edges of the small wound.* **B,** *The angle of the reamer into the acetabulum allows the reamer to clear the skin and reaming to be accomplished without impingement on the skin.* **C,** *The angled reamer can be inserted directly into the acetabulum while preserving visibility of the entire acetabular wall, improving the precision of the reaming and creation of a hemisphere.*

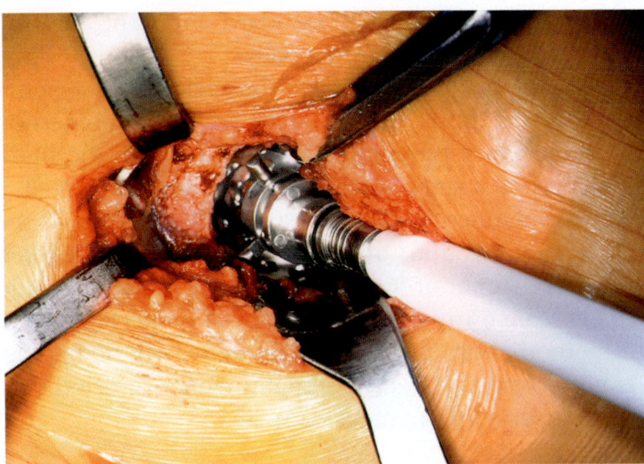

Figure 5–22 *When the straight reamer is used to complete formation of the acetabular hemisphere, its handle must impinge against the distal end of the wound. If the handle is pushed down hard against this skin, as shown, the superior wall of the acetabulum is in jeopardy of being reamed away. The superior edge of the reamer is visible where it has reamed a portion of the superior wall. This technique should not be used.*

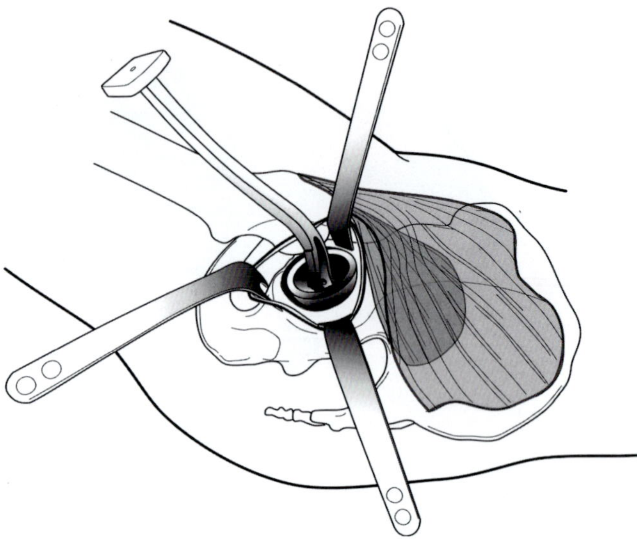

Figure 5–24 *A trial cup is used to determine the stability of the fit for the acetabular component. A curved handle is used for insertion so that the distal edge of the wound does not force the cup into a vertical position. If the trial does not fit snugly into the acetabulum, shows gaps around its periphery, or can be easily pulled out of the bone, the sizing is not correct.*

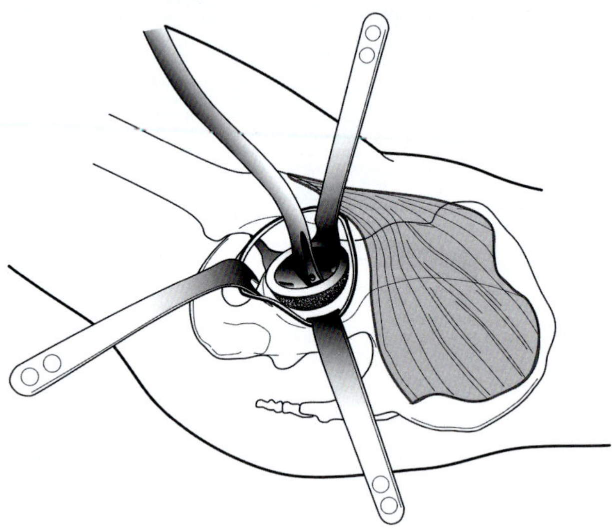

Figure 5–23 *An acetabular cup that is not well fitted into the acetabulum. Over-reaming of the acetabulum has resulted in the anterior wall's being reamed away, and in an attempt to obtain cup stability, a cup too large for the acetabular cavity could be chosen. An oversized cup is lateralized, which can result in increased leg length, increased offset, and pain from impingement.*

cup after reaming, but in my experience this carries the risk of using an incorrectly sized cup that is either too loose or too large and lateralized (Fig. 5–23). The time required to place a trial cup is minimal considering the importance of a correct fit to the comfort and durability of the prosthesis. For a correct fit, the trial cup dome should be against the medial wall of the acetabulum and the anterior peripheral edge, preferably below

bone. The holes in the trial cup can be used to visualize that the cup lies against bone medially and peripherally. If possible, the anterior edge of the cup should lie below anterior bone to prevent postoperative groin pain from irritation of the iliopsoas tendon.

The use of computer guidance allows the size of the acetabulum to be confirmed before reaming so that the correct reamer sizes are selected. If the computer is not used, the size can be judged by the amount of bone cut with the reamer and by insertion of the trial cup. If the trial is loose and easily movable when inserted, the next-size trial is tested; if that fit is too tight, reaming should proceed to the next size so that the correct fit is obtained (Fig. 5–24). If reaming to the next size is done, the surgeon must take extra care to ensure that a hemisphere is created, the reaming is central, and the anteroposterior wall has not been partially reamed away. The most common mistake is to ream too much of the anterior wall, in which case the trial cup will not achieve a tight press-fit. The surgeon then must decide whether to use that size cup and secure it with screws, or to ream to the next size in the hope of obtaining a press-fit. If the anterior wall is reamed away, it is best to use that size cup and secure it with screws.

The posterosuperior edge of the cup may stand proud to the bone by 2 to 4 mm, which ensures that the cup is not too vertical (Figs. 5–25 and 5–26). In our study, the bony acetabulum has an average inclination of 55 degrees, and in the study of D'Antonio and colleagues,[1] the average inclination is 60 degrees. Therefore, a cup buried under the superior wall for its entire

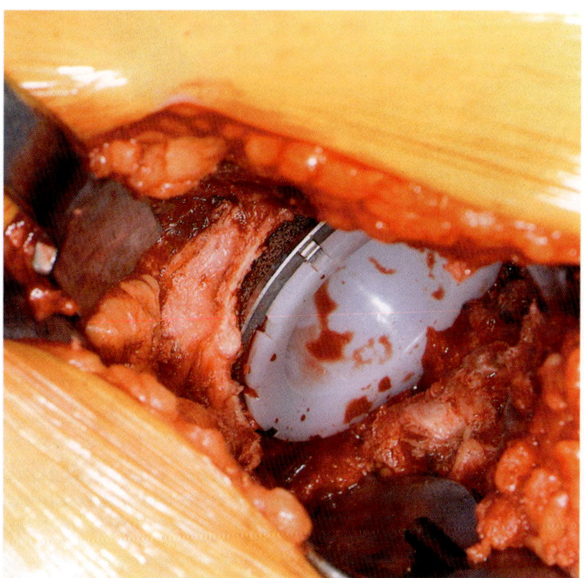

Figure 5–25 *Two to 4 mm of the superoposterior edge of the cup may be uncovered by bone, which ensures that the cup is not too vertical.*

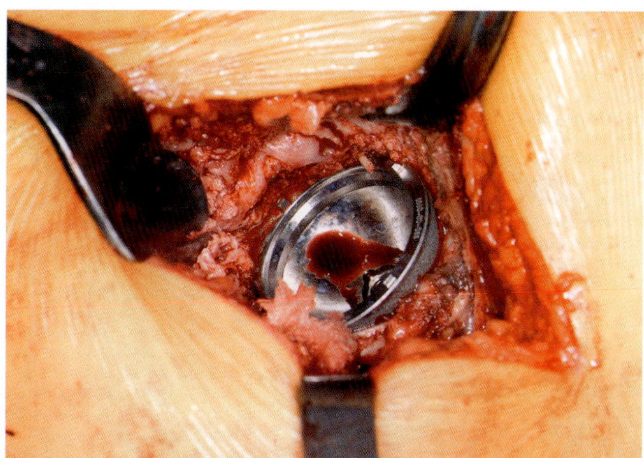

Figure 5–27 *The inclination of this cup is between 40 and 45 degrees as determined by exposure of the posterosuperior edge of the cup; the anterosuperior edge is below the anterior bone. The inferior medial edge of the cup is at the level of the cortical bone of the cotyloid notch. This appearance at operation means that the cup is not too vertical, is well anteverted, and should provide a nearly normal center of rotation for the acetabulum. This cup position also provides good contact areas for the femoral head in the acetabular liner.*

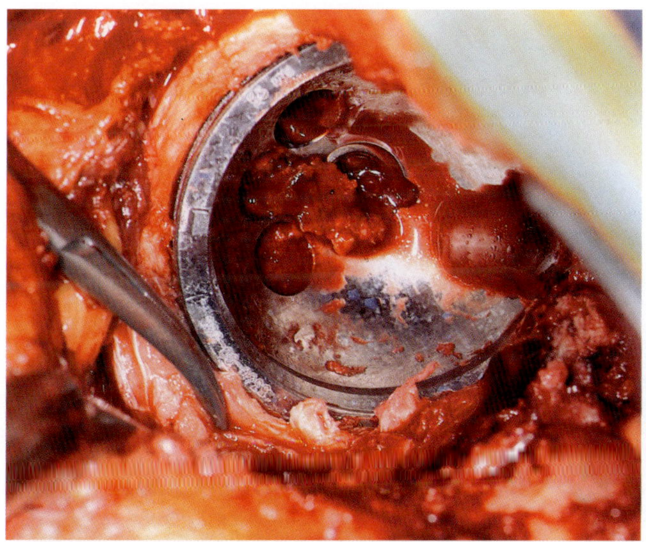

Figure 5–26 *The cup should be positioned in the acetabulum so that its posterosuperior edge stands proud to the bone (as seen here) and its posteroinferior edge lies below the tip of the ischium (which is being touched by the tonsil clamp). With this position, the cup is neither too lateral nor too vertical.*

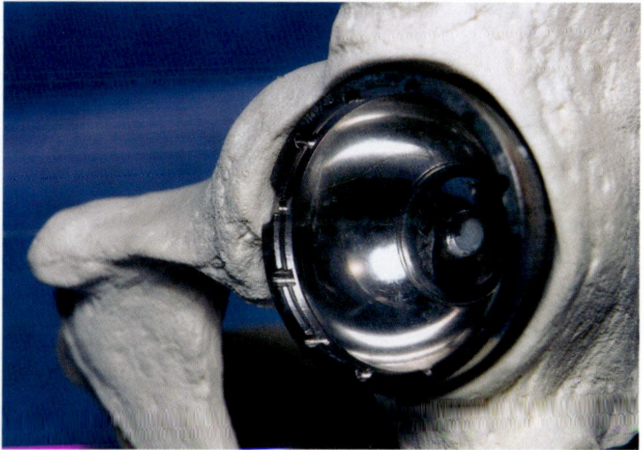

Figure 5–28 *Cup in a sawbone showing the anterosuperior edge lying just below the anterior bone. The anterior medial edge of the cup should be below the pubis, as shown. This usually ensures that the entire anterior edge of the cup is covered so that the iliopsoas tendon does not rub across it.*

circumference will most often have more than 50 degrees of inclination. This is not a favorable position for wear and increases the chances of dislocation. If the posterosuperior aspect of the cup is left slightly proud to the bone, the cup's inclination is generally between 40 and 45 degrees, which is favorable (Fig. 5–27).

The anterosuperior edge of the cup should be against bone or just covered by bone (Fig. 5–28). This is nec-essary to prevent impingement of the metal femoral neck against the edge of the cup in flexion range of motion, and particularly in flexion of more than 90 degrees with internal rotation.

The posterior edge of the cup is always beneath the ischium. If the posterior edge is flush with the ischium, the center of rotation of the acetabulum has not been reestablished or the cup is in excessive anteversion (see Fig. 5–26).

A good landmark for recreating the center of rotation and ensuring correct anteversion is to have the

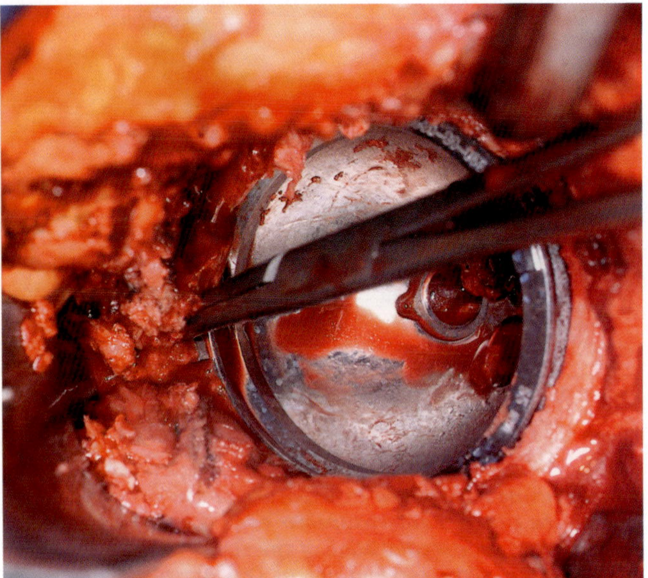

Figure 5–29 *Intraoperative view showing the anterior medial edge of the cup below the pubis, which is being touched by the tonsil clamp. This edge of the cup should be 5 mm below the edge of the pubic tubercle.*

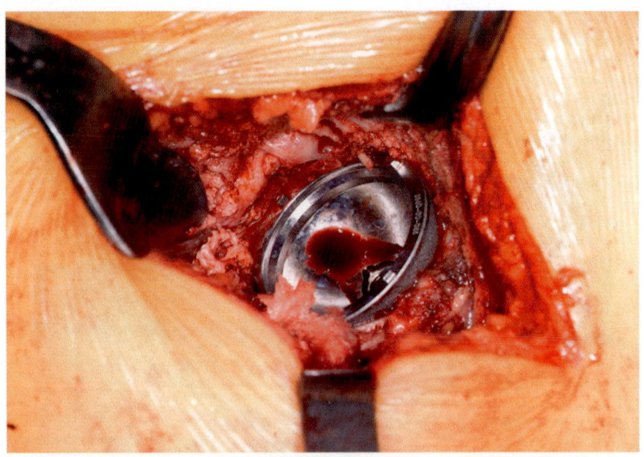

Figure 5–30 *A good position of the cup, with ideal exposure of the acetabulum. The #4 retractor is in the lower portion of the wound, the #5 retractor on the upper right, and the #7 retractor on the left.*

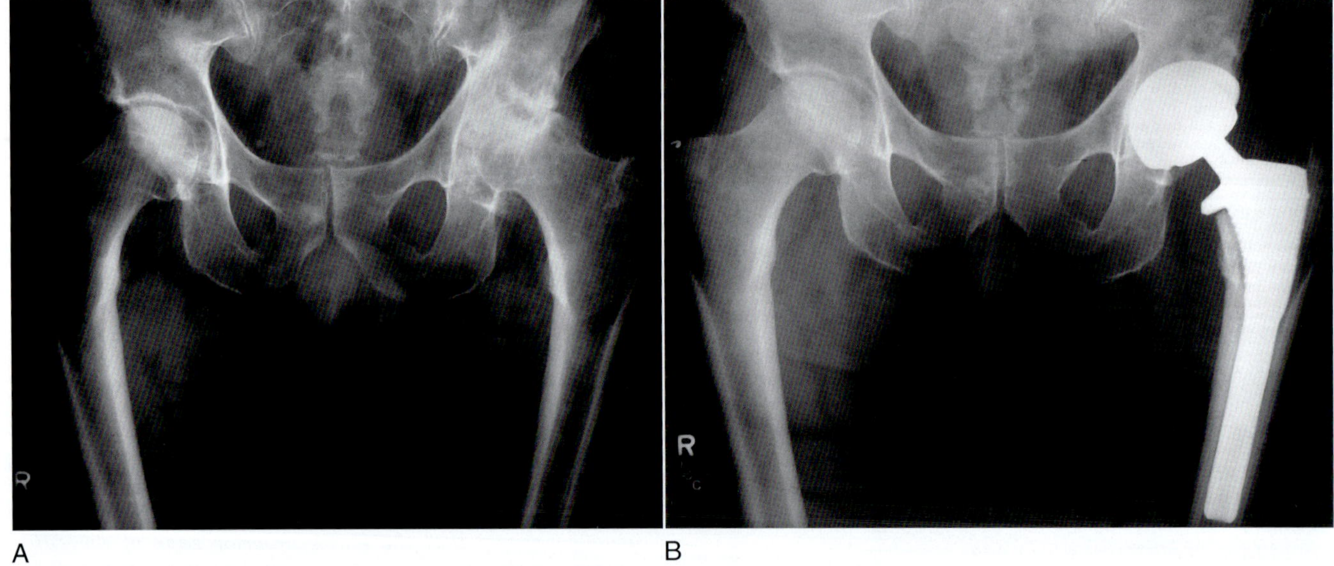

A   B

Figure 5–31 **A,** *Preoperative x-ray showing left hip osteoarthritis and an osteophyte over the transverse acetabular ligament between the pubis and ischium.* **B,** *Postoperative x-ray of correct cup position showing the inferior medial edge of the cup along the edge of the cortical bone of the cotyloid notch between the ischium and the pubis. The osteophyte has been removed.*

anteromedial edge of the cup approximately 5 mm below the palpable border of the pubic tubercle (Fig. 5–29; see Fig. 5–28). The cup is in good position with good protection if the edge of the cup is not more than 2 mm lateral to the cortical bone of the cotyloid notch (Fig. 5–30) and the anteromedial corner of the cup is 3 mm below the pubic tubercle; the anterosuperior edge is at or just below the anterosuperior bone; and the posterosuperior edge is uncovered by no more than

3 mm. The anterior edge of the cup is aligned not with the anterior wall, but with the anterosuperior edge of the acetabulum and the pubic tubercle anteriorly.

An x-ray of this cup position shows that the medial inferior border of the cup is between the ischium and the pubis, is not lateralized, and may be medialized depending on the acetabular anatomy (Fig. 5–31). There are three triangular anatomic geometries of the acetabulum on x-ray: (1) The isosceles triangle does not have

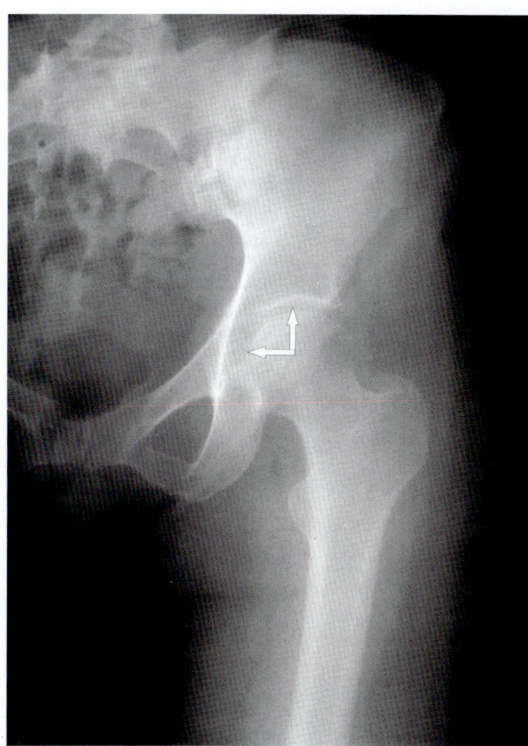

Figure 5–32 *Isosceles triangle acetabular geometry, with the medial wall essentially equal to Köhler's line. In these hips, the medial edge of the cup will intersect Köhler's line on the x-ray. The arrows point to the lucent area above the femoral head in the shape of an isosceles triangle, and to the thin medial wall. The isosceles triangle geometry is more common in women.*

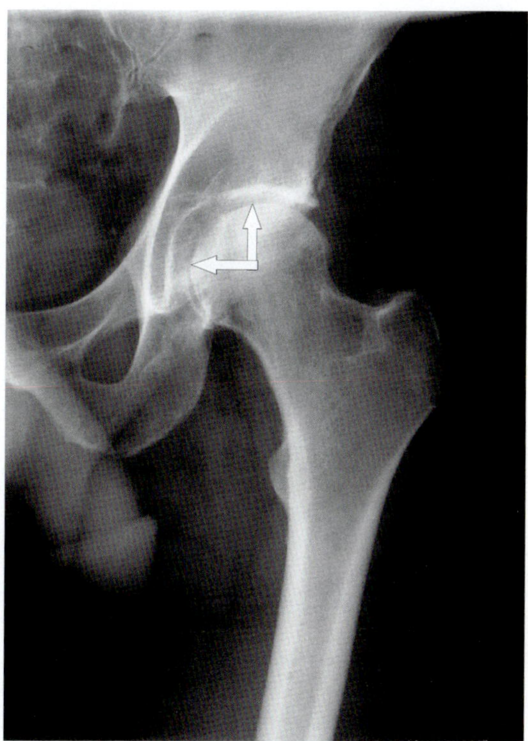

Figure 5–33 *An acetabulum with extended triangle geometry. The medial edge of the cup does not reach Köhler's line, so there is a much thicker medial wall for support of the cup in this type of anatomy. The arrows point to the superior lucent triangle, which extends into the medial wall and forms a thick tear drop. The extended triangle geometry is more common in men.*

a thick medial wall and is more commonly found in women; with this type of acetabular anatomy, the cup may be medialized into or just beyond Köhler's line (Fig. 5–32). (2) With the extended triangle geometry, there is a thick medial wall (thick tear drop) and the medial cup does not reach Köhler's line (Fig. 5–33). The extended triangle anatomy is usually found in men. (3) Finally, a right triangle anatomy is found with dysplastic acetabula (Fig. 5–34).

Insertion of the Permanent Cup

Cup implantation is simple once these decisions have been made with the trial; when the correct position of the trial cup has been obtained, placing the real cup is simply a matter of matching the position of the trial cup. The real acetabular component can be placed without excessive movement, which potentially can change the quality of fit. The same landmarks described for the trial cup should be present for the real cup when it is implanted. If the reaming went smoothly and the acetabulum is formed into a hemisphere, the real Converge acetabular component (Zimmer, Warsaw, Ind.) should have a tight press-fit because it is 1 mm larger than the reamed cavity (and the trial cup). The best test

for stability of the acetabular component is to pull vigorously on the handle used to insert the component once it is seated. If vigorous pulling does not move the cup, the fit into the bony acetabulum is solid enough that no augmentation with screws is necessary. The second test for cup stability is to strike the medial edge of the cup (at the level of the transverse acetabular ligament) with a bone tamp and mallet to determine if the cup tilts. If the cup moves, screws should be used to augment the fixation (Fig. 5–35). Some surgeons use screws routinely, but it is preferable to have a tight press-fit because tightening of the screws may change the position of the acetabular component.

If the acetabular component shows motion on either of the two stability tests, placement of screws for immediate fixation is necessary. When a screw is tightened into a component that is not solidly fixed, the component can move, usually into a more vertical position with less anteversion. To prevent excessive movement while the screw is tightened, a tool should be placed against the inferomedial edge of the cup to maintain the desired position (Fig. 5–36). A long bone tamp is an excellent tool for this maneuver. However, because the cup will change position slightly even when held against the tightening of the screw, it is advisable to

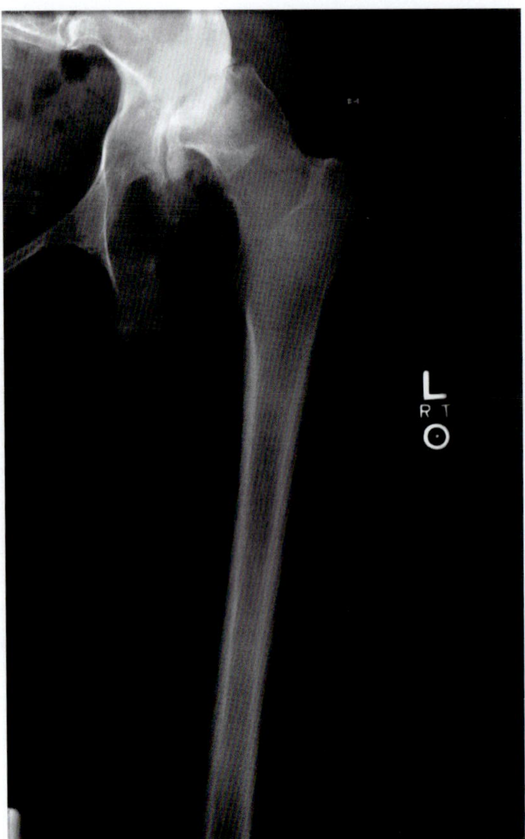

Figure 5–34 *The right triangle acetabular geometry is found only in dysplastic hips, usually Crowe type III or IV. The right triangle always denotes the presence of a dysplastic geometry.*

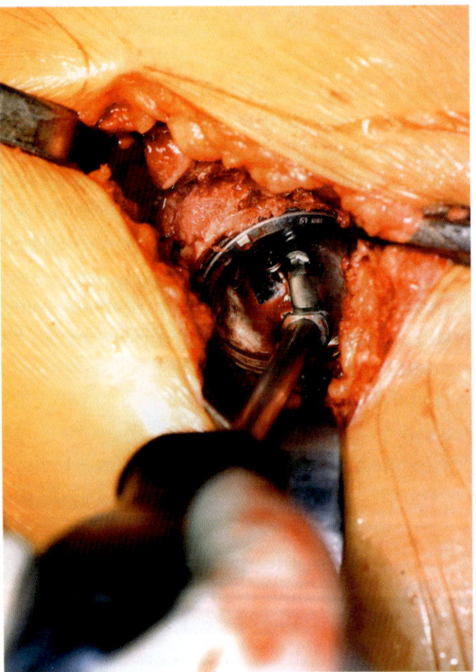

Figure 5–35 *A screw is inserted through the cup into the acetabular bone to augment initial cup stability.*

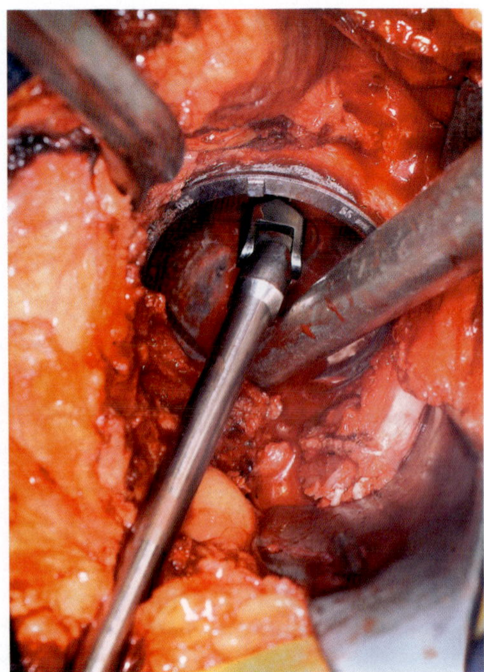

Figure 5–36 *The acetabular cup is stabilized with a long bone tamp held against the edge of the cup while the screw is tightened. This minimizes any change in cup position during screw insertion.*

place the cup with slightly less inclination (a flatter cup) and slightly more anteversion than desired. Then, when the screw is tightened, the cup is brought into a position very close to that originally desired. If the acetabular component is tightly fitted into the bony acetabulum, screw insertion will not change its position and the aforementioned precautions usually are unnecessary. Of course, if the component shifts with insertion of the screw, the screw should be loosened, a tool placed against the inferomedial edge of the component, and the screw tightened.

Insertion of the Acetabular Insert and Inspection

When the acetabular component implantation is complete and fixation is judged to be solid with or without screws, the acetabular insert of choice can be placed (Fig. 5–37). The insert needs to be malleted vigorously to lock it into place. If this visibly changes the position of the cup, the cup was not fixed solidly and the insert needs to be removed and a screw placed into the metal shell; this should not happen if the cup was adequately checked for stability. If computer assistance is used and the anteversion of the insert is known to be correct (approximately 25 degrees), no hood should be used on the plastic because the metal neck can impinge against the hood during extension. Certainly, if a hood is used with adequate anteversion of the metal shell,

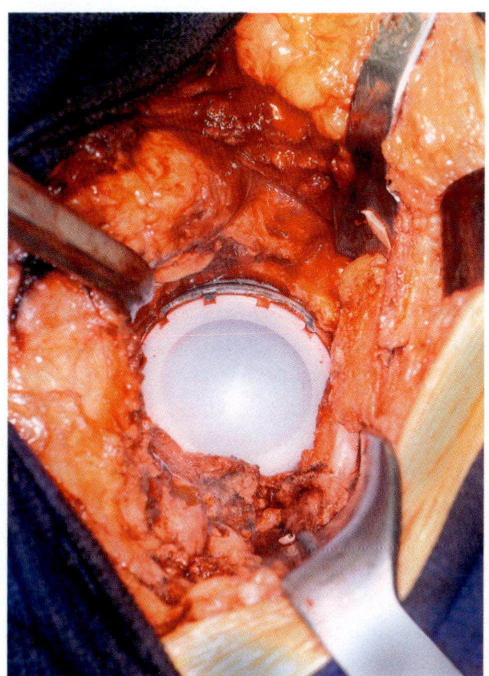

Figure 5–37 *The acetabular insert has been placed. This insert is a highly cross-linked Durasul for a 38-mm head.*

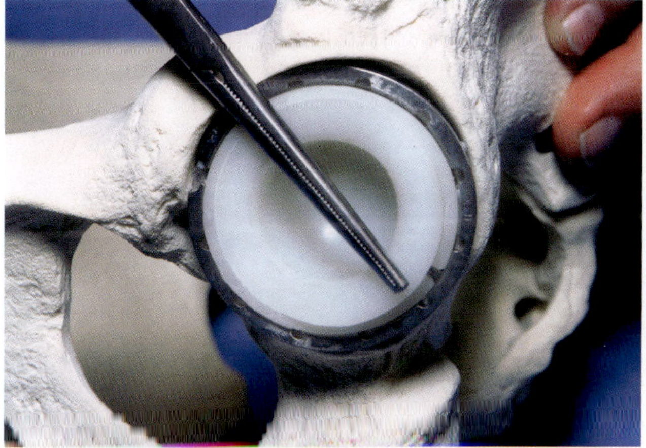

Figure 5–38 *Acetabular cup in a sawbone showing the position of the apex of an extended liner (hood). The apex of the hood is at 4 o'clock in this left hip, as indicated by the Kocher clamp.*

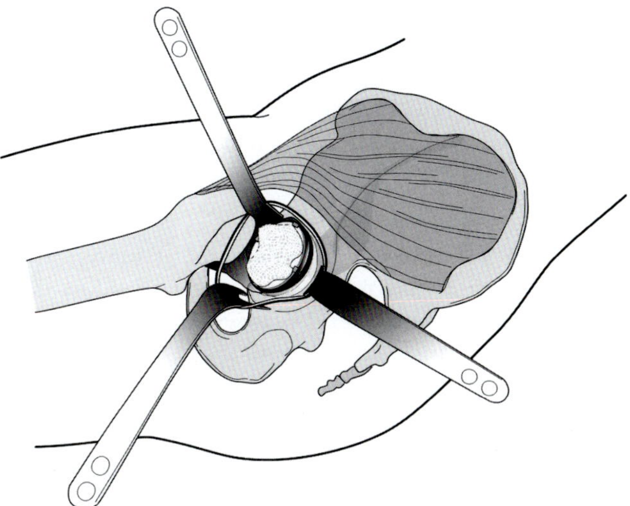

Figure 5–39 *A gauze sponge protects the surface of the cup.*

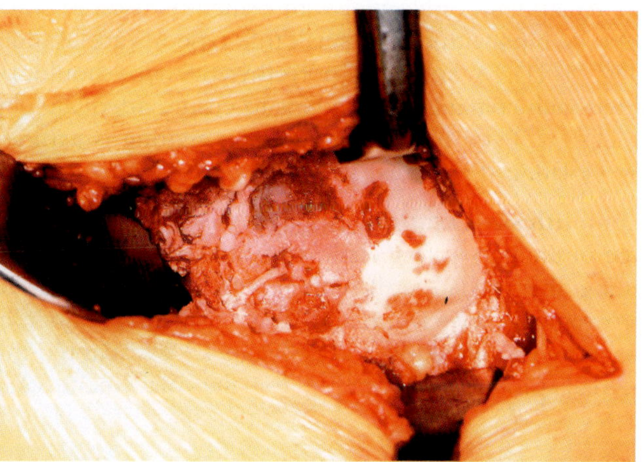

Figure 5–40 *Dysplastic acetabulum in which the femoral head articulated against the superior acetabulum; the acetabular cavity is sloped (not hemispheric). There is no clearly defined cotyloid notch. The acetabular retractors are in position. With the #4 retractor at knee-point, the #5 retractor on the superior edge of the acetabulum, and the #7 retractor on the left.*

the hood should be placed in the posteroinferior position to prevent impingement with abduction and external rotation (Fig. 5–38). This position protects against flexion and internal rotation. With computer guidance and consequent optimal acetabular position, flat inserts should always be used.

Once the insert for the articular surface has been placed, a final inspection of the acetabular component position is done and the articulation surface of the insert is protected with a sponge (Fig. 5–39). This completes the preparation and implantation of the acetabulum.

ACETABULAR PREPARATION OF THE DYSPLASTIC HIP

Reconstruction of a dysplastic hip is the most difficult type of primary hip arthroplasty. The deformed acetabulum has a high posterior wall and a deficient anterior wall; this rotation of the acetabulum gives the impression of excessive anteversion, but in fact the actual anteversion is not much more than 20 degrees. Because the deformed acetabulum has a very long superior slope, a hemisphere is more difficult to construct (Fig. 5–40), and coverage of the acetabular component by bone is more difficult to achieve.

We generally use the Crowe classification of dysplastic acetabula, which identifies four types,[2] whereas Hartofilakidis and associates[3] used a three-type classification. Clearly, however, in both classifications the two most difficult types are those in which the femoral head is subluxed onto the side of the pelvis or is completely dislocated.

Cemented Fixation. With cemented fixation, three techniques are available to cover the cup. Most commonly, a small cup is used because it can be cemented without leaving more than 5 mm of the cup left uncovered by bone.[4] The second technique uses bone cement to fill defects. Johnston and colleagues used this technique and at 15 years reported only a 7% rate of revision.[5] The third technique involves the use of bone grafts to fill defects. With this technique, 20% of cases needed revision and 21% were loose at an average of 12 years.[6]

The modified protrusio technique for placement of an acetabular component with cement is used in some type IV hips with a very small true osseous acetabulum (Fig. 5–41). A small, all-polyethylene cup should be fixed with cement in these hips to ensure adequate cup thickness. Even in these hips, bone grafting is avoided by violating the medial wall if necessary.

Cementlesss Fixation. Another technique for coverage of the cup in dysplastic acetabula consists of weakening the medial wall, either with an osteotome, as recommended by Dunn and Hess,[7] or with a reamer, as done by Hartofilakidis and colleagues.[3] We adapted this medial protrusio technique for the placement of a porous-coated hemispherical acetabular component without cement in patients with dysplastic acetabula.[8]

The principles of cementless fixation of acetabular components in dysplastic hips differ from those of fixation with cement. In some hips with Crowe type I dysplasia, the acetabulum must be reconstructed to a hemisphere for a secure press-fit, and the medial protrusio technique, which involves reaming into or through the medial acetabular wall, is the only technique of which we are aware that permits this (Fig. 5–42). This technique is not needed for all Crowe type I hips, but it is necessary for type II (Fig. 5–43), type III (Fig. 5–44), and type IV (Fig. 5–45) hips.[2] Twenty percent to 30% of the superolateral aspect of the cup can be left uncovered. In our series,[8] in the hips treated with bone grafting, 60% to 84% of the bone graft covering on average 22% of the superolateral aspect of the cup was resorbed. Clearly, the bone graft was unnecessary, and this percentage of the cup can be left uncovered. Garvin and coworkers[2] also suggested that 20% of the superolateral aspect of the cup can be left uncovered.

In our series, the amount of medialization of the center of the femoral head tended to increase with worsening dysplasia, but the average percentage of the cup surface that was left uncovered medially was approximately 40% for all types. In hips with types III and IV dysplasia, medialization of the center of the

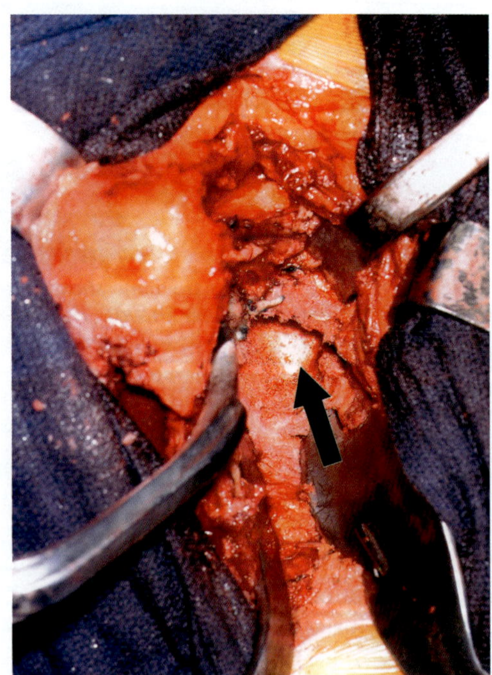

Figure 5–41 *In this acetabulum, a 38-mm Charnley cup was cemented to the bone. With medialization, no bone graft was needed. The acetabulum in Crowe type IV dysplastic hips is very small, but careful technique results in circumferential coverage for 75% of the cup.*

Figure 5–42 *The medial wall of the acetabulum has been reamed to expose its periosteum in the floor of the acetabulum. This medializes the cup sufficiently that a bone graft is not needed.*

femoral head averaged 25 mm. This distance corresponds to the amount of medialization recommended by McQueary, Johnston, and colleagues[9,10] and biomechanically is better than superior displacement of the femoral head.

Technique

First, the surgeon must identify the geometry of the dysplastic acetabulum. The femoral head is usually sub-

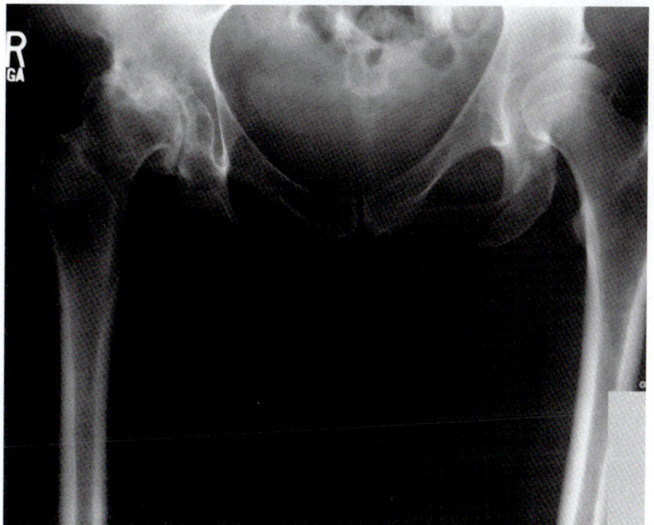

Figure 5–43 *X-ray of Crowe type II dysplastic hip.*

luxed superiorly and laterally, and the greater the subluxation, the more likely it is that the true acetabulum will be covered with fibrous tissue. The procedure performed on the hip shown in Figure 5–46 is described here. This hip is a Crowe type IV dislocation with a previous osteotomy and retained plate. The principles of this reconstruction are illustrated.

Cavity Preparation. In type IV acetabula, the true acetabulum can be covered by a thin cortical shell (Fig. 5–47). The acetabulum is identified by palpating the pubis and ischium and locating the cortical edge of the cotyloid notch. Soft tissue and any bone in the acetabular cavity are removed to expose the cotyloid notch. If the diameter of the acetabular opening is smaller than 40 mm, a high-speed burr is used to open the osseous cavity (Fig. 5–48). The anterior wall is hypoplastic and must be protected during preparation of the bone. After the cavity is opened, reaming begins with a 38-mm reamer and progresses as the size of the osseous acetabulum allows (Fig. 5–49). The sloping superior wall of the acetabulum must be converted to a hemisphere using a small reamer. The direction of reaming is in line with the desired access of acetabular anteversion. The smallest reamer must be used because the formation of a hemisphere with a superior rim requires reaming into the ilium (Fig. 5–50). Initial use of a large reamer can destroy the superior rim, necessitating a bone graft for adequate coverage.

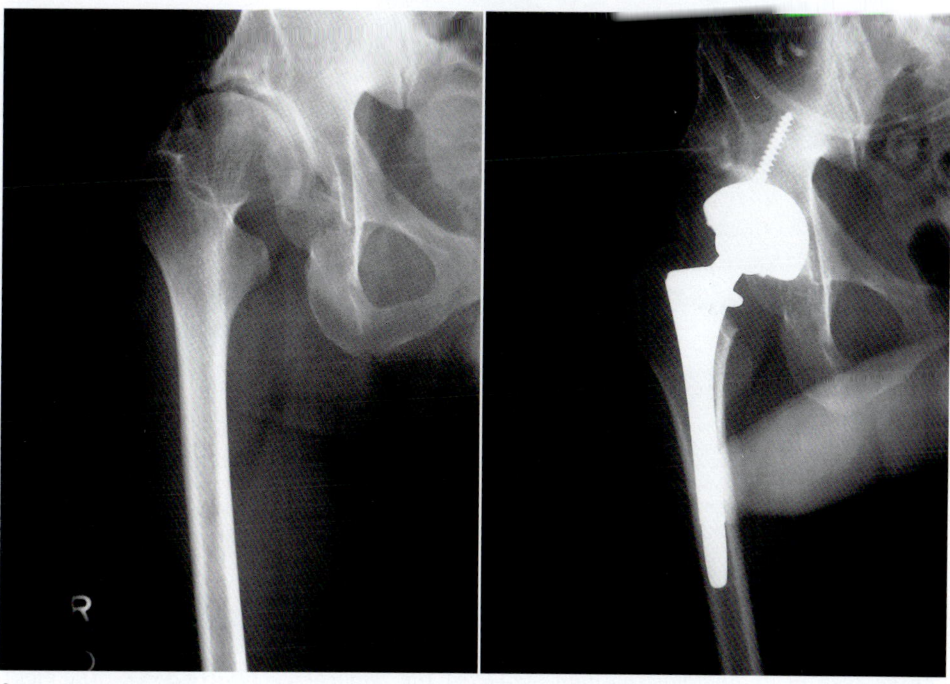

Figure 5–44 ***A,*** *Crowe type III dysplastic hip, in which the center of rotation is elevated 70% above its normal position.* ***B,*** *In a Crowe type III hip, the original acetabulum should be used for implantation of the cup and the inferior osteophyte for the pseudoacetabulum can be used as the superior support for the acetabulum.*

A   B

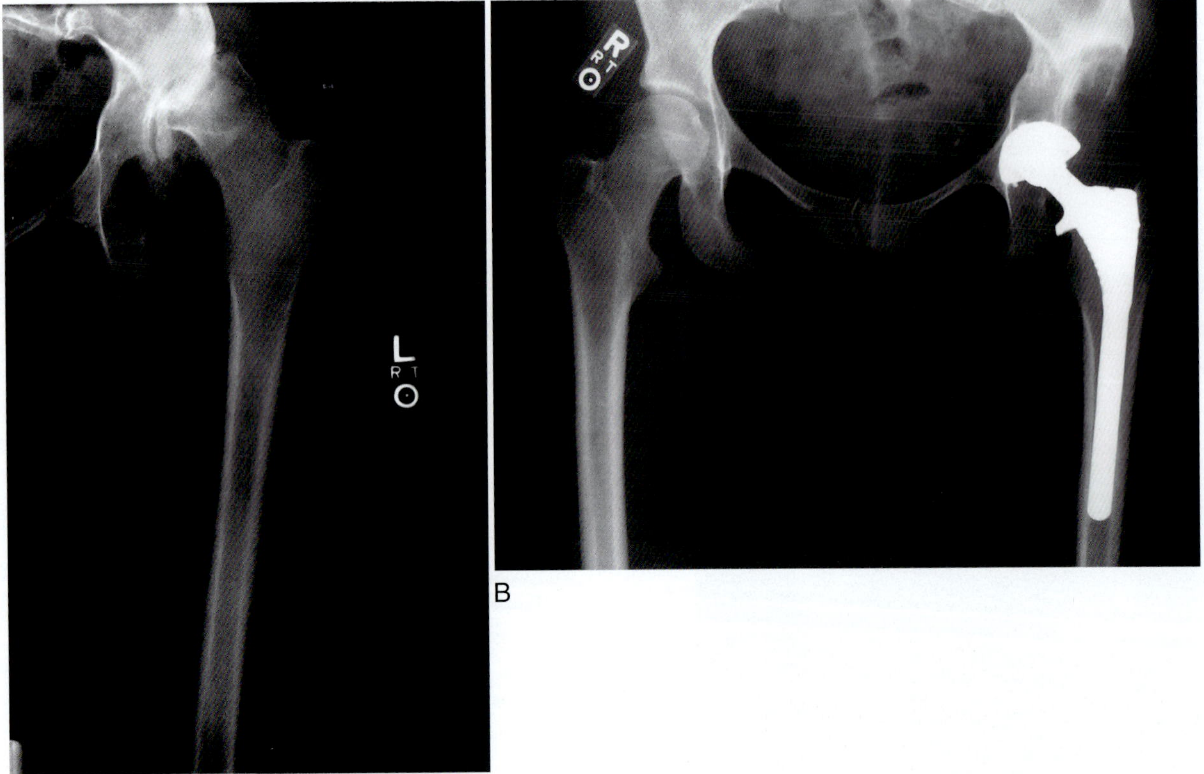

A

B

Figure 5–45 *The Crowe type IV dysplastic hip has a completely dislocated femoral head (center of rotation 100% or more superior).* **B.** *In this reconstructed Crowe type IV hip, the pseudoacetabulum is seen on the ilium. The cup should be placed into the original acetabulum, the size of which is almost always less than 45 mm, which means a 22-mm head is used. Medialization avoids the need for bone grafting. The press-fit was so secure in this hip that a screw was not needed.*

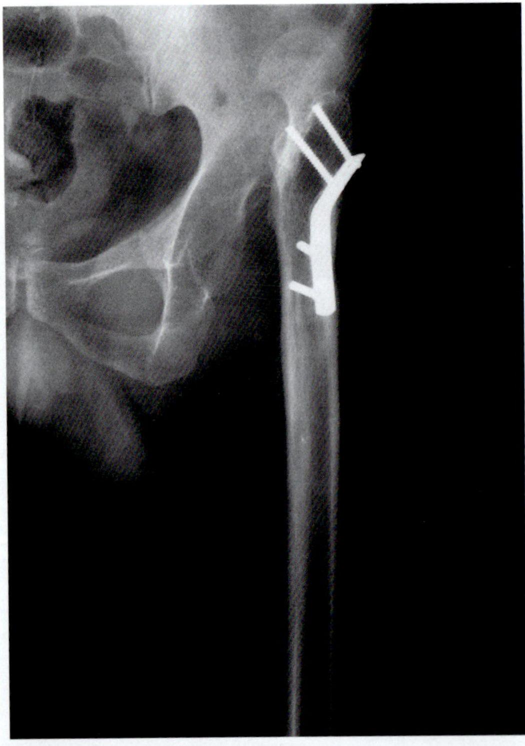

Figure 5–46 *Anteroposterior x-ray of congenitally dislocated hip that underwent osteotomy when the patient was a child. The femoral head sits on the ilium; the true acetabulum can be seen in its anatomic position. Reducing the femoral head of the hip replacement into such an acetabulum will almost always require a subtrochanteric osteotomy to move the femur distally the necessary amount.*

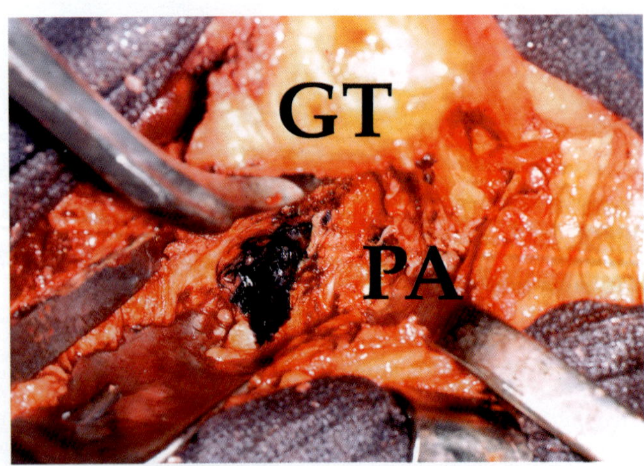

Figure 5–47 *The mouth of the acetabulum has been painted with methylene blue to clarify its geometry and size, as well as to show that the opening is covered with thin cortical bone. GT, greater trochanter; PA, pseudoacetabulum.*

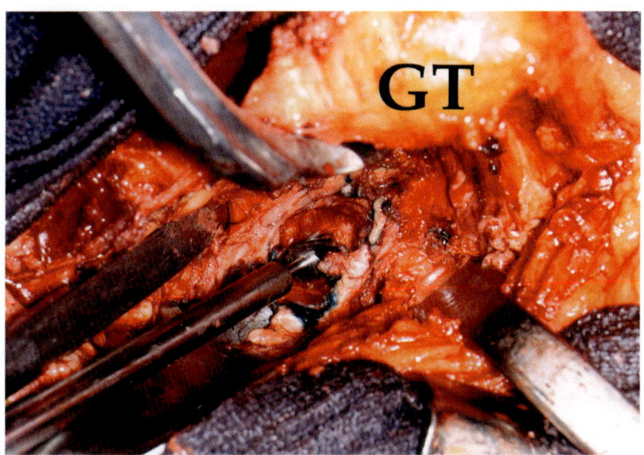

Figure 5–48   *The acetabulum has been opened with a high-speed burr, and its peripheral walls are now clearly visible. The superior wall of the acetabulum is formed by excavating the ilium. The pseudoacetabulum is seen below the greater trochanter (GT).*

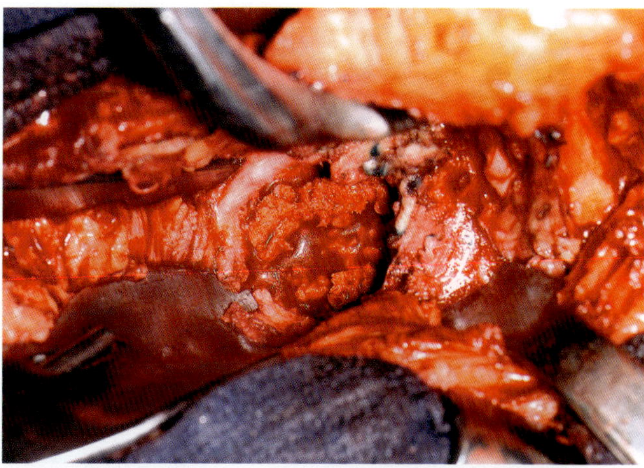

Figure 5–50   *After reaming, the acetabulum shows bleeding cancellous bone with a strong cortical peripheral rim. The superior acetabulum is marked with dots of methylene blue.*

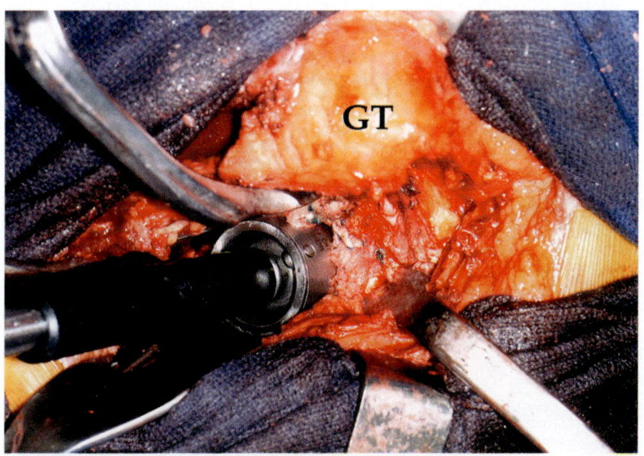

Figure 5–49   *Once the acetabulum has been opened with the high-speed burr and its walls defined, a reamer can be used to form a hemisphere. A 38-mm reamer should be used first, after which the acetabulum can be expanded to allow a press-fit of the acetabular cup, without excessively thinning the anterior and posterior walls. GT, greater trochanter.*

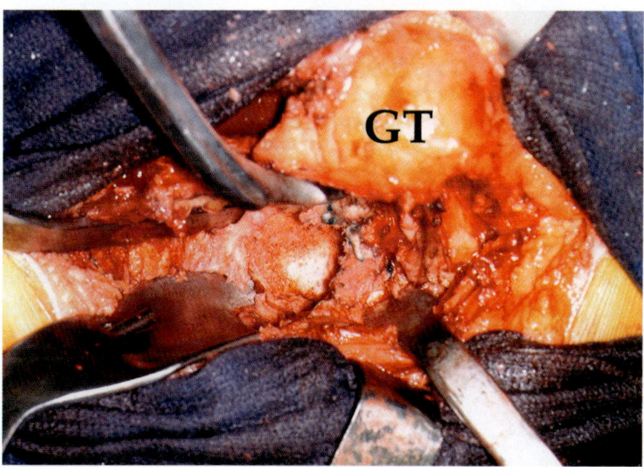

Figure 5–51   *The acetabulum has been reamed into the medial wall to allow a press-fit of the acetabular cup without bone grafting. The periosteum of the medial wall is visible in the floor of the acetabulum. The amount of medial wall exposed should comprise no more than 25% of the acetabular cavity. GT, greater trochanter.*

If the depth of the osseous cavity after this preparation is not sufficient to permit stable press-fit fixation of the acetabular component, the protrusio technique is used to deepen the cavity. Reaming is accomplished into or through the entire medial osseous acetabular wall as needed to provide a stable fit for the metal shell (Fig. 5–51). The medial periosteum is usually left intact, but occasionally we ream through it, and the iliacus muscle is seen in the base of the defect. In cases in which we reamed through the medial periosteum, the medial aspect of the dome was later seen to be medial to both the ilioischial and the iliopubic lines on radiographs (Fig. 5–52). We ream the quadrilateral plate (beyond Köhler's line), rather than creating a controlled fracture with an osteotome, because the hemispherical osseous cavity necessary for cementless fixation of the metal shell can be prepared more accurately with the reamer. With this technique, the anterior and posterior acetabular bone must not be reamed too thin. The defect must be kept medially, with no thinning of the acetabular rim and with no more than approximately 25% of the acetabluar area perforated; more extensive perforation can result in protrusion of as much as 45% of the surface area of the cup

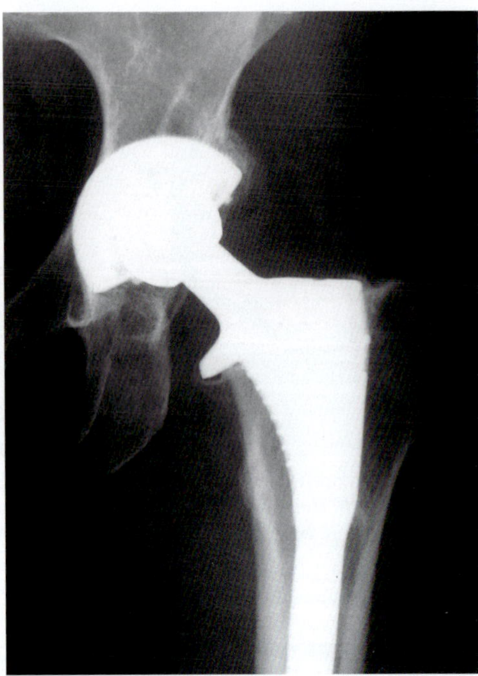

Figure 5–52 *X-ray showing an acetabular cup fitted into the acetabular cavity with medial reaming that extended beyond both the ilioischial and iliopubic lines.*

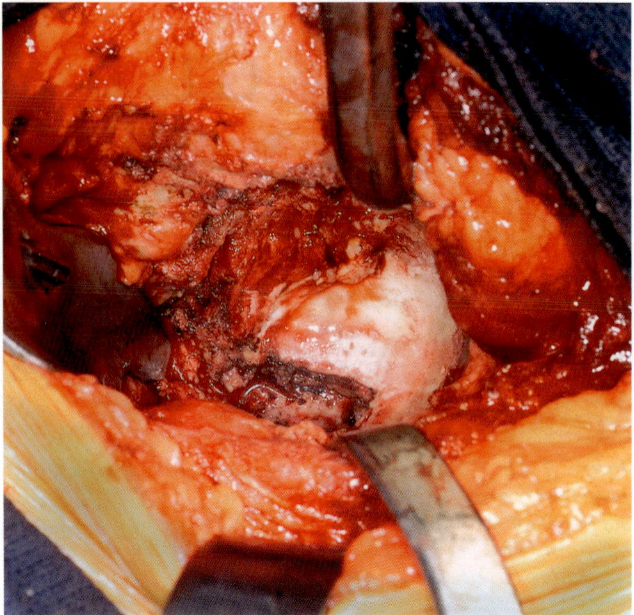

Figure 5–53 *A dysplastic acetabulum from a separate case. The top retractor is the anterior snake (#5). The #4 retractor is at the bottom, and the #7 retractor is on the left. The cotyloid notch of the acetabulum is visible at the base of the #7 retractor. The anterior wall was hypoplastic, and fibrous tissue is evident anteriorly after initial preparation of this acetabulum.*

beyond Köhler's line. Thinning of the anterior and posterior walls or excessive (>25%) removal of the medial wall weakens the hemispherical osseous acetabular cavity, and insertion of the press-fit metal shell can cause fractures through the anterior or posterior column, resulting in an unstable acetabular reconstruction. An example of anterior acetabular wall thinning, which occurred in a separate case, is shown in Figure 5–53.

Insertion of the Acetabular Trial and Cup. The acetabular trial correlating with the last reamer used is inserted. The trial component must have rim fit fixation with no more than 25% of the metal cup uncovered superolaterally (Fig. 5–54). Because of the hypoplastic anterior wall, the anterior edge of the cup may extend beyond the osseous wall, in which case the iliopsoas tendon must be released to prevent abrasive contact of the iliopsoas muscle and tendon with the anterior wall of the cup (which can cause chronic groin pain). Press-fit stability is determined by attempting to move the trial shell manually by tilt or rotation. The surgeon must be aware of the relative sizes of the trial system and the actual cup. With the Converge cup (Zimmer), the cup is 1 mm larger than the trial and gives an even tighter press-fit. With cups that are the same size as the trial, the roughness of the porous surface can provide a sufficient frictional press-fit. Commonly, a 22-mm femoral head size is used in small acetabula (<50 mm), in which case a hooded polyethylene insert is positioned to

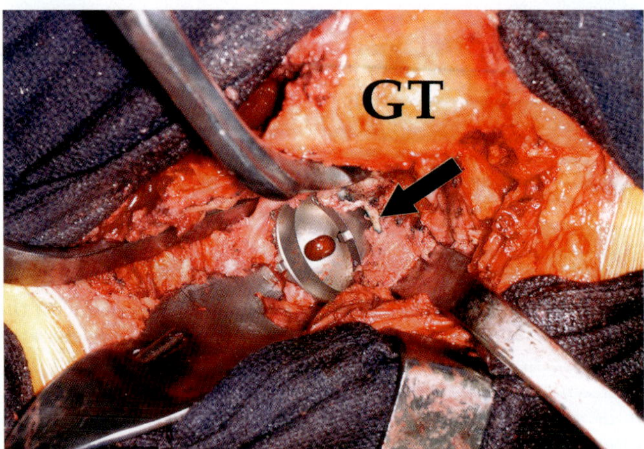

Figure 5–54 *The trial acetabular shell is seated into the acetabular cavity. The arrow points ot the superior lateral cup, as much as 25% of which can be exposed superolaterally while retaining adequate stability. The hole in the acetabular trial shows that the cup is against the acetabular bone. This acetabular preparation affords anterior coverage of the cup, which also contributes to excellent press-fit stability. GT, greater trochanter.*

cover the inner surface of the prominent ischium (3 o'clock for the left hip and 9 o'clock for the right hip; Fig. 5–55).

The osseous fragments produced by reaming the head are collected, and the fat is removed by compressing the fragments in a lap sponge (Fig. 5–56). The

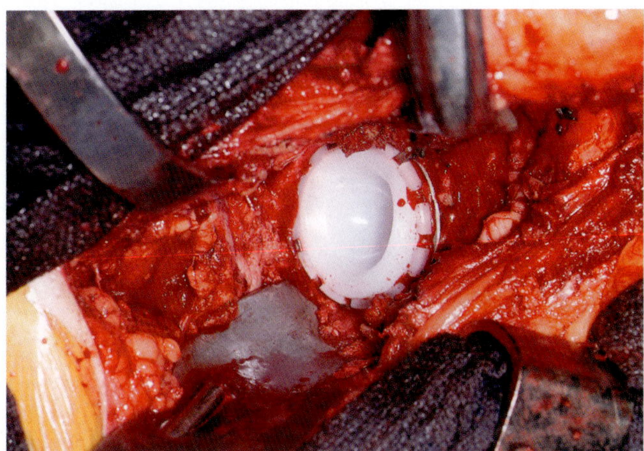

Figure 5–55 *The acetabular liner has been inserted into this left hip with the apex of the hood at 3 o'clock.*

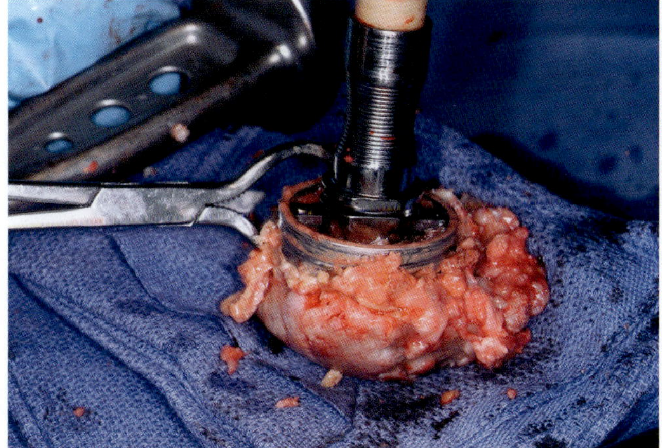

Figure 5–56 *A small reamer is used in the femoral head to obtain cancellous bone for an autograft.*

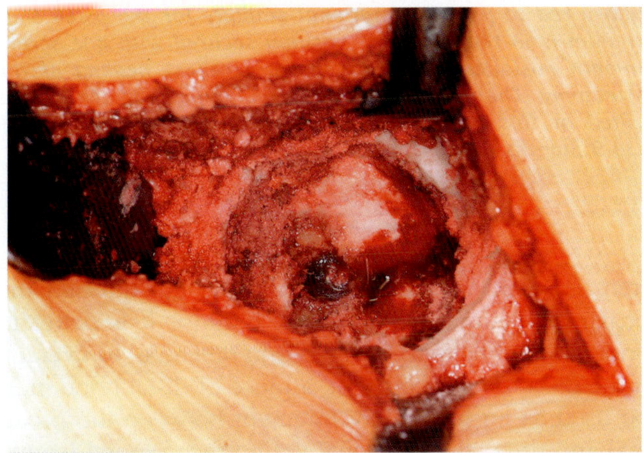

Figure 5–57 *The same acetabular cavity as in Figure 5–53. Reaming of this acetabulum has been completed, and the anterior wall has been grafted with cancellous bone obtained from the femoral head. Because the graft bone was squeezed in a lap sponge to remove the fat, the graft has a compact structure.*

fragments are placed into the defect prior to the implantation of the cup (Fig. 5–57).

The acetabular cup is implanted (see Fig. 5–54). We suggest using a screw for augmented fixation unless a perfect press-fit is obtained (Fig. 5–58; see Fig. 5–45B).

FEMORAL PREPARATION OF THE DYSPLASTIC HIP

Osteotomy

Femoral preparation for completely dislocated hips most often requires osteotomy of the femur because of the distance that the femur needs to be moved to articulate the hip in the original acetabulum. In the hip discussed here, the femoral plate had to be removed (see Fig. 5–46). When a plate has been placed for an osteotomy during childhood, the bone will always overgrow the plate, and the plate must be exposed for removal. I expose the plate using a power burr such as the Anspach (Fig. 5–59), although this sometimes distorts the heads of the plate screws. Where possible, the screws are removed with a screwdriver. If the screwdriver cannot be fitted onto the screw head, the screw head is eliminated with a carbide bit on the Anspach. Once the screw heads have been removed, the plate can be lifted off the bone and the remaining screw shafts exposed using a pencil-tip bit on the Anspach. I then use a small rongeur to grip the shaft and unscrew it from the bone. Removal of the plate often leaves a hole in the bone.

After dislocation of the hip and resection of the femoral head, the femoral canal is opened and sized with reamers. A Charnley awl is useful to open the canal and prepare a track for the reamer, especially if there is a hole in the bone from a previous plate, as in the bone in Figure 5–59. Preparation and sizing of the femoral canal before osteotomy of the femur permits the use of a trial stem for judging the correct length of the femur (Fig. 5–60). A subtrochanteric osteotomy is done. I make an oblique cut from below the lesser trochanter (Fig. 5–61) because a parallel oblique cut can then be made distally, which allows the two surfaces to oppose each other with a large area of contact for good healing. The apposed oblique osteotomies also provide some rotational stability to the femur with a correctly sized femoral stem inserted into the intramedullary canal.

Insertion of the Trial Femoral Stem

After the initial osteotomy is completed, the proximal fragment is mobilized from soft tissue attachments. When it is freely mobile, the trial femoral stem is inserted through the proximal preparation and a trial

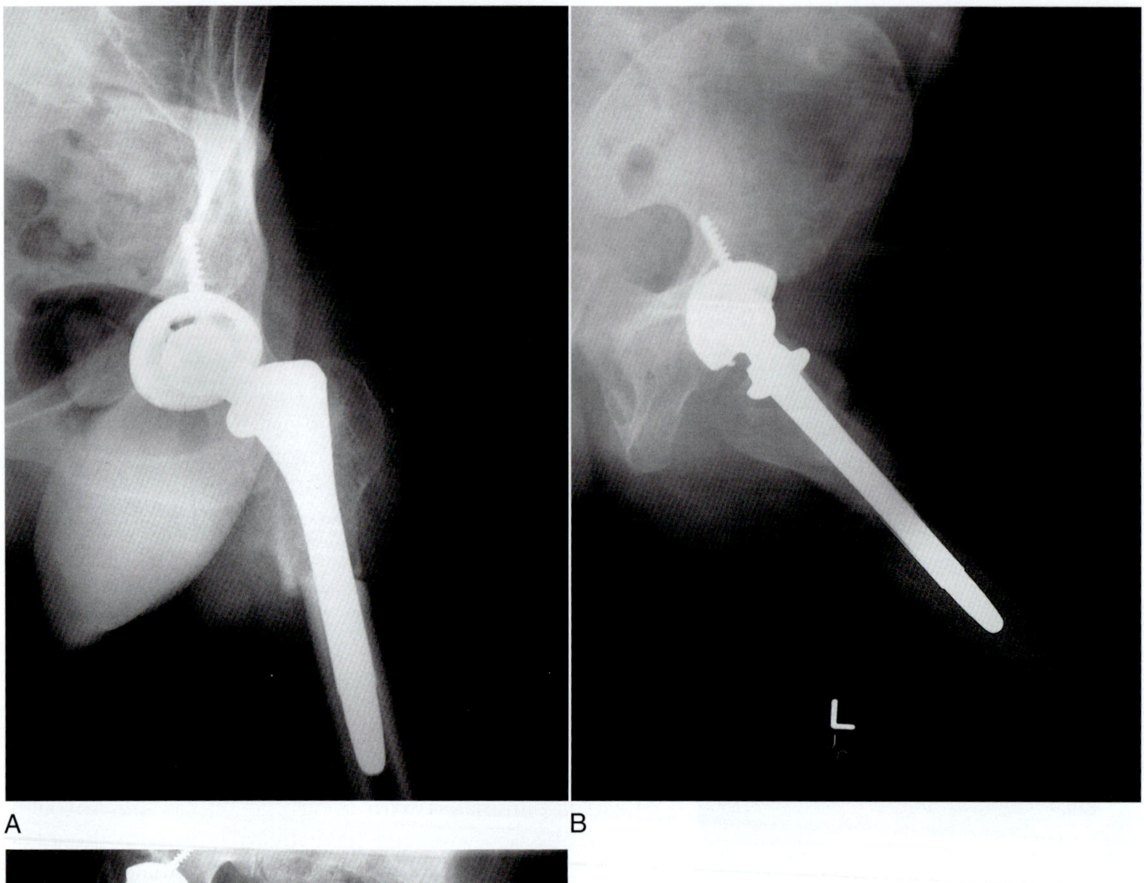

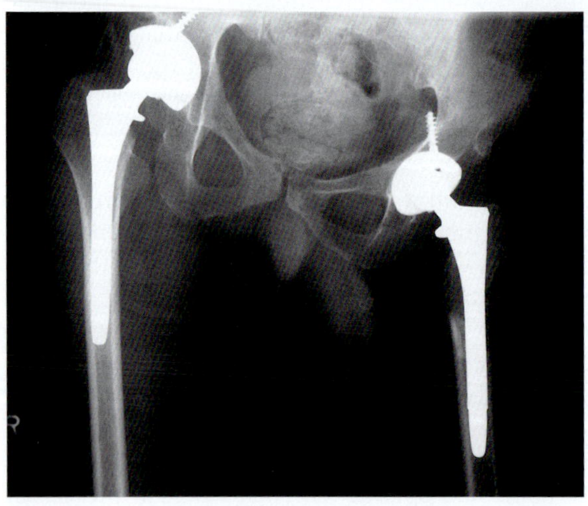

Figure 5–58 **A,** *Postoperative x-ray of congenitally dislocated hip shows the position of the acetabular component in the true anatomic acetabulum and the excellent apposition of the femoral osteotomy after preparation of the femur and insertion of the femoral component. A screw to augment the fixation of the acetabular component is visible through the acetabular cup.* **B,** *Lateral x-ray shows the apposition of the osteotomy and the stem crossing the osteotomy that acts as an intramedullary rod to provide rotational stability for the osteotomy. The acetabulum is in the anatomic position secured with one screw.* **C,** *Three-month postoperative x-ray shows excellent healing of the femoral osteotomy. The cup is in the acetabular position. The pelvis remains tilted at this time from abductor contracture, which will require 6 to 9 months for resolution.*

head and neck are used to reduce the hip into the acetabular cup. With the hip reduced, the distal end of the stem is used to maneuver the proximal fragment so that it lies adjacent to the distal fragment (Fig. 5–62). With the fragments overlaid, the proximal and distal ends of the oblique cut on the proximal fragment are marked with methylene blue where they touch the distal fragment. The trial stem is then removed and the cut is made through the distal femoral bone to remove the required length of distal fragment and allow reduction of the fragment to the proximal fragment when the

stem is in place. I initially make the cut through the proximal methylene blue mark because it is better to undercut and have to cut a second time than to overcut. If the distal bone is overcut, a piece of distal bone must be used as an intercalary fragment between the proximal and distal shafts to give the correct femoral length. The oblique segment removed should have parallel cut ends so that the proximal and distal femoral fragments will have the same angle of cut to allow them to fit closely together (Fig. 5–63). The trial stem is again inserted through the proximal fragment, and the distal

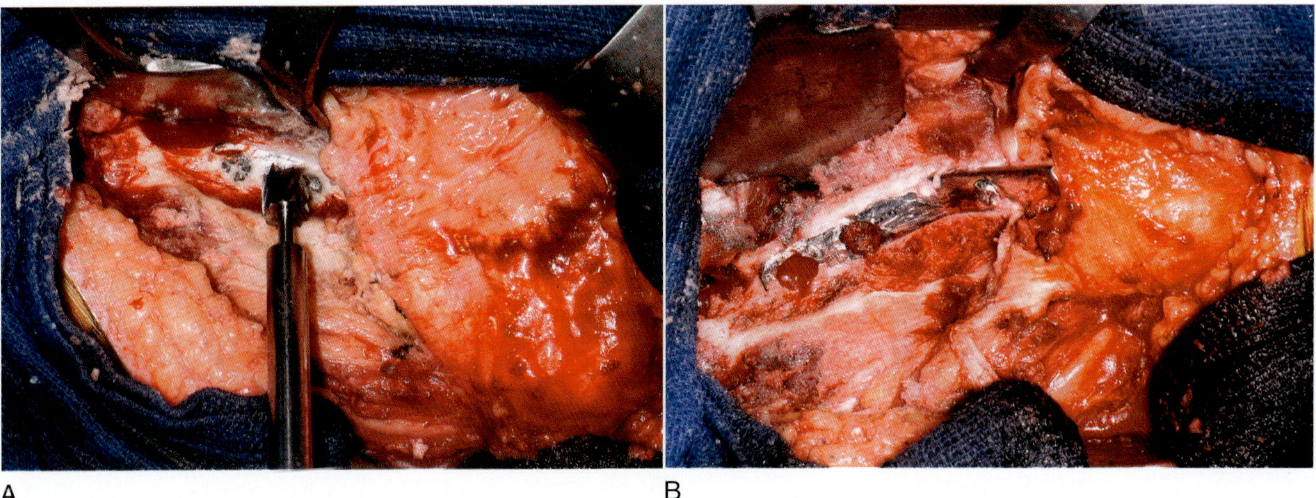

A　　　　　　　　　　　　　　　　　　B

Figure 5–59　**A,** *The high-speed burr removes bone that has overgrown the plate so the plate can be exposed for removal. This process sometimes distorts the plate screw heads, requiring their removal with a carbide bit.* **B,** *The entire plate has been exposed. The bottom two screw heads have been removed using a carbide bit. The top screw has been removed with a screwdriver, as will the remaining screw.*

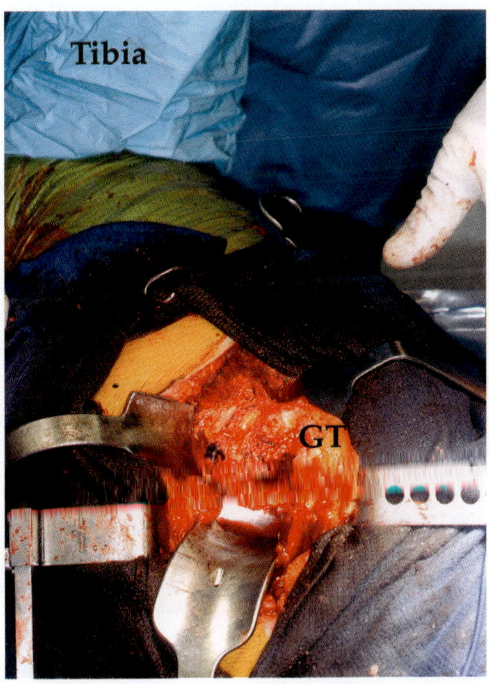

Figure 5–60　*The femoral canal has been opened and prepared first with a Charnley awl and then with reamers. The lesser trochanter is marked with methylene blue. The greater trochanter (GT) and tibia are identified.*

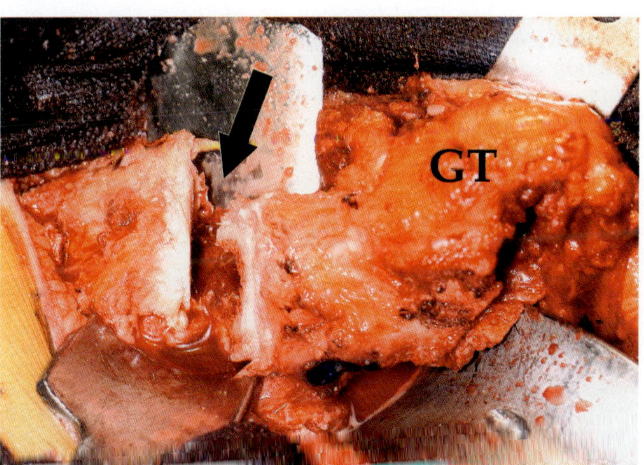

Figure 5–61　*An oblique osteotomy (arrow) has been completed in the subtrochanteric bone. The lesser trochanter is marked with methylene blue. GT, greater trochanter.*

hip joint (Fig. 5–64). With the osteotomy closed, hip stability can be tested with a shuck test. The sciatic nerve should be palpated to ensure that it is mobile and not tense.

Insertion of the Stem

If this reduction is judged satisfactory, the trial is removed and the stem is impacted. Placement of the trial stem will determine whether it is necessary to ream the distal fragment again, in addition to the original reaming done with the femur intact. Sometimes, after removal of the oblique segment of femur, the distal bone needs to be reamed again to ensure that the canal is the correct size. In this patient, the AML bantam stem with a full porous coating (Anatomic Medullary Locking;

end is passed into the distal fragment to provide a union of the two fragments. With a smooth trial stem in place, the two fragments may not be rotationally stable. However, by pushing on the knee and malleting the proximal fragment into the distal fragment, the two fragments can be apposed in a reduced position to determine the contact area of the osteotomy, as well as whether the length obtained provides stability for the

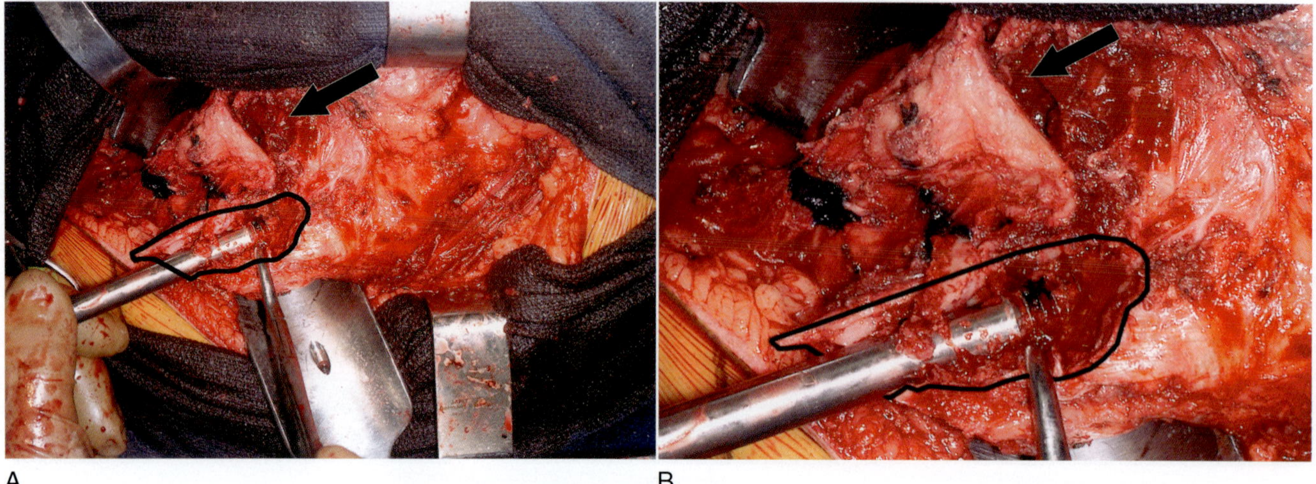

Figure 5–62   **A,** *The trial femoral head has been reduced into the acetabulum and the trial stem is visible protruding from the end of the proximal fragment. The obliquity of the proximal fragment osteotomy is outlined in black. The opening of the distal femoral fragment is identified by the arrow. Two methylene blue marks on the distal fragment identify the levels of the proximal and distal ends of the proximal osteotomy.* **B,** *Close-up view of the overlaid bones showing the proximal fragment adjacent to the distal fragment. The opening of the distal fragment is marked by the arrow, and the methylene blue marks approximate the levels of the proximal and distal end of the proximal fragment against the distal fragment. Initially, the oblique segment removed from the distal fragment should be at the level of the proximal methylene blue mark. When that segment is removed, the trial stem should again be inserted, the two fragments reduced, and a trial reduction of the hip accomplished. If the trial reduction cannot be accomplished because the femur is still too long, a second osteotomy is made through the distal methylene blue mark.*

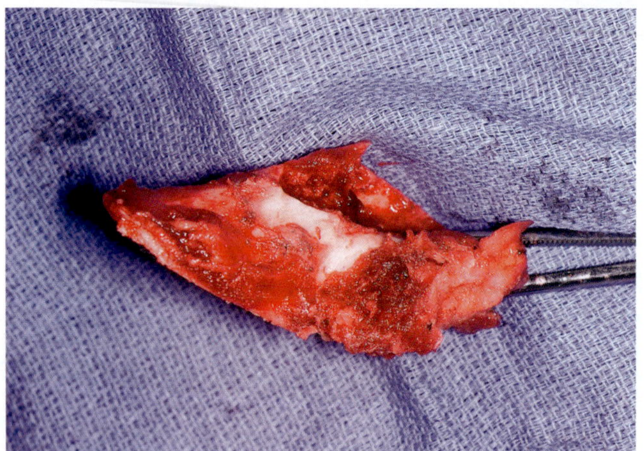

Figure 5–63   *The oblique segment removed from the distal fragment shows that the two cuts are parallel, which will allow good apposition of the proximal and distal segments.*

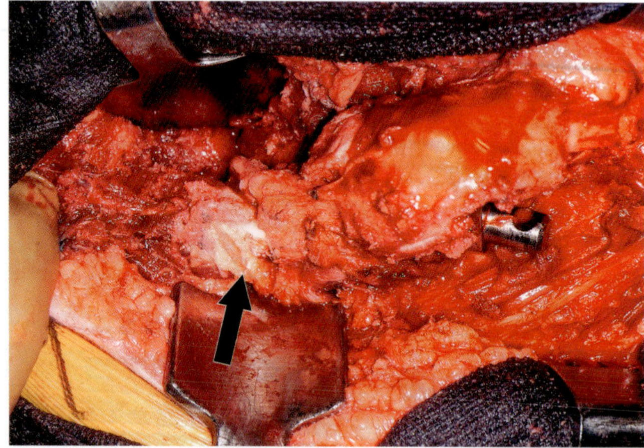

Figure 5–64   *The trial stem is in place and the osteotomy has been reduced, with tight contact along the posterior side of the femur (arrow). A gap is seen anteriorly because some bone is missing from the defect left by the plate.*

Depuy, Warsaw, Ind.) was used because the rough surface promotes rotational stability of the two fragments. As the stem is impacted into the distal fragment, the osteotomy compresses itself (Fig. 5–65). When maximum apposition has been achieved, rotational stability is determined by reducing the hip and rotating the lower leg. If the femur and stem move together, no additional fixation for rotational stability is needed. If rotational instability is detected, a small four-hole fragment plate can be placed with two screws above and two below the osteotomy site to reinforce rotational stability. In this patient, with the hip reduced, the osteotomy is closed posteriorly with an open defect still present from the plate anteriorly (Fig. 5–66).

Sciatic Nerve Testing

One important goal of hip replacement and reconstruction for a dysplastic hip, especially one that is completely dislocated, is to avoid injury to the sciatic nerve;

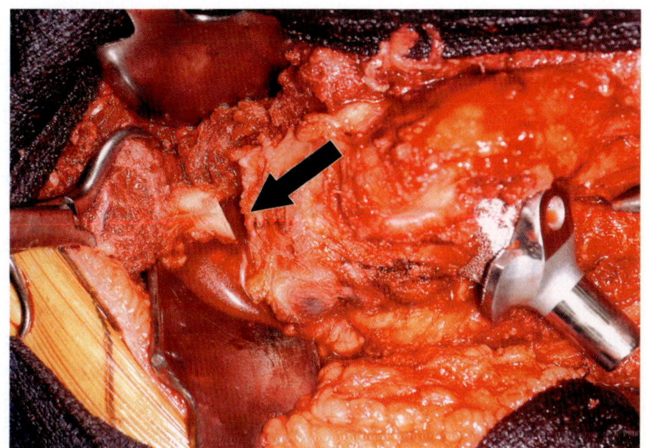

Figure 5–65 *As the real femoral stem with a porous coating is impacted, the proximal and distal fragments are compressed together at the osteotomy site (arrow).*

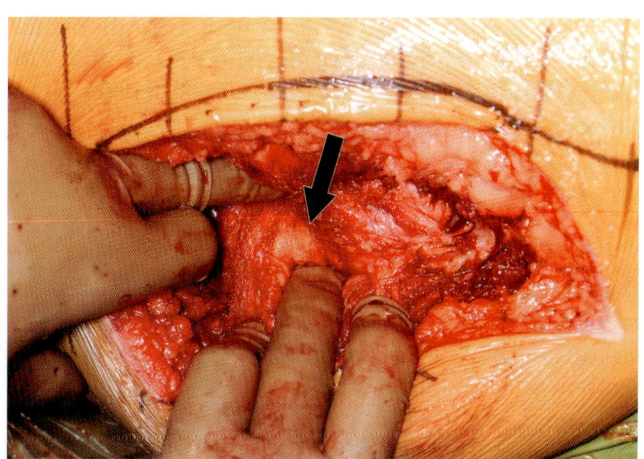

Figure 5–67 *The sciatic nerve (arrow) is palpated in the wound as the knee is flexed and extended. The sciatic nerve should remain soft and malleable during extension of the knee. If the nerve is tight like a banjo string, then the leg is too long.*

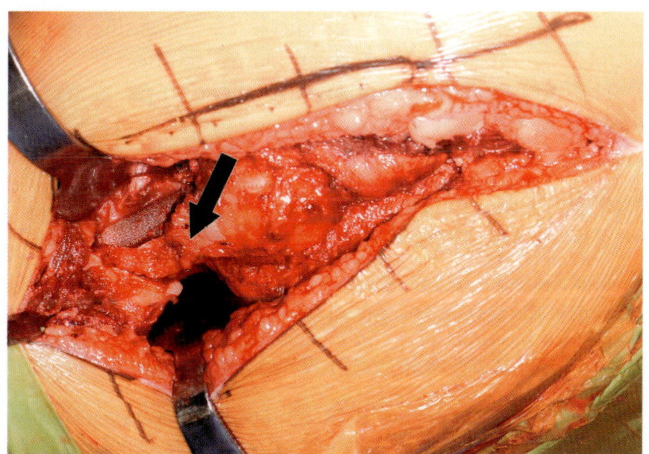

Figure 5–66 *The osteotomy has complete apposition posteriorly (arrow). There is an interior defect from removal of the plate that exposes a portion of the femoral stem. The femoral head has been reduced into the acetabulum, and the leg is rotated to ensure rotational stability of the osteotomy. The stability of the hip is also confirmed by moving the leg through its range of motion.*

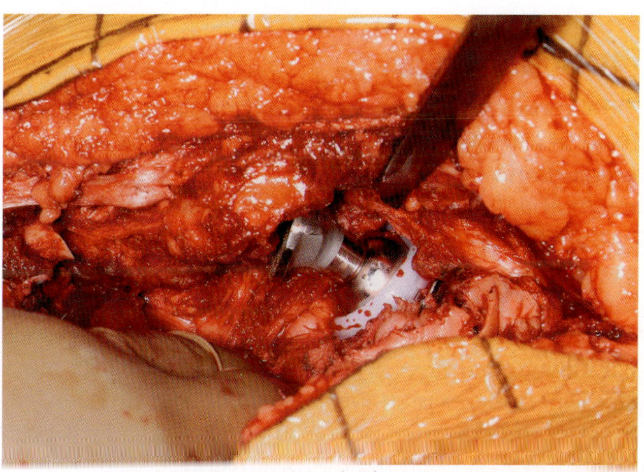

Figure 5–68 *The hip is reduced. The osteotomy site is visible at the far left and shows good apposition. The coverage of the head is nearly symmetrical with the leg held in 30 degrees of internal rotation. In this photograph, the amount of internal rotation can be estimated from the direction in which the collar of the stem points.*

the final length of the leg is comparatively unimportant. It is therefore imperative to test the softness of the sciatic nerve for each hip reduced to ensure its safety. With the hip reduced, the surgeon tests the sciatic nerve for tension by palpating the nerve with his or her finger and moving the leg from a knee-flexed position of 90 degrees to full extension (Fig. 5–67). As the knee is moved from flexion to full extension, the sciatic nerve should remain soft and should not tighten like a banjo string. If the hip is stable throughout its range of motion, with no push/pull laxity, and the sciatic nerve is mobile, then a successful reconstruction of the femoral side has been accomplished. The femoral head should be sym-metrical in the acetabulum with the leg at 30 to 40 degrees of internal rotation (Fig. 5–68).

Postoperative Care

If the rotational stability of the femur is uncertain, a postoperative cast allows the bone to heal before the patient is allowed off crutches and bearing weight. In case of questionable hip joint stability after complete removal of the capsule for the acetabular reconstruction, the patient should be casted or braced for 6 to 8 weeks to allow the capsule to re-form. If the leg remains short, a shoe lift must be prescribed to allow as normal a gait as possible, which optimizes hip joint forces as well as the patient's comfort. Patient education must focus on the importance of the shoe lift so that cosmetic considerations do not overrule its benefits.

ACETABULAR PREPARATION OF PROTRUSIO ACETABULI

The unique geometry of protrusio acetabuli requires adaptation of the acetabular preparation. Primarily, with protrusio acetabuli the acetabular depression is significantly medialized and the walls of the acetabulum can be thinner, especially in rheumatoid arthritis. Preparation of protrusio acetabuli may involve the use of a bone graft to provide medial acetabular support (otherwise the dome of the cup would have a gap behind it). Protrusio acetabuli is better suited to cementless than to cemented reconstruction because there is no cancellous bone for cement interdigitation. I do not recommend cemented reconstruction of protrusio acetabuli.

Technique

The exposure for preparation and implantation of protrusio acetabuli does not differ from that in the usual osteoarthritic acetabulum. Most commonly, protrusio acetabuli is found in patients with rheumatoid arthritis. Protrusio acetabuli develops in some patients with osteoarthritis, particularly medial osteoarthritis. The principle of protrusio acetabular reconstruction is founded on a press-fit of the cup into the bony acetabular cavity regardless of whether it is fully seated medially: a peripheral press-fit is essential, but medially the dome of the cup may not be in contact with host bone because of the depth of the protrusion.

The pattern of acetabular reaming is different from that used for the osteoarthritic acetabulum, in that the medial wall is not initially reamed with protrusio acetabuli. The reaming is done to determine the size of the acetabular cavity. The reamer must touch the peripheral walls of the acetabulum, which are almost always circular, because peripheral wall deformity is rare in protrusio acetabuli. Once the size of the acetabulum has been determined with the reamer, the distance between the medial side of the reamer and the depth of the medial wall can be determined. If this is more than 5 mm, a bone graft will be necessary. If it is 5 mm or less, the acetabulum can be reamed an additional size to allow a full fit of the acetabular component. If the metal edges of the acetabular component sit below the bony edges of the osseous acetabulum when a full fit is present, a protrusio-type acetabular plastic insert can be used to bring the edge of the plastic to the osseous

periphery as well as restore the center of rotation to a more correct position.

If a bone graft is needed, its size should be such that after insertion of the acetabular component, the metal edge of the acetabular component is at the osseous periphery of the acetabulum in the correct acetabular position (25 degrees anteversion, 40 to 45 degrees abduction). The bone graft is best formed by taking from the femoral head a slice that can be impacted into the medial acetabulum and reamed so that the circular dome of the cup will fit into the graft. The acetabular cup should be fixed with at least one screw to provide stability. When the metal edge of the cup sits at the osseous periphery of the acetabulum, a standard acetabular insert can be used, with or without a hood, depending on the anteversion of the cup. The size of the femoral head depends on the size of the cup used. Stability of the construct is tested by striking the edge of the cup with a bone tamp and mallet. The cup should not move with firm but not vigorous malleting of its edge. Malleting the tamp should elicit a metallic ringing sound, which is the sound of secure fixation.

The femoral preparation for these hips is as described in Chapter 6.

References

1. Maruyama M, Feinberg JR, Capello WN, D'Antonio JA: Morphologic features of the acetabulum and femur: Anteversion angle and implant positioning. Clin Orthop 393:52-65, 2001.
2. Garvin KL, Bowen MK, Salvati EA, Ranawat CS: Long-term results of total hip arthroplasty in congenital dislocation and dysplasia of the hip: A followup note. J Bone Joint Surg Am 73:1348-1354, 1991.
3. Hartofilakidis G, Stamos K, Karchalios T, et al: Congenital hip disease in adults: Classification of acetabular deficiencies and operative treatment with acetabuloplasty combined with total hip arthroplasty. J Bone Joint Surg Am 78:683-692, 1996.
4. Garcia-Cimbrelo E, Munuera L: Low friction arthroplasty in severe acetabular dysplasia. J Arthroplasty 8:459-469, 1993.
5. MacKenzie JR, Kelley SS, Johnston RC: Total hip replacement for Coxarthrosis secondary to congenital dysplasia and dislocation of the hip: Long term results. J Bone Joint Surg Am 78:55-61, 1996.
6. Jasty M, Anderson MJ, Harris WH: Total hip replacement for developmental dysplasia of a hip. Clin Orthop 311:40-45, 1995.
7. Dunn HK, Hess WE: Total hip reconstruction in chronically dislocated hips. J Bone Joint Surg Am 58:838-845, 1976.
8. Dorr LD, Tawakkol S, Moorthy M, et al: Medial protrusio technique for placement of a porous-coated, hemispherical acetabular component without cement in a total hip arthroplasty in patients who have acetabular dysplasia. J Bone Joint Surg Am 81:83-92, 1999.
9. McQueary FG, Johnston RC: Cox arthrosis after congenital dysplasia: Treatment by total hip arthroplasty without acetabular bone grafting. J Bone Joint Surg Am 70:1140-1144, 1988.
10. Johnston RC, Brand RA, Crowinshield RD: Reconstruction of the hip: A mathematical approach to determine optimum geometric relationships. J Bone Joint Surg Am 61:639-652, 1979.

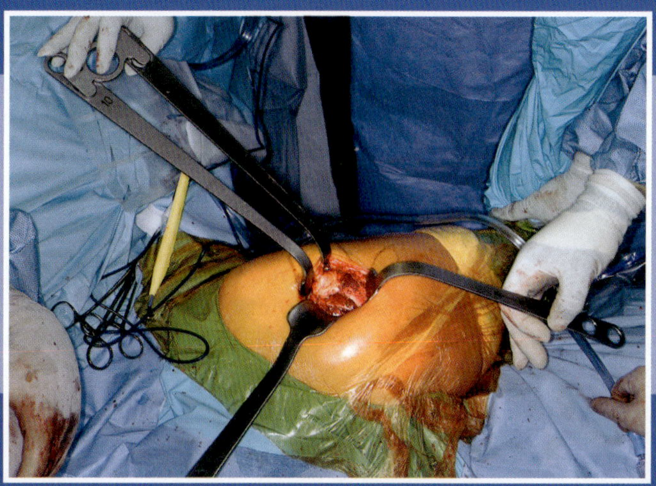

Chapter 6

Posterior Mini-incision: Femoral Preparation*

*In conjunction with this chapter on the DVD-ROM is the video "*Posterior Minimally Invasive Surgery (MIS) Total Hip Replacement.*"

Most orthopedic surgeons find preparation and implantation of the femur easier than the acetabular procedure. Because hip fractures often are treated with hemiarthroplasties, the femoral procedure is more common; in addition, implantation of the stem into the femur involves less complex orientation than is needed for implantion of the acetabular component.

EXPOSURE

With the posterior approach, the femur is exposed by lifting the leg from the table and placing it in flexion and internal rotation. The leg should not be internally rotated to a full 90 degrees (Fig. 6–1). The tissues are more relaxed and the first retractors can be placed more easily if both internal rotation and flexion are approximately 60 degrees. The "jaws" retractor (the #8 retractor in the mini-incision instrument set; Fig. 6–2) is

placed under the anterior side of the cut femoral neck. The jaws retractor is best placed before removal of the "snake" retractor (Fig. 6–3). The snake retractor improves visualization of the femoral neck, particularly when the mini-incision is used, and facilitates engaging the #8 retractor under the anterior neck. Once the jaws retractor is engaged, the snake retractor is removed and the jaws can be fully seated (Fig. 6–4). The #8 retractor is wide enough to depress the posterior wound flap with minimal tension to the skin. The #4 retractor is placed under the quadratus femoris, which is retained in the mini-incision, and on the medial neck to expose the cut edge of the medial neck (Fig. 6–5). The leg now can be placed into a full 90 degrees of internal rotation and usually can be flexed to 70 degrees without difficulty. In men with large muscles and in any obese leg, the leg may be difficult to position because it does not drop easily over the side of the table, and therefore the femur is not lifted as easily into the wound. This requires applying more force with the retractors, and in some patients the mini-incision will also need to be lengthened, although this should involve only the skin and subcutaneous tissue. With an extended incision, the jaws retractor can more effectively depress the posterior wound, thus placing the cut femoral neck more centrally in the wound and making it more accessible.

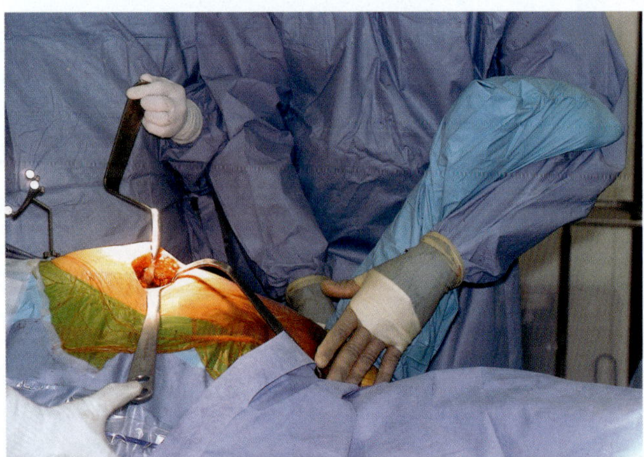

Figure 6–1 *Leg position for initial placement of femoral retractors. The leg is in approximately 60 degrees of internal rotation and 60 degrees of flexion and is resting on the lower leg.*

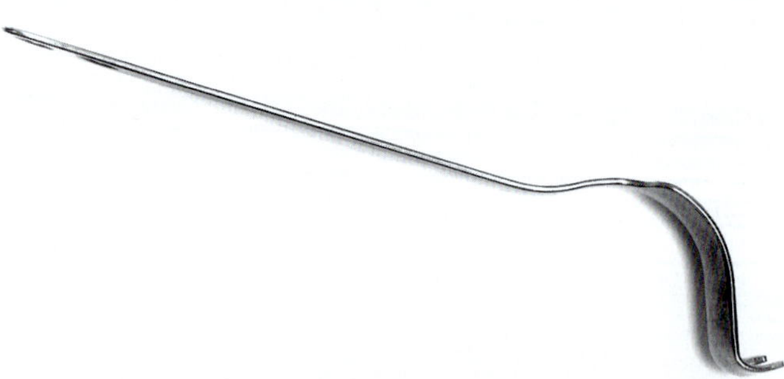

Figure 6–2 *The #8 (jaws) retractor has a radius of curvature that effectively depresses the posterior flap of the wound for exposure of the cut femoral neck.*

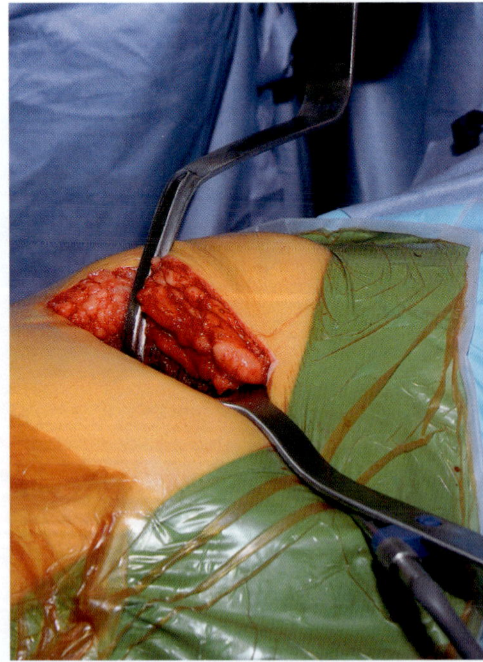

Figure 6–3 *The jaws retractor (on the right) is placed under the femoral neck with the #5 (snake) retractor still in position so that some exposure into the depth of the hip is possible.*

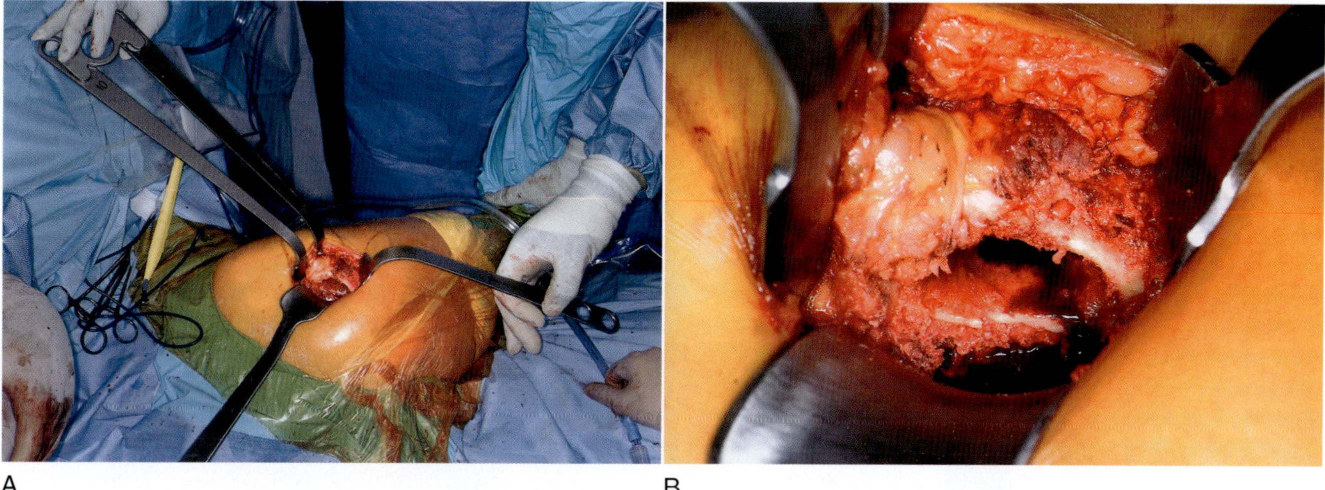

A   B

Figure 6–4   **A,** *The jaws (#8) retractor is engaged under the femoral neck (on the anterior femoral neck) and the paddle of the retractor depresses the posterior wound to expose the cut femoral neck. The long handle of the #8 retractor extends to the bottom of the view. The #3 (or #4) retractor is against the medial femoral neck, retracting the quadratus femoris. The #9 and #10 retractors are placed so that the #9 retractor is over the top of the greater trochanter and the #10 retractor retracts the gluteus medius tendon. These are linked by a joint at their ends that can be held with one finger by the assistant.* **B,** *Close-up view of the hip with the #8 retractor elevating the cut femoral neck into the wound. The #3 retractor is at right, and the #9 and #10 retractors at left.*

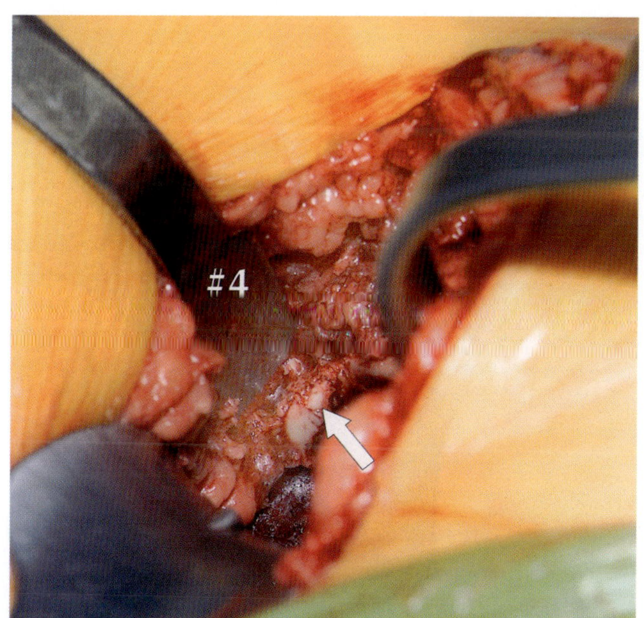

Figure 6–5   *Close-up view of the #4 retractor retracting the quadratus femoris muscle from the cut edge of the medial femoral neck (arrow).*

An alternative #8 retractor is thinner and has a different radius of curvature for wound depression (Fig. 6–6). It works well with thin patients, and its reduced width interferes less with broach and stem insertion.

The final retractor, the #9 retractor in the mini-incision instrument set, is placed superior to the tip of the greater trochanter and retracts the gluteus medius tendon and muscle to protect them from injury during reaming and broaching (Fig. 6–7). In patients with large muscles or obesity, a second retractor sometimes is needed over the tip of the greater trochanter to retract the gluteus maximus muscle and the subcutaneous tissue. If this is necessary, the #9 and #10 retractors from the mini-incision set can be linked together to facilitate manipulation (see Fig. 6–4), and with these retractors in place the cut medial neck is exposed in the wound.

PREPARATION AND IMPLANTATION: CEMENTLESS TECHNIQUE

The preparation of the femur begins with removal of the bone wax from the cut surface of the femoral neck with a curette. Any soft tissue left over the remaining lateral cortical neck also should be removed (Fig. 6–8); this exposes any remaining lateral cortical neck, which can then be cut and extracted with a box chisel (Fig. 6–9). A box chisel is used because sometimes the bone is too strong to be removed with a burr, and if it is left in place it can force the prosthesis into an unwanted varus position (Fig. 6–10). After the remaining lateral cortical neck is removed, the entire elliptical surface of the cut femoral neck is visible (Fig. 6–11). With the posterior mini-incision, the quadratus femoris muscle occludes the remainder of the femoral neck and the

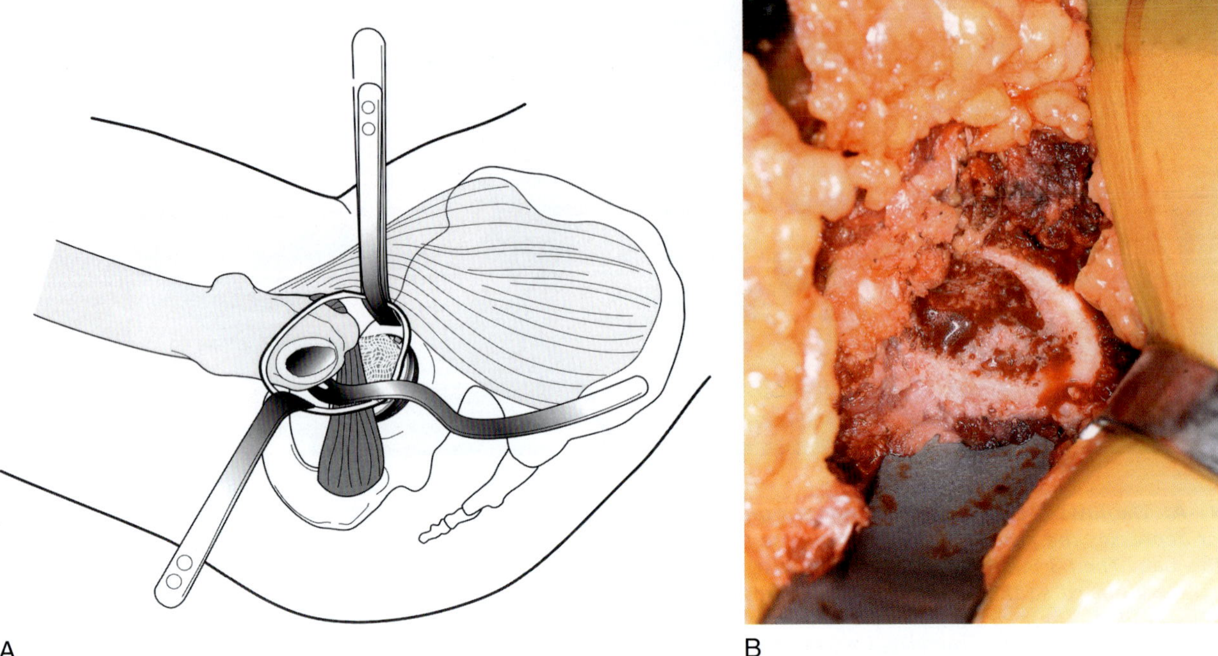

A

B

Figure 6–6   **A,** *The #8b retractor, which also can be used to depress the posterior flap and elevate the cut femoral neck into the wound.* **B,** *Close-up view of the hip with the #8b retractor under the anterior neck and elevating the femoral neck into the wound.*

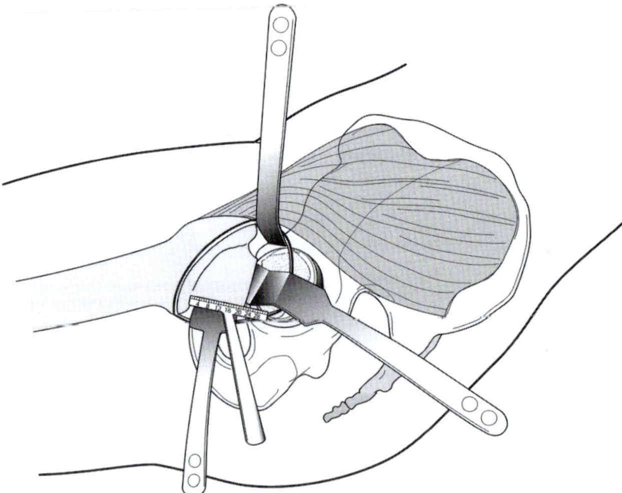

Figure 6–7   *The #9 retractor at the top of the wound retracting the gluteus medius tendon and muscle just superior to the tip of the greater trochanter. The #8 retractor is under the femoral neck, and the #3 retractor is on the medial femoral neck. A ruler measures the cut femoral neck.*

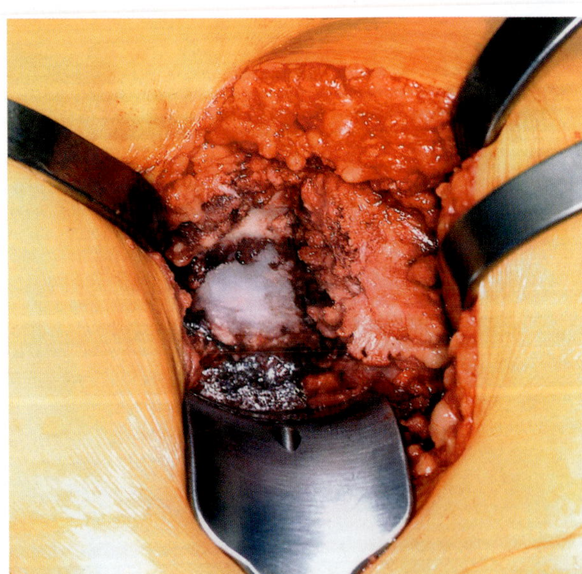

Figure 6–8   *The cut femoral neck is covered with bone wax. Tissue covers the remaining cortical bone of the lateral femoral neck. The tip of the greater trochanter is visible extending above the femoral neck, just to the right of the #8 retractor.*

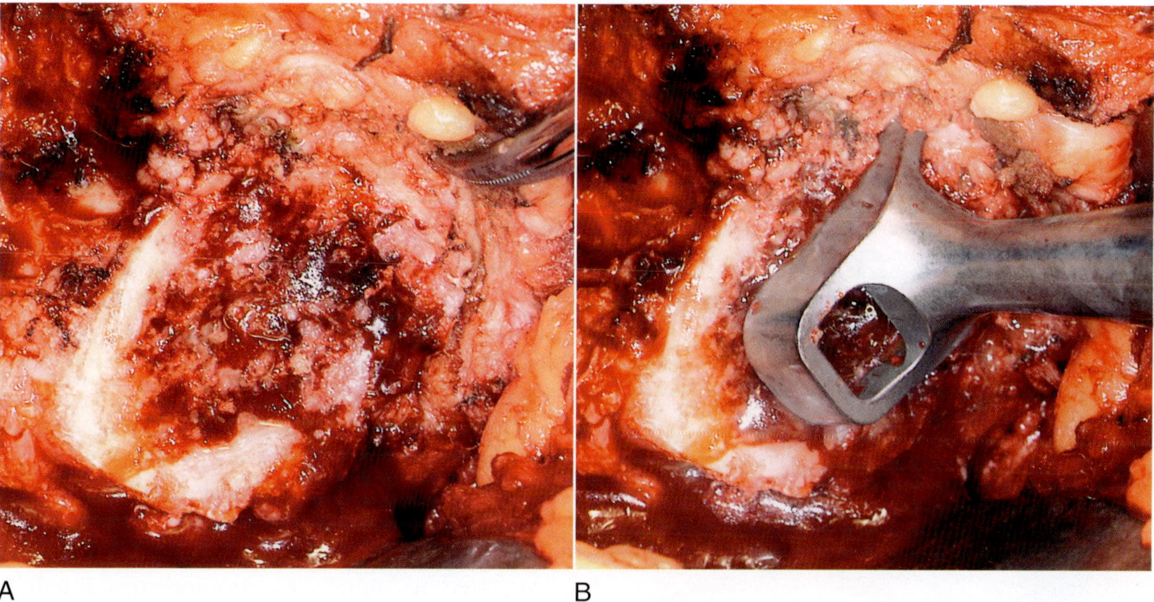

A   B

Figure 6–9 **A,** *The tissue has been removed and the remaining cortical bone of the lateral neck is exposed under the tip of the tonsil clamp.* **B,** *The box chisel has cut the lateral cortical bone so that it can be removed.*

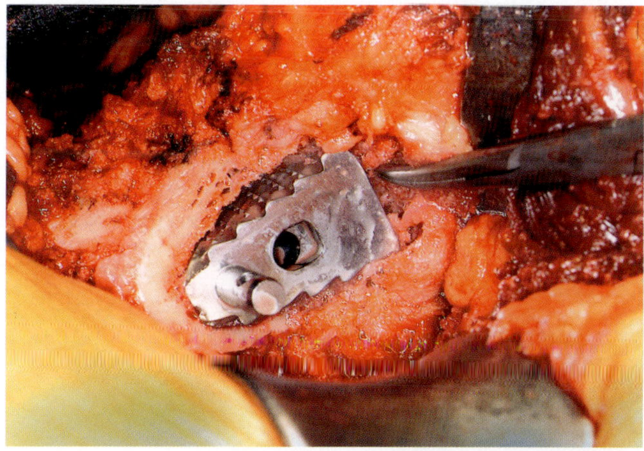

Figure 6–10 *Remaining lateral cortical bone can push the broach into a varus position, potentially to a degree sufficient to fracture the lateral diaphyseal cortex. This bone must be removed with the burr and then with a trochanteric reamer to ensure that it does not impede the safe preparation of the femoral canal.*

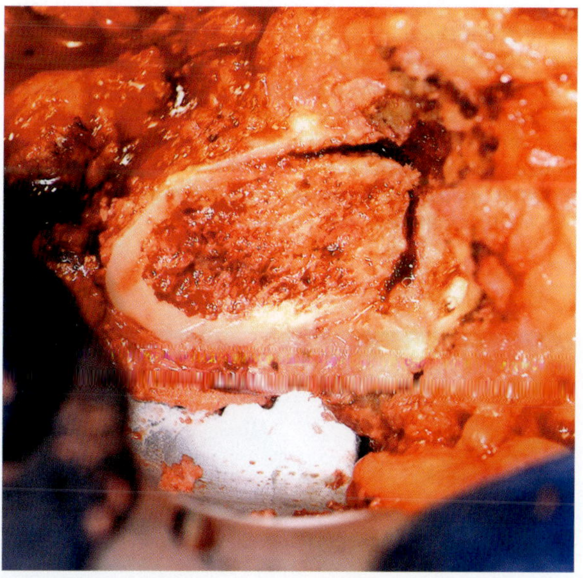

Figure 6–11 *The entire elliptical cancellous bone of the femoral neck is visualized after removal of the lateral femoral neck.*

lesser trochanter; complete familiarity with the instrumentation is necessary for the surgeon to prepare the femur under conditions of limited visibility.

The level of femoral neck cut desired to balance the hip length and offset (and correct the leg length) has been determined from preoperative templates. With a standard posterior incision and release of the quadratus femoris muscle, the greater trochanter and the entire femoral neck, including the lesser trochanter, are visible, and the surgeon has a better all-around view of the proximal femur. In this case, a ruler can be placed against the point where the superior lesser trochanter joins the femoral neck (see Fig. 6–7) to measure the length of the neck cut and match it with the length determined from preoperative templating. Computer navigation can determine the level of the neck cut (see Chapter 7). If the quadratus femoris is retained, however, the lesser trochanter will not be visible and the cut must be made from the base of the femoral head (Fig. 6–12). The correctness of the level of this cut can be determined only when trialing is done with the broach in place, which determines the length of femoral head used and hence the balance

of hip length and offset with the trial components in place.

Tapered Stem with Wedge Fit

This section describes preparation of the femur for a stem such as the Alloclassic/Zweymüller (Zimmer, Warsaw, Ind.), which requires broaching only (Fig. 6–13). This stem has a good record of fixation and durability.[1] The dedicated box chisel for this stem should be used to set the direction of anteversion and remove the lateral neck so that varus is avoided and correct anteversion obtained (Fig. 6–14).

Begin with a broach that is at least three sizes smaller than the size templated; it is not necessary to begin with the smallest broach in the set and move sequentially through each size to the final size. However, if the broach three sizes smaller than the anticipated final size gives excessive resistance or requires too much force for seating, it should be removed and a smaller broach selected. The broach is seated to the stage line, which is the flat surface of the broach where the broad holder connects. The broach is used to rasp the lateral endosteal surface of the femur and the trochanteric bed (Fig. 6–15). By rasping laterally with each successive size, a varus stem position is avoided. Each broach size is malleted sequentially into position. When the final broach is seated, a "cortical" feel and sound will be appreciated. The broach must be stable axially and rotationally.

The broach is removed and a trial stem and head are used to identify the head length necessary for correct

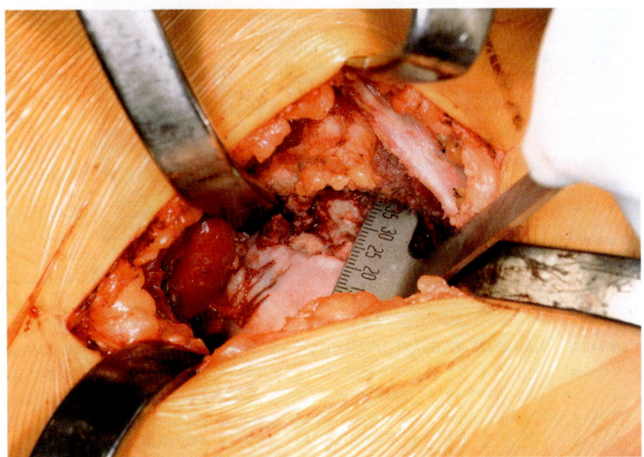

Figure 6–12 *The ruler measures the level of the femoral neck cut from the base of the femoral head. At the distal end of the ruler, the quadratus femoris muscle is being retracted by the #4 retractor, which is under the ruler. The #2 retractor is on the superior femoral neck, retracting the gluteus medius tendon from the field of the femoral neck so it will not be injured while the neck is cut with the saw. The level of the neck cut is measured from the distal femoral head because the lesser trochanter is not visible.*

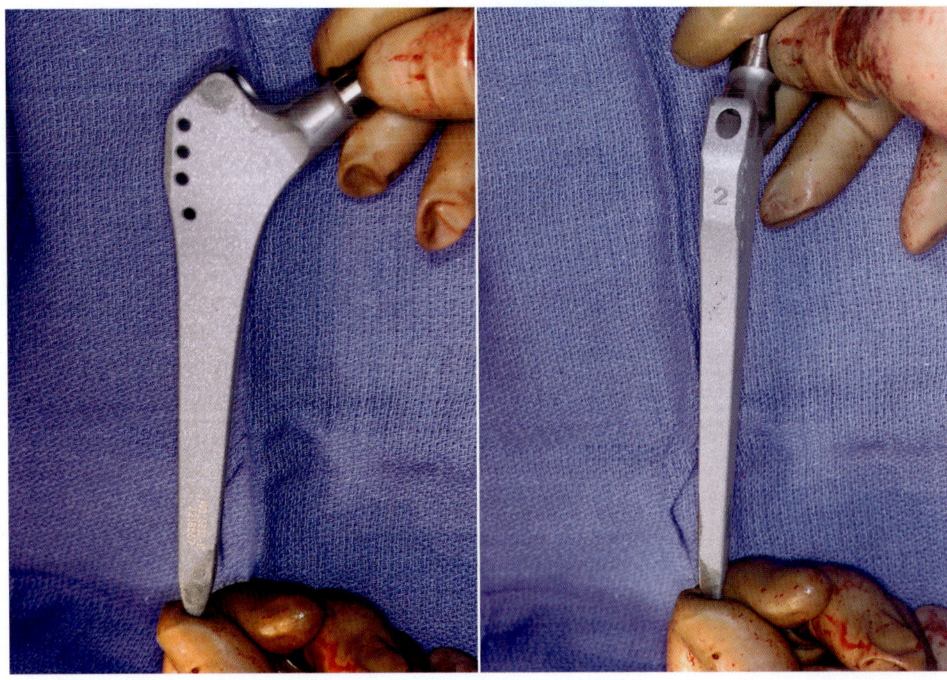

A   B

Figure 6–13 A, *Mediolateral view of the Alloclassic (Zweymüller) stem. This fully grit-blasted stem permits bone fixation over its entire length. **B,** Anteroposterior view of the Alloclassic stem on a lateral x-ray. This profile shows the stem's thin, tapered wedge geometry.*

leg length and offset. The lateral side of the trial should lie under the tip of the greater trochanter for a positive "anti-varus sign" (Fig. 6–16). If it is necessary to reduce offset to balance the offset and hip length, a stem one size larger can be used (Fig. 6–17); conversely, if it is necessary to increase the offset, one size smaller can be used. The final size for the stem should be determined by the fit in the canal and the correct balance of offset and hip length.

Hip length is determined by palpating the relationship of the lesser trochanter to the ischium (Fig. 6–18). Leg length can be confirmed using the surgeon's preferred method; these choices are described later in the chapter. Offset is checked by ensuring clearance of the trochanter from the pelvis by 1 fingerbreadth throughout the range of motion, including extension with external rotation and flexion with internal rotation (Fig. 6–19). The metal femoral neck is palpated to confirm that it does not impinge against the metal edge of the acetabular cup. Finally, the lesser trochanter should clear the ischium by 1 fingerbreadth in extension and external rotation.

The trial is removed and the stem is inserted (Fig. 6–20). The stem can be manually pushed to the last 2 cm and is simply malleted into its rotationally stable position (Fig. 6–21). The stem should feel solid as it is malleted into its final position and should sound as if it is against cortical bone as it is seated. With the stem in position, the femoral head trial is again placed on the stem, and the hip is again taken through the range of motion and the leg length confirmed. The final head is placed onto the stem, and closure accomplished.

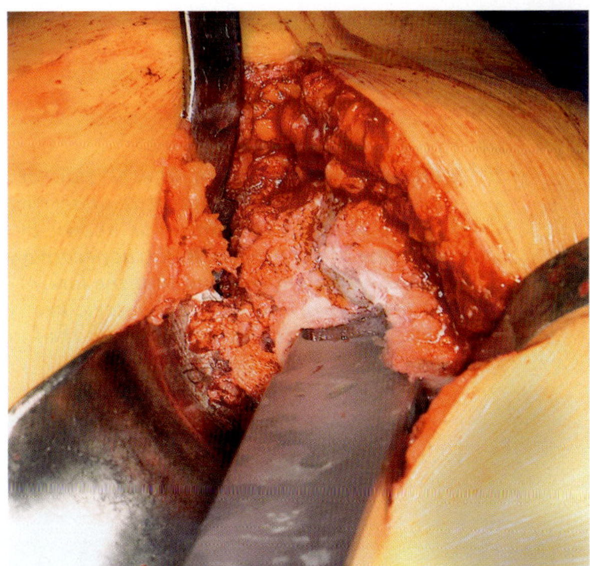

Figure 6–14 *Box chisel for the Alloclassic (Zweymüller) stem is used to prepare the proximal femur for the broach. Note that the chisel is placed parallel to the posterior cortex of the femoral neck so that the femur is not fractured by broaching in an incorrect anteversion angle.*

Anatomic Stem (APR)

The APR prosthesis (Zimmer) is an example of an anatomic stem that uses reaming for preparation of the

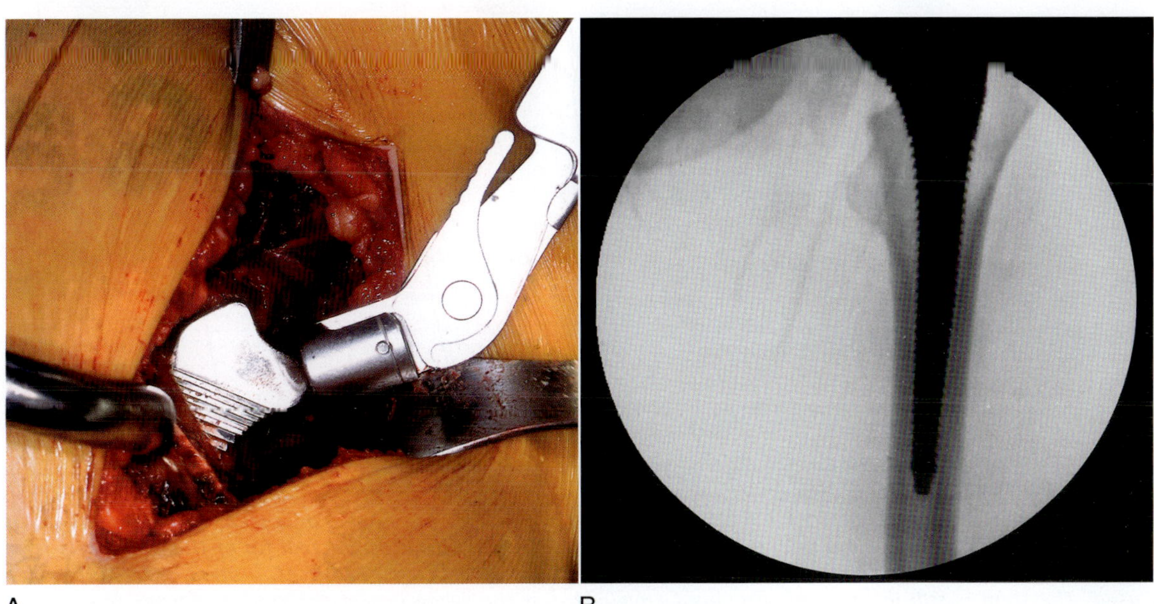

A B

Figure 6–15 *A, The Alloclassic broach is inserted sequentially into the femur until it will no longer seat beyond the stage line, which is the junction of the smooth and rough surfaces. This broach can also be used to rasp the lateral femoral bone to ensure that the stem is not placed into varus. B, Fluoroscopic view of the Alloclassic broach insertion into the femur, demonstrating that the broach is touching cortical bone and is not in varus.*

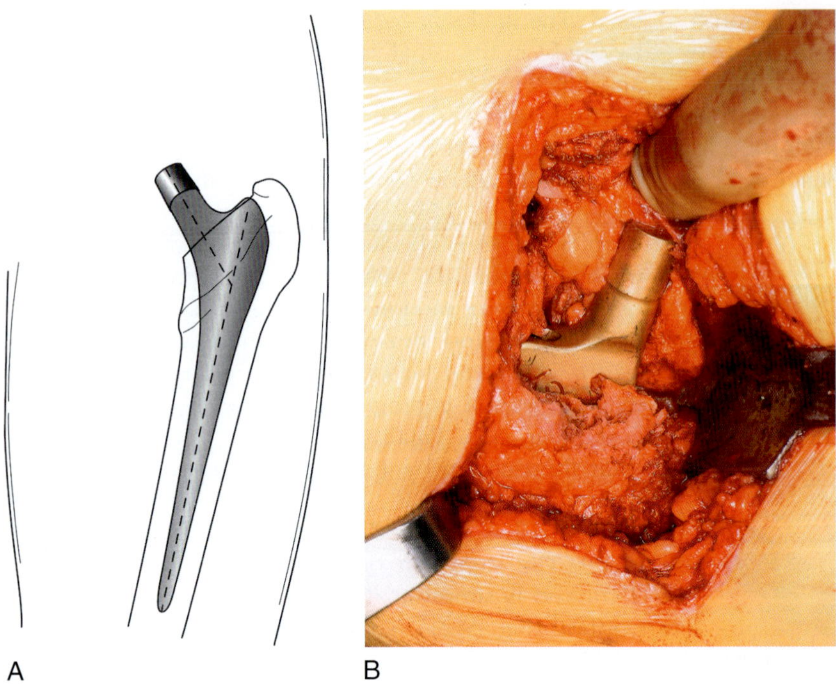

Figure 6–16 **A,** The lateral side of the broach is aligned so that it is under the tip of the greater trochanter, as shown by the axis line of the broach. **B,** Intraoperative view of the trial stem showing that the lateral side of the trial is into the trochanteric bed, with the tip of the trochanter overlying the lateral side of the trial.

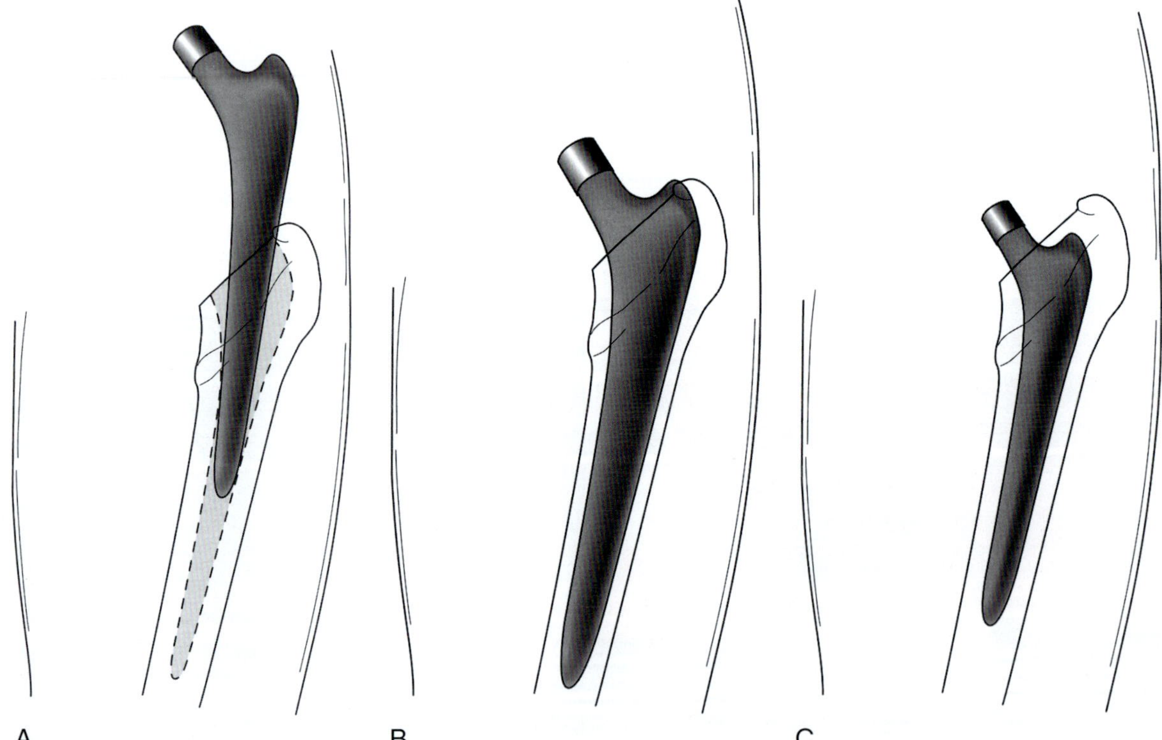

Figure 6–17 **A,** The stem is inserted into the envelope prepared by the broach. **B,** The depth to which the broach is inserted varies according to the size of the stem that will be placed into the prepared envelope. For a stem the same size as the broach, the stem will insert to the same level as the broach, which normally means that the lateral tip of the prosthesis is at the level of the tip of the greater trochanter. **C,** If it is necessary to shorten the hip length or offset, a stem one size smaller than the broach is used. The stem is still in the same prepared envelope, but the stage line of the stem is deeper into the metaphysis, which allows shortening of the hip length and offset when the same head length is used.

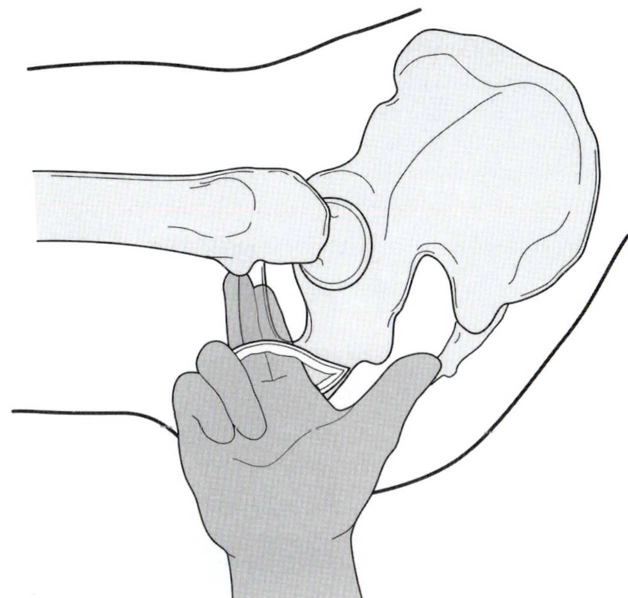

Figure 6–18 *The lesser trochanter is palpated to determine its relationship to the tip of the ischium. The tip of the lesser trochanter should never be below the tip of the ischium because this indicates that the leg has been lengthened.*

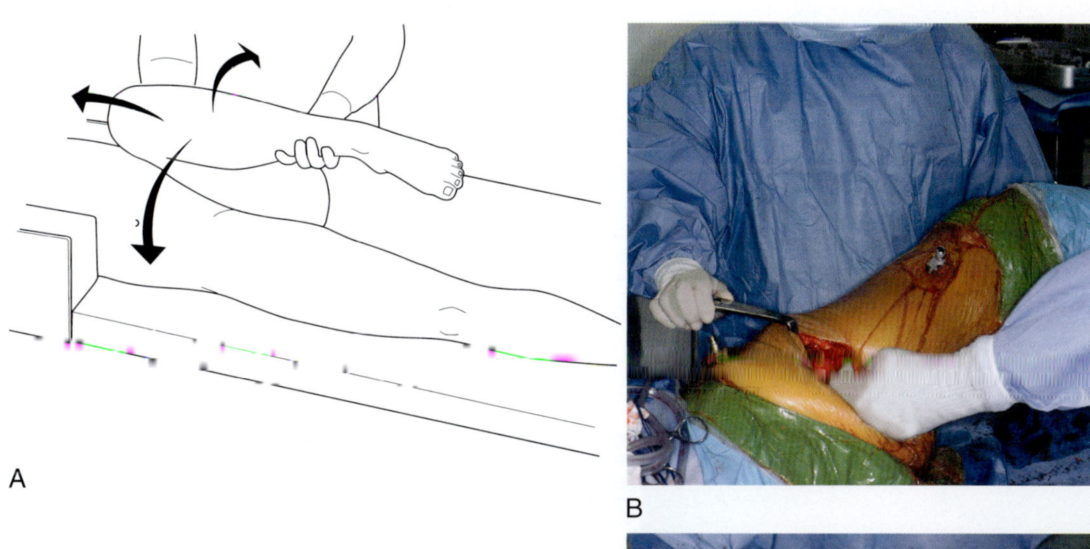

A

B

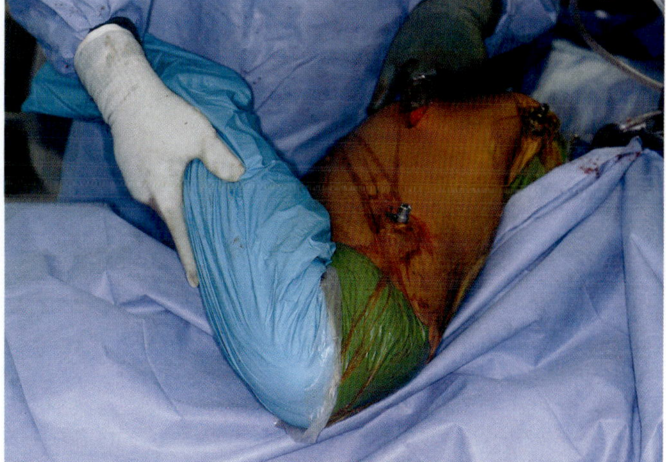

C

Figure 6–19 ***A,*** *The leg is moved through an entire range of motion with the surgeon's left hand, while the index finger of the right hand palpates the clearance of the trochanter from the pelvis and the metal neck from the cup.* ***B,*** *The surgeon's left index finger, visible behind the greater trochanter, palpates the clearance between the trochanter and the pelvis as the leg is brought into extension.* ***C,*** *The surgeon's right hand (white glove) flexes and internally rotates the leg while the left hand (green glove at upper right) palpates the clearance of the trochanter against the pelvis and the metal femoral neck against the cup anteriorly. The metal base for the computer guidance system is attached to the distal femur.*

femoral canal (Fig. 6–22). I use the APR prosthesis because I believe the anatomic shape gives the most stable press-fit with rotational stability. In my experience, the proximal porous coating and distal grit-blasted surface provide fixation that gives the patient an excellent clinical result with long-term durability. However, any type of prosthesis that uses reaming for the canal can be implanted with this hip exposure and approach.

A box chisel is used to remove the lateral cortical bone (Fig. 6–23). A burr can be used to open the femoral canal for insertion of the reamers and broaches (Fig. 6–24). Once the canal has been established, the preparation is sequential and easily accomplished.

Reaming is done sequentially until the bone grips the reamer over approximately a 5-cm length, which will allow a good prosthetic fit (Fig. 6–25). The reamers are "self-centering" by design, which keeps the reamer center in the intramedullary canal. A trochanteric reamer is used to open the trochanteric bed for ease of broaching and proper lateral positioning of the stem (Fig. 6–26).

With the APR, once the femoral canal size is established by reaming, the appropriate broaches are used to prepare the canal for stem implantation (Fig. 6–27). The broach (and therefore the stem) is not in varus if the lateral side of the broach is under the tip of the greater trochanter (Fig. 6–28). The medial side of the broach against the medial neck cannot be taken as an anti-varus sign (Fig. 6–29); the stem portion of the broach is not in varus only if the lateral side of the proximal broach is as lateral as possible—that is, against the bed of the trochanter and under the tip of the greater trochanter.

Inserting the broach with an anatomic stem is not essentially different from inserting the broach with a straight stem. The anatomic stem has a tighter fit and therefore must be malleted harder to achieve a final seat. However, simply aligning the broach with the posterior cortical bone of the femoral neck and inserting it in this plane, as is done with a straight stem, allows a smooth insertion (see Fig. 6–28). How much of the proximal femur the broach fills determines

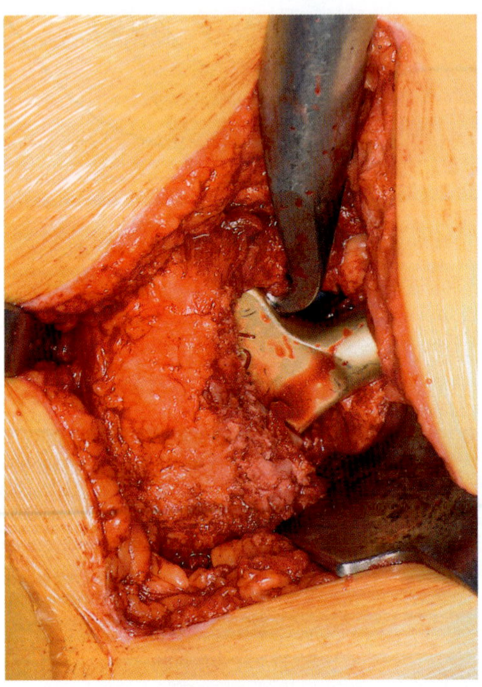

Figure 6–20 *The trial stem is removed by a tool that hooks into an eyelet on the lateral proximal side of the trial.*

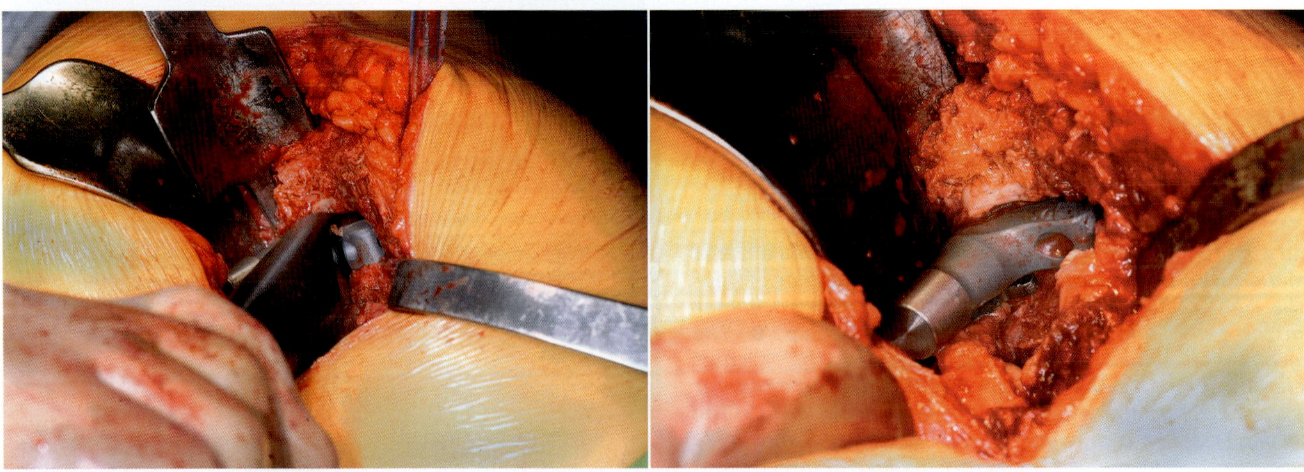

A   B

Figure 6–21 **A,** *A flat impaction tool for the stem can be placed on the lateral shoulder, and a mallet used to drive the stem into the envelope prepared by the broach.* **B,** *The stem has been impacted into its stable position. When it reaches this position, there is a distinct "cortical" sound of the stem against the bone, and the stem will not move any deeper. Note that the posterior surface of the stem is parallel to the posterior neck of the femur.*

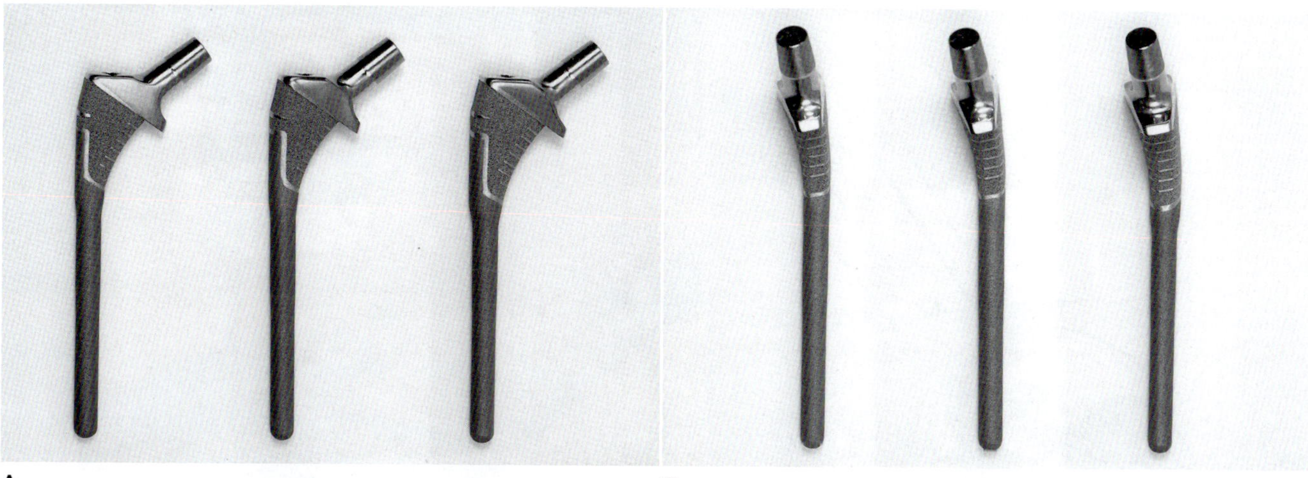

A

B

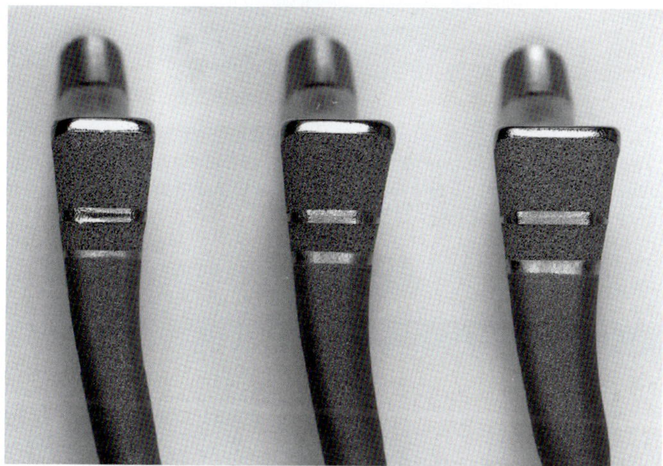

C

Figure 6–22 **A,** *Frontal view of the size 10.5 APR stem, which means that the diameter of the diaphyseal stem is 10.5 mm. Each stem size is available as a standard proximal body, wide proximal body, or oversize stem. The wide body has a wider metaphysis in the anteroposterior plane. The oversize stem means that the metaphysis is one size larger than the diaphyseal size of the stem (e.g., a size 12 standard metaphysis on a 10.5-mm diaphyseal stem). The oversize stem is used in type A bone in which there is a champagne flute femoral geometry.* **B,** *Profile of the size 10.5 stem viewed from the medial side. A 12-degree bend in the proximal stem matches the proximal anatomic bend of the femoral metaphysis. The proximal metaphyseal portion of the stem has porous coating, whereas the diaphysis is grit blasted.* **C,** *Proximal lateral view of the three stem sizes showing the gradual increase in anteroposterior diameter with each size.*

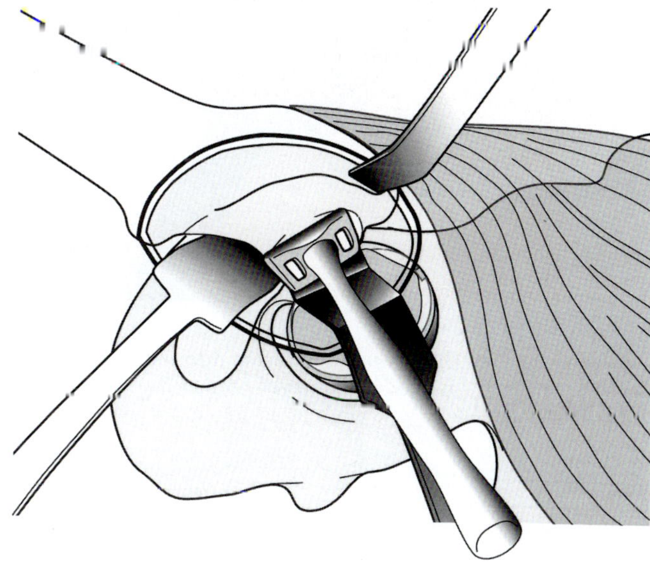

Figure 6–23 *The box chisel is used to remove the lateral femoral neck bone.*

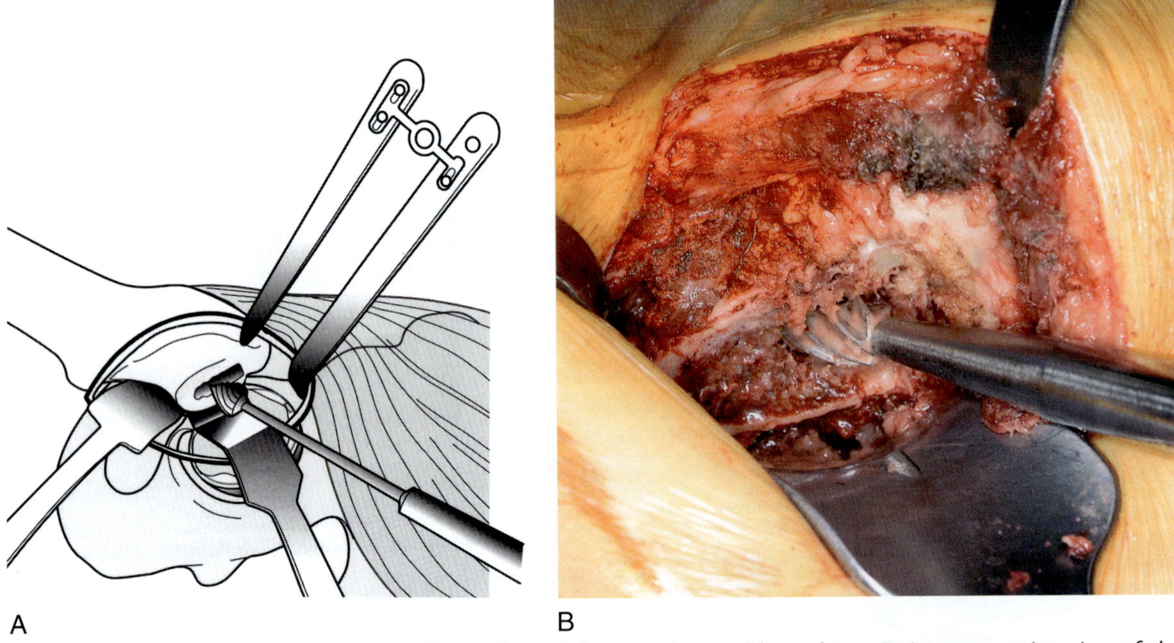

Figure 6–24 **A,** *The burr is used to open the femoral canal for reaming and broaching.* **B,** *Intraoperative view of the burr in correct position for opening the canal. The burr is in the posterosuperior corner of the neck, which will lead directly into the femoral canal.*

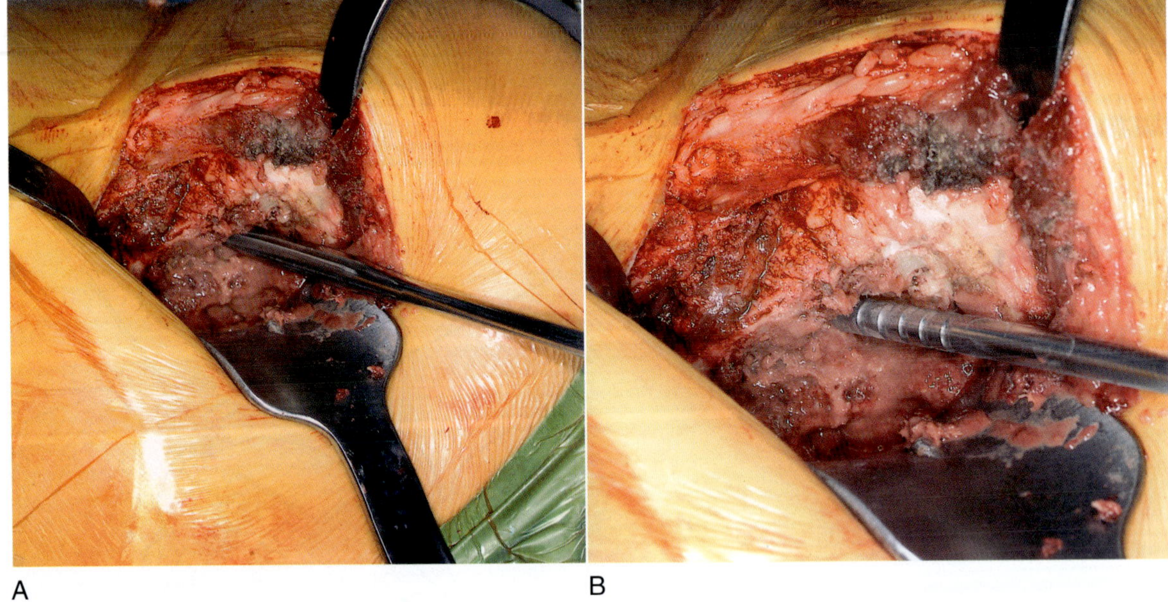

Figure 6–25 **A,** *The reamer is inserted into the opening produced by the burr. The self-cutting flutes of the reamer are visible.* **B,** *The reamer is inserted to the level needed for the length of stem used. The levels are marked by notches on the reamer.*

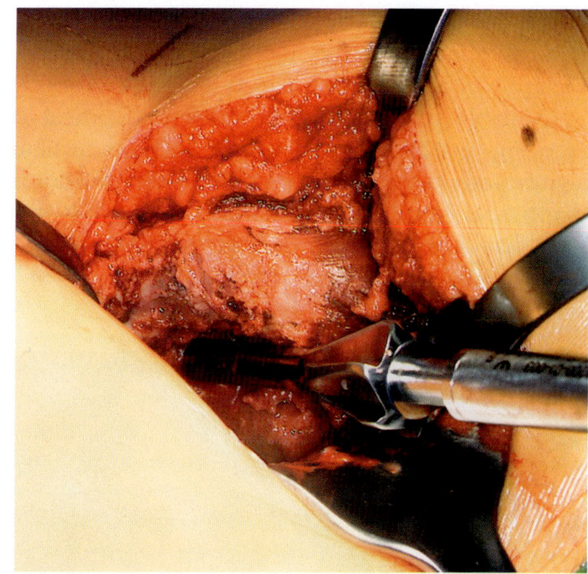

Figure 6–26 *The trochanteric reamer is used to ream the trochanteric bed for ease of broach and stem insertion.*

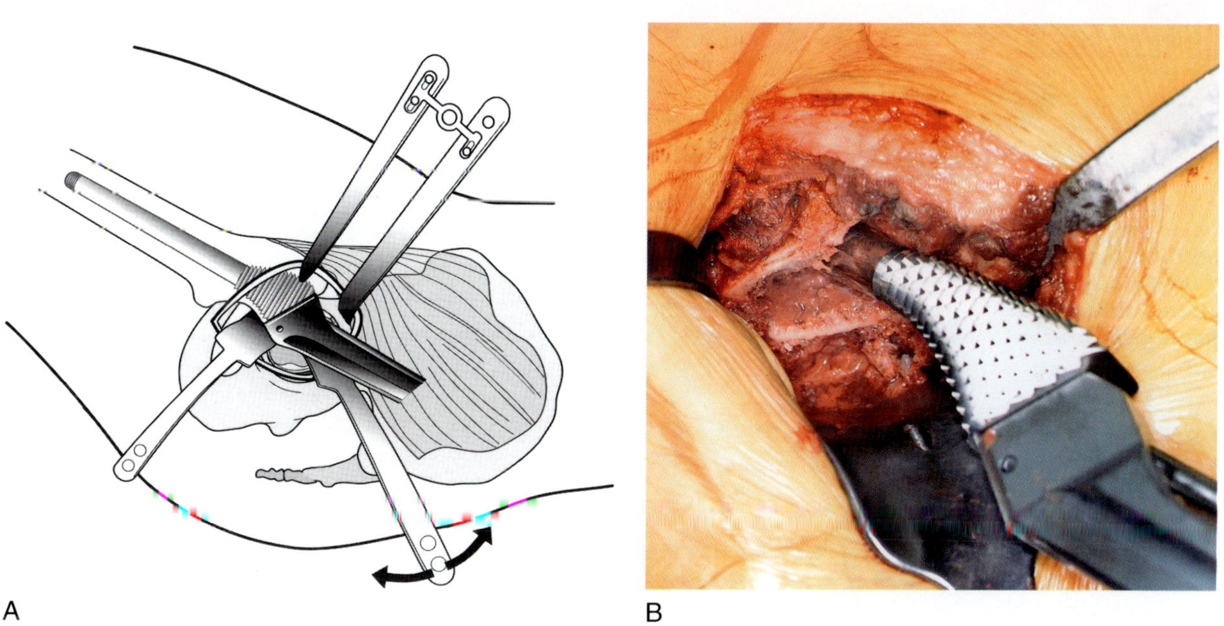

A

B

Figure 6–27 *A, The APR broach is inserted into the canal. The lateral side of the broach should be into the trochanteric bed and ideally under the tip of the greater trochanter. B, Intraoperative view of the APR broach with the stem into the canal. The entrance into the canal is at the posterosuperior corner of the neck, and the broach is crossing the trochanteric bed.*

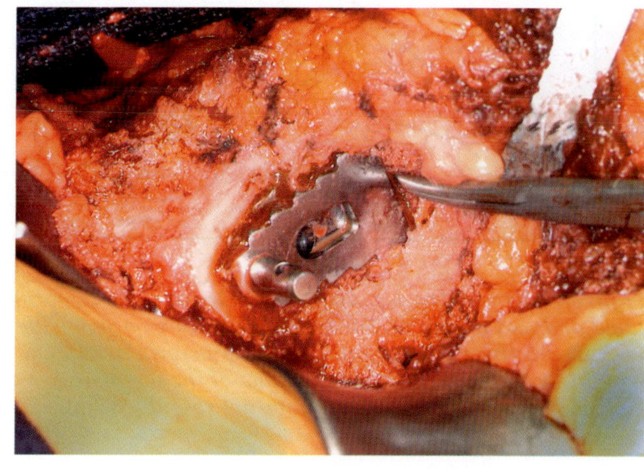

Figure 6–28 *The lateral side of the broach is under the tip of the greater trochanter and into the trochanteric bed (the tip of the tonsil clamp points to the trochanteric bed). Note that the posterior side of the broach is parallel to the posterior femoral cortex and that the broach does not lean into the medial femoral neck. When the lateral side of the broach is under the tip of the greater trochanter, this is the anti-varus sign.*

which stem is selected. The APR stem depends on cortical contact in the metaphysis, so the proximal metaphysis is filled (see Fig. 6–28). A wide-body stem is available to ensure anteroposterior cortical contact (see Fig. 6–22), and an oversize stem is available for significantly tapered (type A) bones that need a narrow diaphyseal stem but a larger metaphyseal stem. If the stem has a good diaphyseal fit but inadequate proxi-

mal fill, the oversized broach should be used to maintain the same diaphyseal size while creating better proximal fill.

With the broach in place, a trial neck and head can be placed and the hip is reduced and taken through its range of motion. Hip length and offset are checked as described previously for the tapered stem (see Fig. 6–19). If the balance of hip length and offset is considered correct, the broach can be removed.

The stem is then inserted into the cut femoral neck at the determined level. The APR stem is available in collared and collarless versions; with the mini-incision, the collarless stem is easier to use and can be left somewhat proud or inserted somewhat deeper. The stem is simply malleted into the "envelope" that has been developed in the femur.

If, as sometimes occurs, the femoral neck impinges against the posterior retractor, there are two choices to seat the femur fully. One option is to internally rotate the leg to clear the femoral neck from the retractor; if this is done, the leg is first lifted from its position over the side of the table and put on the down leg, then internally rotated (Fig. 6–30). If internal rotation is done with the leg over the side of the table, the sciatic nerve can be stretched, causing a sciatic palsy. The second choice is to remove the #8 and #9 retractors (or the combination #9 and #10 retractors, if used) and bury the neck under the skin (Fig. 6–31). With this technique, only the medial neck is left exposed, a disadvantage in terms of visualization during stem implantation. With

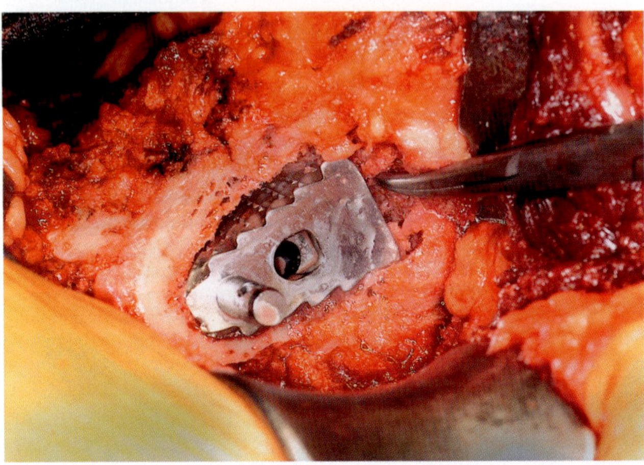

Figure 6–29 *This broach is in varus because its lateral side is medial to the tip of the greater trochanter. The tonsil clamp is against the tip of the greater trochanter, and the lateral side of the broach is medial to the tonsil clamp. The broach also appears to lean into the medial neck, which is another sign that it is in varus.*

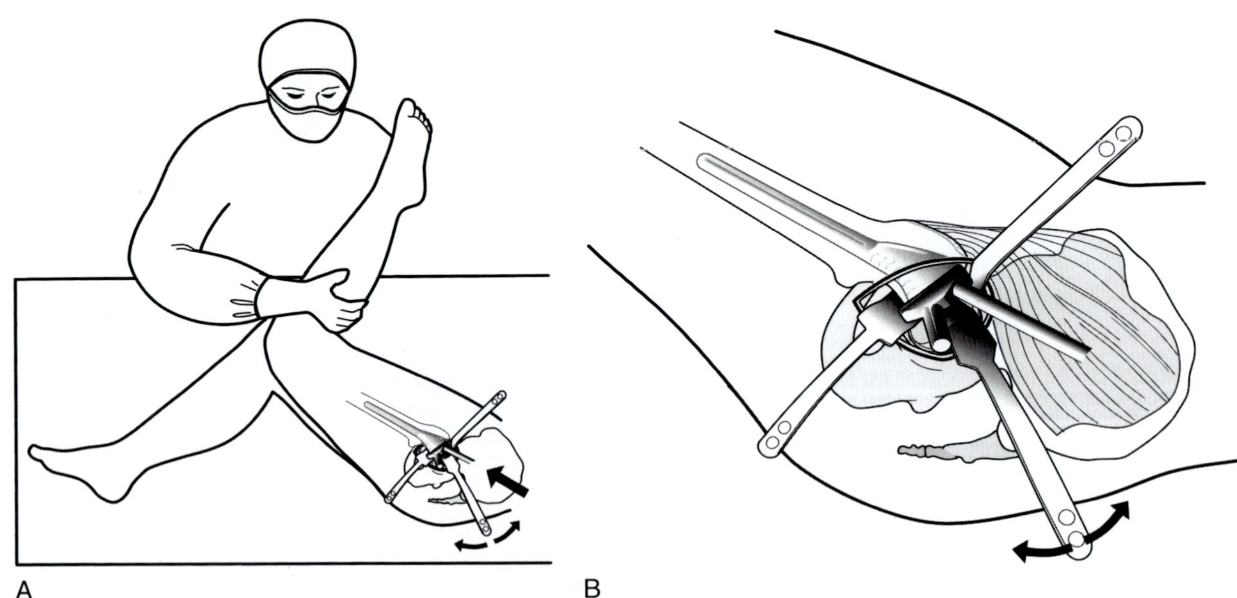

A   B

Figure 6–30 **A,** *The leg position for clearing the femoral neck from the posterior retractor. The leg is brought up onto the table and laid on top of the lower leg. In this position, the leg can be internally rotated by the assistant so that the femoral neck clears the posterior retractor. The arrows at the end of the posterior retractor indicate that this retractor also can be moved back and forth to avoid contact of the metal neck with the retractor.* **B,** *Close-up view of the hip showing the stem clearing the posterior retractor with internal rotation of the leg and movement of the retractor position.*

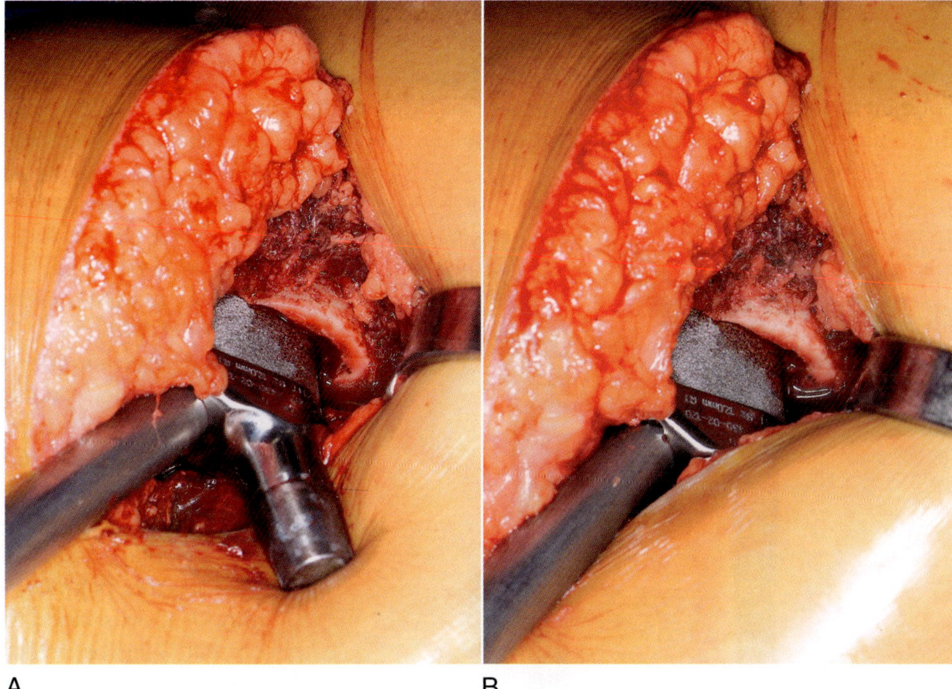

Figure 6–31 **A,** *The femoral neck lies against the posterior wound edge. The #8 and #9 retractors have been removed.* **B,** *The skin and subcutaneous tissue have been lifted over the femoral neck so that the neck is inside the hip. This allows continued impaction of the femoral stem into the femur at the correct anteversion without resistance.*

A   B

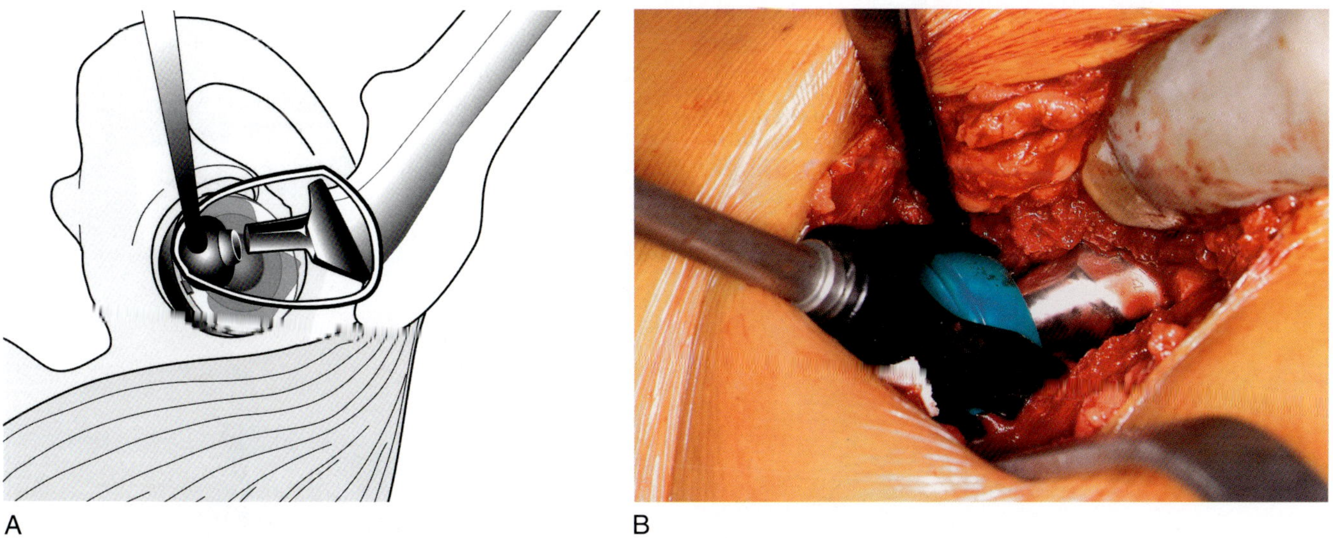

A   B

Figure 6–32 **A,** *The femoral head holder is used to insert the femoral head trial onto the femoral neck inside the confined space of the small incision.* **B,** *Intraoperative view of the femoral head holder inserting the femoral trial onto the femoral neck. The advantage of this tool is that it occupies less space in the wound than the surgeon's hand.*

computer guidance, however, lack of visibility is not an issue, and this is the technique I use with the computer (see Chapter 7).

The trial head is again placed on the femoral stem and trial reduction and range of motion accomplished (Fig. 6–32). The real femoral head then is placed and the hip can be closed. The femoral head used should be as large as possible so that dead space in the hip is reduced after closure. This will accelerate capsular healing and provide better stability and pain relief.

Tapered Stem with Metaphyseal Fill

Implantation of the Natural (Zimmer) tapered hip stem requires both reaming and broaching for preparation of the bone (Fig. 6–33). The stem size as estimated from the template is almost always correct. The surgeon can begin with reamers and broaches two or three sizes smaller; I begin with two sizes smaller, if available. Of course, if the zero and double-zero stems are used, there are no smaller sizes. The box chisel is used for

the lateral cortical neck, and the burr is used to open the femoral canal.

The conical reamers used to prepare the femur can be used sequentially, similar to the self-centering reamers used with the APR stem (Fig. 6–34). The conical reamer has a stop for the cut level of the femoral neck to indicate the correct depth of reaming. The surgeon should be able to feel contact of the conical reamer with cortical bone while reaming.

After reaming to the appropriate size, broaching can be done. Broaching also can begin with broaches one or two sizes smaller than the selected stem; I usually begin with one size smaller (Fig. 6–35). When the final broach is seated, it is tested for rotational stability and axial stability (Fig. 6–36); the smaller broach will not demonstrate stability.

When the broach is seated, the trial neck and head can be placed and the hip taken through range of motion; the balance, offset, and hip length are determined as described for the two previous stems. With correct balance achieved, the broach can be removed and the implant inserted. The implant can be manually inserted except for the last 2 cm, which is malleted into position. The Natural hip is also available as a collared or collarless stem (Fig. 6–37). Trial heads are placed onto the stem and the hip is again taken through range of motion. When the correct length of femoral head is determined, it is inserted onto the stem, the hip is reduced, and closure accomplished. As with any stem, the largest possible femoral head size should be used to minimize hip dead space.

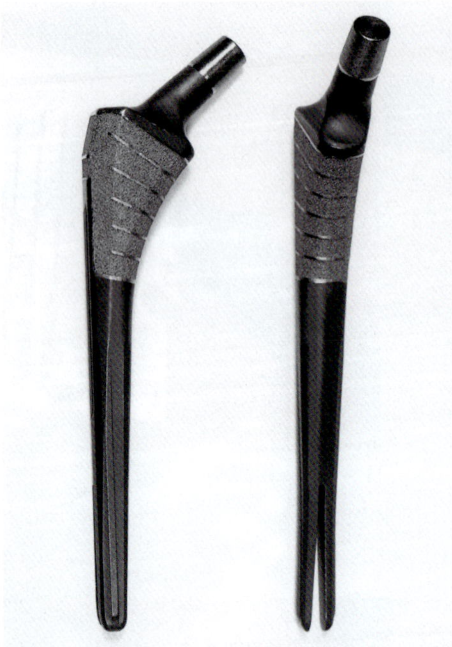

Figure 6–33 *Mediolateral and anterior profiles of the Natural hip stem. Observe the flexible split stem on the anteroposterior profile, which can open or close depending on the width of the intramedullary canal.*

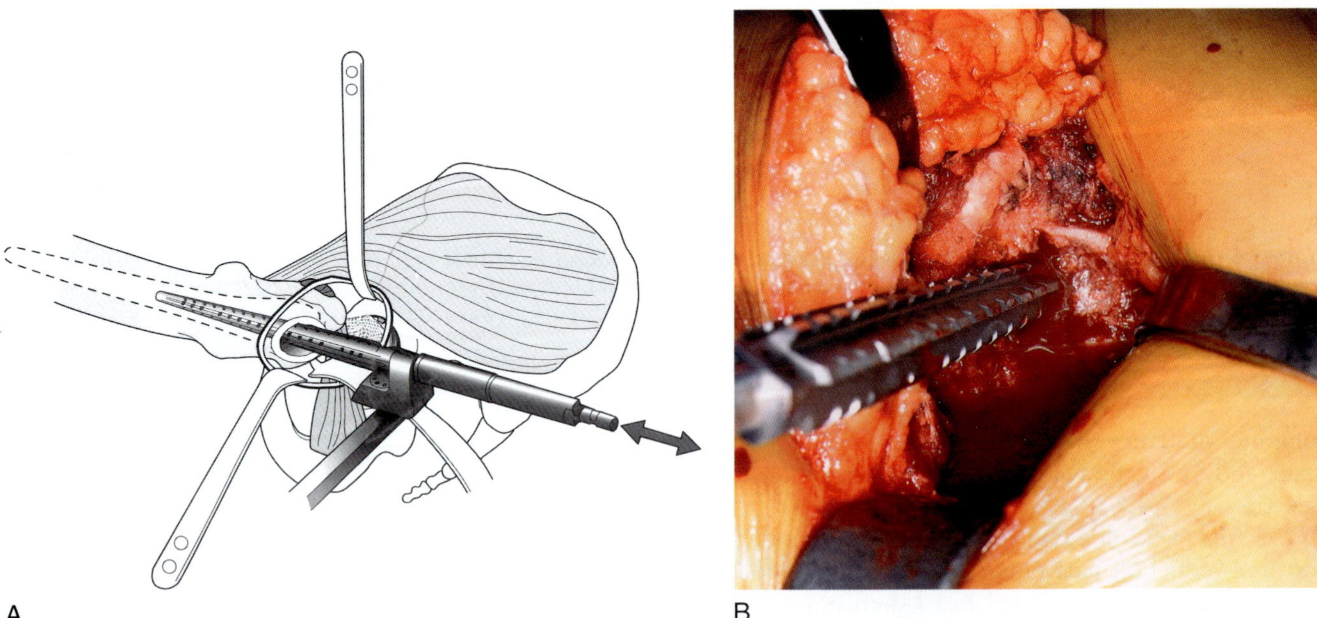

A   B

Figure 6–34 **A,** *The conical reamer is inserted into the intramedullary canal. The stop for the reamer that will contact the cut femoral neck is shown.* **B,** *Intraoperative view of the conical reamer being inserted into the intramedullary canal at the posterior lateral corner of the femoral neck.*

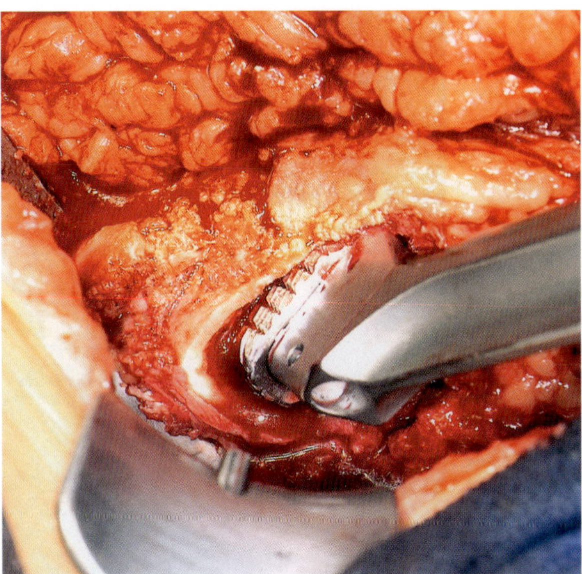

Figure 6–35 *A Natural hip stem broach one size smaller than the actual stem is impacted into the canal.*

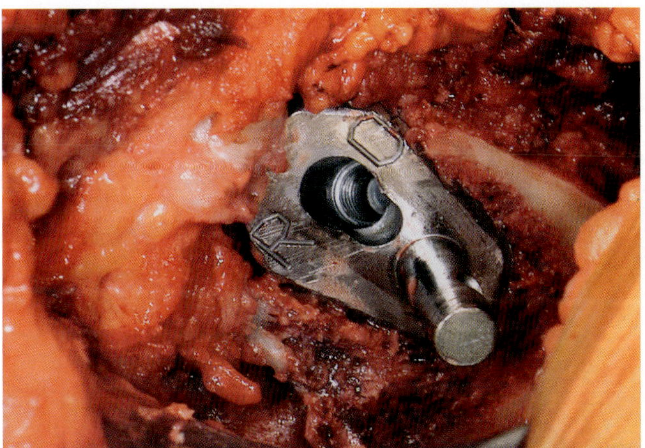

Figure 6–36 *Close-up view of the broach, which is stable in the bone. The broach is not in varus because the tip of the greater trochanter overlies the lateral side of the broach. The broach size is dictated by the intramedullary canal size, so cancellous bone of the neck can still be seen.*

BALANCING LEG LENGTH AND OFFSET

It is appropriate to review the techniques for balancing offset and hip length/leg length. The surgeon can decide whether to do a trial reduction with the trial head and neck with the broach in place, or to wait to determine the trial head to be used with the stem in place. If the surgeon is confident of the stem size and the restored hip length, a trial reduction is not necessary with the broach. However, if there is any question as to whether the hip length and offset have been correctly established with the broach in position, a trial

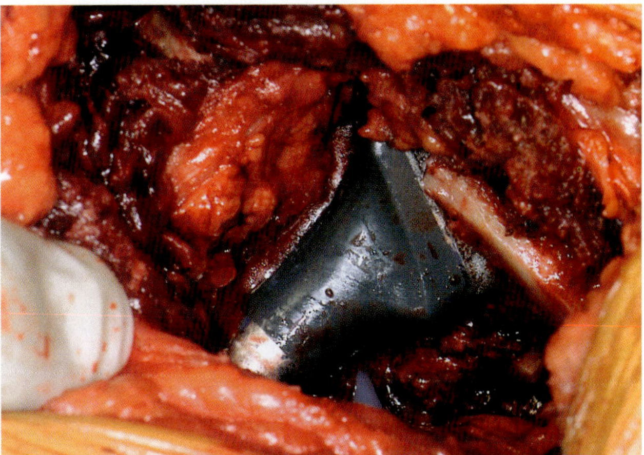

Figure 6–37 *A collarless, noncemented Natural hip stem has been implanted into the envelope prepared by the broach. The lateral side of the stem is in the trochanteric bed. Some cancellous bone of the neck remains, as was seen with the broach in position in Figure 6–36.*

head and neck segment should be added to the broach and a reduction done.

The hip should be cleared through a range of motion during the trialing to ensure that the metal neck does not impinge against the cup and that the trochanter does not impinge against the pelvic bone. The stability of the hip is also judged to ensure that the femoral head does not dislocate out of the cup at the extremes of either extension or flexion with rotation. Using one hand to move the leg and using the index finger of the opposite hand to feel inside the hip is the best way to detect impingement (see Fig. 6–19). Using the index finger, the metal neck can be palpated to determine that it does not impinge against the cup, and the trochanter can be felt to determine that it clears the pelvis. Finally, the Ranawat test can be used to estimate the combined anteversion of the hip. This is done by flexing the hip 30 to 40 degrees and internally rotating the leg by lifting the foot (Fig. 6–38). The combined anteversion is equal to the amount of internal rotation necessary to position the femoral head symmetrically in the acetabulum: if the leg has been internally rotated 20 degrees, the combined anteversion is 20 degrees; if the leg has been internally rotated 40 degrees, the combined anteversion is 40 degrees. The optimal combined anteversion of a hip replacement is 35 to 45 degrees with this test.

The method I use to measure leg length combines palpating the level of the lesser trochanter to ensure that it does not extend below the ischium (see Fig. 6–18) and overlaying the two legs. The positions of the patella of the upper leg and lower leg are used along with the positions of the soles of the feet. With the top leg overlying the bottom leg, these relative positions should be felt before surgery and again after the head is reduced into the cup. Leg lengths are correct if the superior pole of the patella of the operative upper leg is slightly cranial to that of the lower leg (Fig. 6–39),

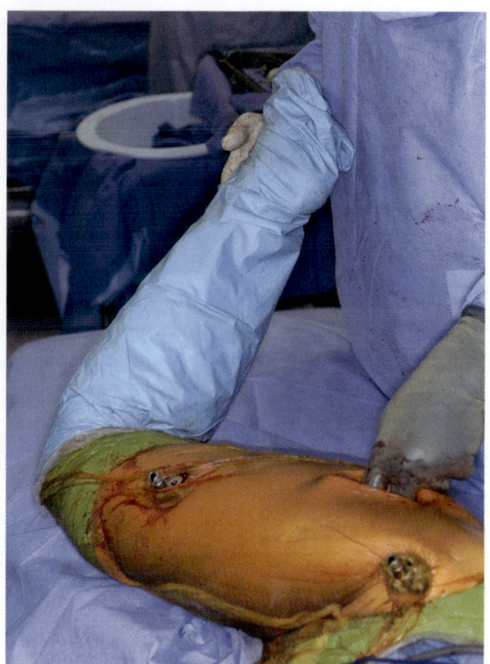

Figure 6–38   *Ranawat's sign is elicited by internally rotating the leg as it lies on the operating table. The surgeon places two fingers of the left hand into the wound to palpate the symmetry of the femoral head in the acetabulum. The amount of internal rotation equals the amount of combined anteversion of the head and cup. The pelvic and femoral bases for the computer guidance system are seen attached to the patient. The computer can give a precise numerical value of combined anteversion (see Chapter 7).*

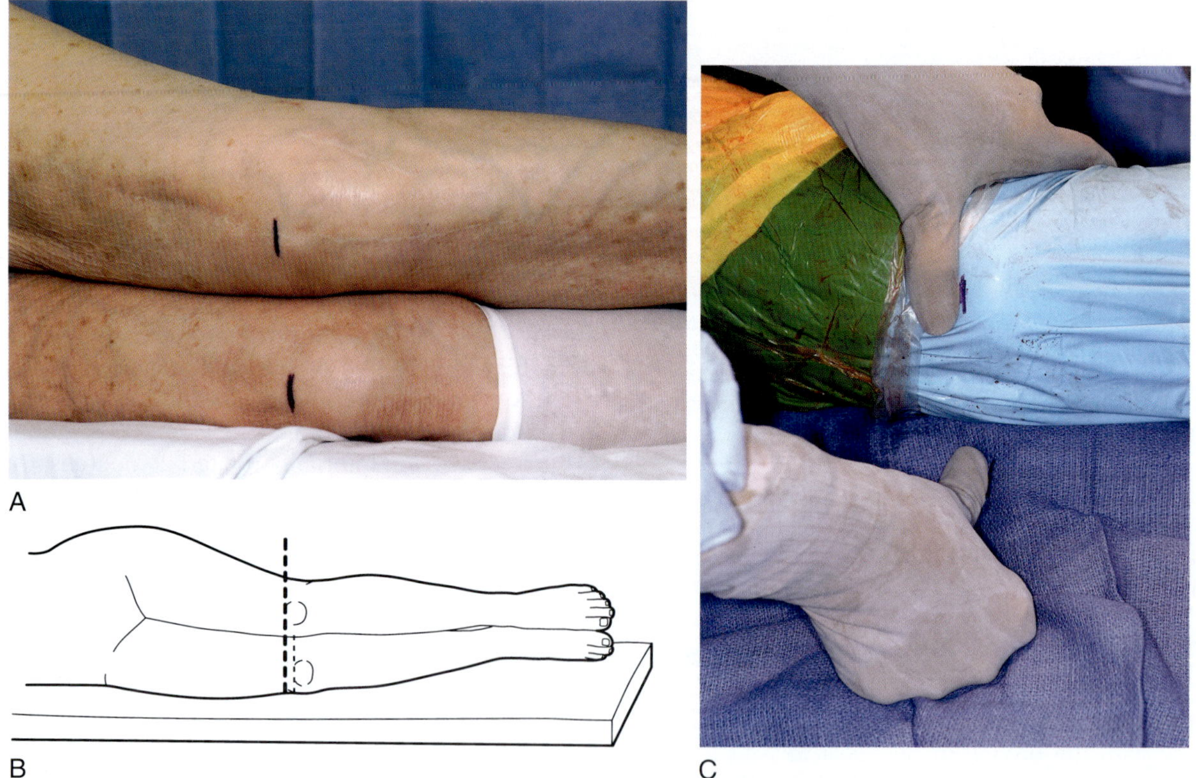

A

B

C

Figure 6–39   **A,** *The legs are overlaid before the patient is draped, which demonstrates that the superior pole of the upper patella is proximal to the superior pole of the lower patella even in legs that are the same length. This is the approximate position for the poles of the patellae in legs of correct length. This patient has a longitudinal scar over the upper knee from previous total knee replacement.* **B,** *Both of the legs, showing the relationship of the patellae to each other.* **C,** *Technique for judging leg lengths intraoperatively by palpating the relationship of the superior poles of the patellae.*

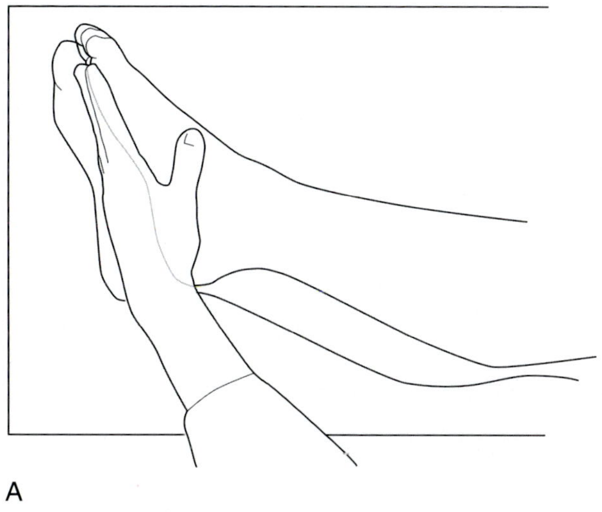

A

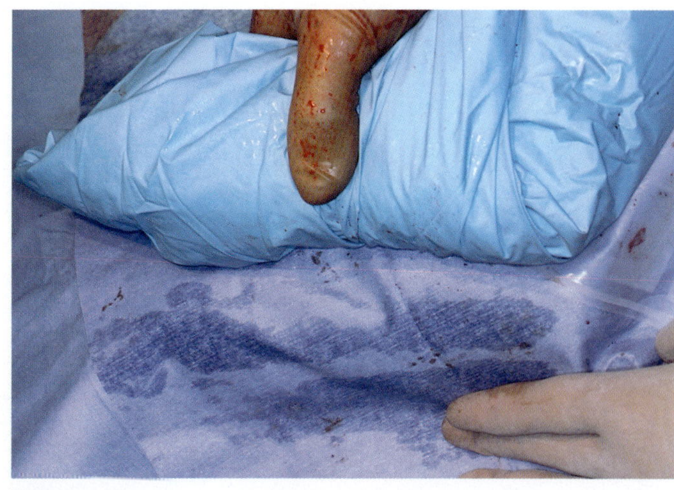

B

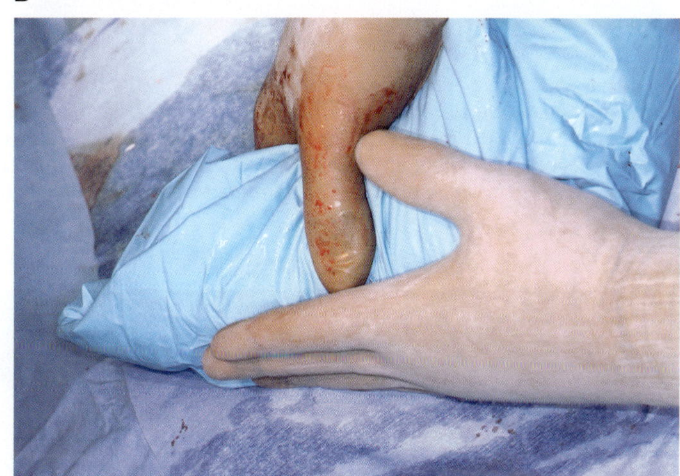

C

Figure 6–40 **A,** *Method for judging leg lengths by the relationship of the feet. With the feet overlaid, the sole of the top foot should be 1 handbreadth superior to that of the lower foot.* **B,** *Intraoperative view showing the lower foot under the drape and the upper foot overlying the lower foot. The upper foot is proximal to the lower foot.* **C,** *Intraoperative view showing a hand placed on top of the lower foot and against the sole of the upper foot.*

and the sole of the operative leg is 1 handbreadth proximal to the sole of the underlying leg (Fig. 6–40). Another technique that can be used with the legs overlaid is alignment of the tibial tubercles instead of the superior poles of the patellae, which is particularly useful if the patient is fat because the tubercles are more prominent and easily felt. As with the patellae, the tibial tubercle of the operative leg should be slightly cranial to that of the underlying leg; the positions of the soles of the feet do not change. The legs should not be completely symmetrical when they are overlaid because the upper leg is adducted onto the lower leg.

Once the correct femoral head length is determined for the stem, the actual head should be locked onto the stem, the final reduction made, and a repeat range of motion performed to ensure clearance of the hip; the leg length is also tested once more. Reduction should never be attempted by pulling on the leg through the knee while rotating the leg, a maneuver that can fracture the leg by resisted rotation. Rather, reduction is

accomplished by pulling on the stem and externally rotating the leg, which involves "hooking" the knee so that the leg can be gently externally rotated while the head is pulled into the acetabulum (Fig. 6–41). The surgeon can push on the head while the assistant pulls on the metal femoral neck. The surgeon can also use one finger to protect the sciatic nerve from being pulled into the hip during reduction.

We test the leg length once more at the completion of the operation, when the patient has been returned to the supine position on the operating table (Fig. 6–42). If the leg lengths are not equal at this time, we reopen the hip and correct the length difference. Patients are always grateful in such cases that we took the necessary measures to ensure that their leg lengths were equal, and when we inform families that we are going to do this, they almost always comment that "he/she would not want a long leg." When judging leg lengths with the patient supine, be sure that the legs are approximated in line with the sternum and not canted

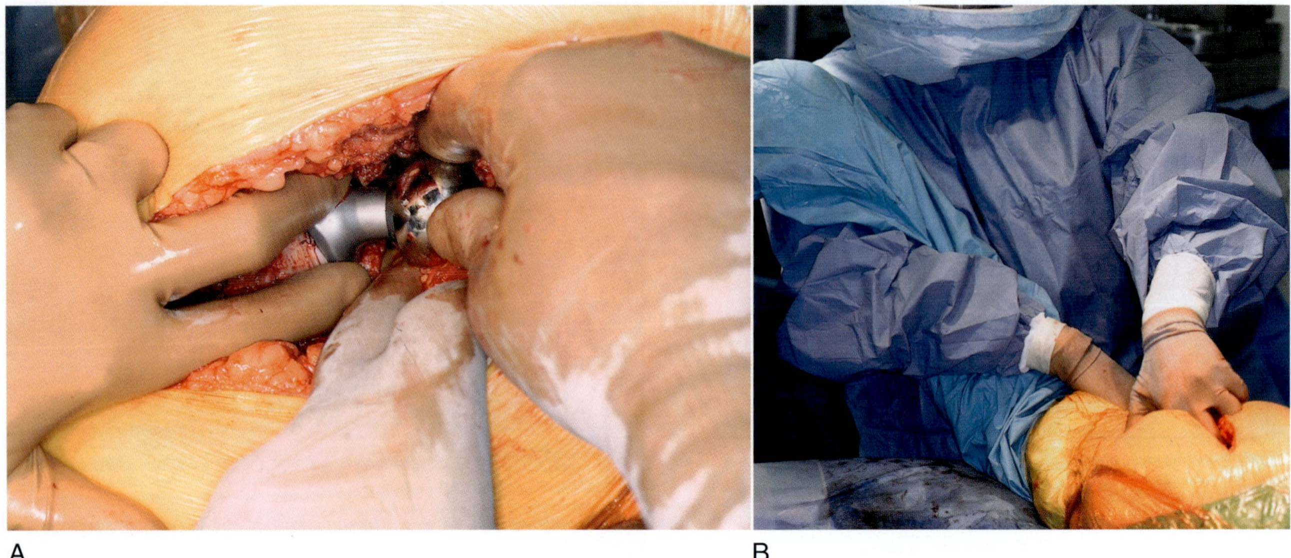

A   B

Figure 6–41 **A,** *To reduce the hip, the assistant grips the femoral neck or the upper end of the femoral stem to pull the femoral head into the acetabulum, rather than pulling on the leg. The surgeon can aid the assistant by pushing the femoral head toward the acetabulum with his or her right hand. The surgeon uses two fingers of the left hand under the femoral head to retract the sciatic nerve and protect it from injury during the reduction.* **B,** *The assistant cradles the leg with his right elbow and the forearm across the knee. The left hand pulls the femoral head into the acetabulum while the right arm gently externally rotates the leg.*

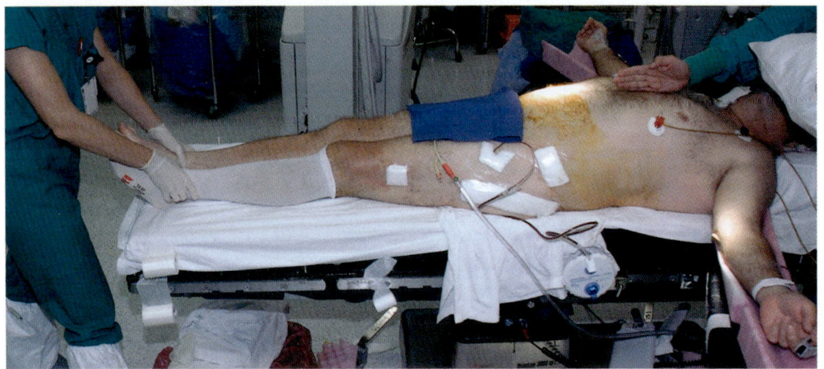

A

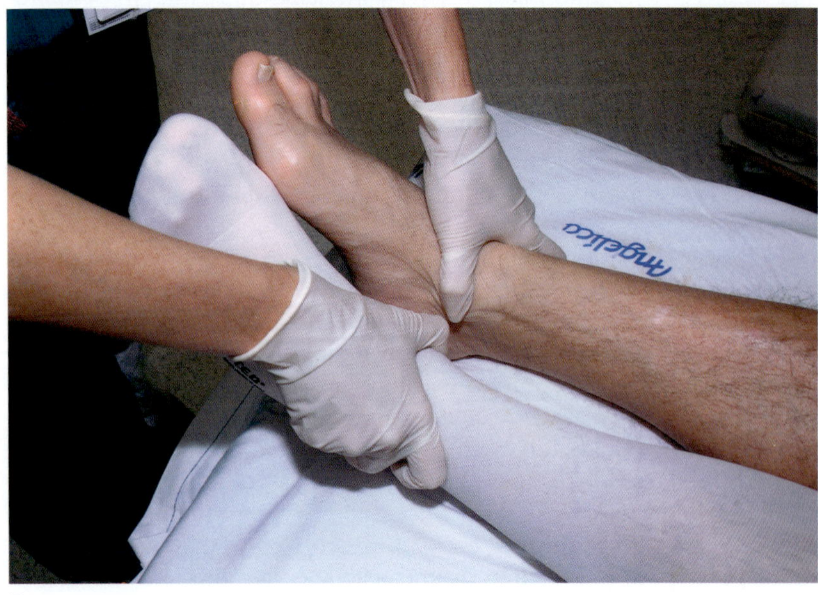

B

Figure 6–42 **A,** *The patient has been returned to the supine position after completion of the operation. The leg lengths are judged by approximating the medial malleoli in line with the sternum, which is marked by the anesthesiologist's hand on the right.* **B,** *Close-up view of the method for measuring the level of the medial malleoli.*

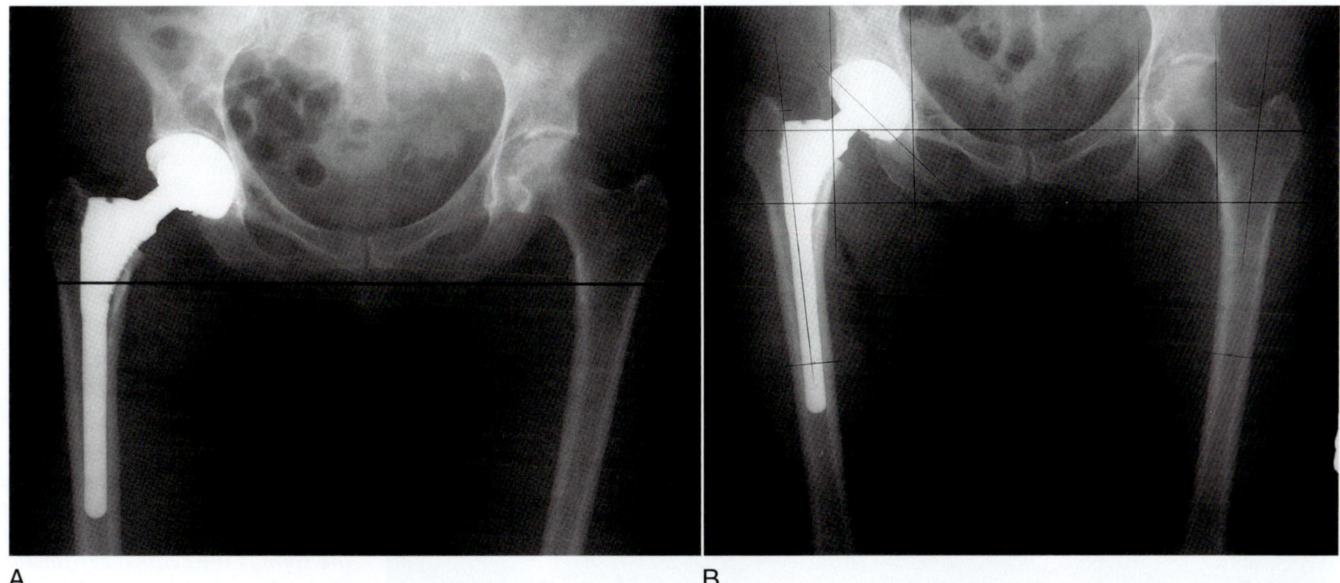

A   B

Figure 6–43 **A,** *Anteroposterior x-ray of the pelvis after the patient has been returned to the supine position. The right leg was almost 1 inch longer than the left leg. This postoperative x-ray shows that the lesser trochanter of the right hip is almost completely below the transischial line (the black line), whereas the left hip is above the transischial line. The offset is also significantly increased in the operative hip.* **B,** *The patient was immediately returned to the lateral position and the hip reoperated on. The femoral stem was impacted deeper into the femur (note the level of the femur in* **A***). A femoral head one size shorter was also used. The x-ray now shows that the lesser trochanters are at the same level and the offsets are essentially the same. The postoperative measurements showed good reconstruction and the leg lengths were clinically equal.*

one way or the other, because this can give a false impression of the lengths. If there is any question as to correct leg length, an x-ray should be taken in the operating room to confirm the positions of the lesser trochanters and the hip lengths (Fig. 6–43).

PREPARATION AND IMPLANTATION: CEMENTED TECHNIQUE

Some surgeons prefer to cement the femoral component. Whereas the exposure and sequence of retraction are the same as for the cementless technique, the differences in canal preparation need to be understood for good cemented fixation.

First, the femoral canal should not be reamed if a cemented stem is used; only broaches are used to prepare the canal. This is a critical difference in canal preparation between cemented and cementless implants. Second, although trialing with a broach is not mandatory with a cementless implant and its various modular heads, a trial should always be done with the broach in place for a cemented implant because of the difficulty with changing a cemented femoral component to correct the depth of insertion. All decisions regarding the implant should be made before the femoral component is cemented.

The goal of proper cemented technique is to obtain a "whiteout" of cement reaching from the well-placed stem to the femoral cortex, with no air or blood bubbles (Fig. 6–44). The canal must be cleared of any debris and blood before cement insertion so that a whiteout is obtained. A whiteout ensures a uniform and strong cement mantle with the least chance of cement failure.

The femur is exposed in the same manner as for cementless stems. The lateral neck is removed with a box chisel, as previously described, and the canal is opened with a burr. A small reamer or a Charnley T-handled canal reamer can be placed into the canal to open the canal (Fig. 6–45). This technique initiates clearance of fat and cancellous bone from the femoral canal.

Once the canal is opened, the femur is prepared with the femoral broach; the size of the broach depends on the size of the cemented stem, which was determined by templating. The broach is inserted into the femur; it can be malleted to a fully seated position if manual insertion is difficult. Once the broach has been fully seated, it should be rotated to loosen it within the canal (Fig. 6–46). The broach is then used as a rasp to remove loose cancellous bone and prepare the lateral trochanteric bed so that the stem can be implanted in a neutral position. If a collar is used, the calcar can be planed with a broach in place (Fig. 6–47).

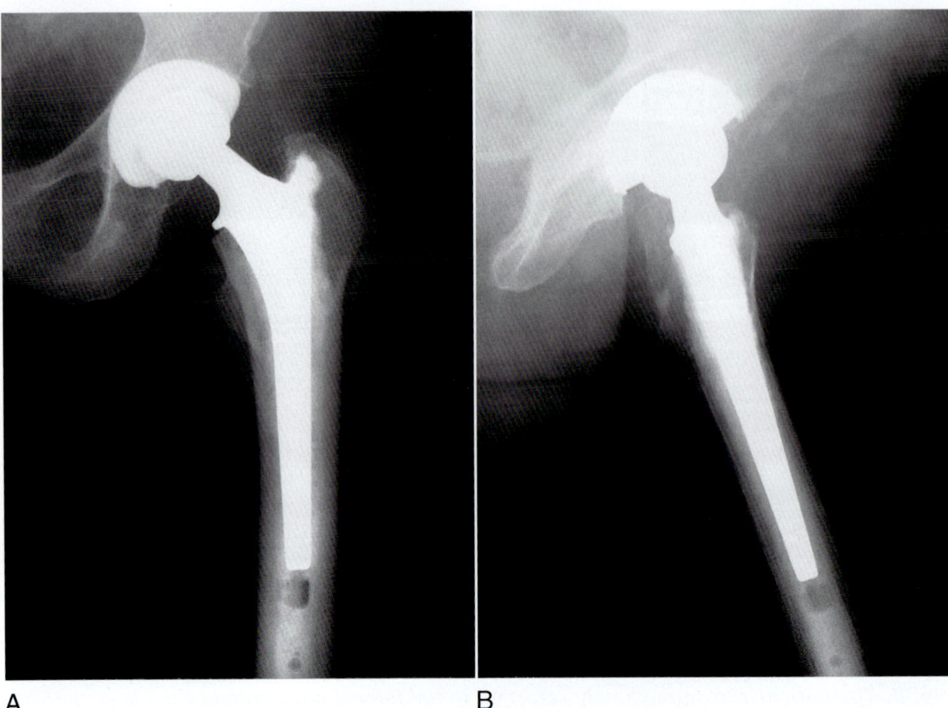

*Figure 6–44 **A,** Anteroposterior x-ray of the hip showing an intact circumferential cement column. The lucency at the tip of the stem is the centralizer for the stem. **B,** Lateral x-ray showing the intact circumferential cement column with the centralizer at the tip of the stem.*

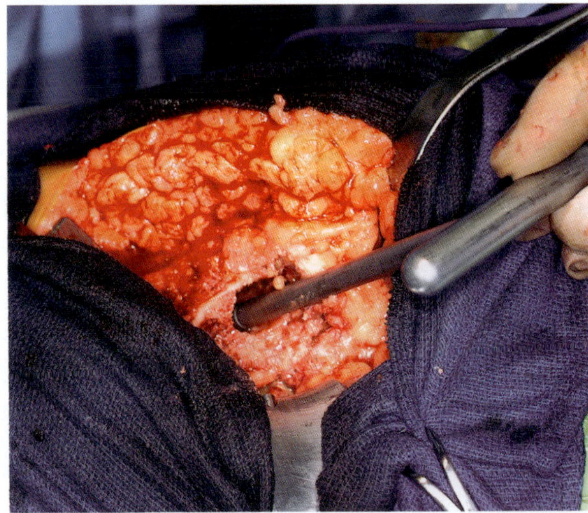

Figure 6–45 A Charnley T-handled canal finder is placed into the canal. After the canal has been opened with a burr, this can be used instead of a reamer to open the intramedullary canal for correct direction of the broach.

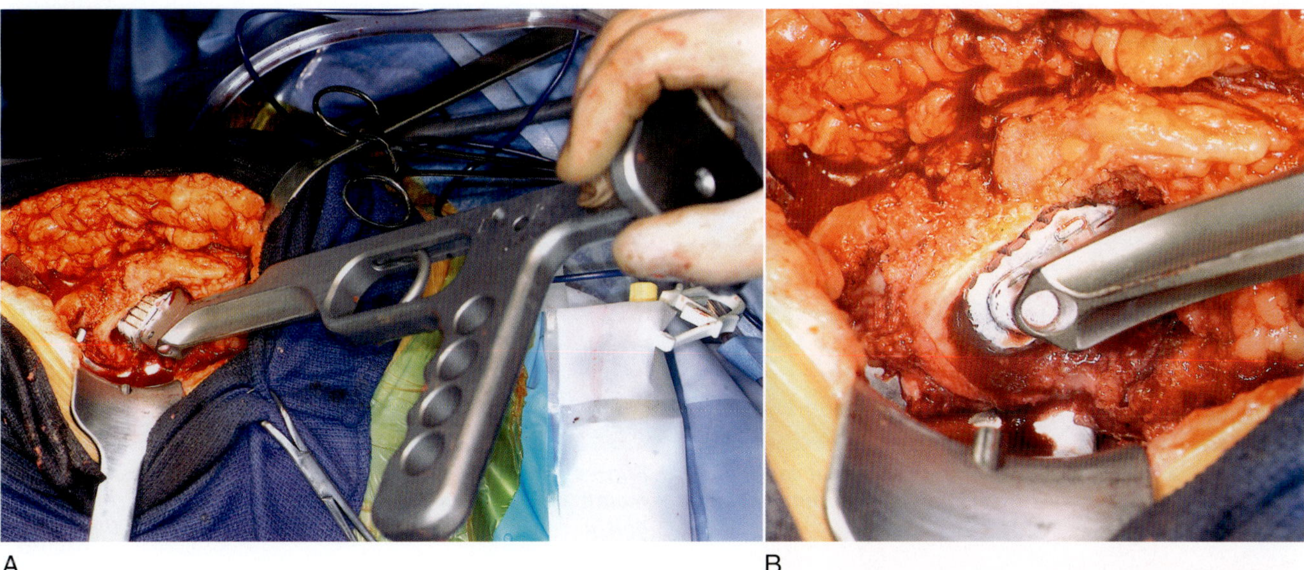

A

B

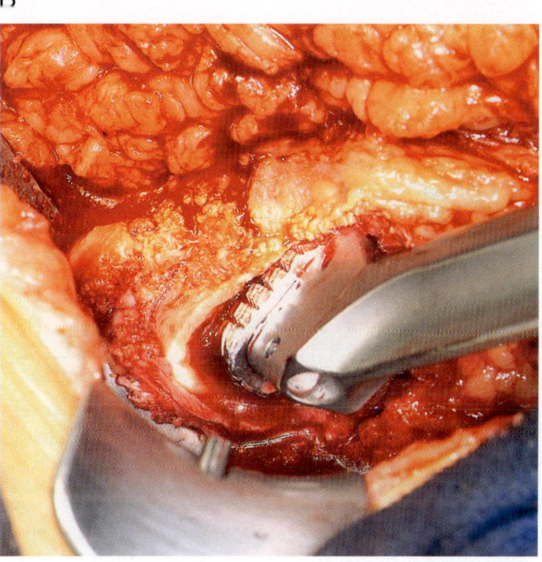

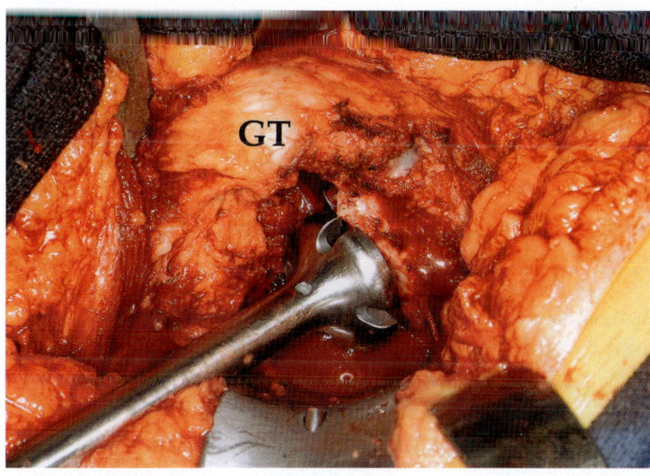

C

Figure 6–46 **A,** *The broach for a cemented stem should be able to be manually inserted into the femoral canal. The initial broach may need to be malleted the final 2 to 3 cm. The broach handle should be used to move the broach up and down against the trochanteric bed to ensure that the lateral side of the femoral canal is cleared of bone.* **B,** *While using the femoral broach as a rasp, it should be rotated within the femoral canal to remove all loose cancellous bone.* **C,** *The broach is rotated within the femoral canal to remove all loose cancellous bone.*

Figure 6–47 *The broach is left in place in the canal and a calcar planer inserted over the broach to plane the calcar. GT, greater trochanter.*

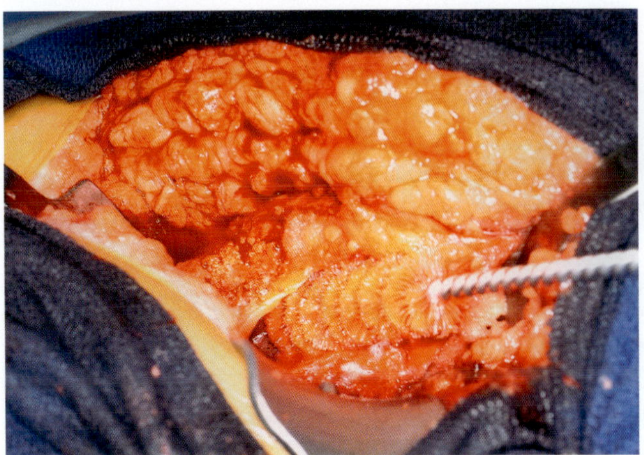

Figure 6–48 *A brush is inserted into the femoral canal and moved up and down vigorously to remove all loose bits of bone and debris.*

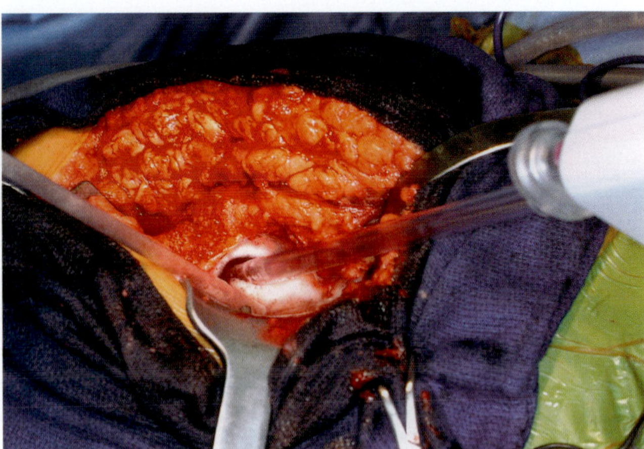

Figure 6–50 *Pulsatile lavage is used until the fluid at the mouth of the femur is clear to ensure that all blood clots and debris are removed from the canal above the cement restrictor.*

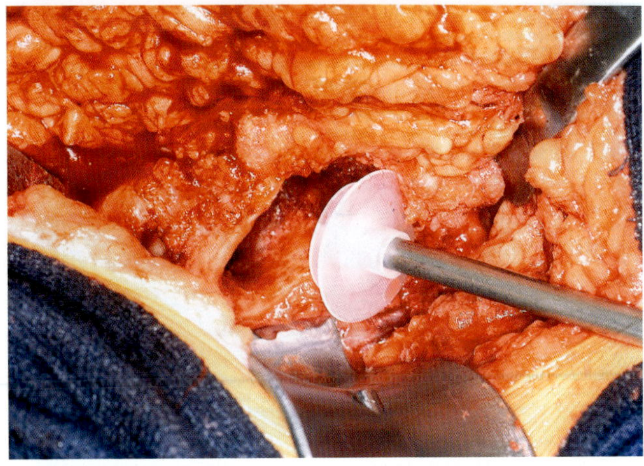

Figure 6–49 *A cement restrictor is placed into the canal at the appropriate depth to allow 2 cm of cement below the tip of the stem.*

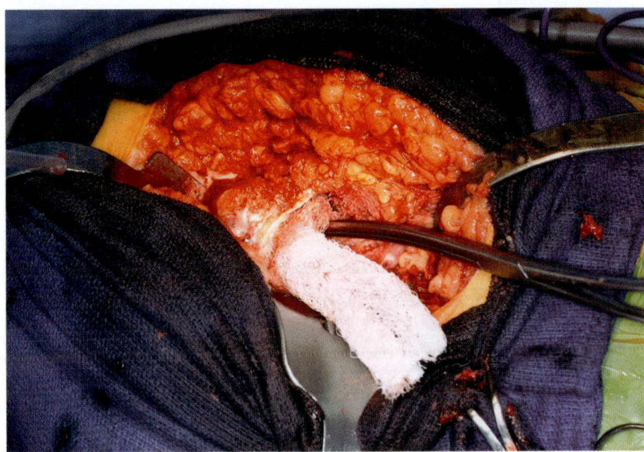

Figure 6–51 *The canal is packed with a Kerlix gauze to absorb blood. Loose debris will also be dragged out of the intramedullary canal with removal of the gauze.*

After the femoral broach is removed, a canal brush is used to remove any small pieces of bone and debris left in the canal (Fig. 6–48). An appropriately sized cement restrictor is placed far enough down the canal to allow for full implantation of the stem with 1 to 2 cm of cement below the stem's tip (Fig. 6–49). A pulsatile lavage system should be used to irrigate the canal until the fluid is clear, ensuring that all blood and blood clots have been removed (Fig. 6–50). The canal is suctioned and a Kerlix gauze is packed from distal to proximal using long forceps (Fig. 6–51). We always mix two bags of Simplex cement (Howmedica-Stryker, Rutherford, N.J.) in a cement gun; it usually takes 10 minutes for the cement to set. We keep the monomer in a sterilizer or hot water to keep it warm. The cement should be inserted when it no longer runs out of the end of the cement gun, but droops (Fig. 6–52). Two to three

minutes after the cement is mixed, the packing is removed from the femoral canal and the cement is inserted from distal to proximal (Fig. 6–53). Placing a moist, gloved thumb over the medial femoral neck helps to pressurize the cement. When the canal is full of cement, remove the gun and use free cement to further pressurize the cement mantle manually until strong back-pressure is felt (Fig. 6–54). The stem is slowly inserted in the desired anteversion (no more than 10 degrees to prevent in-toeing of the foot; Fig. 6–55) and then malleted into final position over the last 2 cm to provide optimal pressurization of the cement (Fig. 6–56). If the cement provides so little resistance that the stem does not need to be malleted the last 2 cm, the cement was too liquid at the time of stem insertion and an optimal whiteout will be difficult to obtain. If a collar is used, try to seat the collar on the

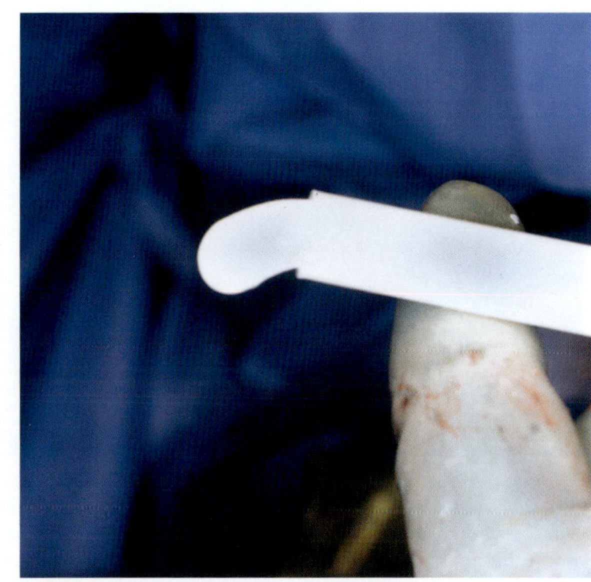

Figure 6–52 *The cement is ready for insertion into the canal when it just droops from the end of the cement gun. If it is runny, it is not doughy enough.*

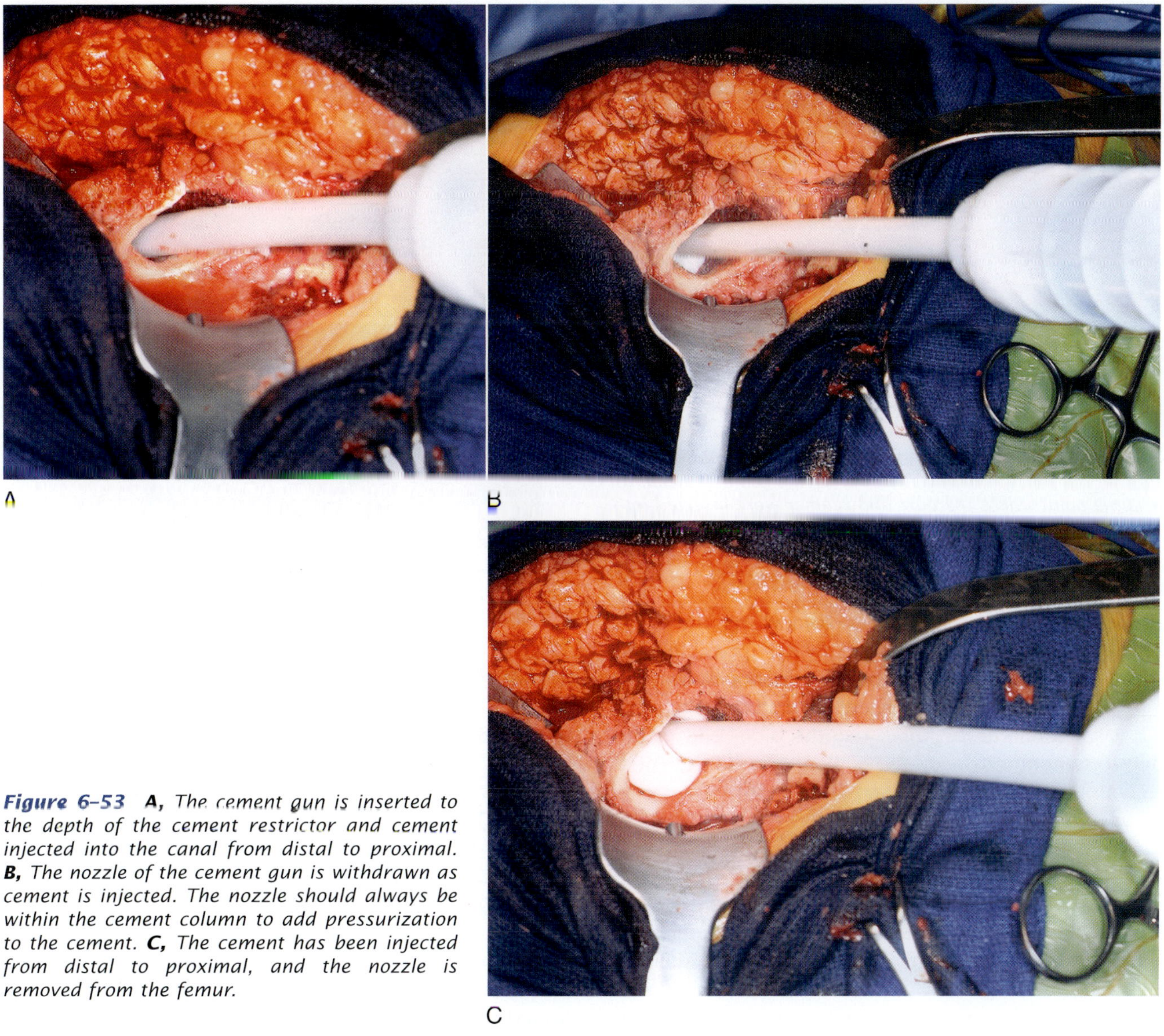

Figure 6–53 **A,** *The cement gun is inserted to the depth of the cement restrictor and cement injected into the canal from distal to proximal.* **B,** *The nozzle of the cement gun is withdrawn as cement is injected. The nozzle should always be within the cement column to add pressurization to the cement.* **C,** *The cement has been injected from distal to proximal, and the nozzle is removed from the femur.*

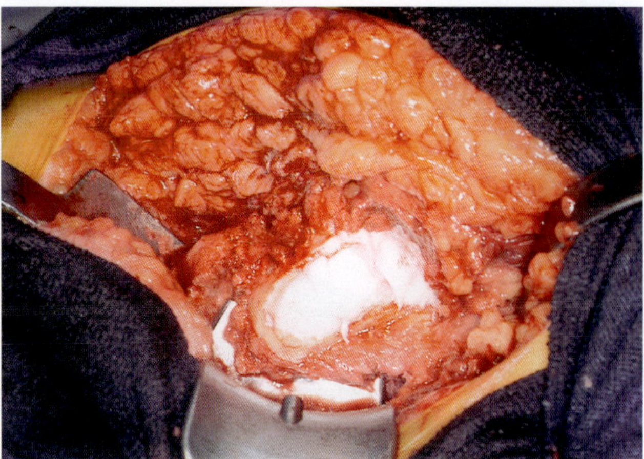

Figure 6–54 *The cement has been manually pressurized into the femoral canal and should have the appearance of a solid cement column with no blood oozing from around it. It should be doughy enough that there is resistance against stem insertion.*

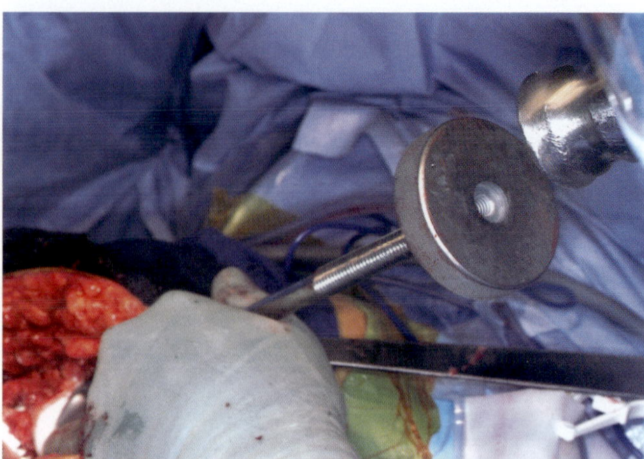

Figure 6–56 *If the cement was in the correct doughy stage, the final 2 cm of the femoral stem should require insertion by malleting. This technique also provides high pressurization within the cement column, which promotes the desired white-out on x-ray.*

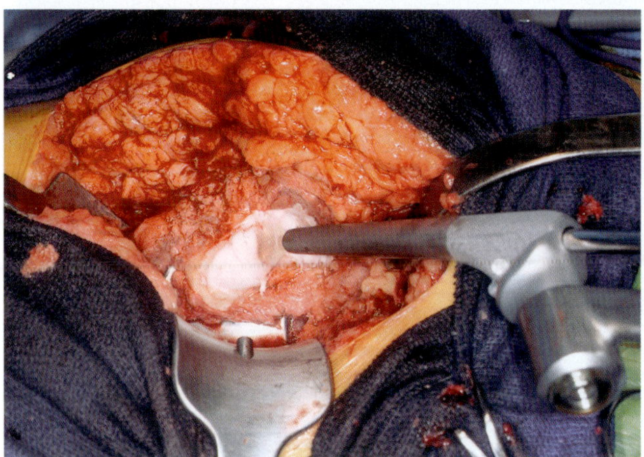

Figure 6–55 *The stem is inserted. The insertion should begin at the posterior lateral corner of the femoral neck, at the same point where the burr and reamer were inserted into the femoral canal.*

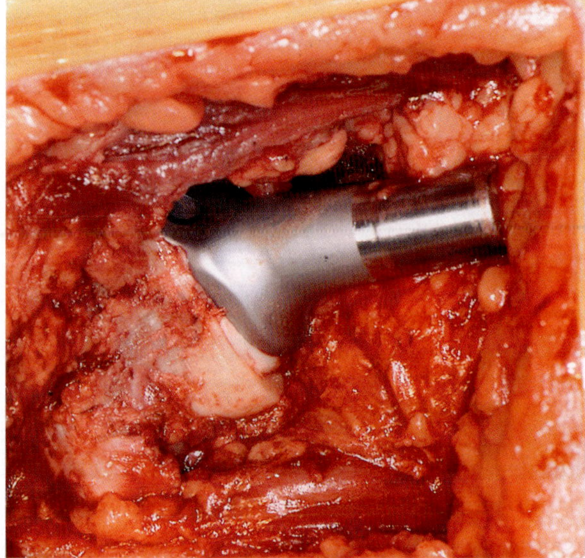

Figure 6–57 *This cemented stem has a collar, but the calcar was not planed and cement is visible between the collar and the calcar bone. It is preferable to plane the calcar to achieve direct contact of metal with bone.*

calcar by removing interposed cement as the stem advances, although this is not always possible and cannot be accomplished if planing was not done (Fig. 6–57). Remove the excess cement from around the stem with a small curette or knife. Use the blunt end of the knife to continue to pack the cement around the prosthesis until the cement is cured (Fig. 6–58).

CONCLUSIONS

Femoral preparation varies depending on whether the stem is to be cemented or cementless. With cemented stems, no reaming, only broaching, should be done. With most of the cementless stems, reaming is done

to size the femoral canal, and the size of stem used depends on the size of the canal, determined by the reaming. Reaming should usually engage the canal over a 5-cm length. Conical reamers are most commonly used for tapered stems, and self-centering reamers are used for stems with a round geometry. The principles of preparation are the same regardless of whether reaming or broaching is done, and the guidelines for determining size depend on the reamer or broach. The anti-varus sign—the lateral side of the implant positioned under the tip of the trochanter—should be

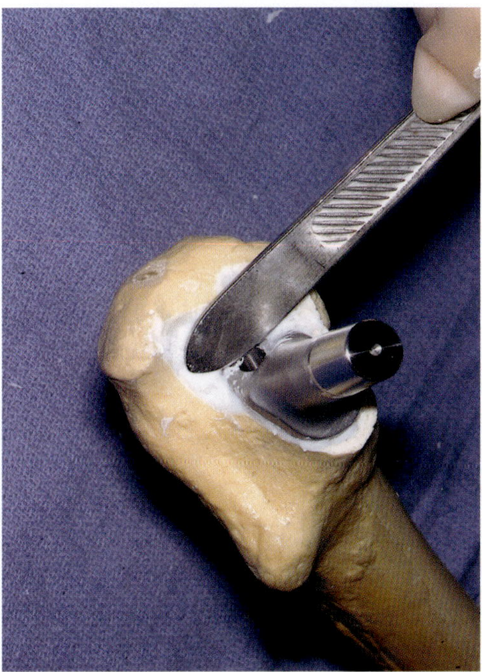

Figure 6–58 *If the stem does not have a full collar, the blunt end of a scalpel is used to pack the cement around the upper end of the cemented femoral stem. If the stem has a collar extending around the entire upper surface, then access to the femoral canal is blocked and this technique is not necessary. If the cement is accessible, packing applies additional pressure on the cement column.*

positive with both cemented and cementless stems. The technique for cemented fixation is the same with different kinds of cemented stems: it is still important to pressurize the cement and promote strong interdigitation between the cement and the endosteal bone of the femoral canal.

The technique for either cemented or cementless fixation can be learned very quickly in cadaver femoral bone (or even sawbone femurs). It is advisable for young surgeons-in-training to practice on cadaver or sawbone femurs to gain confidence in their technique before performing the operation with patients. The technique for femoral preparation is less complex than that for acetabular preparation and implantation and hence can be learned in a predictable and reproducible way with a cadaver or sawbones.

Reference

1. Garcia-Cimbrelo E, Cruz-Pardos A, Madero R, Ortega-Andreu M: Total hip arthroplasty with use of the cementless Zweymüller Alloclassic system. J Bone Joint Surg Am 85:296-303, 2003.

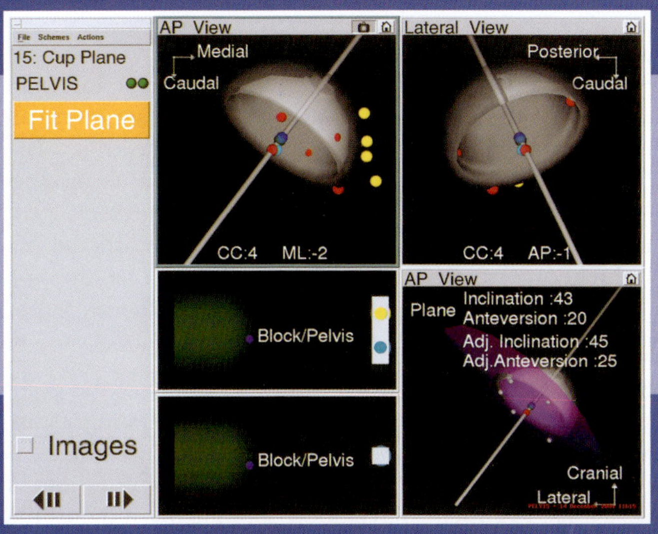

Chapter 7

Computer-Assisted Total Hip Replacement*

*In conjunction with this chapter on the DVD-ROM is the video *"Computer Navigation Total Hip Replacement."*

Computer navigation is the most important technical innovation for the performance of total hip replacement since elimination of the trochanteric osteotomy.

While total hip replacement has been performed successfully for 40 years without computer navigation, there have always been outliers in component position, even in series reporting the results from the best surgeons. In most of these series, the incidence of outliers is 10% to 15%; it probably is even higher in practices in which hip replacement is not performed frequently. Failures are associated with mechanical problems producing dislocation, a painful hip joint, accelerated wear, and early loosening. Most of these failures have been caused by impingement due either to unsatisfactory positioning of components (i.e., impingement of the metal neck on the edge of the cup) or to inadequate reconstruction of the offset/hip length (i.e., impingement of the trochanter against the pelvis). Clearly, patients would benefit from absolute precision in component positioning and soft tissue balance. The computer makes such precision possible.

Outliers can be eliminated by providing the surgeon with more information at the time of the operation. Completely accurate knowledge of the location of osseous anatomy and the relationship of replacement components to bones would allow the correct placement of components, the correct mating of components, the correct reproduction of hip biomechanics, and the avoidance of impingement for all hips. This enhanced knowledge base is available with the use of computer navigation. Precise computer navigation is possible with imageless technology, which means that there is no need for intraoperative fluoroscopy or a preoperative computed tomography (CT) scan.

Expense is the main obstacle to use of the computer. Whether the hospital purchases the equipment depends on the volume of use and the possibility of reimbursement. The cost of the hardware, however, will continue to decrease with time. In the long run, both money and time are saved by using the computer because the number of mechanical complications and therefore the necessity for revision operations are decreased.

BENEFITS OF COMPUTER NAVIGATION

Stress Reduction. To some extent, all operations are stressful for the surgeon because he or she wants to do a perfect job and provide a good result with no complications. The computer reduces this stress because it removes much of the uncertainty during the operation. It allows the surgeon to know the exact positions of the pelvis and femur in three dimensions so that the components can be placed correctly. With better information about the mating of components, the surgeon can avoid impingement and its resultant complications. The computer also allows the surgeon to obtain the optimal leg length and offset, thus providing the greatest possible comfort for the patient. When the components can be mated correctly with confidence at the first attempt, it is never necessary subsequently to lengthen a leg to obtain stability.

Shorter Operating Time. Another benefit of the computer is that it reduces the time in the operating room. With the use of computer navigation, it no longer is necessary to obtain an x-ray to confirm component positions. Computer navigation also greatly reduces the time spent in making decisions regarding anteversion of the acetabular and femoral components, the possibility of impingement, correction of leg lengths, and determination of offset. Because the computer gives numerical measurements of these parameters, the surgeon does not need to agonize over selecting the proper positions. The decision-making time saved in the operating room easily neutralizes the approximately 10 minutes spent setting up the computer before positioning for the operation; during this time, the pelvic registration device is placed and the anteroposterior (AP) plane of the pelvis measured. During surgery, an additional 5 minutes is necessary for measurement of the acetabular and femoral registrations.

Prevention of Impingement. The great advantage of the Orthosoft (Montreal, Quebec, Canada) computer software is that it provides three-dimensional information for the acetabulum, and not just the values for inclination and anteversion. With three-dimensional information, the surgeon always knows the center of rotation of the acetabular cup and the center of head position of the stem. Whether the center of rotation is moved superiorly or inferiorly, medially or laterally, or anteriorly or posteriorly, its relationship with the osseous center of rotation is instantly known. Although the center of rotation cannot be controlled at will with a cementless cup because the cup requires a press-fit, with cemented cups, a smaller cup can be positioned with greater freedom and enhanced control of the center of rotation.

In avoiding impingement, control of the center of rotation is more important than the absolute values for inclination and anteversion. Most commonly, the center of rotation of the osseous acetabulum must be elevated by 2 to 5 mm and medialized by 5 to 6 mm to provide an ideal cup position. The thicker the cup metal, the more elevation and medialization is needed by reaming because the metal's thickness moves the center of rotation distally and laterally.

The placement of the center of rotation must be combined with correct coverage of the cup to avoid

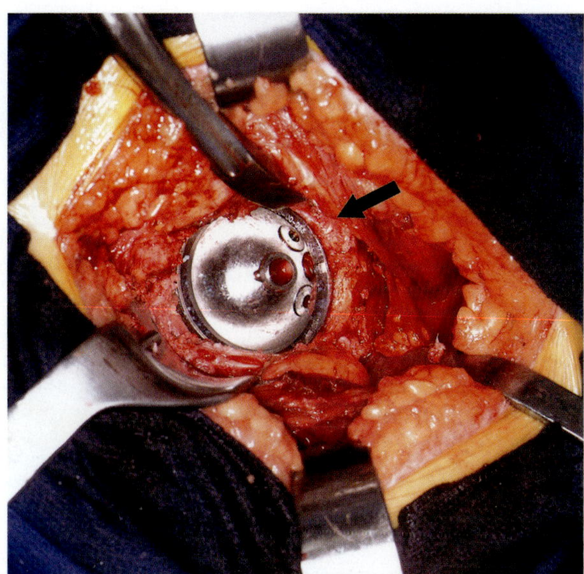

Figure 7–1 *Intraoperative view of correctly placed acetabular component. The metal of the posterosuperior edge of the cup stands proud to the bone, whereas the anterosuperior edge is flush with the edge of the bone (arrow). Inferomedially, the metal edge is below the pubic tubercle and the rim of the ischium and flush with the cortical bone of the cotyloid notch. This is the general principle of metal shell position in the osseous acetabulum; the actual angles of inclination and anteversion are partially determined by the depth of reaming, which changes the center of rotation of the acetabulum.*

impingement. Correct coverage is discussed in detail in Chapter 5 and shown in Figure 7–1. In summary, the superolateral posterior cup may be uncovered, the superoanterior edge is at the edge of bone and should be covered, the anteromedial edge is below the pubic tubercle, the inferomedial edge is at the level of the edge of the cortical bone of the cotyloid notch (or the transverse acetabular ligament), and the posteroinferior edge is below the rim of the ischium.

The inclination of the cup should be no more than 45 degrees to provide an optimal contact area and to minimize wear of the articulation surface. Occasionally, inclination may need to be increased to 50 degrees for correct coverage in patients with a native inclination of 65 degrees or more with an anterior tilt of 15 to 20 degrees.

An anteversion of 25 to 30 degrees is ideal to avoid impingement throughout the range of motion and provide the correct combined anteversion. Anteversion of a cementless stem in men is almost never greater than 10 degrees; if the stem anteversion is 5 degrees, that of the cup must be 28 to 30 degrees. In women, anteversion may exceed 10 degrees, so a cup can be safely positioned at 20 to 25 degrees. I prepare the femur first: I then know the anteversion of the stem, which is fixed, whereas the cup can be manipulated to provide the correct mating and combined anteversion (see X-ray Example 1, at the end of the chapter).

Showing Tilt of the Pelvis. Another significant advantage of using the computer for acetabular positioning is that it shows the tilt of the pelvis. Pelvic tilt can change the position of the cup by as much as 10 degrees, and compensation for this tilt is one of the most valuable assets the computer provides. Before the computer's advent, the degree of pelvic tilt was impossible to gauge, and hence at least 10% of cups deviated from the expected anteversion or inclination by as much as 10 degrees. With the computer, anteversion and inclination can be measured precisely within 3 degrees, ensuring an accurate cup position and reducing the risk of dislocation and impingement.

Accurate Preparation of the Acetabulum. Preparation of the acetabulum is more accurate with the computer because the surgeon knows the reamer's exact position in relation to the anterior, posterior, and medial walls. While reaming, the surgeon is constantly aware of the cup's center of rotation, including any superoinferior and mediolateral changes, and whether the reaming is directed centrally between the anterior and posterior walls. This information allows for precise reaming to reconstruct the acetabular center of rotation such that there is correct elevation and medialization for coverage of the cup by the osseous walls.

Accurate Preparation of the Femur. Three-dimensional information is also provided for preparation of the femur. When a broach or stem is inserted into the femoral bone, using computer navigation the surgeon knows the position of the broach in the canal, the anteversion of the stem, and what the offset of the leg will be. The center of head position of the stem (CH) tells the surgeon how far superior the head is to the original center of rotation of the hip (the cephalocaudal, or CC, number) and therefore how much the leg length would change with that position. The ML number tells the surgeon whether the head is medial or lateral to the original center of rotation. With this information, and knowing the center of rotation of the cup, the surgeon can determine the change in leg length.

Location of the Level of the Femoral Neck Cut. The level of the femoral neck cut can be located exactly with the computer. This information is particularly valuable in the posterior mini-incision, with which the level of the cut in relation to the lesser trochanter is obscured by the retained quadratus femoris muscle, and manual measurement for the level of the cut is made from the inferior rim of the femoral head instead of the lesser trochanter (Fig. 7–2). The computer provides the actual distance in millimeters between the level of the cut and the center of rotation of the acetabular cup. When the neck cut can be related to the cup's center of rotation, the offset can be balanced to the leg length, and the correct length of modular femoral head can be

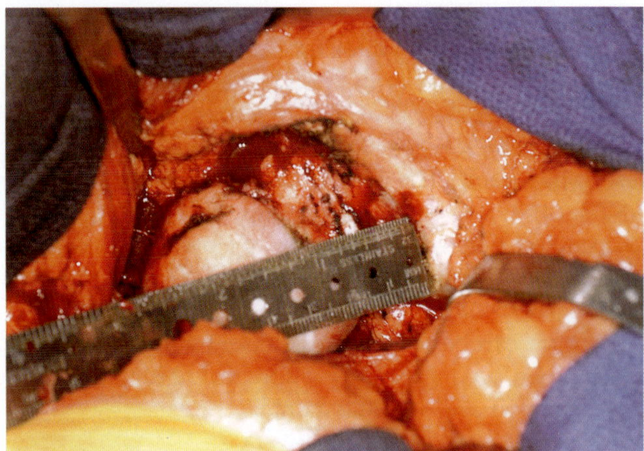

Figure 7–2 *The level of the femoral neck cut is measured from the inferior edge of the femoral head. The average neck cut is 15 mm below the edge of the femoral head.*

Table 7–1
Mean Values of X-ray and Computer Measurements*

Test	Inclination	Anteversion
Computer	41 ± 4.1	27 ± 2.7
X-ray	41 ± 4.3	26 ± 3.0

*All values are in degrees.
For both measurements, the difference between computer and x-ray is 2 degrees. Two degrees is the margin of measurement error for both the computer and the x-ray when compared with computed tomography scans, so these values are within the margin of error.

Table 7–2
Accuracy of Computer Measurements

Measure	Outliers	Accuracy
Inclination	1	97%
Anteversion	1	100%

Precision for measurement of outliers is based on comparison of the computer versus x-ray, with the computer needing to be within ±5 degrees of the x-ray value. Accuracy is based on computed tomography validation of the computer and x-ray measurements. Because the one anteversion outlier had an x-ray source of error, the computer accuracy for anteversion was 100%, and for inclination, 97%.

chosen. Using manual and visual methods, the level of the femoral neck cut must be estimated, and precision is variable.

Calculation of the Combined Anteversion. Knowledge of the absolute anteversions of the cup and femoral component permits calculation of the combined anteversion. From the work of Widmer and Zurfluh,[1] we know that the cup has a greater influence on the overall combined anteversion. In my experience with the computer, the anteversion of the cementless femoral component has very few degrees of freedom. The average femoral anteversion is 7.5 degrees, so 50% of femoral components have an anteversion less than this. Men seldom have as much as 10 degrees of anteversion, and often less than 5 degrees. Therefore, fractures can occur when the surgeon, by rotating the implant inside the femur, attempts to introduce anteversion into the stem that is not present in the femoral bone. Because of the inflexibility in positioning the cementless femoral stem, mating of the stem and cup is controlled by varying the cup anteversion. The anteversion of a cemented stem can be controlled better because the stem is smaller than the intramedullary canal. However, increasing the anteversion beyond 10 degrees with the cemented stem results in an undesirable intoeing gait when the patient walks, so even with a cemented stem the flexibility for adjusting combined anteversion lies with the cup.

CONFIRMATION OF ACCURACY OF COMPUTER RESULTS

Our results using the computer are shown in Tables 7–1 through 7–6. These data demonstrate a close correlation between computer and x-ray results and confirm the precision of the computer compared with radiographs for acetabular component positions (Tables 7–1 and 7–2). The CT scan data (Table 7–3) validate the accuracy of both the computer and radiographic measurements. The femoral component positions cannot be measured radiographically with the same precision as the acetabular component positions. Similarly, the correlation of computer and x-ray results is not as good for leg length and offset measurements as it is for acetabular components, because the rotation that occurs in positioning the leg for radiography affects these measurements (Table 7–4). Therefore, we check the computer readings by the manual methods described in Chapter 6. Clearly, the computer's accuracy is good because the mean difference in leg length measurements comparing both hips in the same patient is 1.4 mm. The computer measurements prove trustworthy when their precision is judged against the results of

Table 7–3
Validation of X-ray and Computer Measurements against Computed Tomography Scans

Test	Inclination	Anteversion
Computer	2.7	2.3
X-ray	2.0	1.7

The values represent the difference in degrees between the computer and x-ray measurements and the computed tomography (CT) scan measurement. Therefore, computer inclination had a mean difference from CT measurements of 2.7 degrees, and the x-ray inclination had a mean difference of 2.0 degrees.

Table 7–4
Leg Length and Offset Measurements by Computer and X-ray

Measurement	Computer	X-ray
Leg length*	5.0 ± 5.1 mm	1.8 ± 5.4 mm
Offset	0.3 ± 9.1 mm	0.3 ± 4.9 mm

*The operated leg length compared with the contralateral leg on the postoperative anteroposterior pelvic x-ray had a difference of 1.4 ± 5.7 mm (leg length difference).

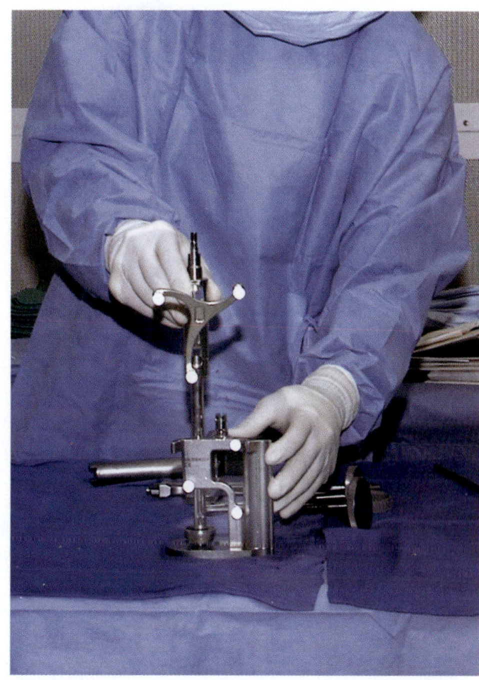

Figure 7–3 *Calibration is performed by the scrub technician before the operation. The tool is secured in a base to eliminate motion. The light-emitting diodes face the optical camera and the tracker on the tool is registered into the computer.*

preoperative physical examination and radiographic planning.

TECHNIQUE OF COMPUTER-ASSISTED TOTAL HIP REPLACEMENT

Calibration and Preliminary Registration

Before the pelvis and femur can be registered, the tools used with the computer need to be calibrated by the scrub nurse or technician with an optical camera (Fig. 7–3). Calibration ensures that the tools will provide accurate information to the computer software. Calibration is accomplished in the operating room while the patient is being prepared for anesthesia, so the process does not add extra time to the operation.

With the patient supine on the operating table, the pelvic registration device is placed on the iliac crest of the operative hip, and the AP plane of the pelvis is registered. We do this while the anesthesiologist is placing some of the intravascular lines used for intraoperative monitoring; our patients have an epidural in place and are sedated with Propofol, so the preparations for computer navigation do not interfere with the anesthesiologist's tasks.

An optical camera locates light-emitting diodes (LEDs) on the pelvic and femoral bases and the surgical tools and transfers these data to the computer (Fig. 7–4). In the future, electromagnetic devices or radiofrequency will be used to obtain measurements, and the need for invasive pins in the placement of registration devices will be eliminated. Regardless of which device is used to transmit measurements to the computer, the principles of computer navigation for total hip replacement will remain as described in this chapter.

The registration device is attached to the iliac crest with three threaded pins (Fig. 7–5) at the thickest portion of the crest (where a bone graft usually is taken). The device is oriented parallel to the iliac crest and is not placed on top of the crest. The pins are placed horizontally, not vertically. To minimize skin damage, a #15 scalpel blade is used to make a puncture wound on the skin and the threaded pin is drilled through this puncture into the iliac crest. The puncture sites can be marked with methylene blue (Fig. 7–6).

With the device fixed to the pelvis, the AP plane is registered using the pointer guide and touching the two anterior superior iliac spines and the pubis (Fig. 7–7).

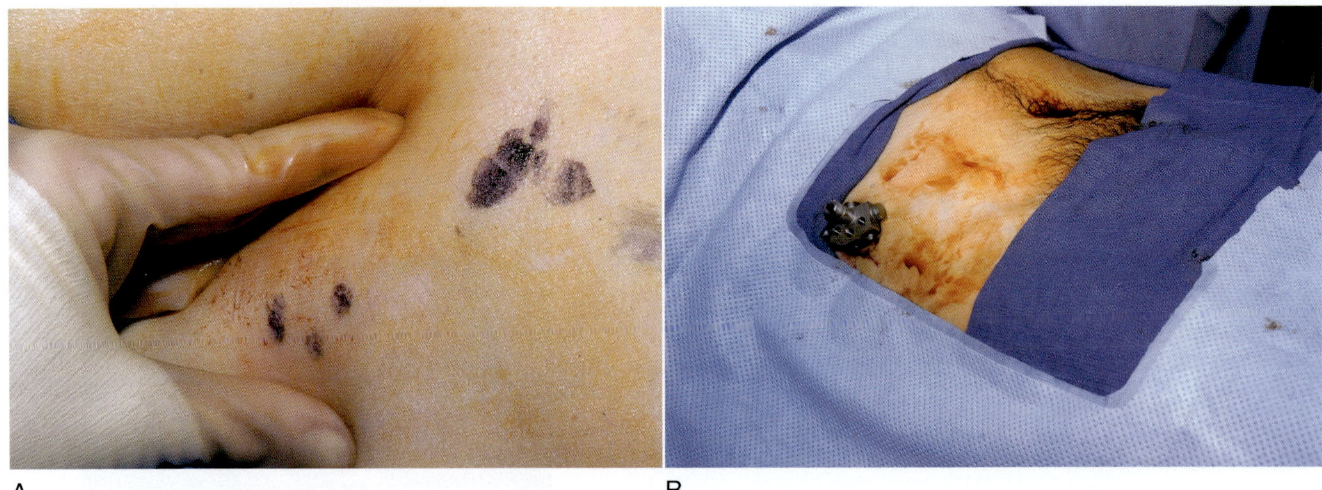

A   B

Figure 7–4 **A,** *The large methylene blue mark on the right is over the anterior superior iliac spine (ASIS). The three methylene marks between the fingers mark the sites for pin placement for the pelvic base. By squeezing along the iliac crest posterior to the ASIS, the thickest portion of the iliac crest can be identified.* **B,** *The base for the pelvic antenna has been pinned to the iliac crest. Three pins fix the base securely and prevent it from vibrating loose during anterior retraction of the femur for acetabular preparation.*

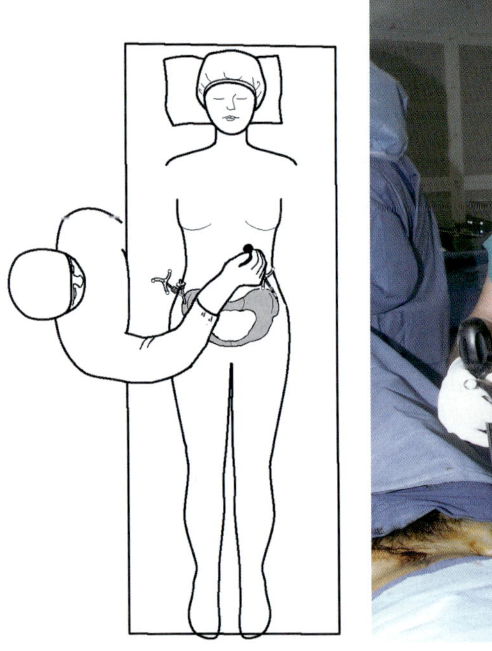

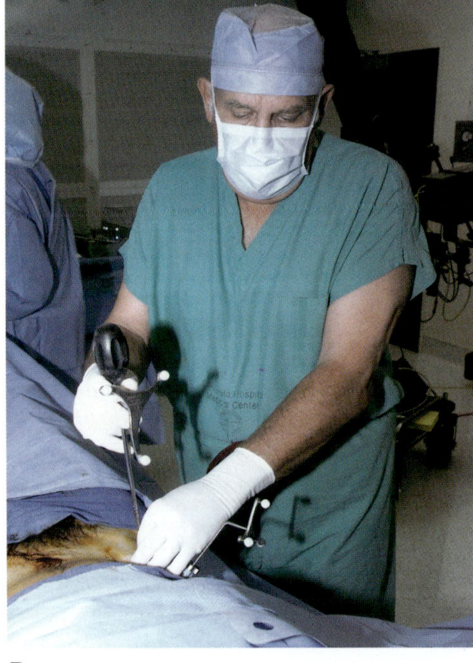

A   B

Figure 7–5 **A,** *Registration of the anteroposterior plane of the pelvis is performed while the patient lies supine on the operating table. The pelvic antenna with light-emitting diodes (LEDs) is seen on the right iliac crest and the pointer guide is touching the anterior superior iliac spine (ASIS) of the left iliac crest.* **B,** *Intraoperative view showing the pointer guide touching the ASIS on the side of the pelvis on which the pelvic tracking guide is based. The LEDs face the optical camera.*

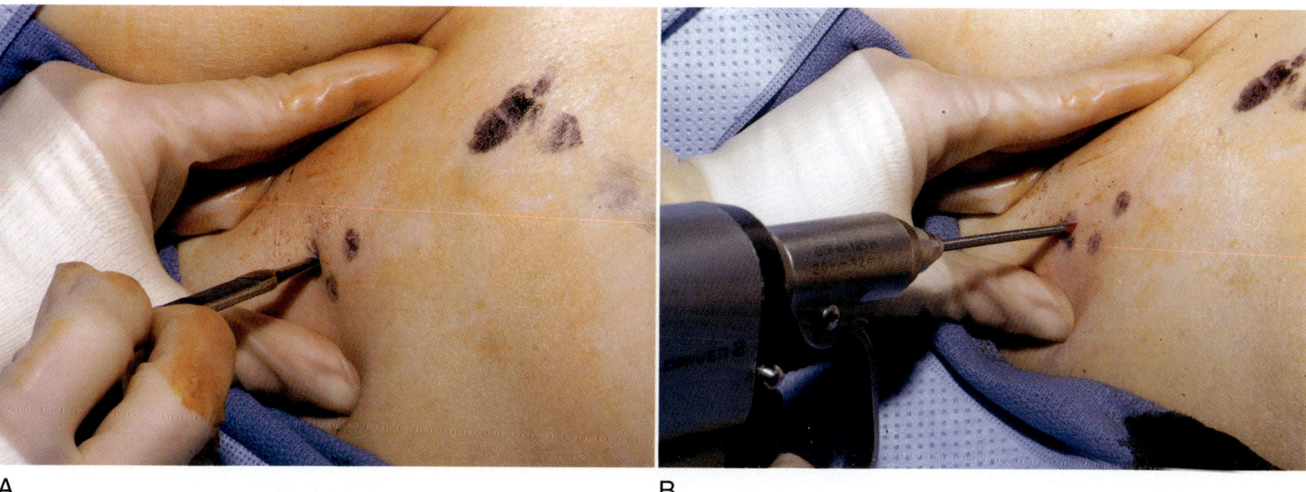

A   B

Figure 7–6   **A,** *The pin sites on the iliac crest have been marked with methylene blue, and small stab wounds (#15 scalpel) are made to facilitate insertion of the threaded pins through the skin into the bone without excessive skin damage.* **B,** *The threaded pin is inserted through the stab wound. Two of the threaded pins are inserted before the base is applied, and the third pin is then placed through the remaining drill hole in the base.*

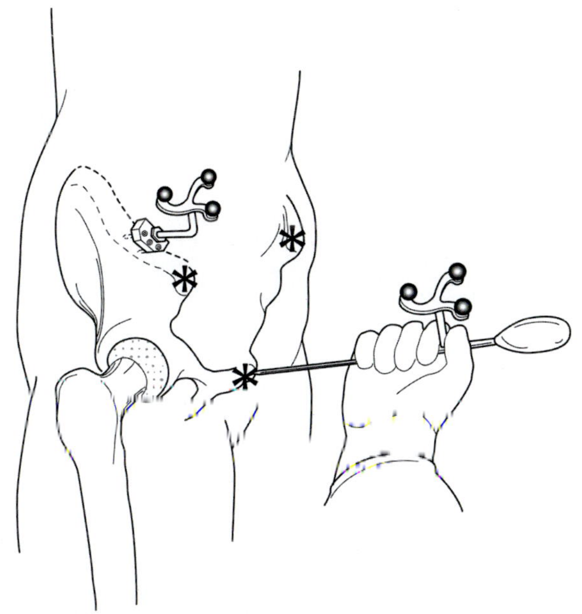

Figure 7–7   *The two anterior superior iliac spines (ASIS) and the symphysis pubis, which are the points touched by the pointer guide to register the anteroposterior plane of the pelvis. The pelvic base antennae are pinned to the iliac crest. It is important that the point of the guide be near or in contact with bone. This requires that over the pubis the point of the guide be pushed through the skin into the symphysis pubis because of the thickness of fat in this area in all patients.*

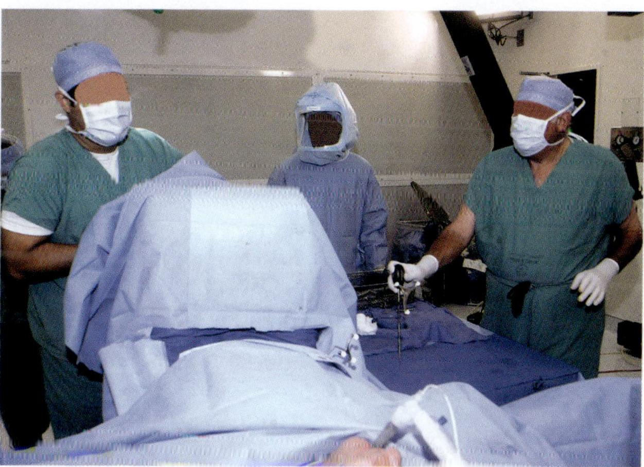

Figure 7–8   *Intraoperative view of the tilt of the pelvis being registered. A metal table adjacent to the operating table is used and a triangle is touched on this metal table to give the computer the information of the plane of the longitudinal axis of the body. Here, the pelvic tilt is being measured with the hips and knees flexed to simulate the sitting position.*

The pointer guide must be pushed through the skin to touch the pubic bone to obtain correct registration of the pubis. It is not necessary to puncture the skin over the anterior superior iliac spines unless there is a thick fat layer between the pointer and the bone. There is always a thick fat layer over the pubis, which is why the pointer must go through the skin to the bone. If the patient is to be operated on in the supine position, pelvic tilt is measured by comparing the AP plane tilt to the longitudinal axis of the body. The longitudinal axis is measured by touching a hard surface parallel to the body, either a table adjacent to the operating table (Fig. 7–8) or a hard surface placed under the patient's legs on the operating table. The operating table itself has soft padding that can be indented and therefore is less precise. Registration is done by creating a triangle of three points on the hard surface because a triangle is most easily recognized by the computer.

I operate with the patient in the lateral position, so once the AP plane of the pelvis is registered with the patient supine, the patient is moved to the lateral position. The hip and leg are prepared and draped as usual; when the hip is draped, the pelvic device must be draped into the field. The leg stockinette should be left at the level of the supracondylar knee because the femoral registration device must be placed into the distal third of the femur (Fig. 7–9). The femoral registration device is placed before application of the Betadine-soaked Vi-Drape, which, when placed, incorporates both of the bases for the trackers (Fig. 7–10). The best position for the femoral device is the anterior distal third of the femur (8 cm above the superior pole of the patella) because it does not interfere with the iliotibial band and there is good bone for firm pin fixation. If the device is proximal to the middle third–distal third junction, the pins can block preparation of the femur for the stem or stem insertion. Once the femoral device is fixed, the Betadine Vi-Drape is applied over the pelvic and femoral devices and then must be lifted off the connections for the tracker guides (Fig. 7–11).

While the femoral base is being pinned into place by the surgeon or assistant, a second assistant can measure the pelvic tilt. The tilt of the pelvis is measured by touching the posterior pelvic and posterior chest supports (Fig. 7–12), creating a triangle between

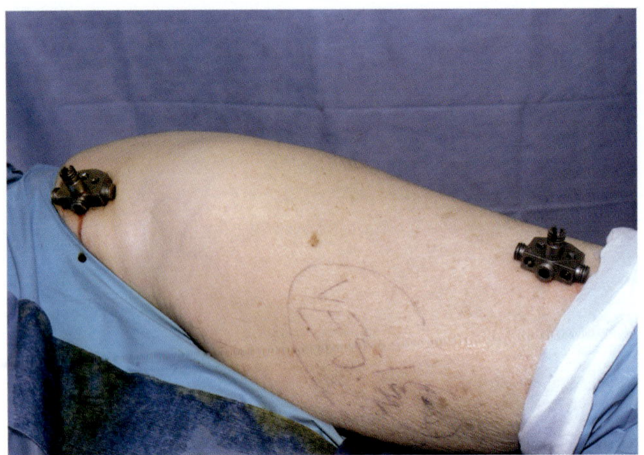

Figure 7–9 *The entire thigh is exposed so that the femoral base can be secured in the distal third of the femur. The base is secured to the femur with two or three pins. This base should be secured anterior to the iliotibial band. As with the iliac crest, methylene blue marks and stab wounds are made in the femur before placement of the threaded pins.*

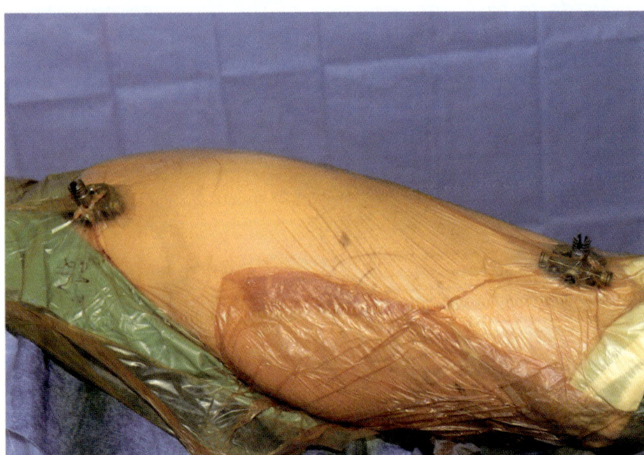

Figure 7–11 *The Betadine drape has been placed over the thigh and then removed from the connections of the bases so that the antennae can be inserted.*

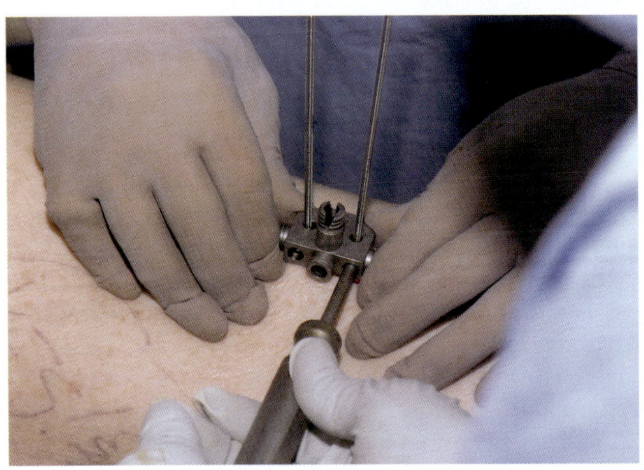

Figure 7–10 *The femoral device has been pinned to the femur and the screwdriver tightens the screws against the pins to fix the base securely to the bone.*

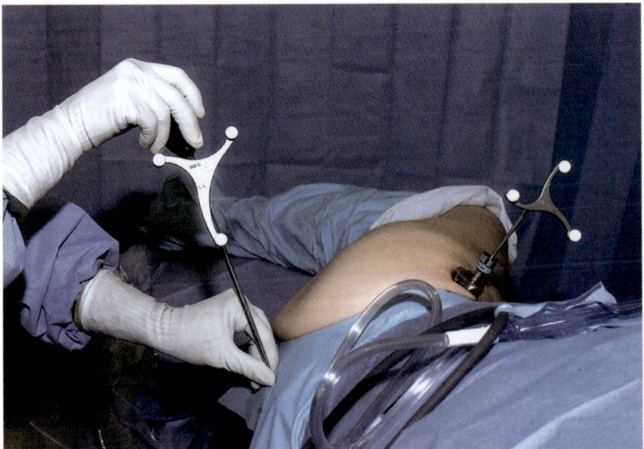

Figure 7–12 *The tracking guide with the light-emitting diode is on the pelvic base. The pointer guide is touched to the posterior support of the pelvis to register the plane of the longitudinal axis of the body with the patient in the lateral position so that the pelvic tilt can be calculated by the computer software.*

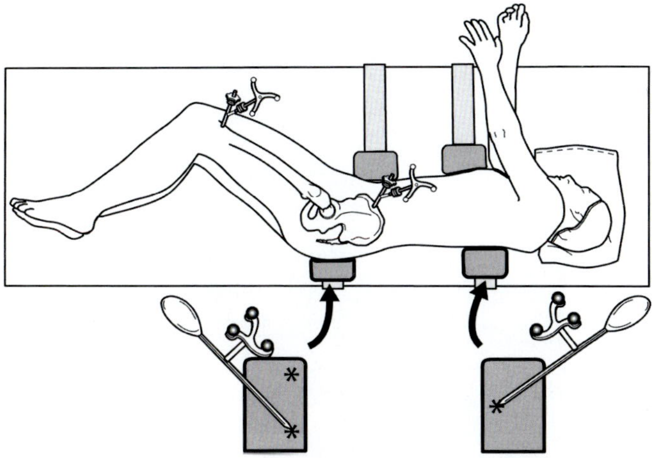

Figure 7–13 *A triangle is formed using the posterior supports of the pelvis and the chest to register the longitudinal axis of the body. This is illustrated with two points on the pelvic support and one on the chest support.*

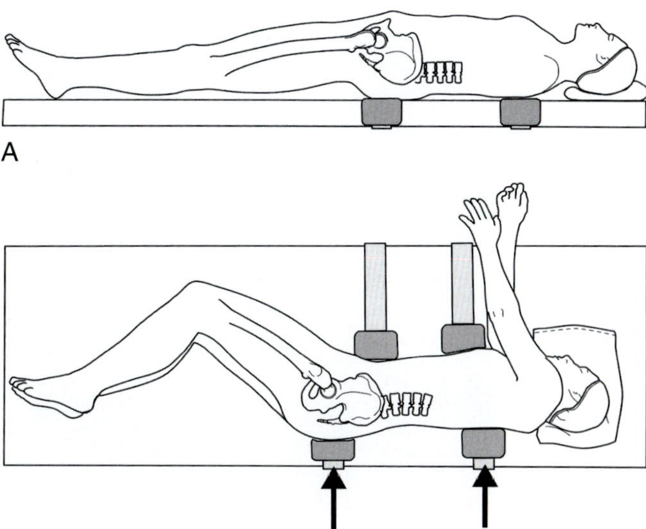

A

B

Figure 7–14 **A,** *The patient in the supine position most commonly has an anterior pelvic tilt, as illustrated by the coccyx pointing anteriorly. This anterior tilt in the supine position affects the anteversion of the cup by giving a false impression of excessive anteversion. The adjusted anteversion for an anteriorly tilted pelvis shows the acetabular component to be in less anteversion than is thought to be present based on visualization. **B,** When the patient is turned to the lateral position, the pelvis extends from the anterior position seen in the supine position, as reflected by a change in the position of the coccyx compared with **A.** This means that the pelvis takes on a posterior tilt. Eighty percent of patients have extension from the anterior position while supine; 50% extend 5 degrees or more, and 30% have absolute posterior tilt. With posterior tilt of the pelvis, the adjusted anteversion means that the anteversion of the cup is actually greater than appears visually.*

the supports to register them (Fig. 7–13). The computer can now calculate the pelvic tilt because it knows the AP plane of the pelvis and the relative position of the pelvis to the longitudinal plane of the body (Fig. 7–14). Pelvic tilt is one of the most critical measurements for computer navigation because the correct interpretation by the software of all measurements of pelvic data depend on it. As with calibration of the tools, any error in determining the pelvic tilt can invalidate all adjusted acetabular measurements.

Preoperative Measurements of Anatomy

The operation begins with the incision to the greater trochanter. The computer provides precise information with any long incision and provides superb assistance with mini-incisions.

Establishing Baseline for Offset and Leg Length Measurement

The baseline for offset and leg length measurement is obtained when both the femoral and pelvic trackers are in place. To establish the baseline, the leg is lifted under the knee and at the ankle so that it is separated from the lower leg (Fig. 7–15). The computer then registers the leg's position. After the reconstruction, and with the hip relocated, the leg will be lifted into the same position. The preoperative leg position must be exactly duplicated postoperatively, and the position of the leg for flexion/extension, internal/external rotation,

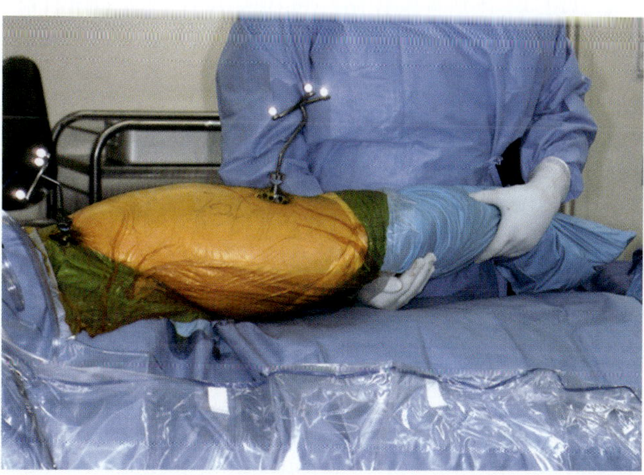

Figure 7–15 *Both the pelvic and femoral bases have been placed and have antennae with light-emitting diodes. The leg is lifted to register the baseline value for leg length. It is best to lift the leg because it is easier to reproduce the abduction position of the leg if it has been lifted instead of left lying on the table.*

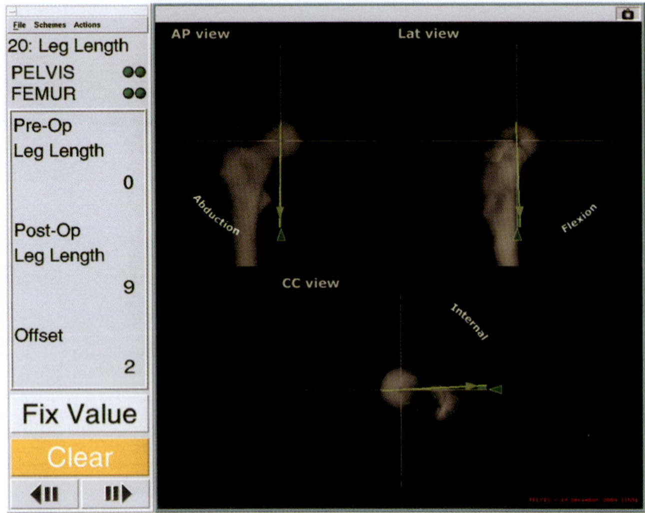

Figure 7–16 *Computer screen showing postoperative leg length and offset. The change in leg length from preoperative is 9 mm longer, and the change in offset is 2 mm greater. The screen shows that the leg has been placed back into exactly the same position as it was preoperatively by alignment of abduction/adduction, flexion/extension, and internal/external rotation.*

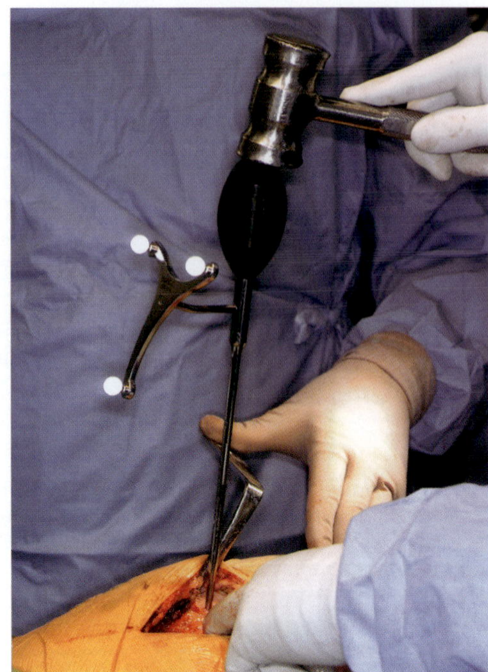

Figure 7–17 *The pointer guide is in contact with the greater trochanter and a mallet is used to make a small divot in the greater trochanter so the same point can be found after the hip replacement is completed. It is important to insert the pointer guide gently into this divot after the reconstruction so that it does not puncture further through cancellous bone. If the pointer guide is pushed farther through cancellous bone than the depth created with the initial divot, the offset measurement can be affected.*

and abduction/adduction is shown on the computer screen. When the postoperative leg has been placed into the preoperative position, the *change* in leg length and offset will register on the computer screen (Fig. 7–16).

The leg length and offset can also be measured if only acetabular, and not femoral, registration was done. The greater trochanter is touched with the LED pointer guide (Fig. 7–17). To ensure that the same point will be used in the postoperative measurement, a divot is made in the greater trochanter and marked with methylene blue (Fig. 7–18). When the reconstruction is complete, the marked point is touched with the LED pointer guide, and the computer calculates the difference in leg length and offset (Fig. 7–19). The leg must be in the same position after reconstruction as it was when the initial registration was done; I ensure this by overlaying one leg on the other, just as we do for measuring leg length (Fig. 7–20).

Determining Femoral Anteversion and the Position of the Stem in the Bone

With the greater trochanter exposed, the plane of the leg is registered so that the computer can give the anteversion of the femoral component, as well as the position of the stem within the bone (Fig. 7–21). The leg should be bent to nearly 90 degrees flexion at the hip and 90 degrees flexion at the knee for registration of the malleoli. The plane of the leg is measured by touching the short pointer guide to the trochanter, the two

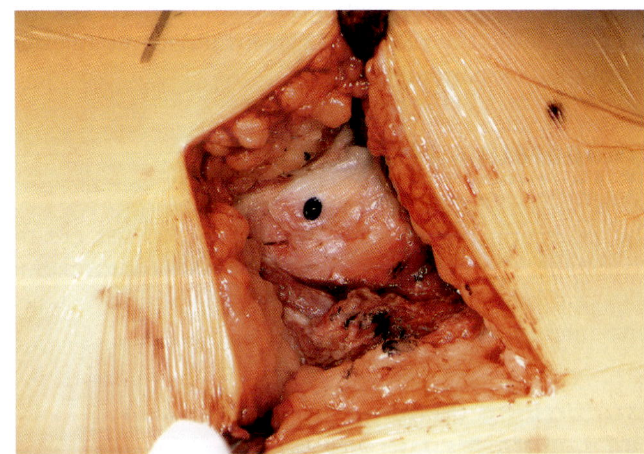

Figure 7–18 *The divot in the greater trochanter is marked with methylene blue.*

epicondyles of the femur at the knee, and the two malleoli of the ankle.

Once the plane of the leg has been registered, registration of the anatomy is complete and precise intraoperative measurements for component positions can be done.

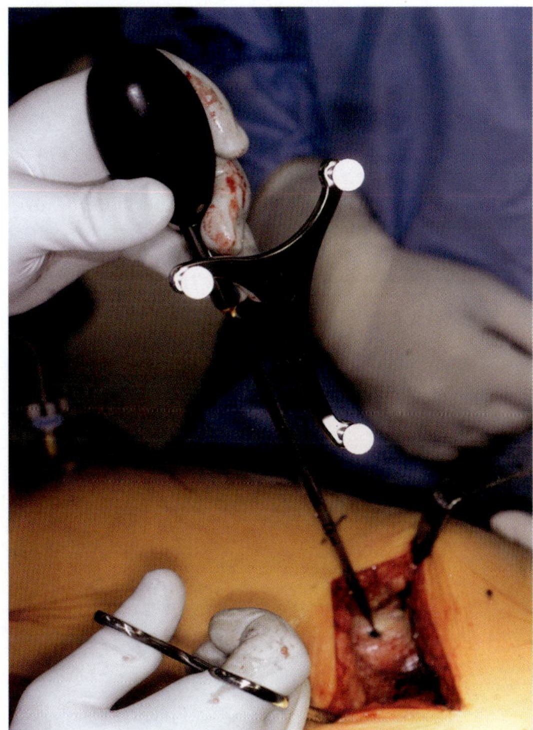

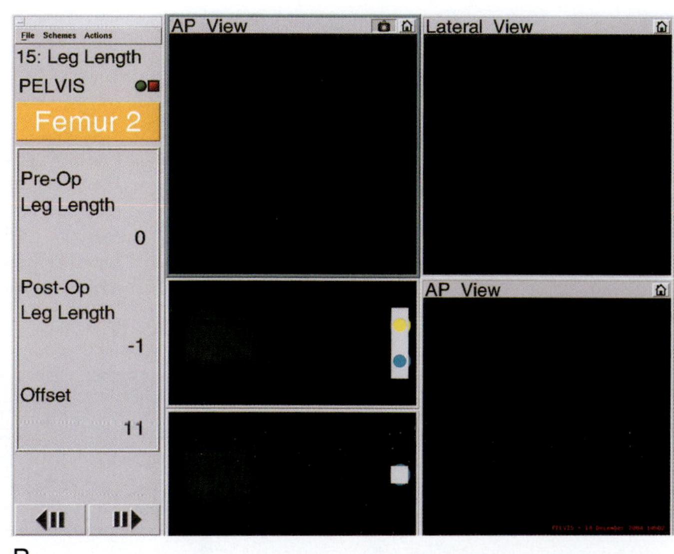

A

B

Figure 7–19 **A,** *After completion of the hip replacement and with the hip reduced and the leg in the same position as it was with the initial measurement (I overlay the two legs), the pointer guide is put into the divot with the light-emitting diode facing the camera.* **B,** *The change in leg length and offset is calculated by the computer software and is seen in the left column.*

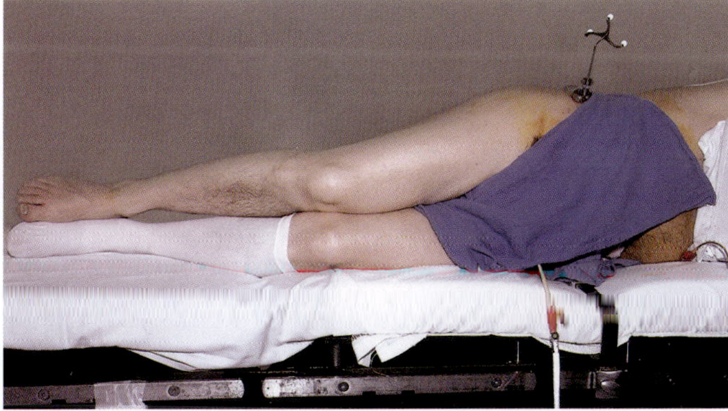

Figure 7–20 *The leg position we use for measurement on the trochanter for leg length and offset. The legs are overlaid. Obviously, for an operation the legs are draped.*

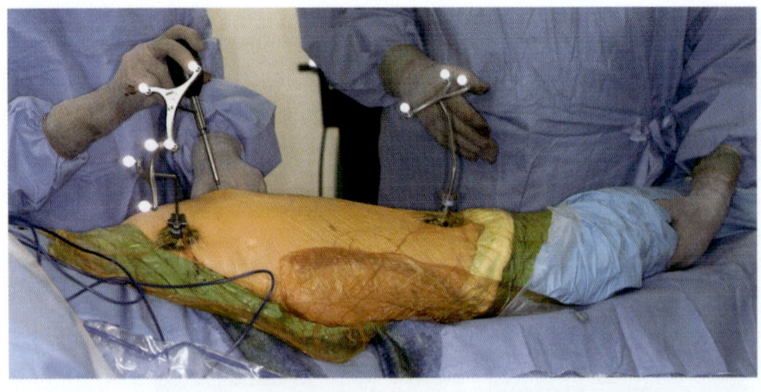

A

Figure 7–21 **A,** With the femoral and pelvic trackers in place, the plane of the leg is registered by initially touching the greater trochanter with the short pointer guide. **B,** The medial and lateral epicondyles of the femur are touched with the short pointer guide. **C,** The medial and lateral malleoli of the ankle are touched with the short pointer guide. The hip and knee should be in 90 degrees of flexion for this malleoli measurement.

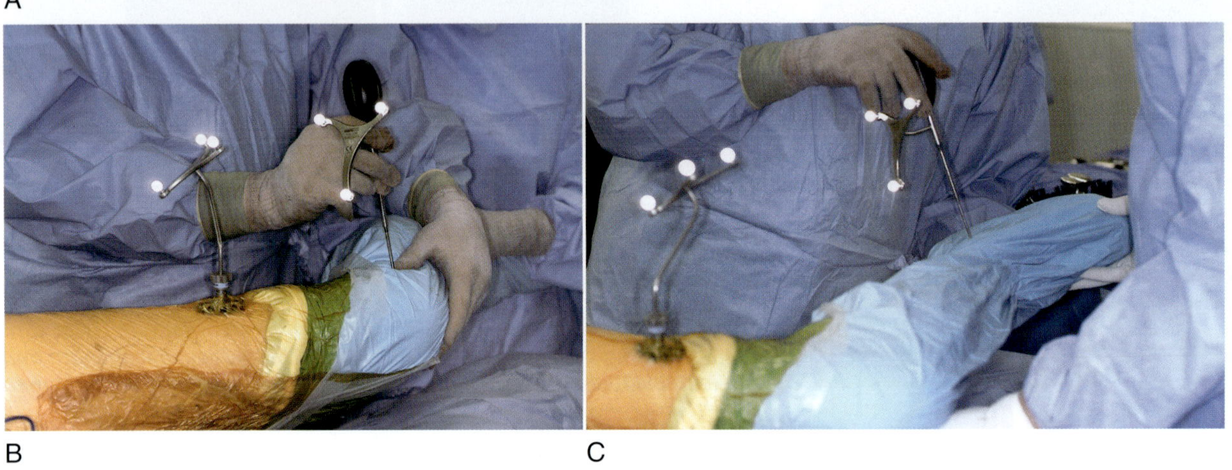

B

C

First option

Femoral preparation
    Ream and broach
    Determine anteversion

Acetabular preparation
    Center of rotation
    Reaming
    Cup placement

Femoral implantation
    Check neck cut
    Implant stem

Control change in leg length and offset
    Depth of stem implantation
    Head length

Second option

Acetabular preparation
    Center of rotation
    Reaming
    Cup placement

Femoral preparation and implantation
    Open canal
    Broach or ream
    Implant stem

Control change in leg length and offset
    Depth of stem implantation
    Head length

Figure 7–22. Algorithm showing two possible sequences in performing total hip replacement.

Intraoperative Measurements and Procedure

Figure 7–22 shows the sequence I follow in total hip replacement (first option). I prepare the femur (see discussion below) before the acetabulum to obtain the femoral anteversion so that I can correctly position the cup to mate the stem and provide a correct combined anteversion of approximately 35 degrees. The femur is exposed with retractors, as shown in Chapter 6. The canal is opened with the burr and reamed to the correct size. The canal is registered with five points (see Fig. 7–40). The broach is inserted to determine the anteversion of the stem (see Fig. 7–41). Once I know the femoral anteversion, I proceed to acetabular preparation.

Alternatively, the surgeon could follow the steps in the second option (see Fig. 7–22).

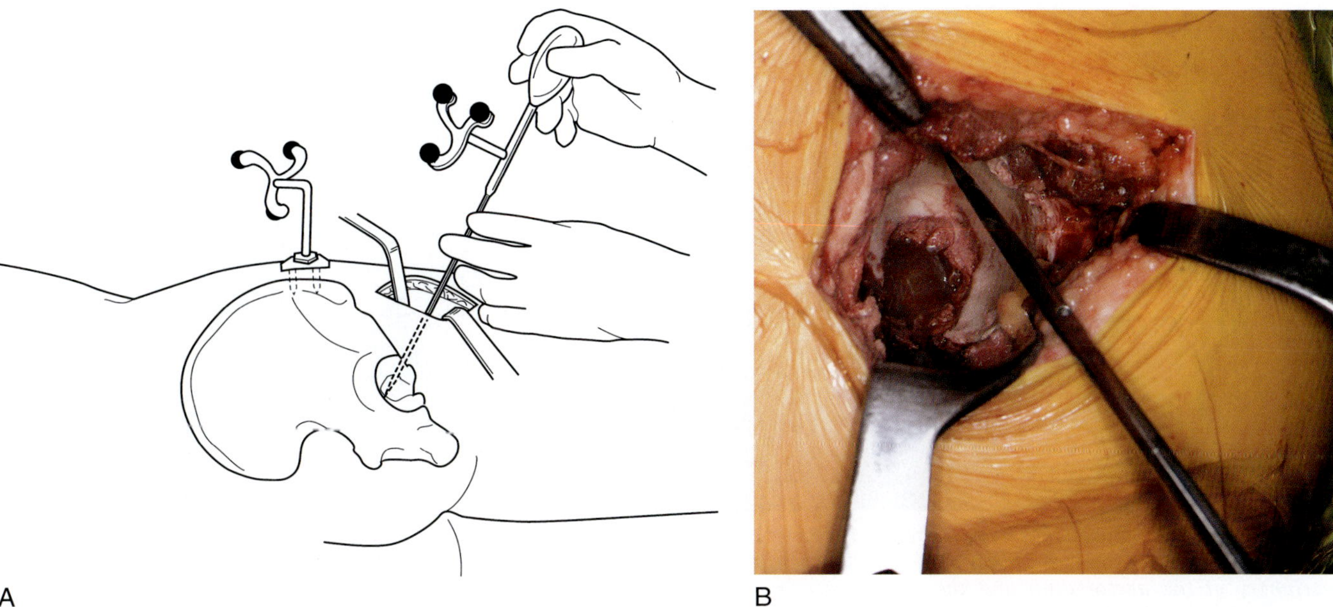

A   B

Figure 7–23 **A,** *The long pointer guide is used to touch the acetabular bone. For registration of the center of rotation, 16 points are made on the acetabular bone, avoiding the medial cotyloid notch and osteophytes.* **B,** *Intraoperative view of the pointer guide touching the periphery of the acetabulum. The central cotyloid notch is avoided for this measurement, as are osteophytes.*

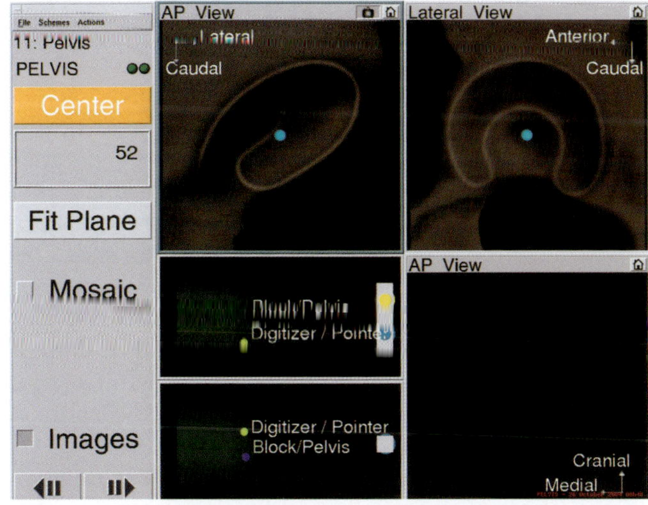

Figure 7–24 *After the 16-point registration of the acetabulum, the computer screen shows the acetabular center of rotation in the two planes. The center of rotation is located in the area of the cotyloid notch. On the left side of the screen, in the box under the word "center," the diameter of the acetabulum is given (52 mm in this patient). The size of the cup used is usually 2 mm larger than the size of the osseous acetabulum because it is necessary to ream the acetabulum into a hemisphere for fixation of a hemispheric cup.*

Acetabular Preparation with Computer Navigation

Center of Rotation, Mosaic, and Fit Plane. The acetabulum is exposed and retractors placed. The pulvinar is excised from the cotyloid notch. It is important to expose the cotyloid notch so that the medial wall of the acetabulum can be registered. The pointer is used to make 16 points on the acetabulum for a determination of the acetabular *center of rotation* (Fig. 7–23). When the 16 points have been recorded, the computer screen shows a dot that indicates the center of rotation of the acetabulum (Fig. 7–24). The diameter of the osseous acetabulum is also displayed on the screen, and this can be compared with the preoperative templated size. In my experience, the size of cup that will be used is usually at least 2 mm bigger than the osseous acetabulum; therefore, if the osseous acetabulum is 52 mm, the cup size would be expected to be 54 or 55 mm.

A second set of points is then made to create a *mosaic* of the acetabular anatomy. The peripheral wall is displayed on the computer screen in both the sagittal and coronal planes (Fig. 7–25). In Figure 7–25, the peripheral wall is indicated with red dots and the medial wall with yellow dots. The medial wall is outlined by touching the cortical bone of the cotyloid notch (Fig. 7–26).

Once more measurement is taken from the acetabulum by making six points along the acetabular periphery. This is called the *fit plane* of the acetabulum, and it is displayed in the lower right quadrant of the computer screen. (Fig. 7–27). From the fit plane, the software calculates the inclination and anteversion of the native acetabulum and displays the adjusted anteversion and inclination.

Although I generally do not use the information on the native acetabular angles during implantation of the

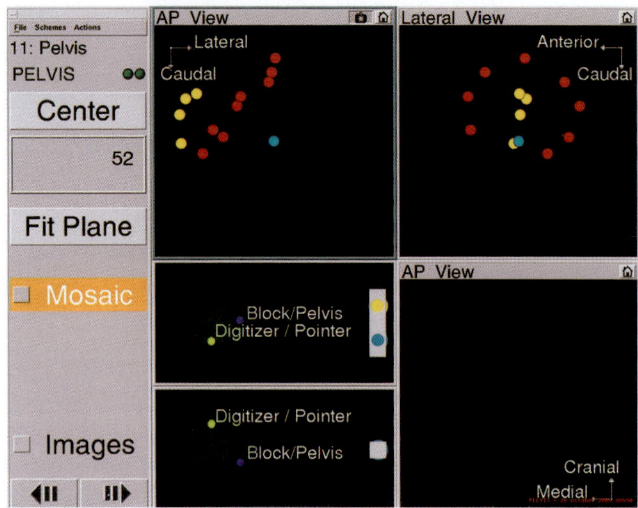

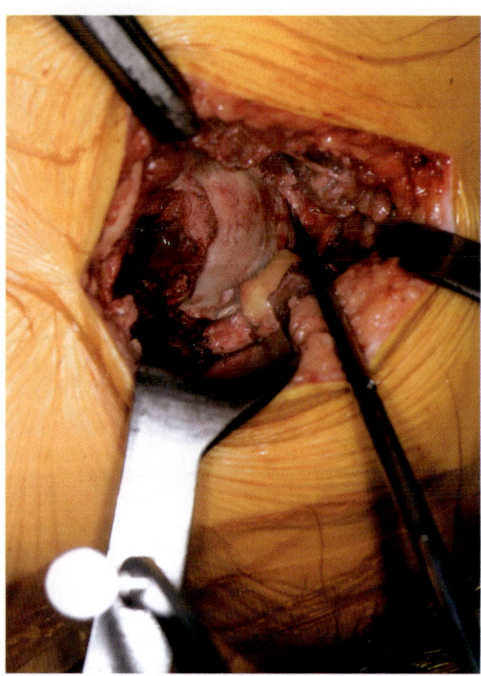

Figure 7–25   *The mosaic of the acetabulum is shown on the computer screen in the two planes. The red dots outline the periphery of the acetabulum and the yellow dots represent the medial wall. The blue dot is the center of rotation of the acetabulum. Again, on the left, the size of the osseous acetabulum is given (52 mm).*

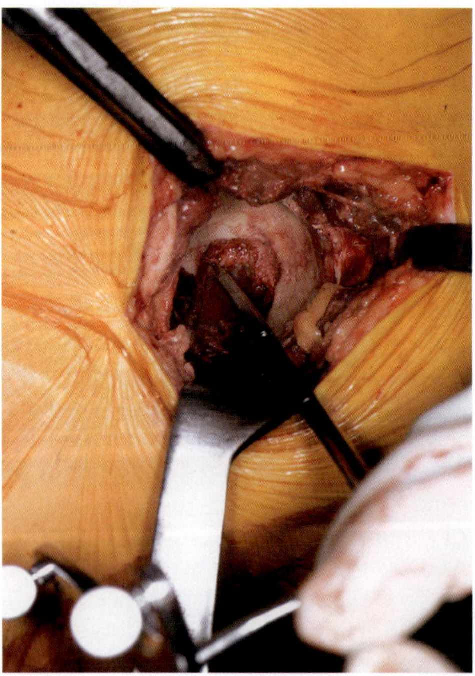

Figure 7–26   *Intraoperative view showing the pointer guide touching the medial wall in the cotyloid notch. This gives the yellow dots seen on Figure 7–24. The yellow dots represent medial wall, which is the medial end point for reaming.*

Figure 7–27   *Intraoperative view showing the pointer guide touching the periphery of the acetabulum. The fit plane is registered by touching six points on the periphery of the acetabulum. The fit plane gives the inclination and anteversion of the osseous acetabulum. This measurement can also be used to measure the position of the metal shell, as described later.*

acetabular component, it does tell the surgeon that the component cannot be placed in accordance with the native anatomy because so placing it would not result in optimal component position. The inclination is almost always too steep; the mean inclination is 55 degrees, and 40% of acetabula are inclined greater than 55 degrees. The mean average anteversion is 12 degrees, with 52% at 10 degrees or less and 12% in absolute retroversion (i.e., negative degrees of anteversion). The steepness of the native inclination is the reason the posterosuperior edge of the cup is almost never covered by bone, with 5 mm of metal left exposed (Fig. 7–28). If the metal were entirely covered by the native acetabulum, the inclination of the cup might be too great. The metal of the cup will be entirely covered by bone only if the cup has been reamed superiorly (i.e., the center of rotation elevated 5 mm or more).

Registration of the three acetabular measurements (center of rotation, mosaic, and fit plane) requires 2 to 3 minutes. Once this information has been recorded, the remaining technical parameters relevant to the acetabular procedure are quantitatively expressed on the computer screen.

Reaming. The reaming of the acetabulum can be monitored on the computer screen. The reamer has three silver LEDs attached to it so that the camera can record its position (Fig. 7–29). The reamer position is fully outlined on the computer screen (Fig. 7–30), which displays the number of millimeters the reamer has changed the center of rotation medially, anteriorly, or posteriorly, as well as superiorly or distally (see Fig. 7–30). It is important that the reamer be kept centrally, as determined by anteroposterior placement, so that the anterior or posterior walls are not reamed away. The reamer should not deviate by more than 5 mm either anteriorly or posteriorly. The depth of the reamer determines the center of rotation measurement. The medialization should have been estimated from preoperative planning (Fig. 7–31). It is critical to remove all floor osteophytes before registration of the medial wall, or the medial wall will be falsely represented by the floor osteophyte (see X-ray Example 2). There should be 4 to 5 mm of medialization to allow the metal of the cup to be fit against the acetabular bone and the center of rotation of the cup to be near normal. The center of rotation of the cup is rarely the center of rotation of the osseous acetabulum, because to obtain coverage of the cup, the reaming must be 2 to 3 mm superior and 5 to 6 mm medial. If a depth of at least 4 mm is not achieved, the cup will be lateralized. In some acetabula, the medial wall is 10 to 11 mm deeper than the osseous center of rotation. In a dysplastic acetabulum the cup is often reamed 5 to 10 mm superiorly and 10 mm or more medially (see X-ray Example 3). During reaming, it is more important to know the three-dimensional position of the cup than the inclination and anteversion of the reamer, which are relevant only for preparation of the bone. Obviously, the inclination and anteversion of the cup are critical.

Trial Cup Placement. The trial cup is placed when reaming has been completed. The position of the trial cup is recorded through the silver LEDs on the cup

holder (Fig. 7–32), and the computer screen lists the medialization, center of rotation, and anteroposterior position of the cup (Fig. 7–33). The screen also exhibits the inclination, adjusted inclination, anteversion, and adjusted anteversion. The adjusted values should be selected because they are adjusted for the patient's pelvic tilt.

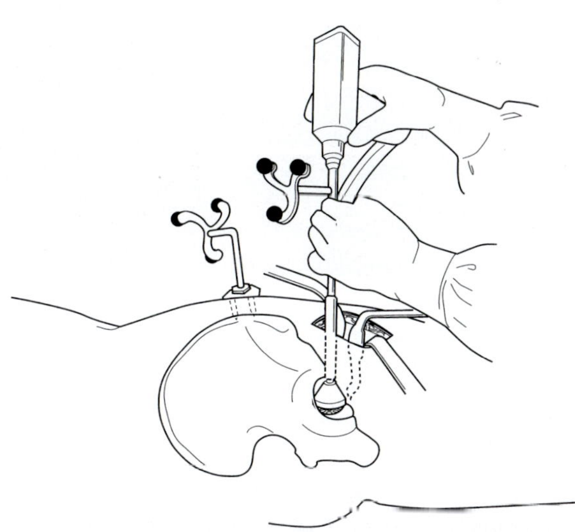

A

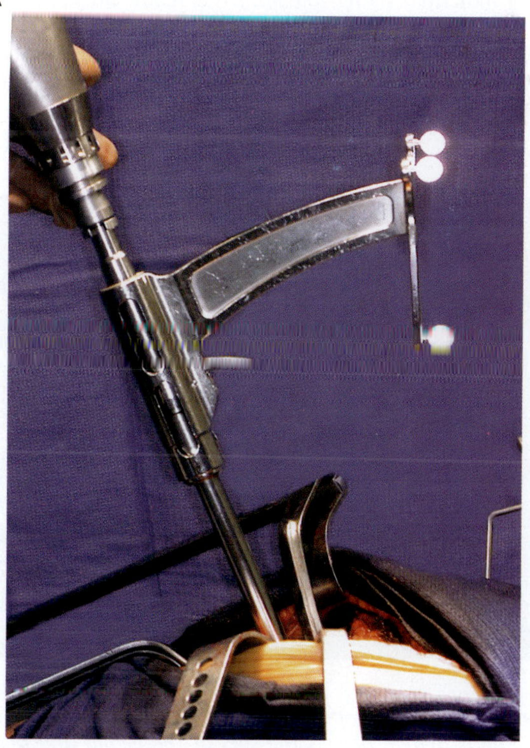

B

Figure 7–29 **A,** *The initial reaming of the acetabulum is done transversely to remove the acetabular ridge. Reaming is performed to the level of the cortical bone of the cotyloid notch, which means that by watching the computer screen the surgeon can advance the reamer until it touches the yellow dots.* **B,** *Intraoperative view showing the light-emitting diode on the reamer the computer uses to register the position of the reamer in the osseous acetabulum.*

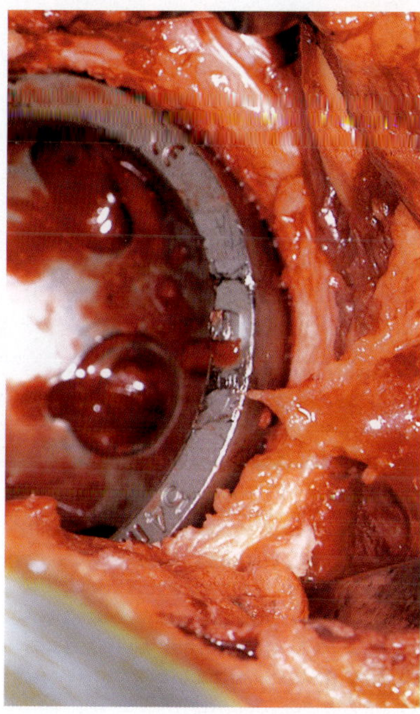

Figure 7–28 *The posterosuperior edge of the cup stands proud to bone. Because the average inclination of the acetabulum is 55 degrees, this metal edge needs to clear the bone to ensure that the cup is not too vertical.*

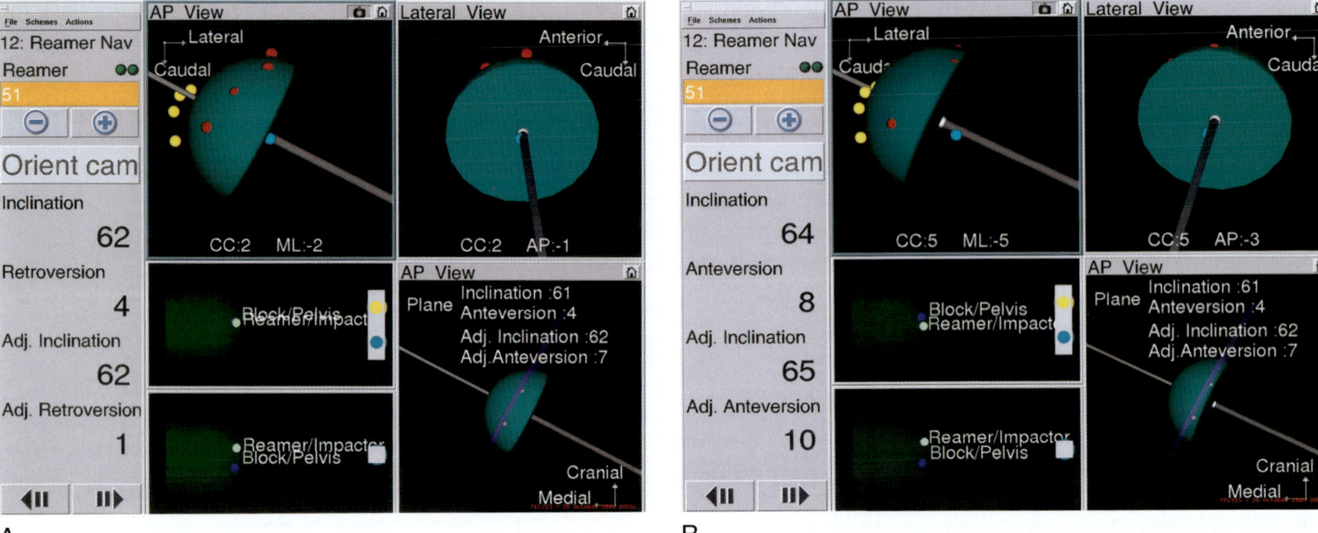

A   B

Figure 7–30 **A,** *A computer screen showing the information available during reaming. In the left column, the angles of the reamer are given. Because this reaming is being done transversely, the inclination is steep. The reamer can be adjusted into anteversion as desired. There is relatively little anteversion in the reamer during the transverse removal of the ridge. The upper two quadrants show the reamer and its position in the acetabulum. The CC number (2) means that the reamer is 2 mm superior to the center of rotation of the osseous acetabulum. The ML number (–2) means the reamer is 2 mm medial to the osseous center of rotation (CR). In the upper right quadrant, the CC number (2) means that the reamer is 2 mm superior to the CR, and the AP number (–1) means that the reamer is 1 mm posterior from the center. This gives the surgeon complete information with regard to the change in the acetabular CR induced by reaming.* **B,** *The reamer has been advanced to the level of the medial wall, as indicated by its touching the yellow dots. Reaming is now being done in greater anteversion to keep the reamer from going too posteriorly. In the upper right quadrant, the AP number indicates that the center has been moved 3 mm posteriorly. The upper left quadrant shows that the center of rotation has been elevated 5 mm and medialized 5 mm. The lower right quadrant provides a graphic illustration of the coverage of the cup with the reamer in its current position compared with the values of the native acetabulum.*

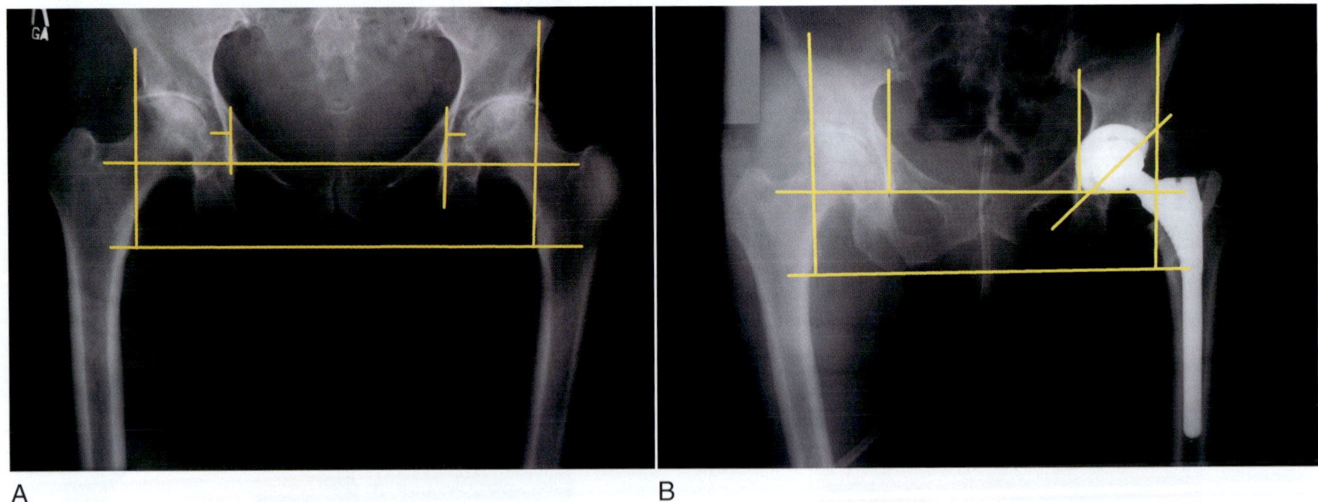

A   B

Figure 7–31 **A,** *Preoperative x-ray of patient having a left total hip replacement showing the measurements taken. A transverse line is drawn across the tips of the ischia and across the bottom of the tear drops. Vertical lines are drawn through the base of the junction of the lesser trochanter to the femoral neck and through the tear drop. The measurement between the tear drop and the lateral vertical line gives a measurement for the offset. The measurement from the tear drop vertical line to the edge of the femoral head gives an approximation of medialization, which is usually 5 to 6 mm. The leg length can be measured by a line that is placed at the junction of the lesser trochanter to the neck in both hips and then measuring the changes required to equalize the reconstructed hip to the contralateral hip.* **B,** *Postoperative x-ray of hip replacement with the same lines drawn and an additional line for inclination of the acetabulum. The anteversion of the acetabulum is calculated mathematically by determining the ellipse of the acetabular opening (this method can be reviewed in Wan and Dorr[2]). The lines on this x-ray allow the changes from preoperative to postoperative measurements to be compared, and these radiographic measurements to be compared with the computer measurements.*

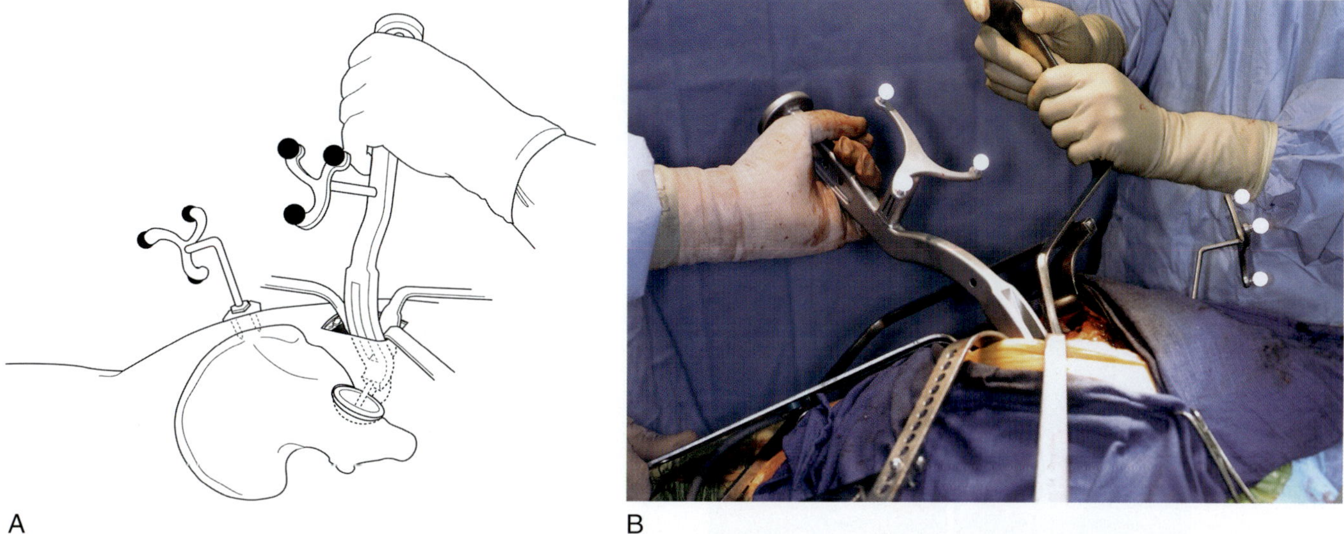

Figure 7–32 ***A,*** *The curved cup holder inserting the acetabular component with the light-emitting diode (LED) antenna. The computer can register the position of the component in the acetabulum. The tracker guide on the cup holder must be absolutely secure or a false reading can result. To check the cup holder, we do a fit plane measurement after removal of the cup holder.* ***B,*** *Intraoperative view showing the cup holder with the LED. Note that the antenna with the LED is placed in a solid base so that it cannot easily vibrate loose.*

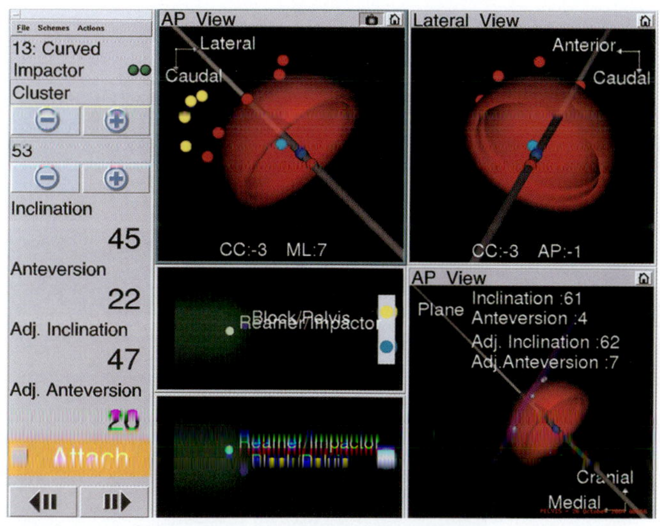

A

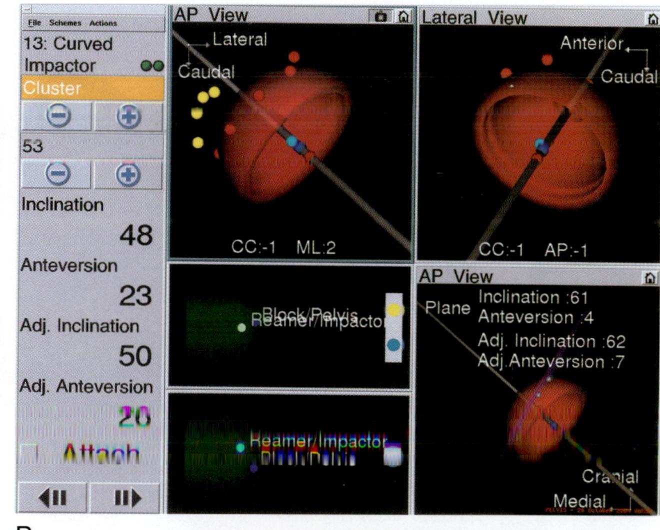

B

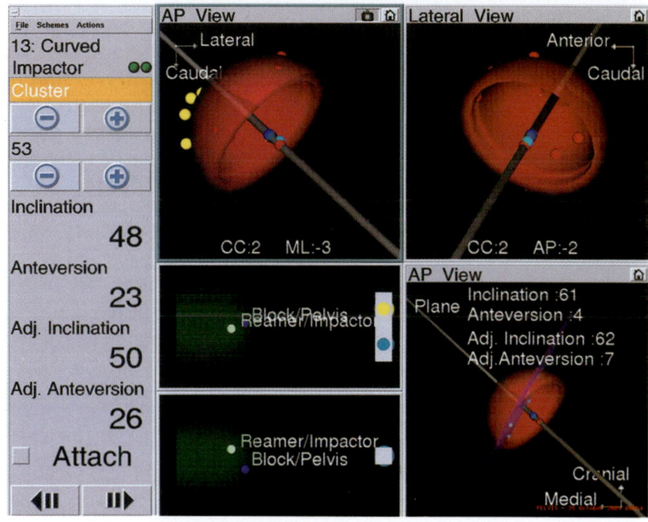

C

Figure 7–33 ***A,*** *The information available to the surgeon from the computer during insertion of the cup. The left column gives the absolute inclination and anteversion and the adjusted inclination and anteversion according to the pelvic tilt. This pelvis had a posterior tilt, so the adjusted anteversion is greater than the absolute anteversion. In the upper left, the cup is just being placed into the mouth of the acetabulum, and the center of rotation (CR) is 3 mm lateral (CC –3) to the osseous CR and 7 mm lateral (ML +7). In the upper right, it can be seen that the cup is 1 mm posterior (AP –1). The lower right gives a graphic representation of the position of the cup relative to the inclination of the osseous acetabulum.* ***B,*** *The acetabular component is advanced into the osseous acetabulum. It now is at a position where the center of rotation is 1 mm caudal (CC –1), 2 mm lateral (ML 2), and 1 mm posterior (AP –1). The adjusted inclination of this acetabular component is 50 degrees, with an adjusted anteversion of 26 degrees.* ***C,*** *The acetabular component has been seated into the osseous acetabulum. The final position of the center of rotation is 2 mm superior (CC 2), 3 mm medial (ML –3), and 2 mm posterior (AP –2). The adjusted inclination is 50 degrees and the adjusted anteversion, 26 degrees. The graphic illustration with the fit plane in the lower right shows why the posterior superior edge of the cup needs to be proud. The final inclination and anteversion are shown in Figure 7–34.*

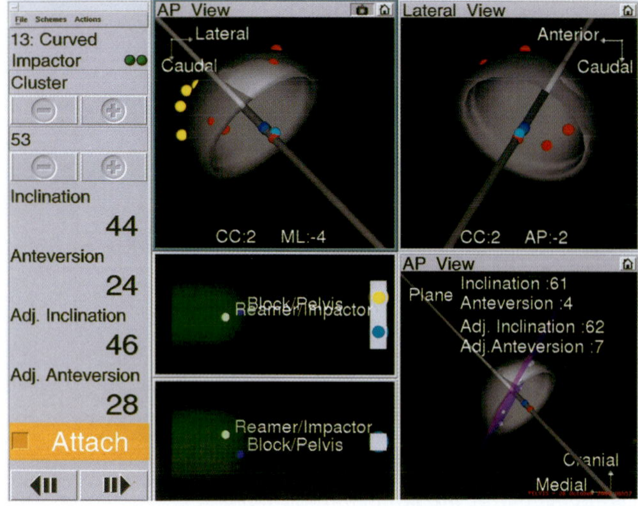

Figure 7–34 *Computer screen showing the seating of the acetabular cup with position of the center of rotation (CR) 2 mm superior, 4 mm medial, and 2 mm posterior. The adjusted inclination is 46 degrees and the adjusted anteversion, 28 degrees. The fit plane in the lower right is that of the osseous acetabulum.*

Table 7–5
Fit Plane Measurements*

Fit Plane	Adjusted Inclination	Adjusted Anteversion
Cup holder[†]	41.4 ± 3.4	23.6 ± 3.8
Cup	41.3 ± 3.5	25.8 ± 4.5
After one screw	42.5 ± 3.5	24.2 ± 3.2
After liner	42.7 ± 4.0	25.1 ± 3.5

*All values are in degrees.
[†]The cup holder values are those obtained with the cup holder and are listed for comparison with the values obtained with the fit plane measurements.
The fit plane adjusted inclination and anteversion for each maneuver with the cup are listed, showing the mean change that occurs with each maneuver.

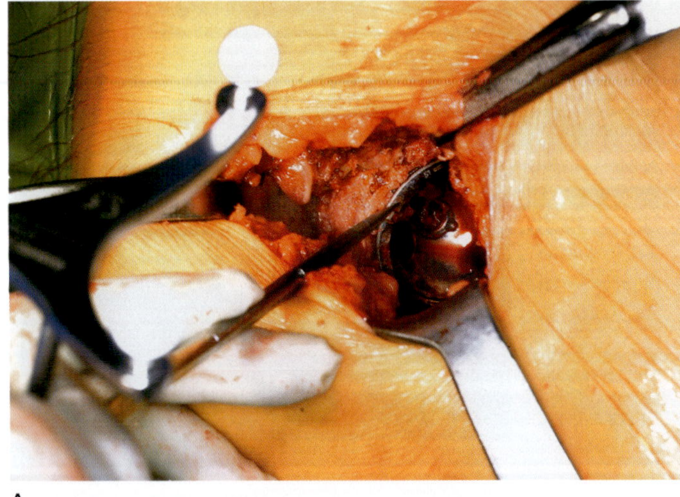

A

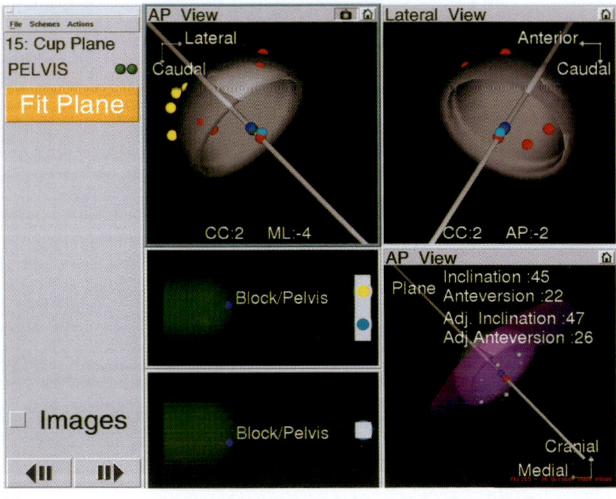

B

Figure 7–35 **A,** *The fit plane of the cup is measured by touching the edge of the metal shell in six places with the pointer guide. The fit plane registers the inclination and anteversion of the cup.* **B,** *The fit plane values are seen in the lower right, with an adjusted inclination of 47 degrees and an adjusted anteversion of 26 degrees. Compare these with the cup holder values (see Fig. 7–33) of 46 degrees inclination and 28 degrees adjusted anteversion. The 2-degree difference between the cup holder and the fit plane can result just from the vibration of removing the cup holder. Two degrees also seems to be the measurement error of two different measurements with the computer.*

The most critical parameters for the trial cup are its center of rotation, inclination, and anteversion. Once these are ascertained, the trial component is removed and the acetabular component implanted. If screws are necessary, the screw holes should have any covers removed. Once again, LEDs on the cup holder permit the software to determine cup position (see Fig. 7–31), and the cup's center of rotation, medialization, and anteroposterior position are known (Fig. 7–34).

The inclination is influenced by the center of rotation because correct coverage of the cup depends on depth of reaming. If a screw is added, the inclination and anteversion of the cup may change, and these positions should be checked after screw insertion by using the fit plane program (Table 7–5; also see X-ray Example 2). The edge of the cup is touched six times with the guide, and the inclination and anteversion are displayed in the lower right quadrant of the computer

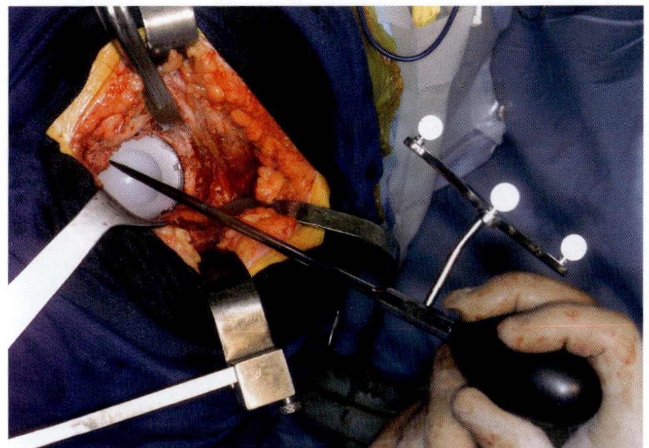

Figure 7–36 *The fit plane measurement can be repeated once the plastic liner has been inserted into the metal shell by touching the periphery of the liner at six points. In our experience, insertion of the liner changes the inclination/anteversion numbers by up to 3 degrees, but this is of no clinical significance, especially with a margin of measurement error of 2 degrees.*

Table 7–6
Pelvic Tilts by Pelvic Position*

Position	Pelvic Tilt
Supine	5.0 ± 6.0 (range, –8 to 17)
Lateral	–0.4 ± 8.0 (range, –19 to 17)
Sitting	0.2 ± 7.8 (range, –28 to 18)
Standing[†]	Not available

*All values are in degrees.
[†]The standing anteversion averages 3.4 degrees more than the supine anteversion based on radiographic measurement, and this value was used to interpolate standing anteversion.
The sitting and lateral positions were essentially within 0.5 degrees of each other, whereas the supine position differed from both of these by 5 degrees anterior.

screen (Fig. 7–35). This also can be done after the cup liner has been placed (Fig. 7–36).

There is no ideal numerical position for a cup. The inclination and anteversion will vary somewhat depending on the reamed center of rotation. The key point for inclination and anteversion is that the cup position should allow clearance during hip range of motion so that impingement is avoided. As a general rule, the anteversion is usually 25 to 30 degrees and the inclination 40 to 45 degrees. The range of acceptability for anteversion is 20 to 30 degrees, and for inclination, 35 to 45 degrees (in a few rare hips, 50 degrees of inclination may be needed to provide coverage of the anterosuperior edge of the cup). If the acetabulum has been reamed superiorly by 5 mm or more and medially by 10 mm or more, the inclination of the cup will be between 35 and 40 degrees (see X-ray Example 4).

The average best number for anteversion was investigated by combining measurements of the pelvic tilt when the patient was supine, in the lateral position, and with the hips flexed to 90 degrees, such as a sitting position (see Fig. 7–8). When the patient is standing, the anteversion of the cup is 4 degrees more than when supine (determined by comparing standing x-rays with supine x-rays). The combination of these values is shown in Table 7–6. Based on these values, we could judge an average position of the cup for anteversion that would give coverage of the femoral head in all positions. This average position could vary, however, according to the position of the reamed center of rotation. The single number for mean anteversion that would provide the best stability for all positions was 25 degrees.

When the cup is in 25 to 30 degrees anteversion, a polyethylene hood should not be used because there will be impingement in extension.

As mentioned, the cup anteversion depends on the femoral anteversion, and therefore it is best if the femoral anteversion is known before the cup anteversion is finalized. If the femoral anteversion is less than 5 degrees, the cup should be anteverted 30 degrees (see X-ray Example 4). This variability of cup anteversion controls the combined anteversion. A combined anteversion of 30 to 35 degrees provides mechanical stability and avoids impingement, which are further enhanced by using the largest femoral head possible.

The leg length and offset can be determined without performing femoral registration. The pointer guide is placed into the divot that was made in the trochanter for registering leg length and offset before dislocation of the patient's native hip (see Fig. 7–18). The change in the leg length and offset will be displayed on the computer screen (see Fig. 7–19).

Femoral Preparation with Computer Navigation

I determine the anteversion of the femoral component, then prepare the acetabulum (see Fig. 7–22). With the cup positioned and the liner inserted, I can return to the femur confident that the cup is in the correct position for this femoral anteversion.

Determine Anteversion
Measure the Neck Cut and Adjust. The first step, on return to the femur, is to measure the neck cut so that it can be accurately placed in relation to the center of rotation of the cup. The cup center of rotation must be known before the correct level of neck cut can be finally determined because the center of rotation may be medialized or lateralized from the original osseous center of rotation.

The leg is positioned in flexion and internal rotation so that the tibia is vertical, and retractors are placed to

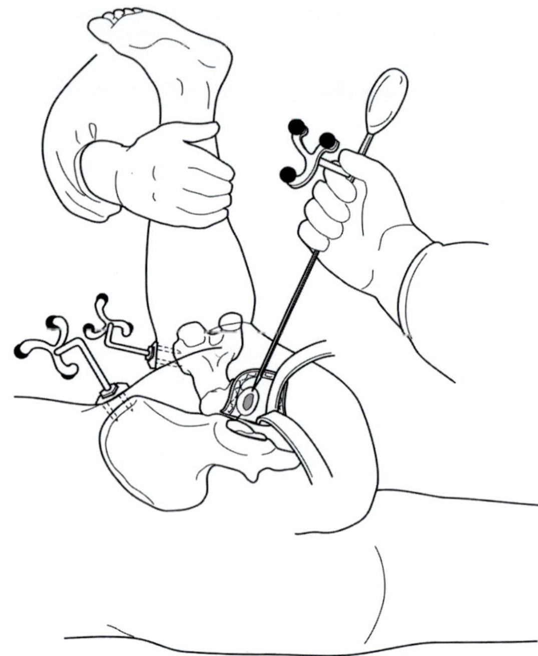

Figure 7–37 *The cut femoral neck is touched with the pointer guide at six points to identify the position of the cut neck. The medial neck cortical bone is touched to register the level of the cut point in comparison with the center of rotation of the cup. The number given for this distance will be determined according to the femoral neck and head length the surgeon inserted into the computer (see Fig. 7–39).*

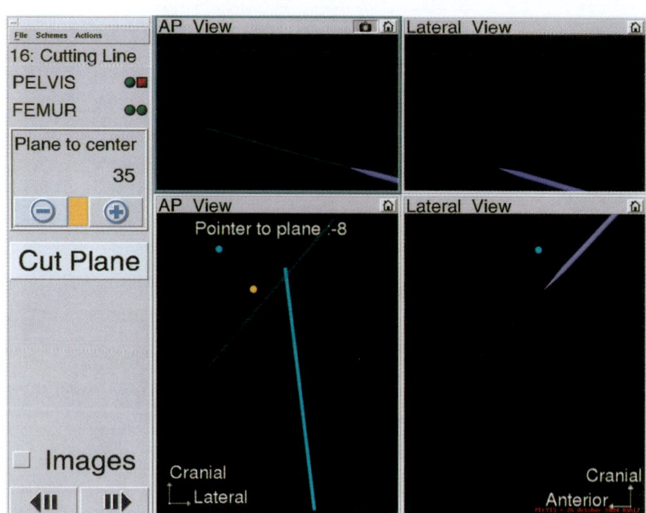

Figure 7–39 *Computer screen showing the information obtained by touching the medial neck bone. The surgeon has told the computer that 35 mm is the desired head length (plane center distance). The computer displays this in the lower left quadrant. The blue dot represents the center of rotation of the cup and the orange dot represents the neck cut level. The oblique line represents the desired cut level of the neck from the center of the cup (35 mm). The vertical light blue line represents the intramedullary canal. For this hip, the orange dot is 8 mm from the desired neck cut length (pointer to plane equals −8). This means that for the orange dot to be at the desired cut level, an additional 8 mm would need to be removed from the bony neck.*

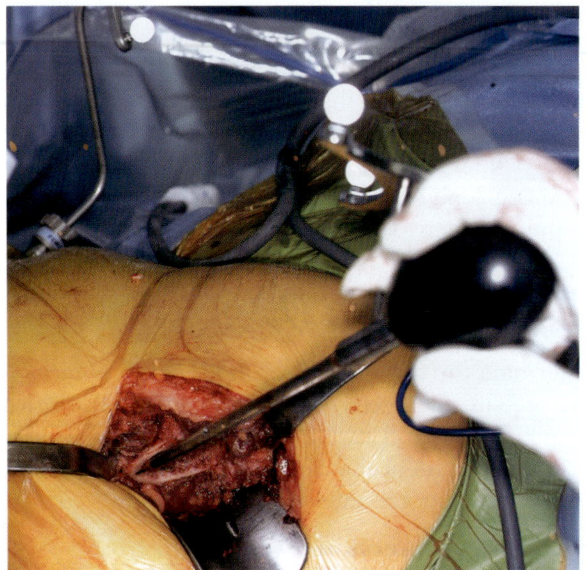

Figure 7–38 *Intraoperative view of the pointer guide touching the medial bone of the cut femoral neck.*

expose the cut femoral neck (Fig. 7–37). The medial cut surface of the neck is touched with the pointer guide (Fig. 7–38); the medial surface is used because this is the level with which the medial broach will align. When the broach is inserted to the level of the neck cut, the plane of the superior surface of the broach is measured by the computer at the point where the broach holder is attached to the broach. This plane of the broach may not match the plane of the cut surface of the neck, which is why the most medial bone of the neck cut is the most reliable point for registering the neck cut (see Fig. 7–38). The level of desired neck cut, which was input into the computer before the operation, is displayed graphically on the computer screen, and this is used to measure the actual neck cut (Fig. 7–39). The computer screen also displays the difference between the actual and desired neck cuts (i.e., whether the actual neck cut is shorter or longer than desired). Most commonly, the desired level of femoral neck cut is set for a 35-mm neck and head length, which is a neutral head and neck length for most hip systems. If the preoperative templating suggested that an increase or decrease in head length was needed, the length would be changed accordingly. For instance, if a +4 head length is templated as providing the correct balance of offset and hip length, then the neck cut would be listed as 39 or 40 mm.

Adjust Hip Length Measurement for the Center of Rotation of the Cup. The hip length measurement must be adjusted for the center of rotation of the cup. The usual templating of a cup position places the medial edge of the cup just at or just above the level of the transverse acetabular ligament. When the Converge cup is flush with the ligament (or the cortical edge of the cotyloid notch), its center of rotation will be 3 to 5 mm superior to the original osseous center of rotation (CC = 3 to 5) and 4 to 6 mm medial (ML = −4 to −6). The thickness of the metal shell can vary with different brands of cup, and this value must be known so that the reaming can be guided to bring the center of rotation back to a correct position. The neck length cut desired was based on the templated cup position. If a neutral ball was anticipated for a head and neck length of 35 mm, the computer will determine whether the neck cut needs to be adjusted.

When the center of rotation is adjusted with acetabular placement, the computer can calculate the distance in millimeters between the acetabular center of rotation and the neck cut. The surgeon must understand the interplay of center of rotation and femoral neck cut level to obtain the correct balance of offset and hip length. The computer provides the necessary numbers, but the surgeon must decide the level of the stem/neck cut according to the head length needed to provide stability with correct soft tissue balance of leg length and offset. If the center of rotation has changed by 5 mm or more, the surgeon will probably need to adjust the femoral neck length. Perhaps the neck would need to be recut; perhaps a longer modular head would give satisfactory clearance, offset, and leg length; or perhaps leaving the stem proud to the neck cut to correct the leg length and offset would be best. The surgeon can decide which of those options is best once computer measurements of center of rotation of the cup and level of neck cut are known (see X-ray Example 5).

Once the decision about the neck cut has been made, if the femur has not been broached, the femoral (intramedullary) canal is opened with a burr or canal finder. If the femur has already been prepared and the neck cut has been accurately adjusted, the stem is inserted (see Fig. 7–22).

Broach or Ream the Intramedullary Canal. The first step of femoral preparation of the "envelope" for the stem is to open the intramedullary canal (Fig. 7–40). Five points are registered in the intramedullary canal so that the software can show a straight line representing the canal's center (Fig. 7–41). Reaming or broaching is then done.

The broach handles have silver LEDs so that the broach's position in the canal can be monitored by the computer (Fig. 7–42). As broaching is performed, the computer lists the anteversion of the broach in the femur, the broach's varus/valgus position in the femur, and the offset of the leg with that stem position (Fig. 7–43). The broach's position in the intramedullary canal is also visualized by its relationship to the straight line representing the canal. The computer screen graphically displays the broach as it advances. The relationship of the stem to the desired hip length and anteversion, varus/valgus position, and offset are all displayed. The computer screen displays the relationship of the center of head position (CH) of the stem as it relates to the

center of rotation of the original hip; this is the CC measurement (see Fig. 7–43). The CC measurement is given as an increase or decrease in the length of the femur from the original center of rotation of the hip. If the CC number for the CH is 5, and the CC number for the acetabulum is 1, this means the leg length change is an increase of 4 mm. The leg length change is the sum of the CC numbers for the CH of the stem and the center of rotation of the cup.

Insert the Stem Into the Femur. Once broaching is complete, the stem is inserted into the femur. Like the broach, the stem holder also is equipped with LEDs. The stem should be advanced into the envelope prepared by the broach (Fig. 7–44), and the same anteroposterior, varus/valgus, and mediolateral positions should be seen with the stem as with the broach. The anteversion cannot be forced beyond what the femoral bone will accept, at the risk of fracturing the bone or jamming the broach.

As with the broach, the computer displays the advance of the stem (Fig. 7–45), along with the anticipated increase or decrease in leg length as the stem advances. If the surgeon wants to increase the leg length by 10 mm, then the best position would be the one indicated by +10 mm on the display. The surgeon, however, must still decide on the stem position in relation to both leg length and offset, and the depth of the stem must be combined with a correct head length to balance leg length and offset. Therefore, for example, the surgeon may decide that a +5 leg length stem depth with a +5 femoral head provides the best combination of leg length and offset (see X-ray Example 5).

By combining the leg length measurement and the offset number displayed in the left column of the computer screen, the surgeon can determine which head length will best balance the hip length and offset. If either the offset or the hip length is not what is wanted, adjustments will have to be made in the neck length of the femur or the position of the stem relative to the neck cut. For instance, if the offset were 10 mm, and stem position indicated that the leg length would be increased by 10 mm with a neutral head length, and this leg length was acceptable but the offset was not, then a change would need to be made. If an offset of 5 mm was desired, the femoral component could be left above the neck cut, which would decrease the offset, and the modular head would need to be changed to a −4 mm head length. This change would still leave a 10-mm increase in leg length but would reduce the offset. This example demonstrates that the surgeon still is faced with important decisions in correctly balancing hip length and offset, but the computer provides the information necessary to make a choice that achieves as near perfect a result as possible.

The anteversion of the stem is displayed on the computer as the stem is inserted (see Fig. 7–45). The

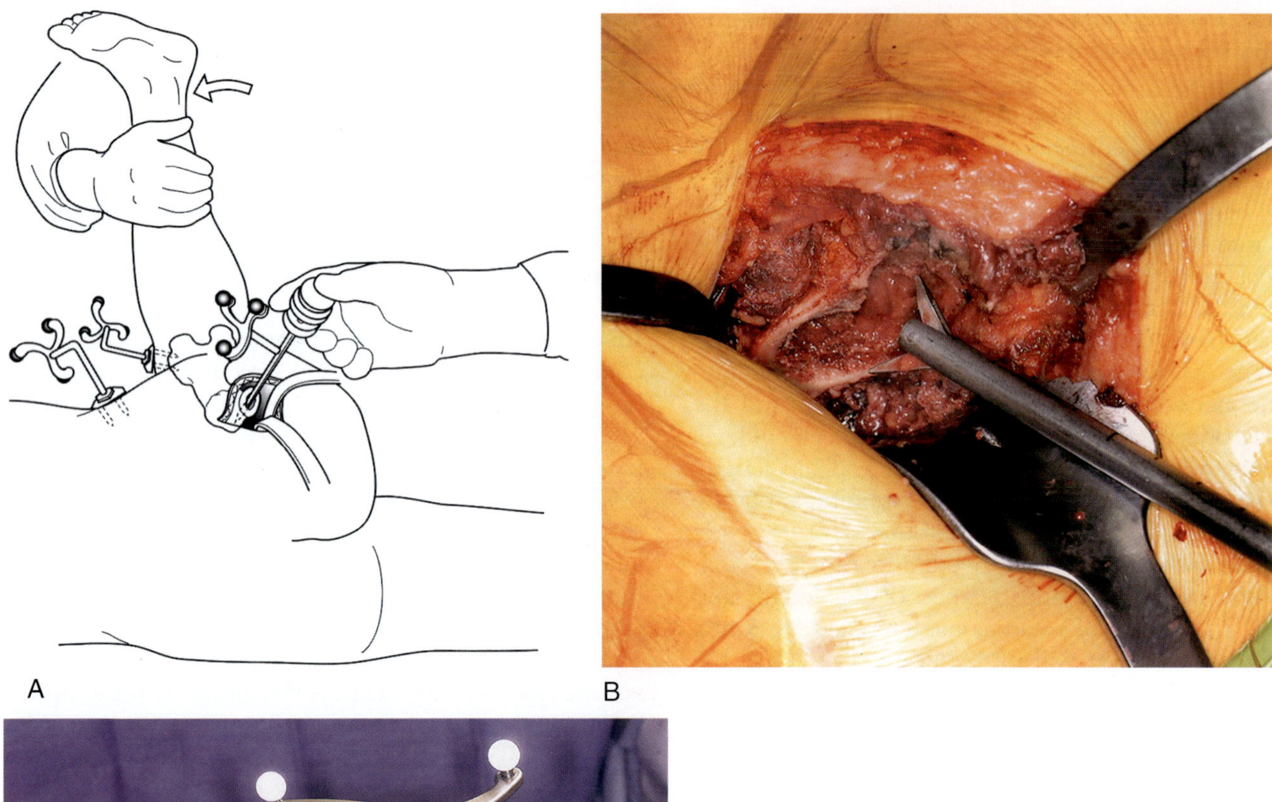

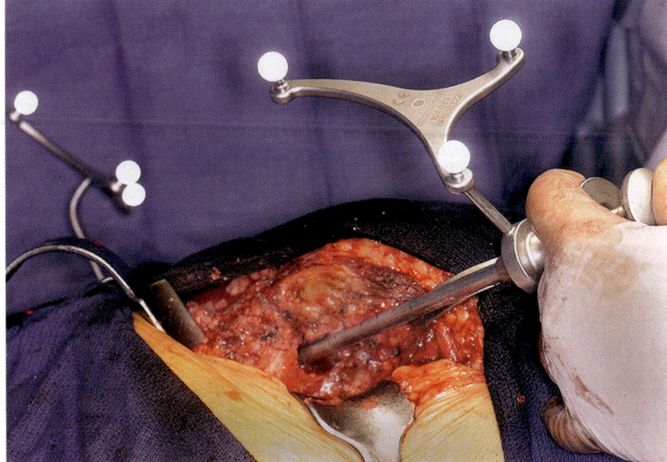

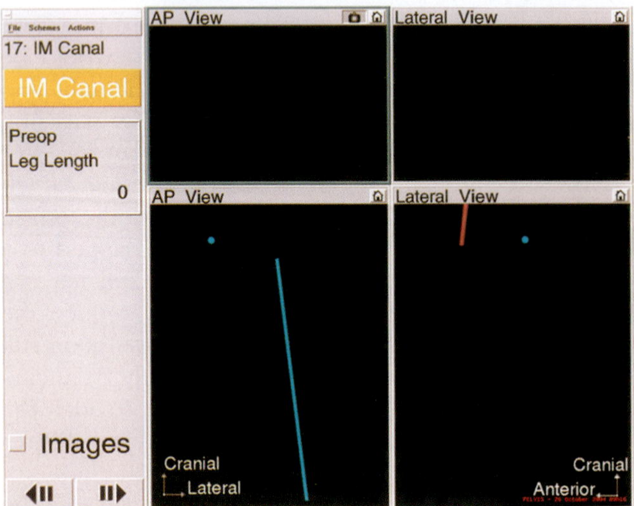

Figure 7–40 **A,** *Registration of the intramedullary canal. The registration tool is placed into the canal and the light-emitting diode on the tool transfers the information to the computer.* **B,** *The open wings of the registration device touch the interior of the intramedullary canal to provide registration when the tool is inserted into the intramedullary canal.* **C,** *The registration tool is touched to the intramedullary canal five times to register the canal's direction.*

Figure 7–41 *The light blue line in the lower left represents the intramedullary canal, which has been registered; when the stem is inserted, the angle of the stem in the canal is represented adjacent to the blue line.*

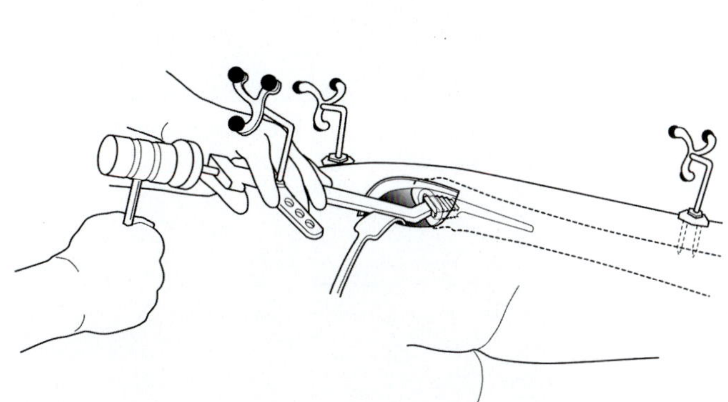

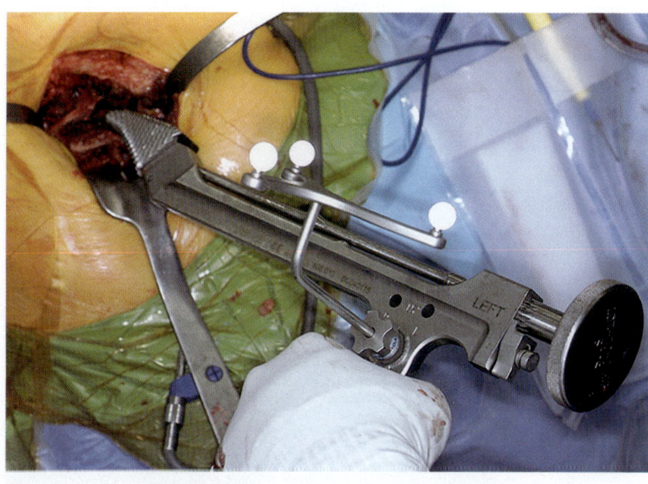

A

B

Figure 7–42 **A,** As the broach is inserted into the femur, the light-emitting diode (LED) on the broach handle allows the computer to recognize the broach's position in the intramedullary canal. **B,** Intraoperative view of the broach being inserted into the femur, with antenna and LED on the broach handle transferring this information to the computer.

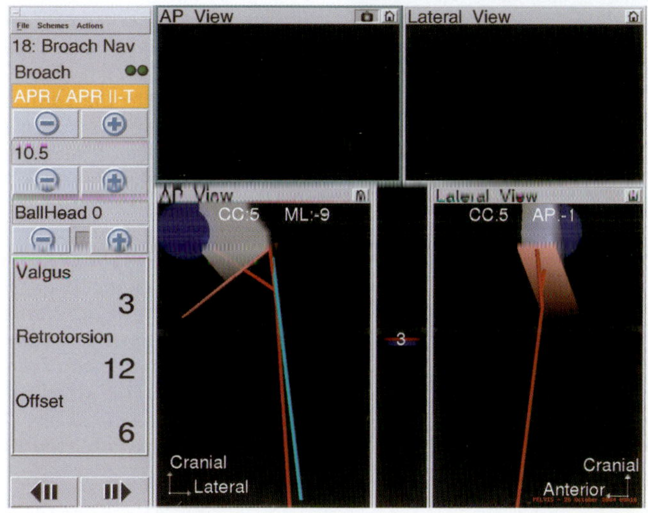

Figure 7–43 The broach is inserted into the femoral canal ("Broach Nav" at top left). The broach is in 3 degrees of valgus in the intramedullary canal and in 12 degrees of retroversion; the offset of the femur from the center of rotation of the cup is 6 mm. The CC number means that the center of the femoral head (dark blue ball in lower left quadrant), in its present position, is at a distance from the center of rotation of the cup that would increase the hip length by 5 mm. The ML number means that the center of the femoral head has been medialized 9 mm. The AP number means that the center of the head is posterior to the intramedullary canal by 1 mm, which is consistent with retroversion of the broach. Normally, the center of the femoral head should be anterior to the intramedullary canal with anteversion of the broach. The number "3" in the center column means that the current distance from the center of rotation of the cup to the stage line of the broach would result in an increase in leg length of 3 mm.

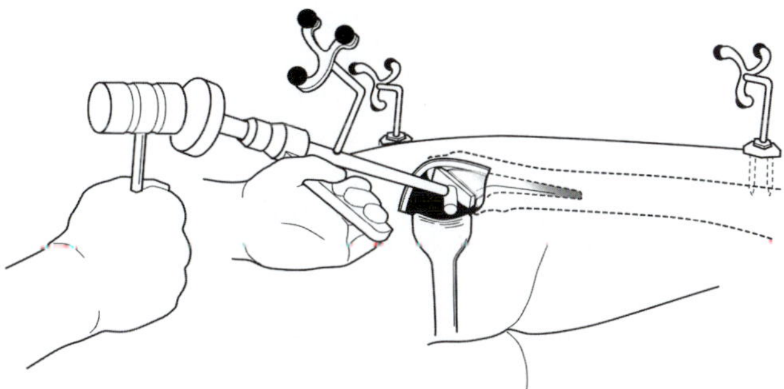

Figure 7–44 Insertion of the femoral stem. The light-emitting diode on the stem inserter allows the computer to monitor the stem position in the bone.

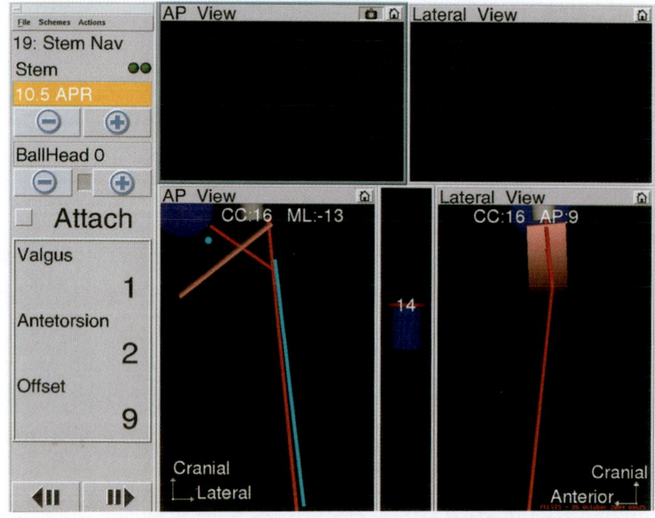

A

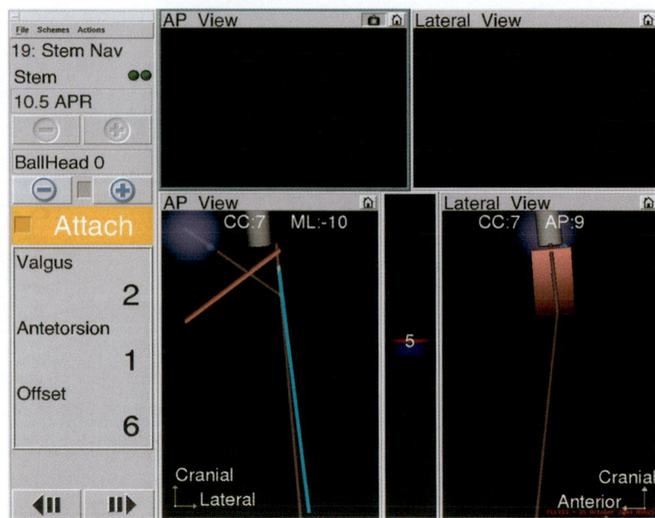

B

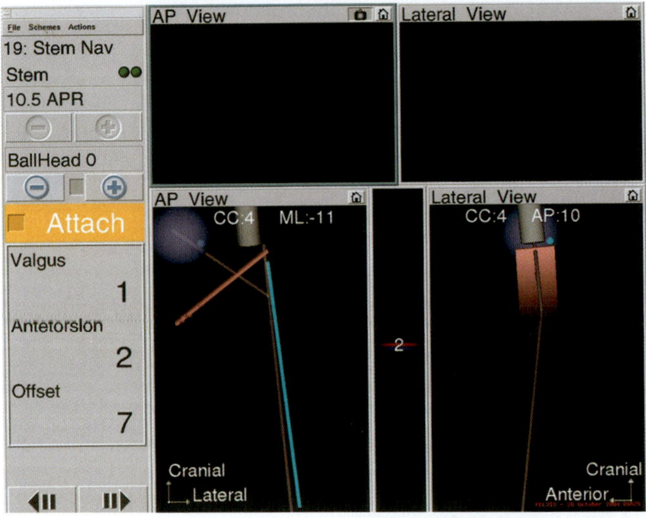

C

Figure 7–45 **A,** *Stem insertion. The left column shows that the stem is in 1 degree of valgus and 2 degrees of anteversion and has an offset increase of 9 mm. This stem is not fully seated, so the femoral head would increase the leg length by 16 mm. The center of the femoral head (CH) would be 13 mm medial and 9 mm anterior to the center of the intramedullary canal. The center column shows that if the stem were left in this position, the leg length would be increased by 14 mm because the cup position is elevated 2 mm. **B,** With the stem advanced, the valgus position is 2 degrees, the anteversion is 1 degree, and offset is 6 mm and 9 mm anterior to the intramedullary canal. The medial position of the CH supports offset, and the anterior position of the CH supports anteversion. The center column shows that the leg length difference would be 5 mm. **C,** The stem is fully seated, and CC is 4 mm, ML is –11 mm, and AP is 10 mm. The central column shows that the leg length would be increased to 2 mm (+4 mm CH stem, –2 mm center of rotation of the cup). The stem is in 1 degree of valgus and 2 degrees of anteversion, and the offset is increased by 7 mm.*

anteversion of a cementless stem cannot be greater than the bone will accept. If the femoral bone anteversion is 5 degrees, then the anteversion of the stem must be 5 degrees. In our experience, the anteversion varies from 5 to 20 degrees and averages 7.5 degrees. In men, the anteversion is almost always below 10 degrees and often below 5 degrees. As mentioned earlier, it is worthwhile to measure the femur before acetabular implantation to determine the degree of femoral anteversion. With this knowledge, the cup can be anteverted correctly to provide a good combined anteversion. I suggest that the femur be measured before the final positioning and fixation of the cup; if the femur is not measured first, it is important not to add screws to the cup or insert the real liner, so that adjustments can be made based on subsequent femoral measurement.

The surgeon cannot obtain the correct combined anteversion with femoral position alone; the cup position provides the variability for obtaining a correct combined anteversion of 30 to 35 degrees. If the surgeon tries to force femoral anteversion with a broach, the broach may become stuck in the femur, or the femur may fracture (Fig. 7–46). If the broach does become stuck, it must be removed through a vertical cut in the femoral bone, and then cables will be necessary to repair this iatrogenic fracture (Fig. 7–47). To avoid the intraoperative complication of a wedged broach or fractured femur, it is simplest to measure the femoral anteversion first so that the cup position can be adjusted to provide the correct combined anteversion. This is the technical routine I currently use.

CONCLUSIONS

The use of computer navigation during total hip replacement gives the surgeon accurate and comprehensive measurements of component positions and soft

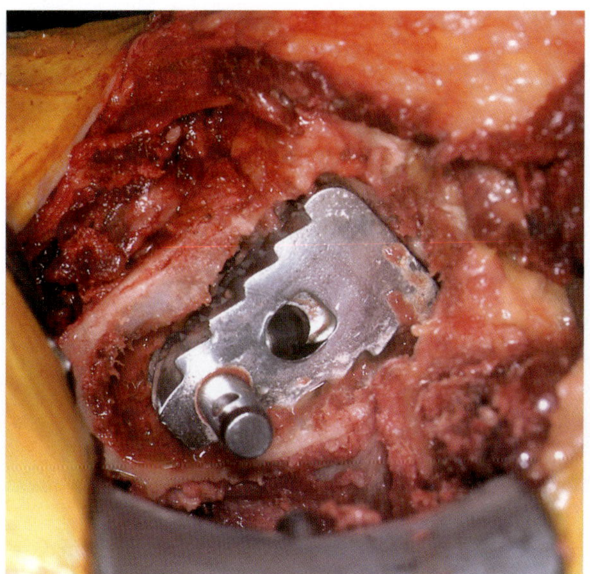

Figure 7–46 *An attempt has been made to increase the anteversion of the femoral stem by anteverting the broach across the femoral head instead of keeping the posterior edge of the broach parallel to the posterior femoral neck. This has resulted in the broach being jammed. A vertical cut in the femur was necessary to remove this broach, and two cables were used to secure the vertical cut (see Fig 7–47).*

tissue balance that, if used correctly, will provide as perfect a hip replacement as possible. The computer cannot make the final decisions for the surgeon, but it provides the knowledge necessary for making correct decisions. The surgeon still must choose correctly among the various options so that the hip replacement is aligned as perfectly as possible. The advantage for the surgeon is that more information reduces the stress inherent in making these decisions; the advantage for the patient is that with increased precision of component placement and soft tissue balance, the hip replacement has the potential for optimal durability.

CASE EXAMPLES OF USE OF COMPUTER NAVIGATION FOR TOTAL HIP REPLACEMENT

The patient is a 65-year-old man with osteoarthritis of the right hip (Fig. 7–48). A posterior mini-incision was performed. Pelvic and femoral trackers were used. The pelvic tilt was 8 degrees posterior. After exposure of the greater trochanter, the plane of the leg was registered.

The acetabulum was exposed and there was no osteophyte over the cotyloid notch that required removal. The pulvinar was removed. From the acetabulum, three data were recorded: the center of rotation

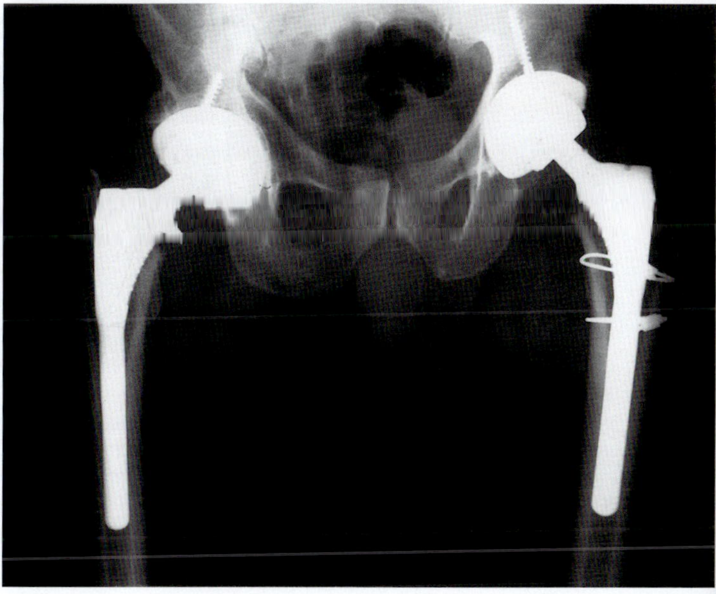

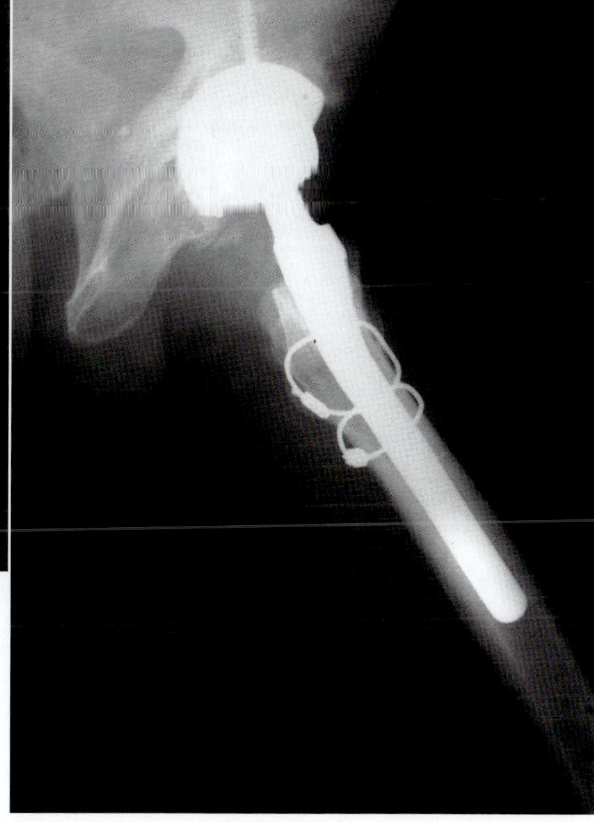

Figure 7–47 A, *Anteroposterior pelvic x-ray showing cables around the left femur to secure the cut made to remove a jammed broach (see Fig. 7–46). The right hip was operated on later, and because we had learned that we could not force increased anteversion, there was no breakage of that femur. The collar of the right total hip replacement was not fully seated to keep leg lengths and offset correct.* **B,** *Lateral x-ray of the left total hip replacement showing no disruption of the femoral anatomy by the vertical saw cut made to remove the jammed broach.*

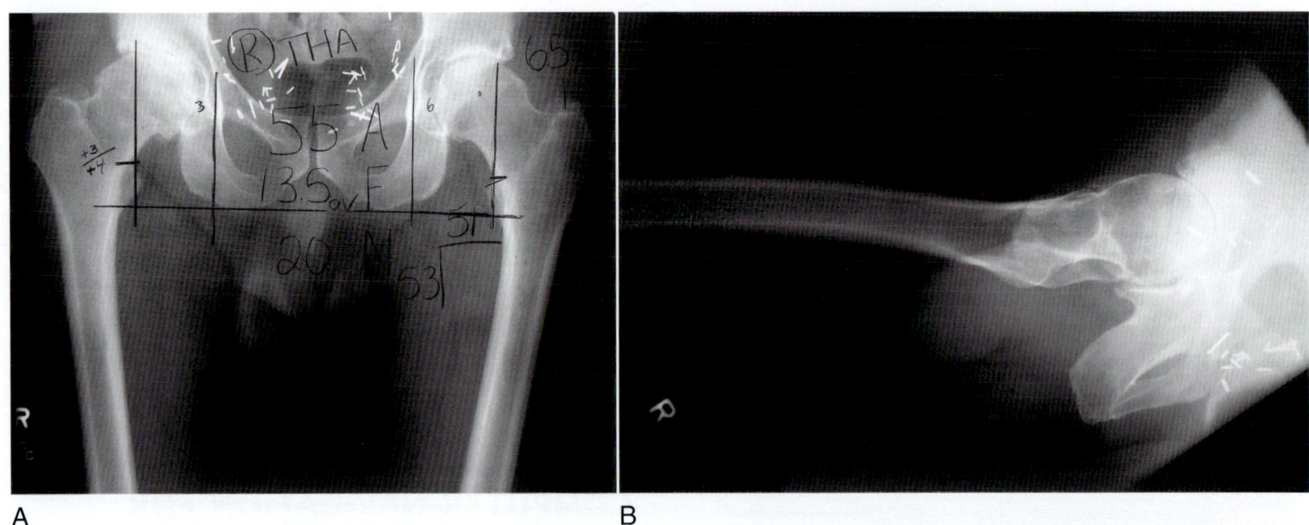

A   B

Figure 7–48 **A,** *Anteroposterior pelvic x-ray showing preoperative planning. The acetabulum is anticipated to be a size 55. The femur templates to a size 13.5, and a neck cut of 20 mm was expected from the lesser trochanter. The neck cut would be 15 mm from the bottom of the femoral head. As indicated in the upper right, the patient is a 65-year-old man. A right total hip arthroplasty is being performed. On the right metaphysis of the femur, the number "3" means the leg length needs a 3-mm increase and the number "4" means the offset needs a 4-mm increase. The numbers "3" and "6" to the medial side of the femoral heads are the measurements of the medialization from the edge of the femoral head to the medial wall.* **B,** *Lateral x-ray of the right hip showing type B bone. The size of the acetabulum is determined from this x-ray by measuring the diameter of the acetabular mouth. This modified Lauenstein x-ray gives a clear outline of the subchondral bone of the acetabulum, which allows the diameter to be measured most accurately.*

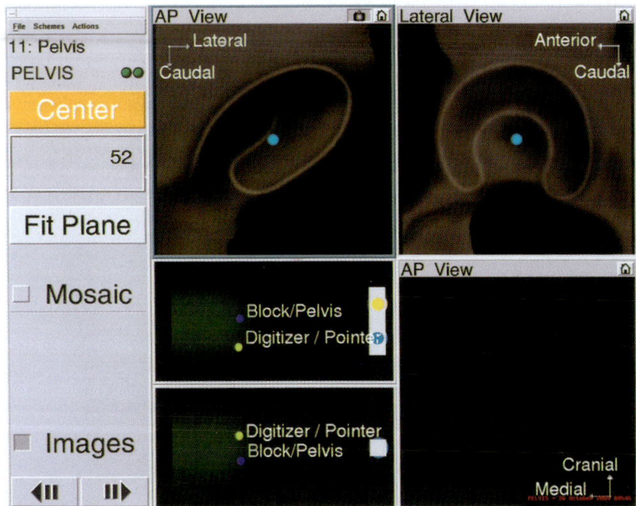

Figure 7–49 *The blue dots represent the position of the acetabular center of rotation as determined by 16 points measured on the osseous acetabulum.*

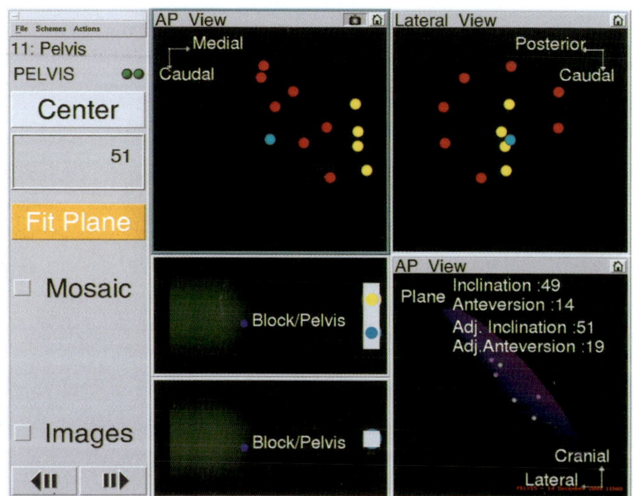

Figure 7–50 *Measurement of the mosaic outlines the acetabulum, with the periphery indicated by red dots and the quadrilateral plate (medial wall) by yellow dots. The blue dot is the acetabular center of rotation. The size of the acetabulum is listed in the left column as 51 mm. In the lower right is the fit plane, which measures the inclination and anteversion of the osseous acetabulum (the adjusted inclination was 51 degrees and the adjusted anteversion, 19 degrees).*

(CR; Fig. 7–49), the mosaic (Fig. 7–50), and the fit plane of the osseous acetabulum. Reaming was done to the medial wall (Fig. 7–51; yellow dots). The CR was moved 3 mm superior, 3 mm medial, and 1 mm posterior. (It is necessary to move the CR at least 3 to 4 mm superior and 3 to 6 mm medial to accommodate the 3.5-mm wall thickness of the Converge shell. Otherwise, the cup [and the CR of the cup] will be lateralized, which risks

an increase in leg length and increases the risk of impingement.)

Reaming was initially done for a 53-mm-diameter acetabulum (the osseous acetabulum was 51 mm). Line-to-line reaming was done, so a size 53 reamer was used. The cup was press-fit (Fig. 7–52) but not secure without screws. When two screws were added, the position changed from 25 degrees adjusted anteversion to 20 degrees adjusted anteversion as determined by the fit plane (Fig. 7–53). This cup position was not visually acceptable, and 20 degrees anteversion is at the lower end of the acceptable range. Furthermore, in this male

patient with osteoarthritis, I knew that the femoral anteversion would be less than 10 degrees, so I needed 25 degrees of acetabular anteversion at a minimum to achieve a combined anteversion of 30 to 35 degrees. I removed this cup and reamed to 54 mm for a 55-mm cup.

The reaming for a 55-mm cup allowed a secure press-fit that did not need screws. The CR position of this cup center of head was CC 4 mm, lateralized 1 mm, and posterior 2 mm (Fig. 7–54). The adjusted inclination was 40 degrees, and the adjusted anteversion was 28 degrees. The coverage and stability of the cup were good (Fig. 7–55). The position of the cup changed with fit plane measurement by 2 degrees after the insert was impacted into place. A change of 2 to 3 degrees with insert impaction is normally expected.

Femoral preparation was done with the box chisel, burr, and reamers for the femoral size of 13.5 mm. The size matched the templating for a size 13.5 stem. The preoperative measurements were an increase in leg length of 5 mm and an offset of 3 mm. Medialization was 3 to 6 mm (6 mm on the contralateral hip and 3 mm on the operative hip, but there were rotational differences).

The intramedullary canal was registered (Fig. 7–56) and shown on the computer screen (Fig. 7–57). The size 12 broach and then the size 13.5 broach were inserted (Fig. 7–58). The size 13.5 stem was implanted (Fig. 7–59). The anteversion of the stem was 6 degrees, as anticipated, so the combined anteversion was 34 degrees (the cup anteversion was 28 degrees). With a

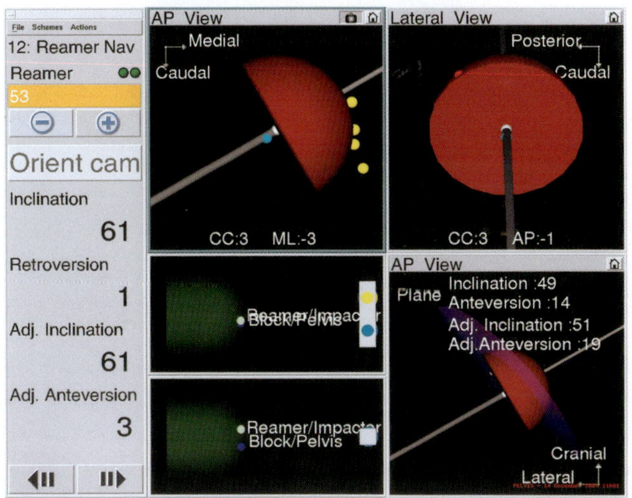

Figure 7–51   *The upper left corner of the screen shows that the reamer (in red) has advanced to the medial wall (yellow dots). The angle of the reamer (which is in a transverse position) is shown in the left column and is of no consequence for the final inclination and anteversion of the cup. CC 3 means the center of rotation is elevated 3 mm, ML −3 means the center is medialized 3 mm, and AP −1 means that the center is moved posteriorly 1 mm. The inclination and anteversion of the osseous acetabulum are depicted at lower right.*

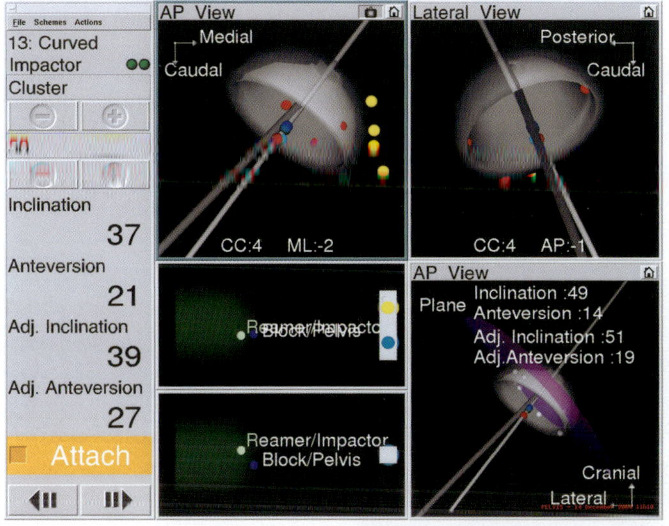

A

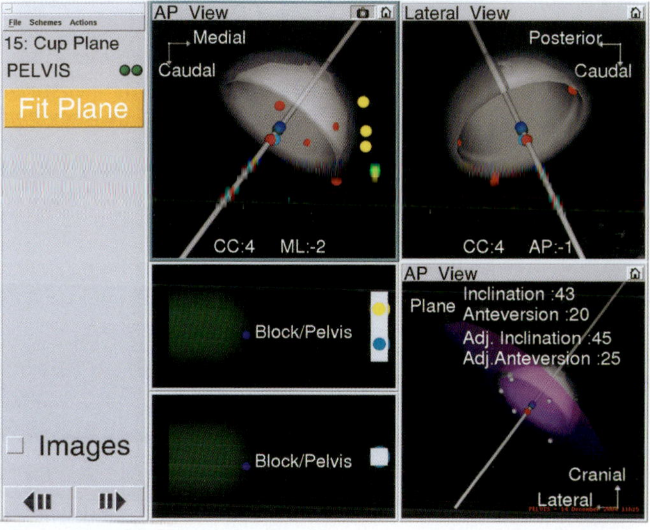

B

Figure 7–52   ***A,*** *A 53-mm cup was placed first and positioned at an adjusted inclination of 39 degrees and an adjusted anteversion of 27 degrees. The cup was 4 mm superior, 2 mm medial, and 1 mm posterior to the original acetabular center of rotation. The osseous fit plane is shown in the lower right.* ***B,*** *The fit plane of this cup after removal of the cup holder showed an inclination of 45 degrees and an anteversion of 25 degrees, compared with 39 degrees and 27 degrees, respectively, with the cup holder* ***(A).*** *The 6-degree change from 39 degrees to 45 degrees of inclination suggests that the press fit of the cup is not secure.*

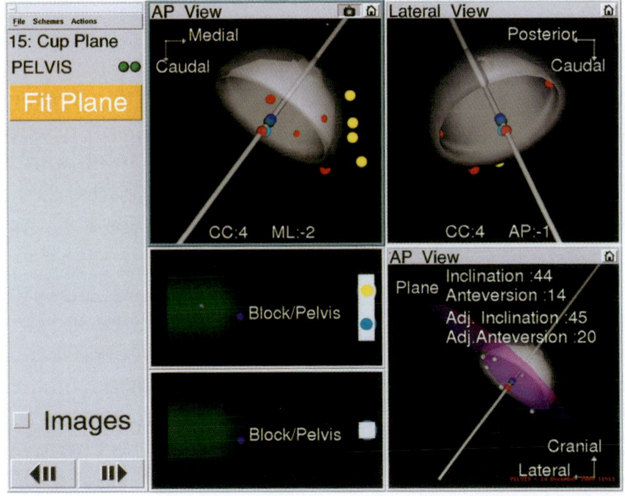

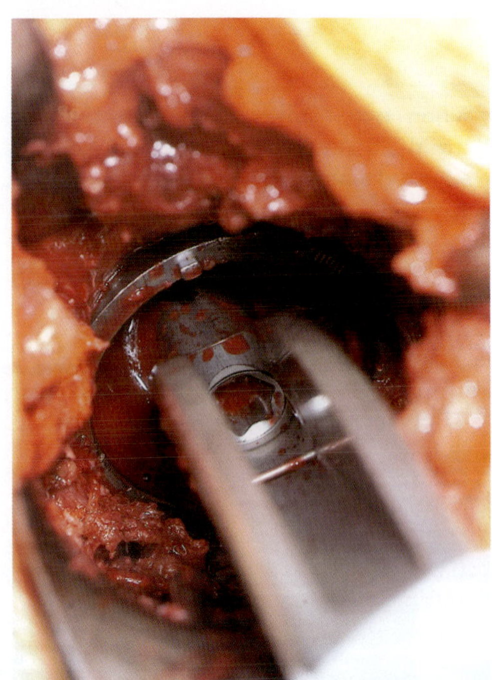

Figure 7–53 *Position of the cup after addition of two screws, as measured by the fit plane (lower right quadrant). The anteversion has been reduced to 20 degrees, which was unacceptable considering that the anteversion of the femur would be less than 10 degrees. For a combined anteversion of 30 to 35 degrees, the adjusted anteversion of the cup must be 25 to 30 degrees.*

Figure 7–55 *Intraoperative view of the trial placement with the cup holder attached, showing the visually accepted position of the trial cup.*

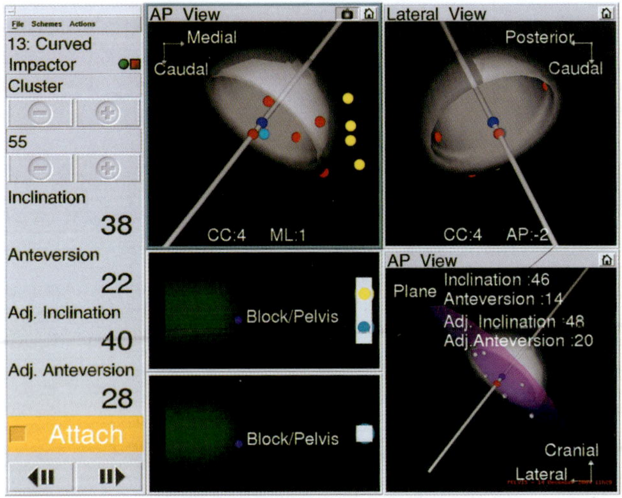

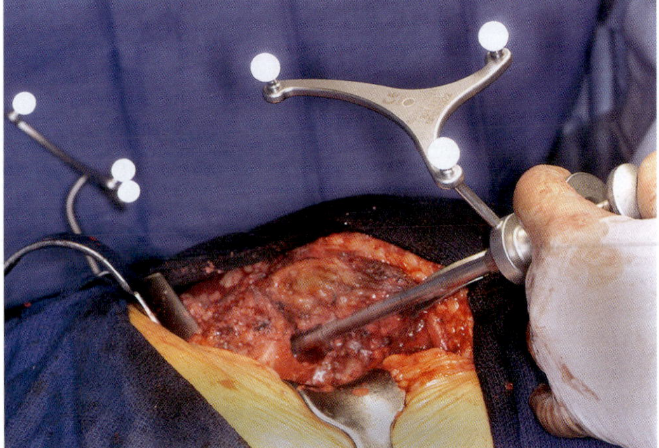

Figure 7–54 *Final position of the 55-mm cup as measured by the cup holder. The adjusted inclination is 40 degrees and anteversion, 28 degrees. The cup is 4 mm superior, 1 mm lateral, and 2 mm posterior. The fit plane numbers in the lower right are left over from the fit plane measurement of the 53-mm cup.*

Figure 7–56 *The intramedullary canal is registered into the computer by five points in the canal.*

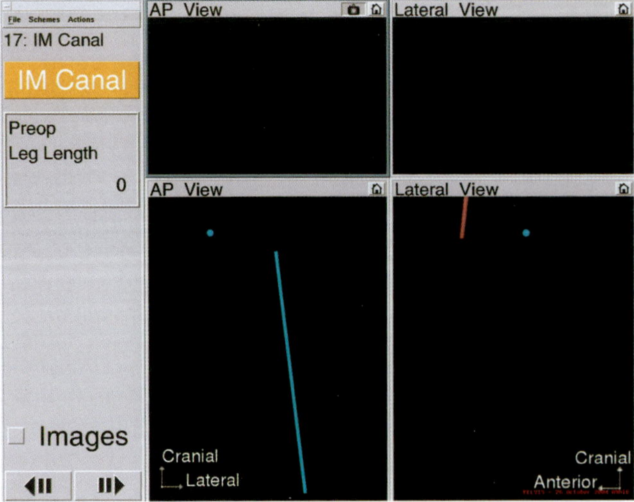

Figure 7–57 *The intramedullary canal is shown on the computer screen as a straight blue line in the lower left.*

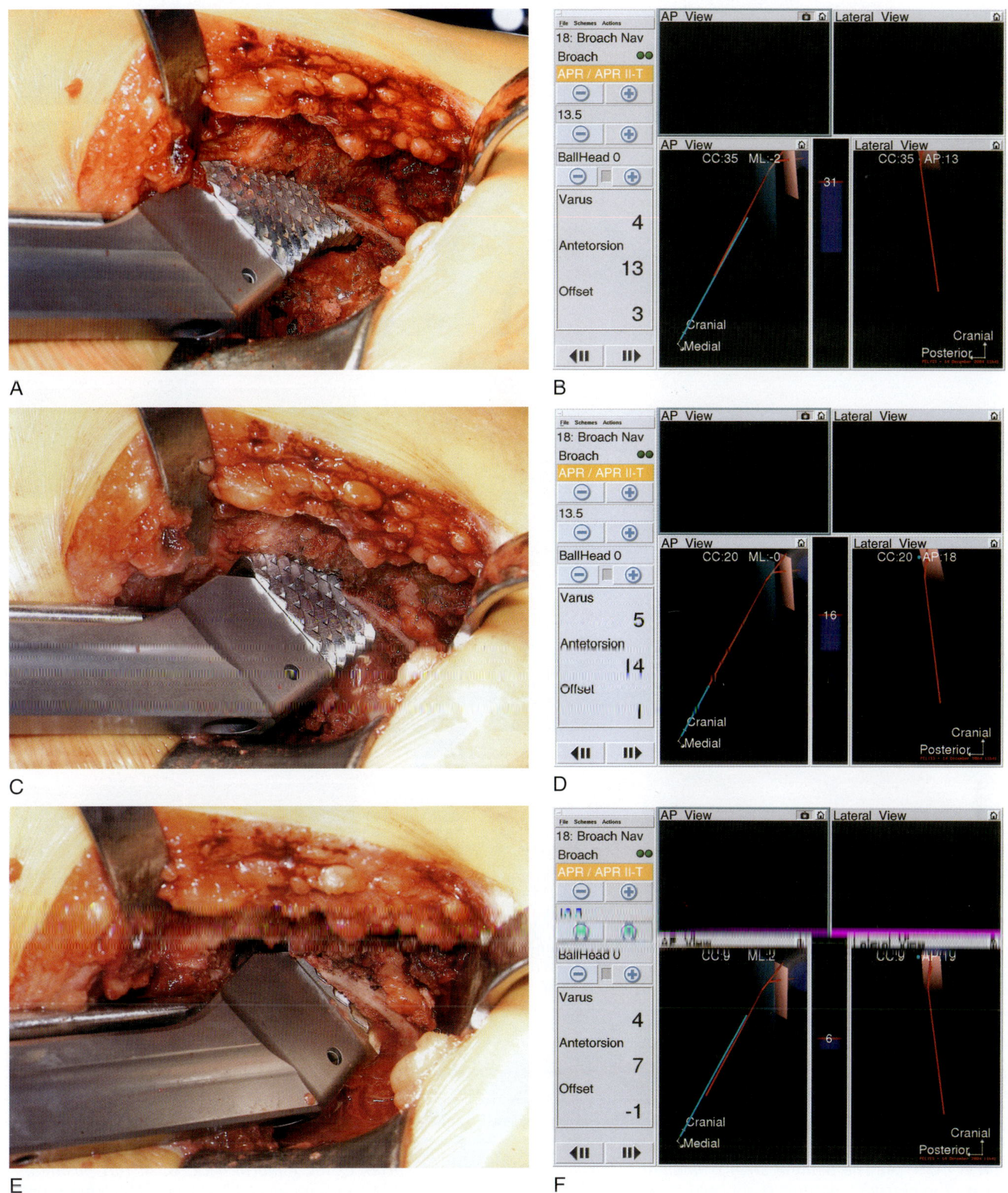

Figure 7–58 ***A,*** *The broach is inserted into the femur parallel to the posterior cortex of the femoral neck.* ***B,*** *With the broach in this position, it is 31 mm from being in the position where no leg length change would occur (center column). The CC is 35, ML −2, and AP 13. The broach at this position has 13 degrees of anteversion. The numbers with the broach in this position are important only to ensure that the broach is advanced into the canal in a correct position so that fracture does not occur.* ***C,*** *The broach is advanced further into the femur.* ***D,*** *The broach is now 16 mm from 0 leg length change (center column). The broach is at 14 degrees of anteversion and the center of the femoral head (CH) is changing as the broach advances.* ***E,*** *The broach is fully seated in a stable position and is resistant to further advance.* ***F,*** *This broach position indicates that the leg length would increase by 6 mm (preoperatively, 3 mm was predicted; see Fig. 7–47A). The anteversion is 7 degrees. The broach is in 4 degrees of varus and the offset is decreased by 1 mm. Four degrees of varus is acceptable with this anatomic stem because the size for this type A femur is determined from the lateral x-ray. The CC of 9 means a leg length increase of 9 − 4 mm (center of cup position) = 5 mm, which is consistent with the 6 mm in the center column. The CH is 2 mm medial and 19 mm anterior.*

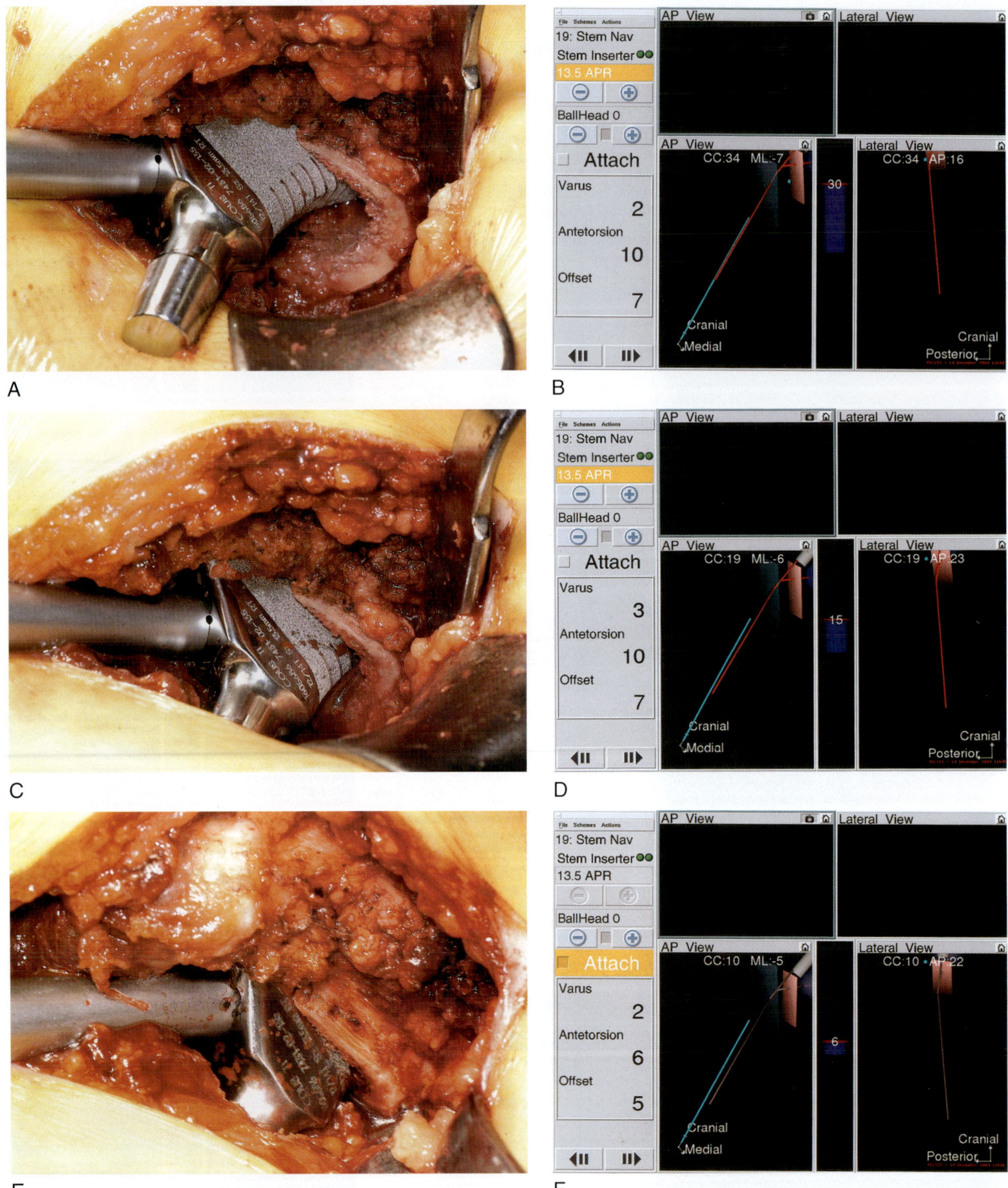

Figure 7–59 *A, The femoral stem is implanted parallel to the posterior cortex of the femoral neck. B, At this position, the stem is 30 mm from a position that would result in no leg length increase, with an anteversion of 10 degrees. The other numbers are meaningless at this point. C, The stem has been advanced. D, The stem is now 15 mm from a zero leg length increase, with an anteversion of 10 degrees. E, The stem is implanted to the same level as the broach and is stable. F, The stem is at the same level as the final broach position (see Fig. 7–58E), resulting in a 6-mm leg length increase, and the center of the femoral head (CH) is 5 mm medial and 22 mm anterior to the intramedullary canal. The CH is anterior to the intramedullary canal because the anatomic stem has an anterior head position (as does the femur itself). The anteversion is 6 degrees, which with the final cup position of 28 degrees gives a combined anteversion of 34 degrees. The anteversion of 6 degrees is the reason the 53-mm cup could not be accepted. With the 53-mm cup, the combined anteversion would have been 26 degrees. There was just sufficient clearance for impingement in flexion and internal rotation with the combined anteversion of 34 degrees, so there would have been impingement with the 53-mm cup. The offset is increased by 5 mm; the change predicted from preoperative planning was 4 mm (see Fig. 7–48A). The stem is in 2 degrees of varus, consistent with the postoperative x-ray (see Fig. 7–61A).*

neutral head length, the leg length would be increased 6 mm (central column), and this was consistent with the CC measurement of 10 mm and a cup CR of 4 mm (10 − 4 = 6 mm). The leg length measurement was an increase of 9 mm, and the offset was increased 2 mm (Fig. 7–60). A 38-mm head was used with Durasul poly-ethylene. The clinical leg lengths determined by overlaying the legs were equal. There was no impingement throughout the range of motion, although the clearance was small at full flexion and internal rotation, suggesting that any lower value for combined anteversion would have resulted in impingement. The hip replacement was performed with full knowledge of all the measurement numbers, and the decisions made were based on the measurements. The result was a well-mated hip replacement with a combined anteversion of 34 degrees and no impingement throughout the range of motion. This result, combined with an articulation surface of Durasul, predicts long-term durability for this patient.

The postoperative x-ray shows an increase in leg length from preoperative of 5 mm and an increase in offset of 5 mm (Fig. 7–61), compared with the computer-measured change in leg length of 9 mm and in offset of 2 mm. Rotation of x-rays makes measurement of leg length and offset less accurate than with the computer. The radiographically measured inclination was 39 degrees, and anteversion was 24 degrees, which corresponded to the computer measurement of 40 degrees inclination and 28 degrees anteversion. The stem was in slight varus on x-ray, which correlated with the computer measurement of 2 degrees varus. The APR stem can have slight varus on the AP x-ray with type A bone because with this type of bone the fit is determined by the fit on the lateral x-ray (the true AP plane). Tapered stems always are fitted mediolateral, as seen on the AP

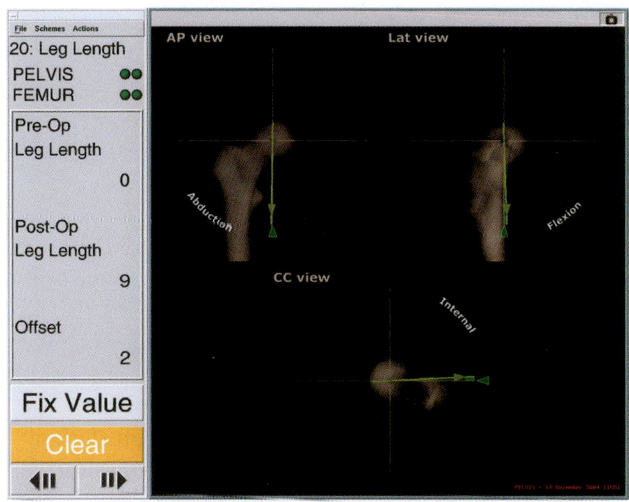

Figure 7–60 The actual leg length increase was 9 mm (3 mm greater than predicted from the stem holder, and of no clinical significance). The actual offset increase was 2 mm rather than 5 mm; again, this is of no clinical significance. The screen shows that in all planes, the leg position has been duplicated from the position used to make the preoperative predictions.

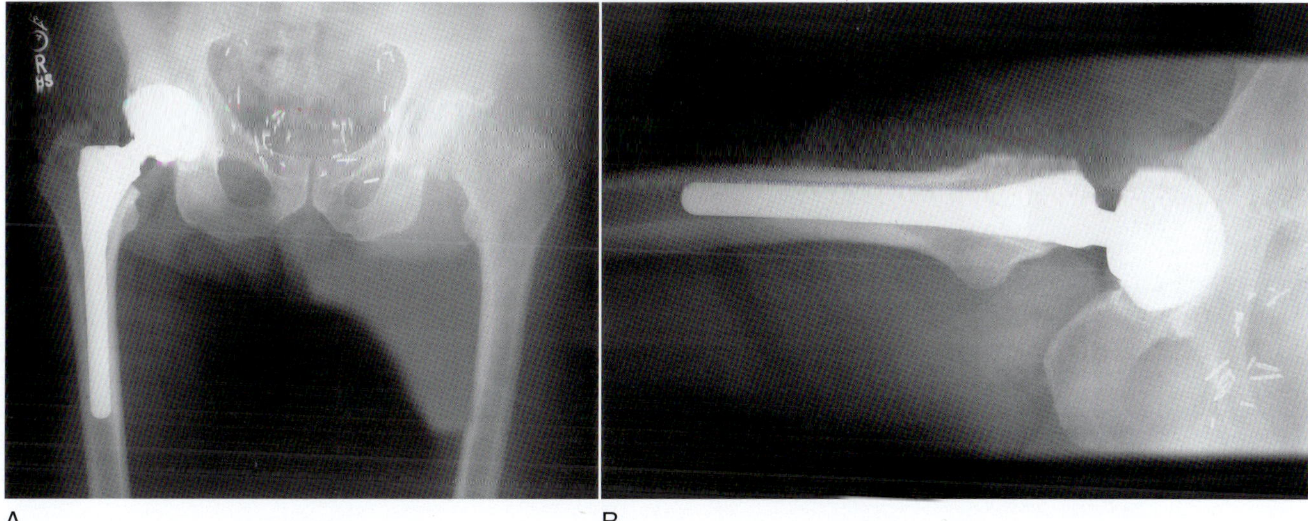

Figure 7–61 A, On the postoperative x-ray, the measured inclination is 39 degrees compared with the computer's 40 degrees, and the anteversion is 24 degrees compared with the computer's 28 degrees. The computer had the stem in 2 degrees of varus, and it is in slight varus on the x-ray. The offset and leg length are nearly perfect, as determined by the position of the right and left lesser trochanters. B, The lateral x-ray shows why the size of an anatomic stem is determined on this view. This anatomic stem fills the lateral intramedullary canal and the tip is against the anterior cortex. Any larger stem to prevent varus on the anteroposterior x-ray would have fractured this femur. The size can be predicted by preoperative templating and confirmed by the reamed size of the intramedullary canal.

x-ray, whereas the fit of an anatomic stem like the APR varies by bone type.

The accuracy of the computer is demonstrated by this case report. The x-ray, though not necessary, confirmed my intraoperative knowledge; the assistance to the surgeon rendered by the computer can be readily understood. With the size 53 cup, cup size and position were unsatisfactory. I knew that the femoral component anteversion would be approximately 5 degrees, and a cup anteversion between 14 and 20 degrees would not be enough. The level of stem insertion was known and could be correlated to an expected leg length change of 5 mm and an offset change of 5 mm (which were exactly as seen on x-ray), and therefore the neutral head size could be selected with confidence. The stress of decision-making was removed, and even in the operating room we knew that we had a superb arthroplasty.

X-ray Example 1: This patient has osteoarthritis of the hip (Fig. A). There is no significant destruction of the acetabulum, so acetabular reconstruction should be able to be accomplished without great difficulty. The medial edge of the femoral head is 6 to 7 mm from the medial wall, so the medialization should be at least that much. As measured by the lesser trochanters, there is very little difference in leg lengths. The postoperative x-ray is shown in Figure B. A cementless APR stem has an excellent fit. The cup is in good position, as demonstrated by the position of its caudal edge between the ischium and the pubis. The adjusted inclination of this cup with the cup holder was 38 degrees, and 36 degrees after the liner was impacted. The adjusted anteversion with the cup holder was 30 degrees, and 27 degrees after the liner was impacted. The femoral anteversion was 5 degrees, which required that the cup have this much anteversion to give a combined anteversion between 30 and 35 degrees. The CC of the cup showed 5 mm superior, and the ML of the cup showed 9 mm medial. The offset change was −10 mm, and the leg length change was 0. Comparison of the preoperative and postoperative x-rays shows very little difference between the preoperative and postoperative offset, which demonstrates the difficulty of taking into account rotation of the x-ray for measuring offset. Preoperatively, the leg lengths needed little correction, and none was done; on the postoperative x-ray, the leg length of the operative leg measured 2 mm longer.

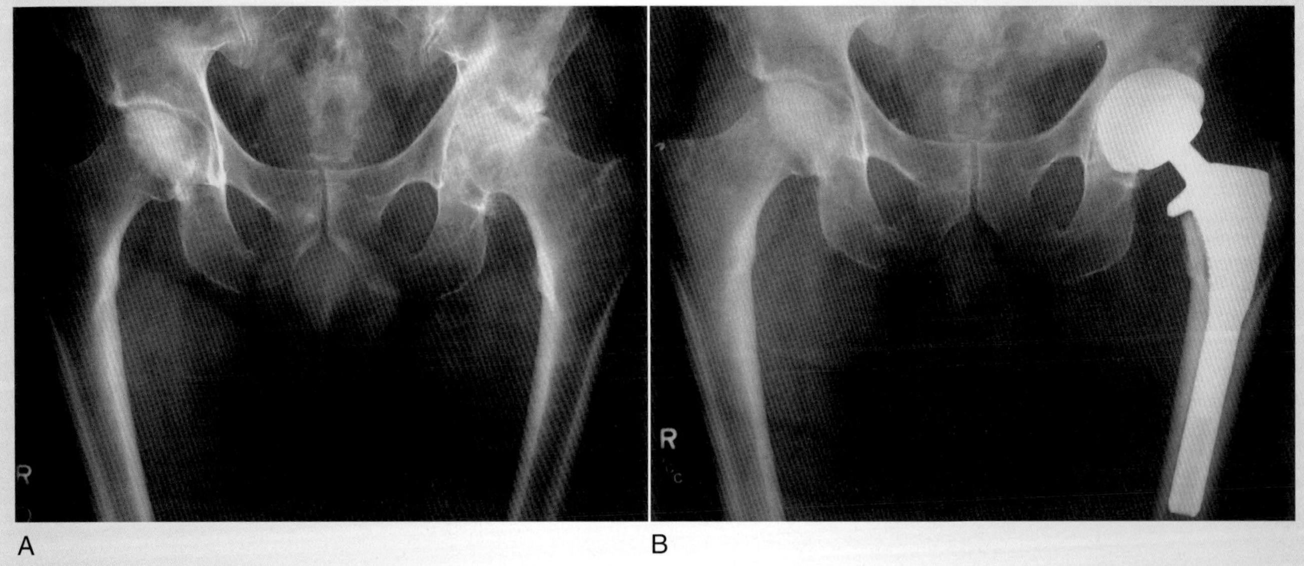

A   B

X-ray Example 2: Figure A is the preoperative x-ray of a patient scheduled for bilateral hip replacement. There are floor osteophytes in both acetabula. The postoperative x-rays are seen in Figure B. The acetabulum on the right hip is in good position, with an inclination of 36 degrees and an adjusted anteversion of 21 degrees. The cup in the left hip, however, is not in ideal position because it is not fully medialized. The acetabular osteophyte clearly was not completely removed, and the cup is implanted against the osteophyte rather than the medial floor of the acetabulum. This lateralizes the cup, as is clearly shown by the inferior edge of the cup lateral and caudal to the tear drop. The consequence of this is that the hip offset is increased (relative to the opposite hip) compared with the preoperative offset. Lateralization of the cup is probably the most common cause of increased leg length. The leg lengths were clinically equal in this patient, although on the x-ray the left leg is longer than the right by the position of the lesser trochanter. Because this cup was placed on the osteophyte, it did not have sufficient inherent stability and required a screw.

This case also illustrates the change in cup position that can occur with the use of a screw. With the cup holder, the inclination was 44 degrees and the adjusted anteversion was 21 degrees. After the placement of the screw and on the basis of the fit plane measurement, the inclination was 50 degrees and the adjusted anteversion was 13 degrees. This operation was performed during our early experience with the computer, and the technical error of not placing the cup against the medial wall was the consequence. It provides a perfect example of incorrect technical placement of the cup and the change in component position that can occur with the use of screw fixation. This change in component position could result in such poor mating of the femoral and acetabular components that dislocation occurs.

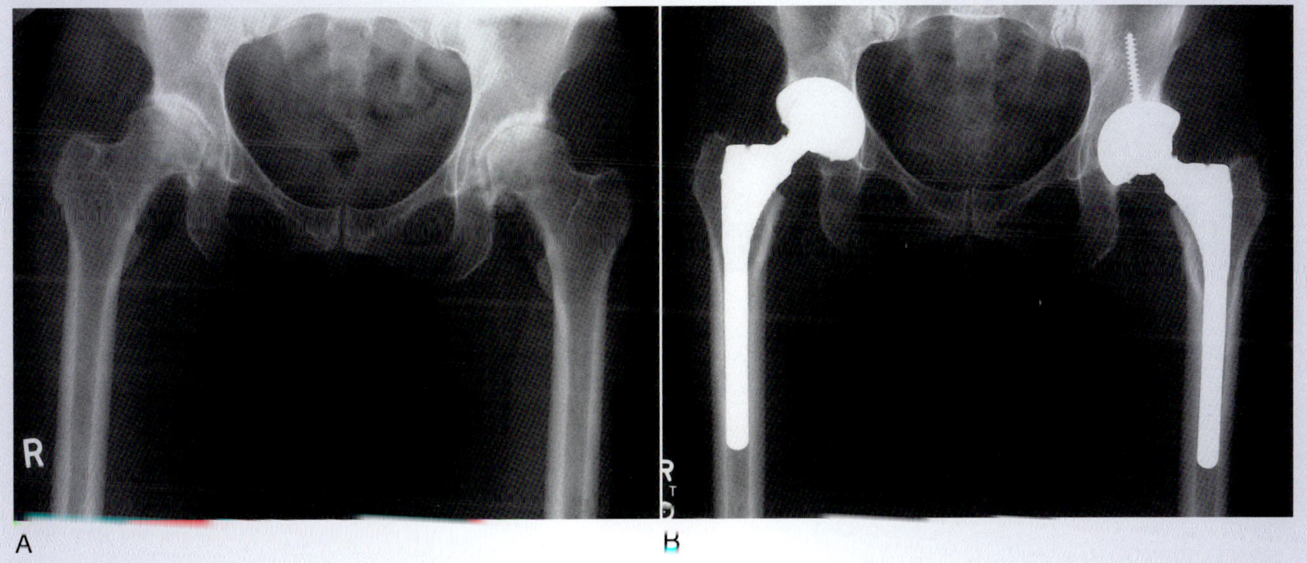

X-ray Example 3: The preoperative x-ray shows severe dysplasia with superorlateral subluxation of the femoral head (Fig. A). When presented with hips such as this, the surgeon can anticipate that the cup will require significant medialization and that it will be in a superior position. In fact, as seen in the postoperative x-ray (Fig. B), the medialization of the right cup was 19 mm and of the left cup, 17 mm. The right cup had a CC of 6 mm superior and the left cup had a CC of 2 mm superior. The adjusted inclination of the right cup is 46 degrees, with an adjusted anteversion of 27 degrees. The adjusted inclination of the left cup is 51 degrees, with an adjusted anteversion of 26 degrees. Femoral anteversion was not being measured at the time these operations were done. It is important to observe the amount of femoral neck that was retained in this patient. When the surgeon knows that the cup is going to be medialized and superior, high femoral neck retention is necessary because the center of rotation will be elevated and medial. Comparison with the preoperative x-ray shows that the offset of the hips was maintained and the leg lengths are equal.

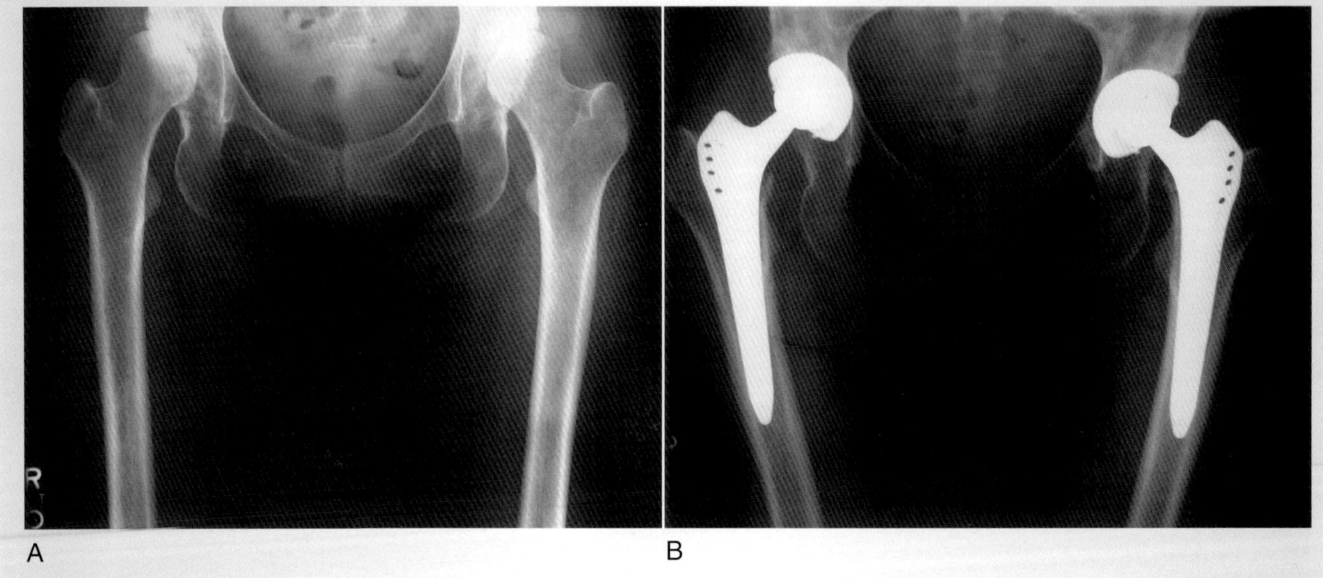

A   B

X-ray Example 4: The femoral head in this patient is displaced significantly laterally, and a floor osteophyte is present. This hip will require medialization of at least 10 mm (Fig. A). The postoperative x-ray is shown in Figure B. The computer is clearly a big help in reconstructing this acetabulum. The cup is in excellent position, with its caudal edge between the pubis and the ischium. The adjusted inclination of the cup is 38 degrees and the adjusted anteversion is 30 degrees. After the liner was impacted, the fit plane–adjusted inclination was 36 degrees and the adjusted anteversion was 27 degrees. The medialization was 9 mm and the CC was 5 mm superior. This example shows the correlation between inclinations of 35 and 40 degrees when medialization of nearly 10 mm occurs. The femoral anteversion in this patient was 5 degrees, which means that the cup anteversion needs to be nearly 30 degrees to result in a combined anteversion near 35 degrees.

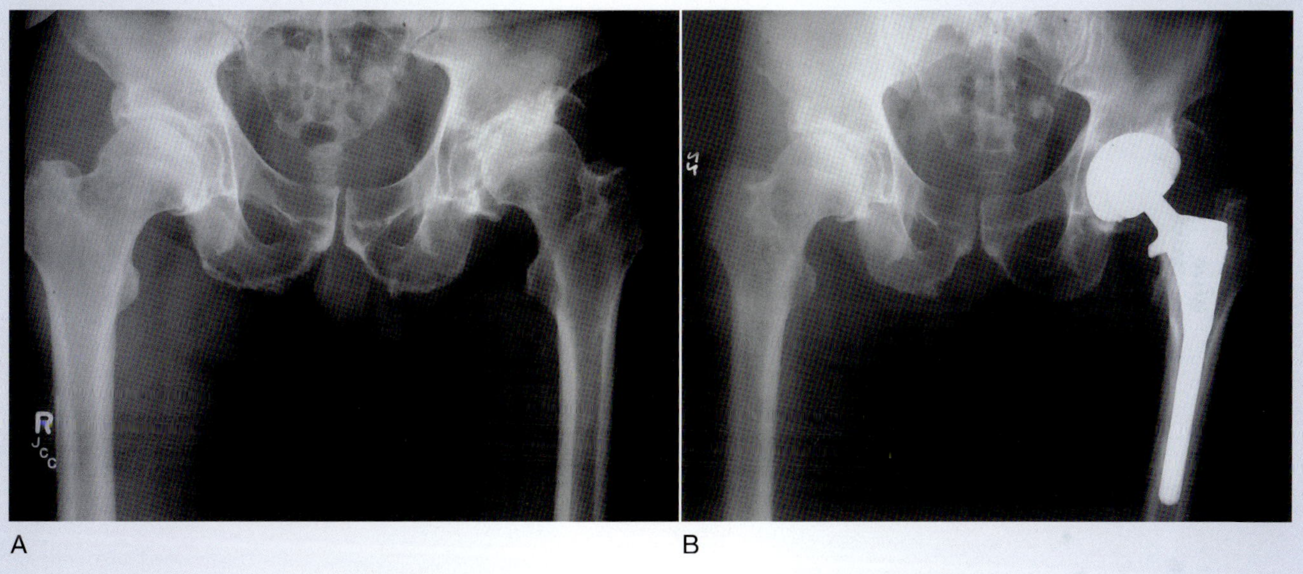

A B

X-ray Example 5: This x-ray shows an example of adjustment of length and offset by positioning of the femoral component. In the left hip, the collar was not seated, and the right hip was not completely seated without coverage of all of the porous coating. This is one technique used for adjustment of hip length and offset if the neck cut is not at the perfect position.

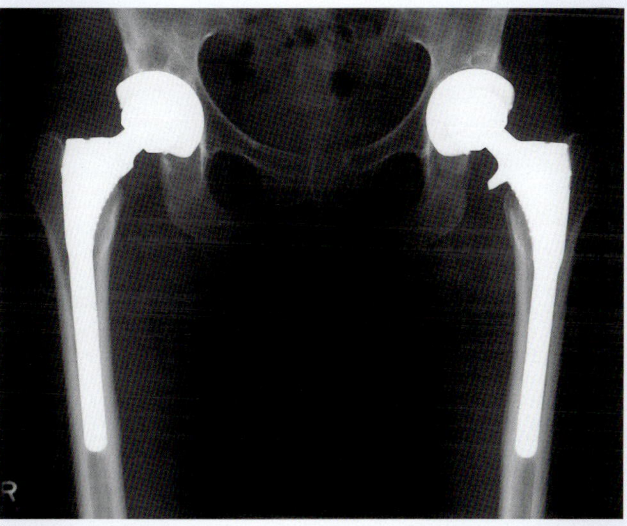

References

1. Widmer KH, Zurfluh B: Compliant positioning of total hip components for optimal range of motion. J Orthop Res 22:815-821, 2004.
2. Wan Z, Dorr LD: Natural history of femoral focal osteolysis with proximal ingrowth smooth stem implants. J Arthroplasty 11:718-725, 1996.

Preoperative Planning for Computer-Assisted Total Hip Replacement

Preoperative planning for computer-assisted total hip replacement primarily involves identifying the acetabular deformity, which will determine the technical methods to be used for reconstruction. Second, preoperative planning determines the necessary changes in leg length and offset for correct biomechanical reconstruction of the hip.

I. Acetabular Implantation

Because femoral anteversion is a fixed quantity for each patient, adjustments must be made in cup implantation to obtain the correct combined anteversion, avoid impingement, and set the cup's inclination for good contact areas and bony coverage. The geometric deformity of the acetabulum influences the depth of reaming, cup anteversion (based on anticipated femoral anteversion), and anticipated offset of the hip reconstruction (offset in particular in type IV deformity).

Use of the Dorr functional classification of geometric arthritic acetabular deformities permits the surgeon to anticipate the technical maneuvers that will be necessary in reconstructing the acetabulum. In viewing the x-rays shown here of types I through IV acetabular deformities, observe how correct preparation of the acetabulum and implantation of the cup result in a reproducible cup position, so that the postoperative x-rays of the acetabular reconstruction all closely resemble each other.

Type I: The type I acetabular deformity (Figs. 7A–1 and 7A–2) is characterized by either symmetrical loss (inflammatory arthritis), maintenance of the joint space (avascular necrosis), or in osteoarthritis, early superolateral migration of the femoral head. The common denominator with this arthritic acetabulum is that the superior subchondral bone is intact. With osteoarthritis, there may be an osteophyte over the cotyloid notch or between the pubis and ischium.

Types II and IIa: In type II deformity (Figs. 7A–3 and 7A–4), the femoral head has migrated superiorly and laterally into the subchondral bone. This is seen in osteoarthritis with migration or the final stage of avascular necrosis. In type IIa, the femoral head migrates through the sourcil subchondral bone and is flattened.

Type III: In type III deformity (Figs. 7A–5 and 7A–6), femoral head migration is inferior and medial, the opposite of that seen in type II. The cartilage loss is seen best on the lateral x-ray. There commonly is an osteophyte between the ischium and the pubis. This type can progress to protrusio.

Type IV Type IV deformity (Figs. 7A–7 through 7A–10) is a dysplastic hip that differs from type II in that the neck–shaft angle is 140 degrees or more. There is superolateral migration of the femoral head, which can progress to destruction of the subchondral bone (type IVa; see Fig. 7A–9). Type IV requires the most medialization of reaming and cup placement. The postoperative offset of the femur is commonly increased because of the very narrow preoperative offset that accompanies the valgus neck–shaft angle. If the offset is increased more than 5 mm, the iliopsoas tendon should be at least partially released to prevent iliopsoas tendinitis due to stretch.

II. Planning the Reconstruction of Hip Biomechanics

Preoperative planning for total hip replacement by templating assumes correct cup placement when judging the level of femoral neck cut to provide the correct leg length and offset (*see "Templating for Total Hip Arthroplasty"*).

If the cup is correctly placed (as shown in the postoperative x-rays of geometric deformities I through III; see Figs. 7A–2, 7A–4, and 7A–6), the stem simply needs to be implanted at the level planned preoperatively for correction of leg length and offset, and the reconstructed hip biomechanics should then be correct. If the cup is superior (see Fig. 7A–10) or lateralized (Fig. 7A–11), the femoral stem insertion depth or the femoral head length will need to be adjusted for this cup position. The surgeon must know the cup position to make adjustments on the femoral side. The cup is superior if its position as measured by the computer (cephalocaudal, or CC number) is +5 mm or more (or if there is palpable bone between the inferior edge of the cup and the edge of the cotyloid notch); the cup is lateral if the medialization and CC position are each not at least 0 (see Fig. 7A–11). The cup also is lateralized if its edge is palpable beyond the cotyloid rim of the acetabular notch by more than approximately 5 mm.

During surgery, biomechanical reconstruction is controlled by the femoral stem. The depth to which the stem is implanted and the length of femoral head used (combined with the knowledge of the acetabular center of rotation) determine the hip length and offset (and therefore the leg length as well, unless there are extra-articular influences on leg length).

The change in leg length and offset can be judged from the computer by the sum of the CC of the cup and the CC of the femoral head. For example, if the center of rotation of the cup is superior by 2 mm (CC = +2) and the center of head of the femoral head is superior by 7 mm (CC = +7), the leg length is increased by 5 mm (increased 7 mm on the femoral side and reduced 2 mm on the acetabular side for a total 5 mm increase). The leg length change is also shown by repositioning the leg into its preoperative position (as demonstrated in Chapter 7). Finally, the leg length can be confirmed by whatever manual method the surgeon prefers to use.

Before surgery, the leg length difference can be measured clinically by lifting the legs together (to eliminate the effect of

Text continued on page 173

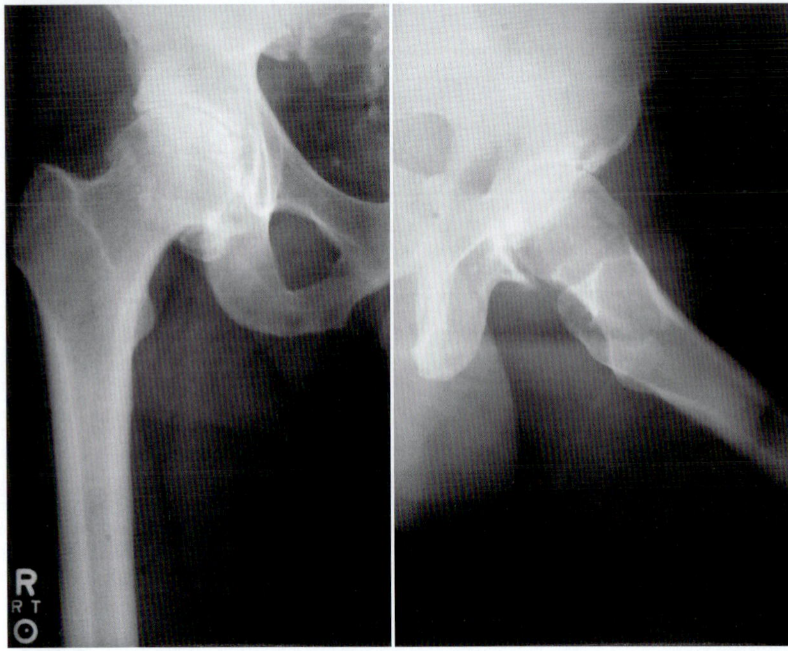

Figure 7A–1 *Type I osteoarthritis with incipient superolateral migration. The average reaming depth on x-ray is 7.5 mm. In our experience with type I deformity, the mean medialization of the acetabular center of rotation is 4 mm and the mean CC (superior displacement of the center of rotation) is 0. The mean femoral anteversion is 7.5 ± 4.5 degrees. The average anatomic inclination is 53 degrees (range, 41 to 63 degrees) and the average anteversion is 12 degrees (range, –8 degrees retroversion to 27 degrees anteversion).*

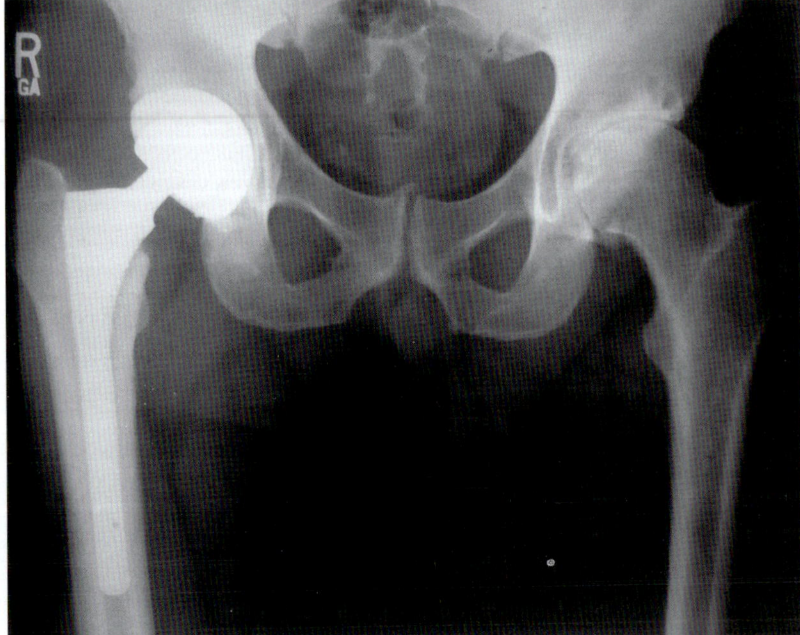

Figure 7A–2 *Postoperative x-ray of the hip in Figure 7A–1 shows the inferomedial edge of the cup at the level of the transverse acetabular ligament (which means it lies between the ischium and the pubis), medial edge of cup at Köhler's line, and with superolateral coverage permitting no more than 5 mm of the cup to be exposed. In this hip, inclination is 48 degrees, anteversion is 30 degrees, and femoral anteversion is 5 degrees. The offset and leg lengths are well reconstructed.*

Figure 7A-3 Left, *A type I deformity. Right, The same patient 18 months later with migration of the femoral head into the sourcil, as well as flattening of the femoral head (type II deformity). The average reaming depth on x-ray for a type II deformity is 9.5 mm. The average anatomic anteversion is 50 degrees (range, 37 to 64 degrees), and anatomic anteversion is 12 degrees (range, –2 degrees retroversion to 23 degrees anteversion). Reaming is deeper than for type I because the acetabular cavity is enlarged, so that usually a one size larger cup is needed for a press-fit. A bigger cup requires more medial reaming to prevent lateralization of the cup. By computer, the mean medialization of cup is 5 mm and the CC (superior) is 3 mm. The average femoral anteversion is 5.2 ± 3.6 degrees. The cup anteversion needs to be approximately 30 degrees to obtain a combined anteversion of 35 degrees.*

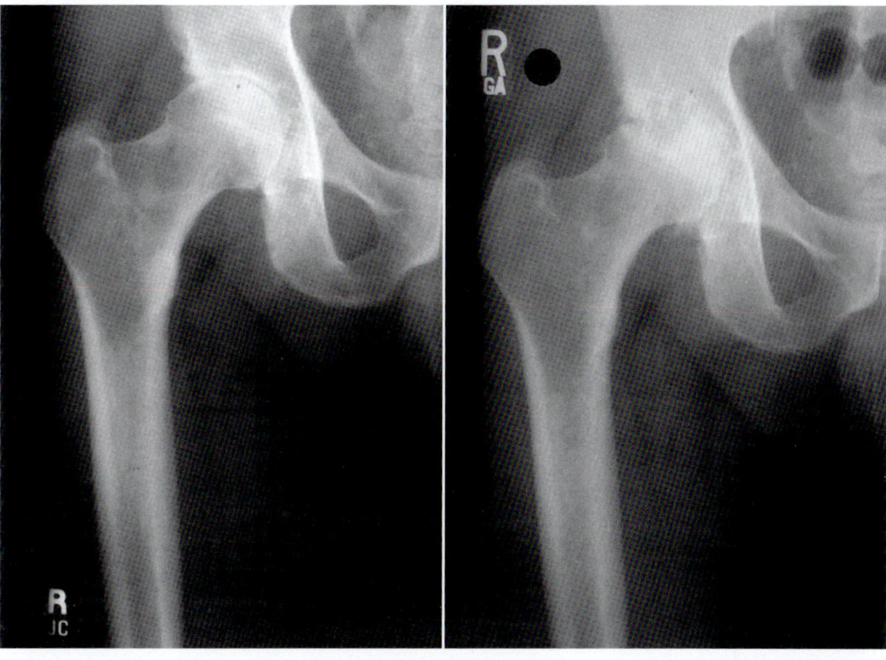

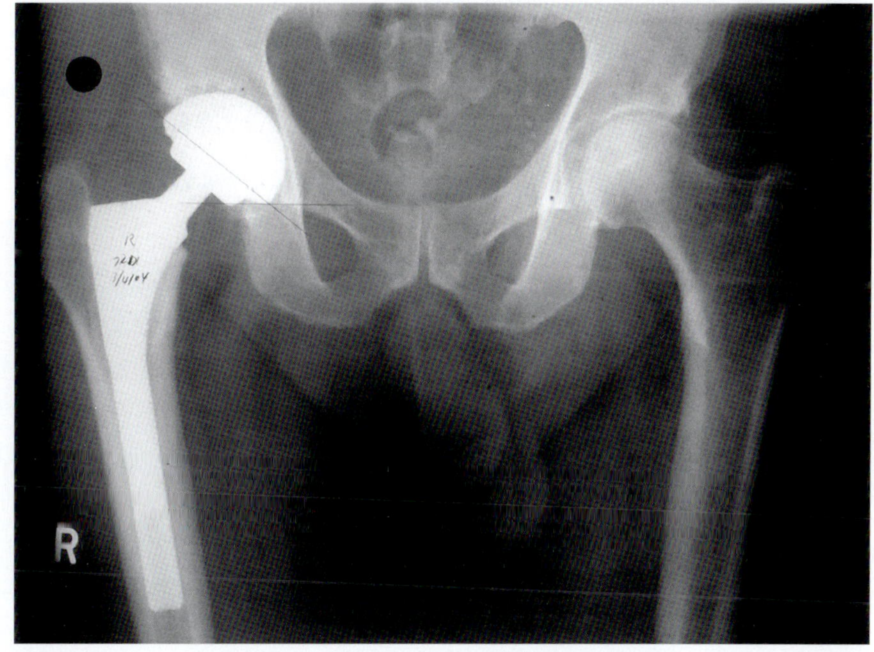

Figure 7A-4 *Note that the cup position appears the same as that in the hip in Figure 7A-2. Inclination is 30 degrees; anteversion is 23 degrees (this operation was done before we incorporated measurement of femoral anteversion into our procedure). The offset and leg length are correctly reconstructed.*

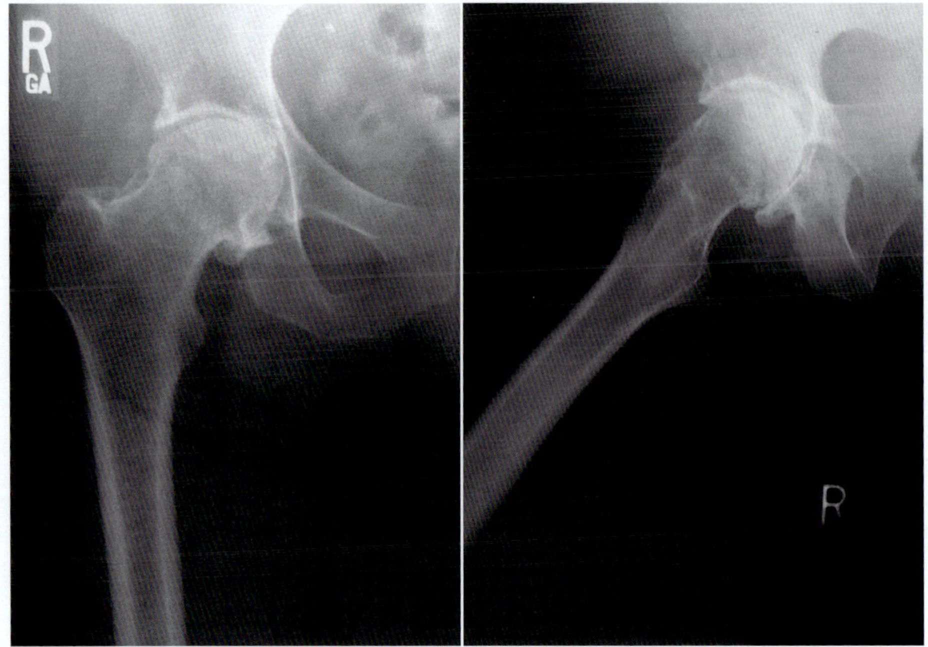

Figure 7A–5   *The diagnosis of a type III deformity is confirmed on the lateral x-ray. There will always be a narrowing of the joint space in zone 3 without loss in zone 1. In this x-ray, there is complete loss of the joint space inferomedially, whereas the superior joint space remains intact. There is an osteophyte between the pubis and ischium. The average x-ray depth of reaming is 3 mm (P = .0001 for being statistically less reaming than for the other types of deformity). The mean computer cup medialization is 2 mm and the CC is 0 mm. The anatomic inclination averages 57 degrees (range, 42 to 66 degrees) and the anatomic anteversion is 8 degrees (range, −15 degrees retroversion to 26 degrees anteversion). The average femoral anteversion is 10.1 ± 5.1 degrees. The cup anteversion can be 20 to 25 degrees because the femoral anteversion is usually 10 degrees or more.*

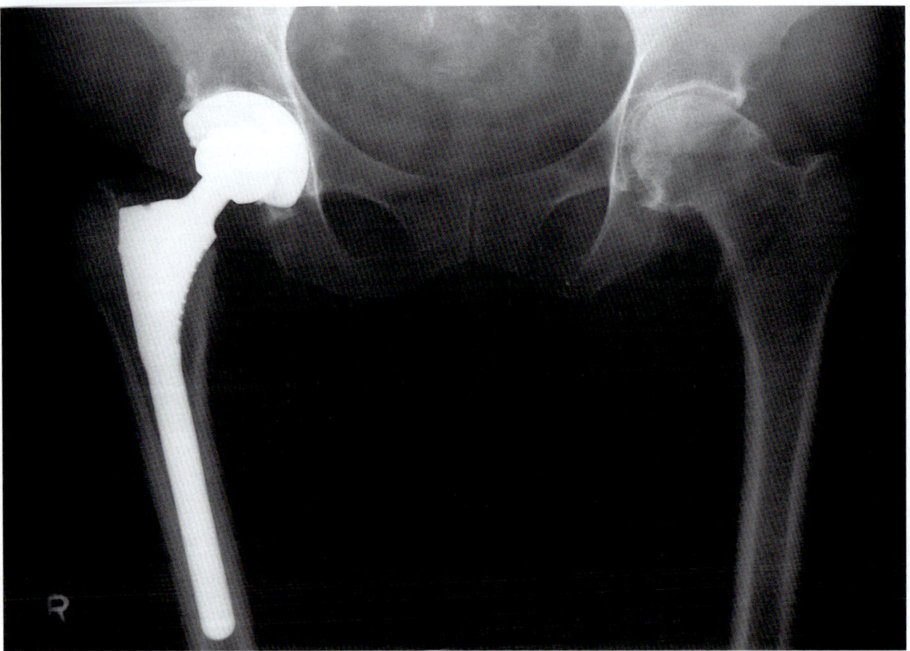

Figure 7A–6   *Postoperative x-ray, type III deformity (same hip as in Fig. 7A–5). Observe that the cup position appears identical to that in types I and II hips. The cup position should be the same regardless of the acetabular deformity to provide good stability and contact areas, and to avoid impingement. In this hip, inclination is 41 degrees, cup anteversion is 22 degrees, and the femoral anteversion was not available.*

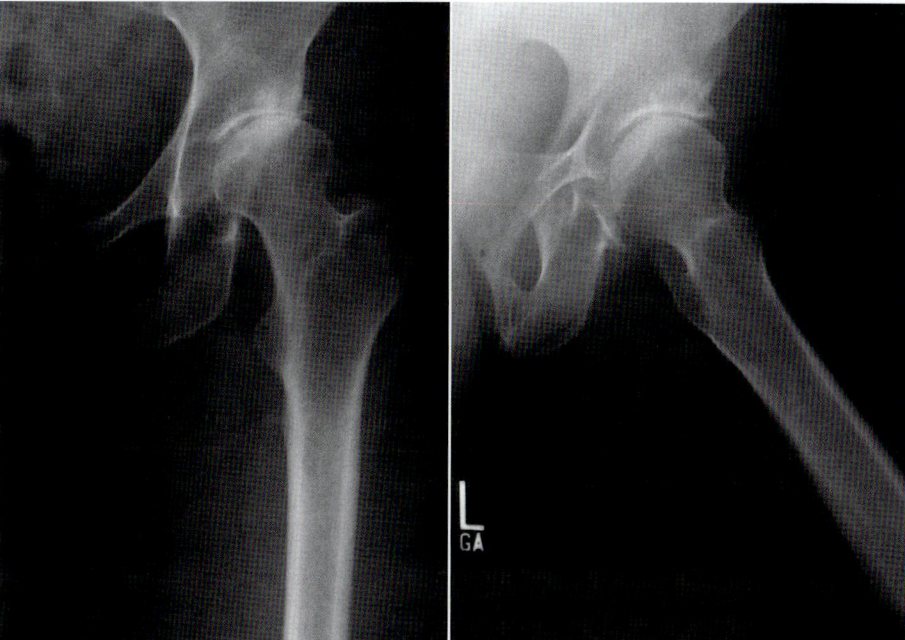

Figure 7A–7 *Type IV deformity with a steep neck–shaft angle and superolateral migration of the femoral head. The average x-ray reaming depth is 11 mm. The average computer cup medialization is 10 mm, and the CC is 3 mm. The anatomic inclination averages 50 degrees (range, 40 to 67 degrees), the anatomic anteversion averages 10 degrees (range, −10 degrees retroversion to 24 degrees anteversion), and femoral anteversion averages 6.8 ± 4.8 degrees. The cup anteversion needs to be at least 25 degrees because femoral anteversion seldom is more than 10 degrees.*

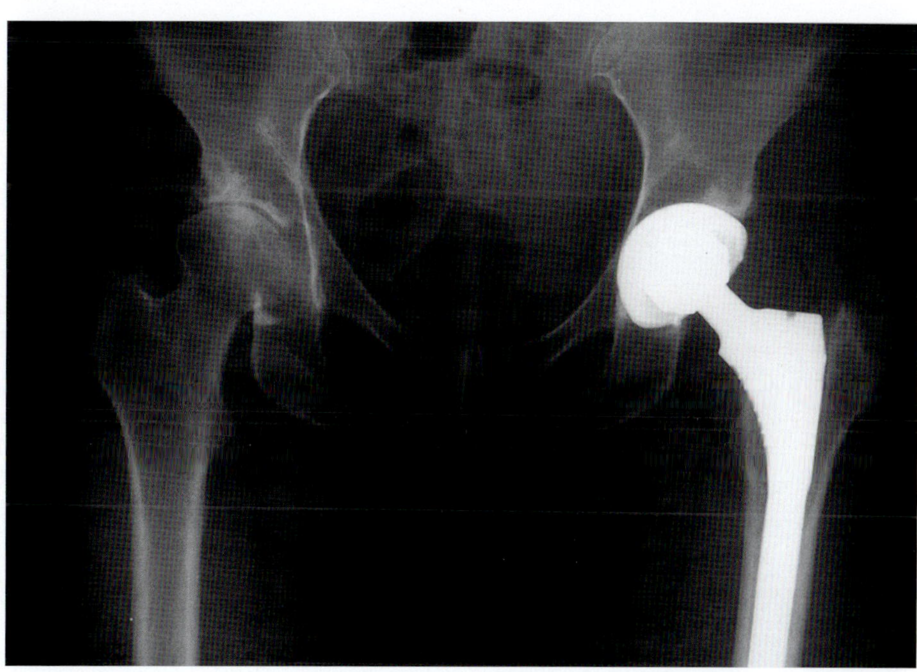

Figure 7A–8 *The cup position in this postoperative type IV hip (same hip as in Fig. 7A–7) again appears the same on the x-ray as with the other types of hip deformities. The femoral offset is increased in this hip, which is not uncommon with type IV because of the very narrow preoperative offset. If the offset is increased by more than 5 mm, the iliopsoas tendon must be at least 50% released from the lesser trochanter to avoid stretch-induced iliopsoas tendinitis. In this hip, inclination is 46 degrees, cup anteversion is 29 degrees, and the femoral anteversion was not available.*

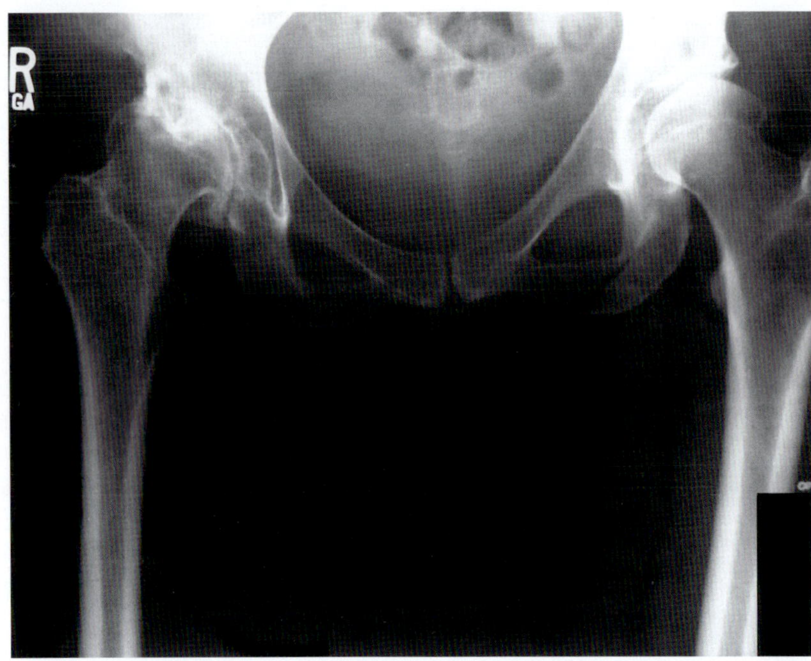

Figure 7A–9 *Type IVa deformity with significant superolateral displacement of the femoral head, migration of the head into subchondral bone, and a thick medial acetabular wall.*

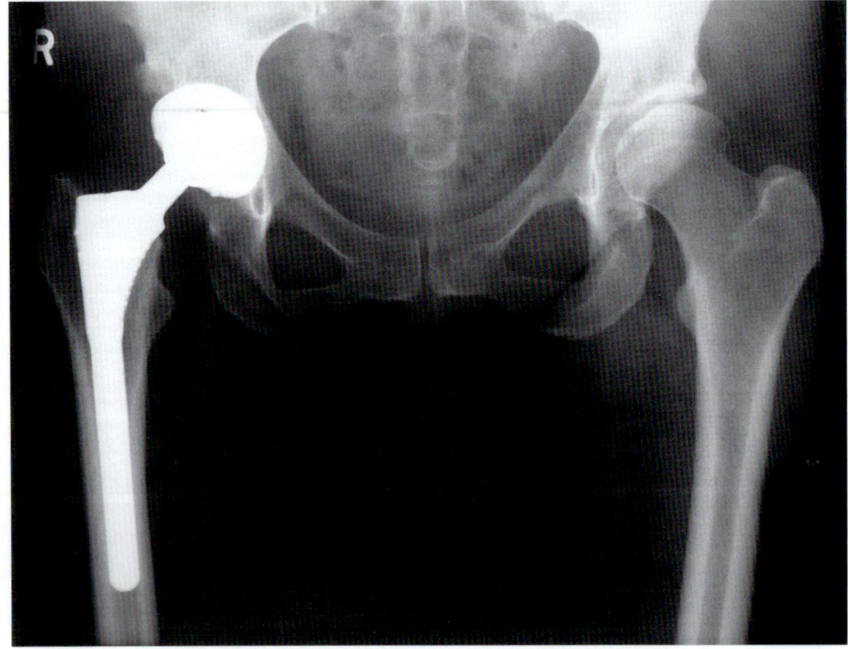

Figure 7A–10 *The cup position in this postoperative type IVa hip (same hip as in Fig. 7A–9) again has the same x-ray appearance as the other hips, despite the preoperative deformity. In this hip, inclination is 46 degrees, anteversion is 30 degrees, and femoral anteversion is 6 degrees. With this cup the medialization was 29 mm and the CC 10 mm, which gives the cup a superior position. The offset and leg length are correctly reconstructed by the level of stem implantation and head length used. A superior cup requires the surgeon to adjust the plan of the femoral reconstruction.*

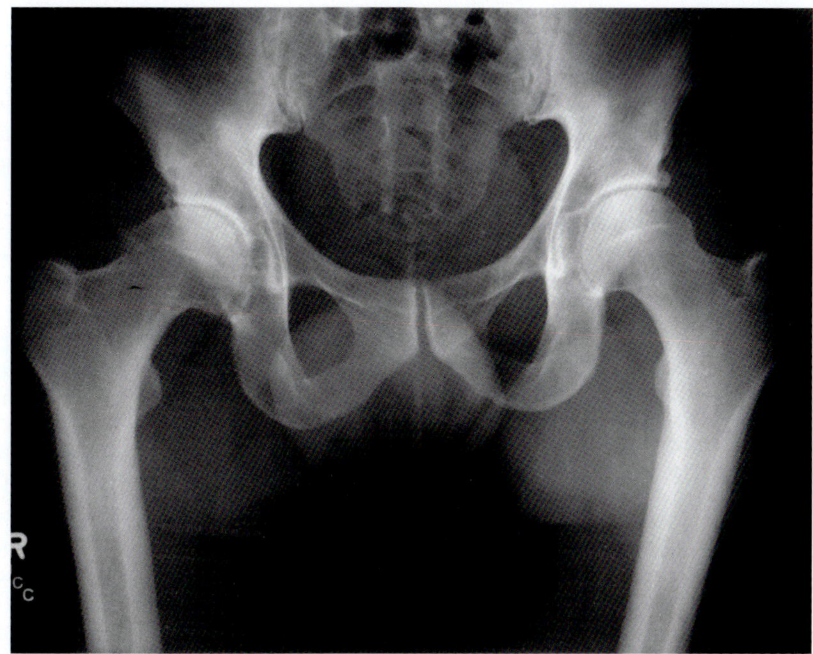

A

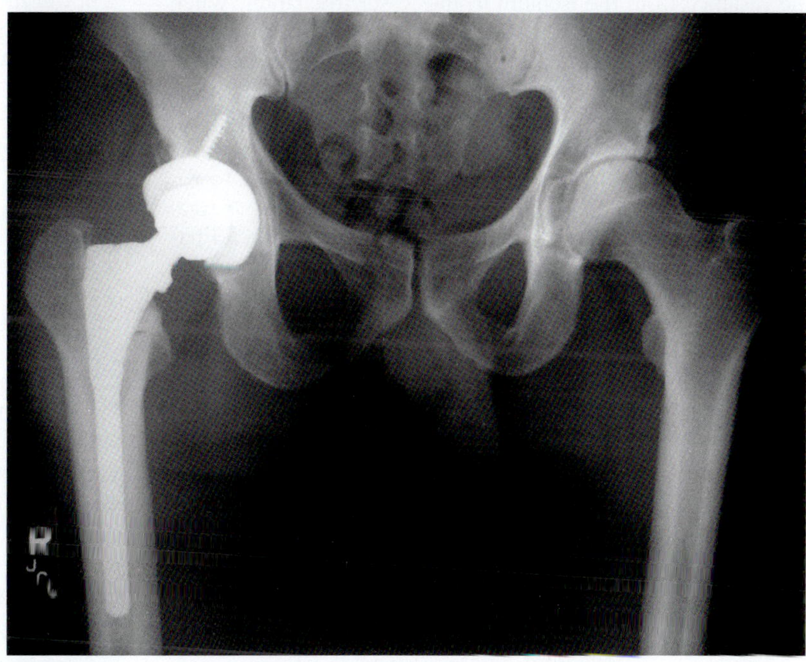

B

Figure 7A–11　**A,** *In this hip, there was plenty of medial wall to ream because this hip has an extended triangle structure, which means that there is a thick tear drop.* **B,** *The failure to ream sufficiently medially results in the cup's being lateralized, with a medialization of –4 mm (lateralized 4 mm) and CC of 0. The cup inclination is 40 degrees and anteversion, 20 degrees. This was the only hip in the computer series to dislocate, which highlights the danger of lateralizing the cup.*

a flexion contracture) and measuring the vertical difference between the medial malleoli. It is important to ensure that the legs are in the line of the body (lined up with the sternum) and not angled to either side.

The CC of the stem is directly related to its depth of implantation into the femur. The depth of implantation is referenced from the neck cut. The level of the neck cut is known when the medial cut surface of the neck is touched with the pointer guide. The computer then calculates the distance of the neck cut from the acetabular center of rotation. If, before surgery, the surgeon calculated that the center of rotation of the acetabulum would be zero, and placement of the stem with a neutral head at the level of the neck cut would reconstruct the hip length and offset, then he or she can calculate the necessary parameters for the current level of neck cut. Most implants have a 35-mm neck length and a neutral head. If the center of rotation of the cup is superior by 5 mm, the surgeon knows from the preoperatively determined level of neck cut that a total of 40 mm is needed to equalize leg length and offset. However, if the level of neck cut created by the surgeon shows a difference of 35 mm from the acetabular center of rotation, the surgeon will need to remove 5 mm more of neck to create a 40-mm gap, and a +5 mm head length will need to be used to reconstruct the correct hip length and offset. If the stem were implanted at the measured level of neck cut and a neutral head used, this would fill the gap of 35 mm, but the offset would be reduced. The offset can be calculated by adding the medialization of the cup and the mediolateral position of the center of the femoral head. For example, if the cup medialization is 5 mm medial and the position of the center of the femoral head will lateralize the femoral head 3 mm, the sum is −2 mm medialized, so the hip offset is reduced by 2 mm.

III. New Method of Planning Biomechanical Reconstruction Using the Radiographic Center of Rotation of the Acetabulum and Femur

The traditional method of measuring the leg length difference involves measuring the height of the lesser trochanter from the transischial line on preoperative radiographs. Rotation of the x-ray can affect this measurement, as well the measurement of offset difference, which is traditionally measured by the distance from the ischium to the lesser trochanter. When templating just before the operation, these x-ray measurements can be used to make a good estimation of the change needed to reconstruct leg length and offset.

A more accurate measure of the change needed in leg length and offset is obtained by measuring the migration of the center of the femoral head away from the center of rotation of the acetabulum. In a normal hip, these centers of rotation should overlay. In an arthritic hip, the femoral head has migrated from the original center of rotation of the hip (which is now just the center of rotation of the acetabulum). Measurement of the difference in the centers of rotation of the acetabulum and the femoral head allows an accurate estimate of the necessary change for length and offset because the femoral head is round and rotation has little effect on these measurements. This technique is least accurate with a severe external rotation contracture of the femur, which causes a false-positive valgus femoral neck alignment on the radiograph and therefore a falsely elevated center of rotation of the femoral head.

The normal neck–shaft angle of the hip is nearly 125 degrees. With this neck–shaft angle, the anatomic center of the head is where a line drawn tangent to the cortex of the superior neck crosses the line of the neck axis (Fig. 7A–12). In arthritic hips, the center of the head is superior or inferior to this point of interception, depending on the neck–shaft angle (Table 7A–1). The R value of these measurements is 0.93, so their accuracy is excellent.

The technique for measurement of the acetabular center of rotation does not vary by geometric type of arthritic deformity. The center is always found by first drawing a vertical line perpendicular to the horizontal line connecting the tear drops, and tangent to the lateral margin of one of the tear drops (see Fig. 7A–12). A horizontal line perpendicular to this vertical line is drawn tangent to the superior subchondral bone of the acetabulum, and a point is marked two thirds of the distance to the lateral margin of the acetabulum (the lateral margin is defined here by the cortical indentation on the

lateral margin). From this point on the superior subchondral line, a perpendicular vertical line is directed down for two thirds of the vertical distance of the acetabulum. This point marks the center of rotation of the acetabulum with a standard deviation of ±3 mm.

A second and simpler method for determining the acetabular center of rotation and the change in the femoral center of rotation consists of first drawing a line across the mouth of the acetabulum from the midpoint between the tear drop and ischium to the superior lateral corner of the acetabulum. The center of rotation of the hip is 7 mm lateral to the midpoint of this line on a perpendicular to this line (green dot in Fig. 7A–13). The coordinates of the center of rotation of the acetabulum and the femur are now drawn as shown in Figure 7A–13. The red box shows the method for obtaining the coordinate of the femoral center of rotation, and the yellow box the method for the coordinate of the acetabular center of rotation. In a normal hip these two are the same because the hip has a single center of rotation. The centers of rotation separate in an arthritic hip because the femoral head migrates. The right hip in Figure 7A–13 is arthritic, and the migration of the femoral head is shown by the red dot. The vertical and horizontal measurements between the red and green dots represent the required changes in leg length and offset to equalize these parameters between the two hips. The postoperative x-ray (Fig. 7A–14) shows a near-perfect reconstruction, with the acetabular and femoral centers of rotation 1 mm apart and ideal cup coverage, with the inferior edge of the cup at the level of the transverse ligament and the superolateral cup covered.

Figures 7A–15 and 7A–16 illustrate a second example in which the cup was placed too far superior, so the femoral center of rotation and reconstructed hip center of rotation (blue dot) are therefore superior to the anatomic center of rotation (green dot).

A combination of preoperative planning, including the use of the largest head–neck ratio possible, and the intraoperative information provided by the computer navigation system allows the surgeon, predictably and reproducibly, to avoid impingement when implanting the acetabulum (because the combined anteversion is known), and to create the correct

Table 7A–1
Position of Center of Femoral Head According to Neck–Shaft Angle

Neck–Shaft Angle (degrees)	CH Position (mm)
120	−3.0
125	0
130	+2.0
135	+4.5
140	+4.7

CH, center of femoral head.
The technique and measurements for this center of head position were researched by Dr. Yutaka Inaba.

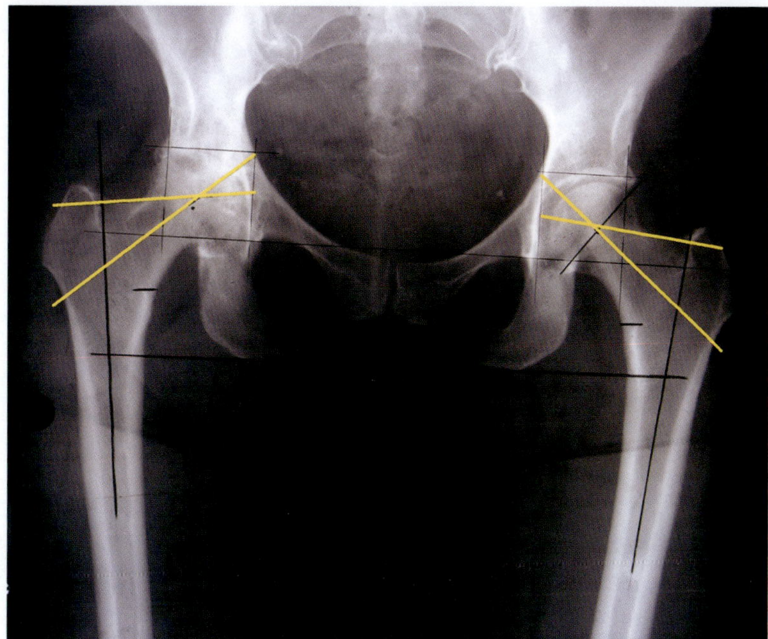

Figure 7A–12 *These hips have a neck–shaft angle of 125 degrees. The two yellow lines represent the axis of the neck and the line tangential to the superior cortex of the femoral neck. The intersection of these lines is the center of the femoral head. This center of the femoral head moves with migration of the femoral head. The distance the center of the femoral head migrates from the acetabular center of rotation defines the change needed in femoral leg length and offset. The arthritic right hip shows the migration of the femoral head center from the black dot, which is the acetabular center. This distance is close to that obtained by measuring the distance from the lesser trochanter to the transischial line, a measurement indicated by a mark at the superior edge of the lesser trochanter; this distance is 7 mm. The distance from the changed center of rotation of the femoral head to the acetabular center of rotation is also 7 mm. The femoral head offset change was 5 mm, which would require an increase in offset of 5 mm. The box outlining the acetabulum is used to locate the acetabular center of rotation. See text for description of the method.*

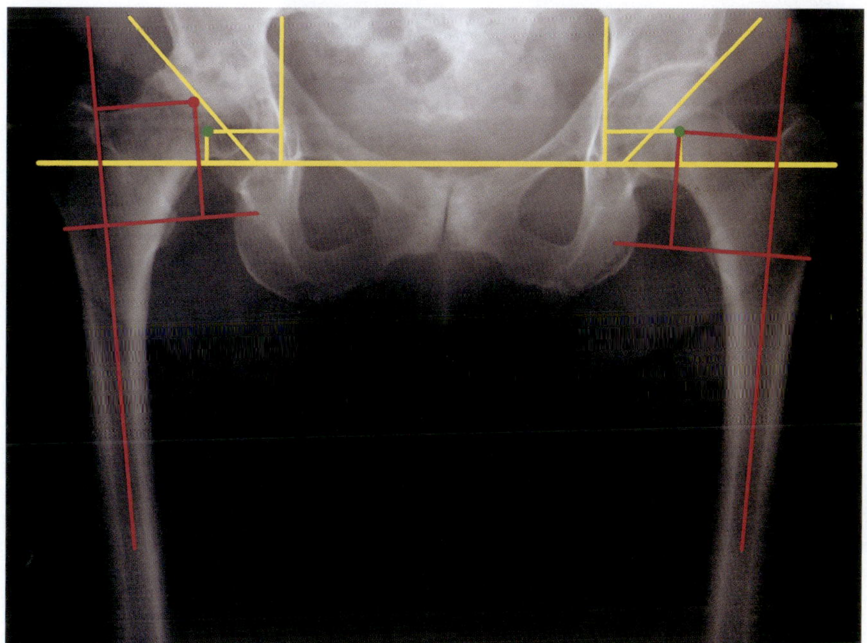

Figure 7A–13 *The center of rotation of the hip can be found by drawing an oblique line across the mouth of the acetabulum from the midpoint between the pubis and the ischium to the lateral edge of the acetabulum. The center of rotation of the hip is 7 mm lateral on a perpendicular line drawn to the midpoint of this line (the ruler is not magnified). The center can also be estimated by using a line 5 mm from the old epiphyseal line in the center of the compression trabeculae (the ruler is not magnified), but the epiphyseal line and compression trabeculae are not always easily seen. A box is constructed to measure the point of the center of rotation of the acetabulum (and the normal hip) (yellow box) by drawing a vertical line from the trans–tear drop line to the green dot and a horizontal line from the vertical inner tear drop line to the green dot. The vertical and horizontal distances to the center of rotation of the hip can then be reconstructed in the arthritic hip (right hip). Reconstruction of this box in the preoperative hip allows accurate measurement of the correct center of rotation of the hip. The center of the femoral head in the normal left hip is measured by the coordinates in red (red box). The box is constructed by drawing a line that bisects the intramedullary canal and perpendicular lines through the apex of the lesser trochanter and to the center of the hip (green dot). The vertical distance from the green dot to the line through the lesser trochanter is the height of the center of the femoral head. Reconstructing this box with lines of the same length, both horizontal and vertical, on the arthritic (right) hip marks the migrated position of the femoral head. Therefore, the change in leg length and offset required at surgery are the vertical and the horizontal differences between the red and green dots on the right hip.*

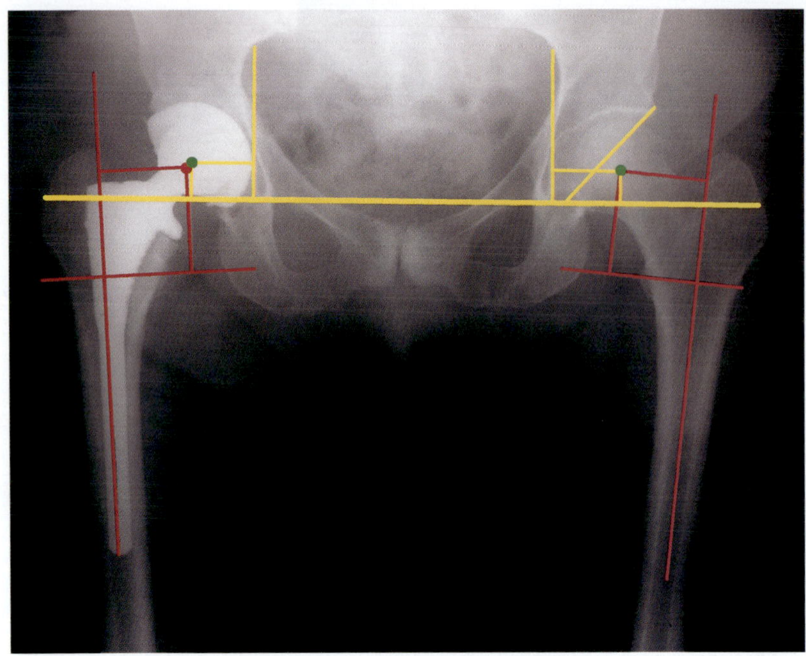

Figure 7A–14 *Postoperative x-ray of the hip in Figure 7A–13. Reconstruction of the leg length and offset was accurate within 1 mm, as shown by the position of the center of rotation of the hip* (green dot) *and the center of rotation of the femoral head* (red dot).

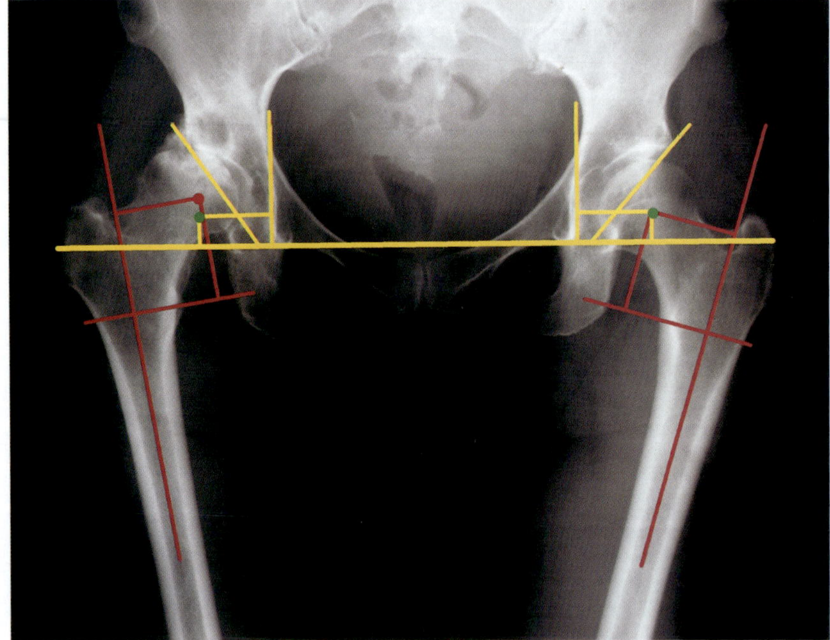

Figure 7A–15 *Another example of measurements of the normal center of rotation and, in the arthritic right hip, the migrated center of rotation of the femoral head, with the difference between the red and green dots representing the changes necessary to reconstruct leg length and offset.*

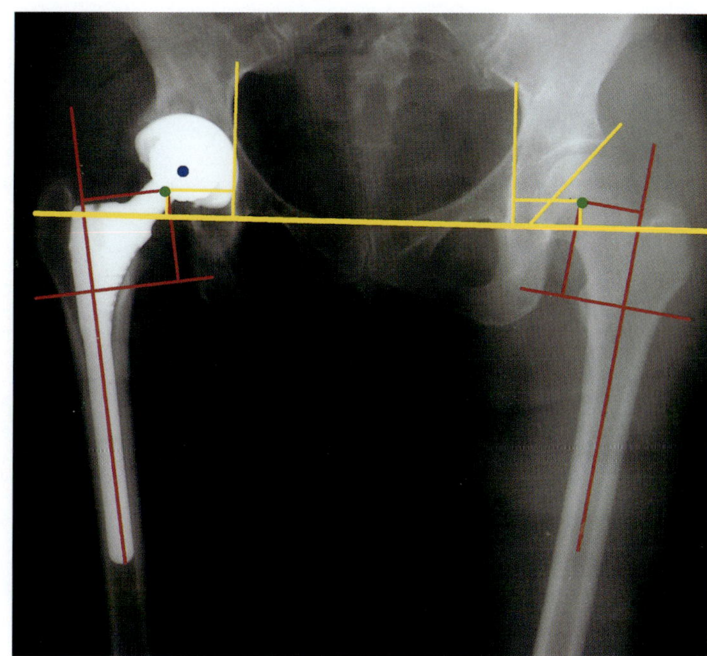

Figure 7A–16 *Postoperative x-ray of the hip in Figure 7A–15 shows superior cup placement, which moves the center of rotation of the hip superior and medial to the normal center of rotation, so the biomechanical reconstruction is not accurate.*

bony coverage of the cup with an inclination that gives good contact areas (which depends on the amount of medialization), thus virtually guaranteeing stability. The biomechanical reconstruction of the hip is controlled by the femur, and can be adjusted by the surgeon based on his or her knowledge of the neck cut level. The level of the neck cut can be read on the computer, so the stem can be implanted at a level that puts the center of the head at the correct position for the necessary change in leg length and offset according to the numerical position of the acetabular center of rotation. If the acetabular center of rotation is precisely reconstructed, the center of the femoral head will be at the anatomic center of rotation of the hip (see Fig. 7A–14).

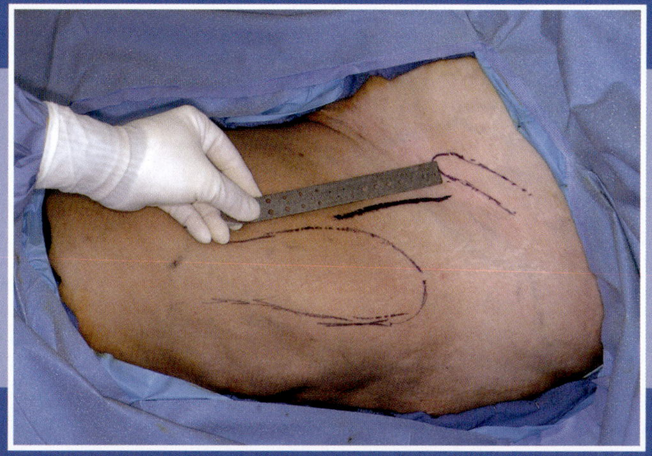

The Anterior Mini-incision Intermuscular Approach: A Single Incision*

ANDREW G. YUN

*This chapter is the technique for the anterior intermuscular and internervous technique that uses the PROfx table, as performed by Dr. Yun. In conjunction with this chapter on the DVD-ROM is the video "*Anterior Approach for Total Hip Replacement*," showing the anterior intermuscular internervous approach without use of a particular table, as performed by Dr. Clive Duncan of Vancouver, British Columbia, Canada.

The single-incision anterior approach provides predictable surgical exposure with comparatively minimal muscle dissection (Fig. 8–1). The anterior approach, originally described by Smith-Peterson, has a historical basis. It is also known as the "distal window of the iliofemoral approach." It is to be differentiated from the better known anterolateral and modified lateral approaches. Until relatively recently, the anterior approach has been used sparingly for pelvic osteotomy and acetabular and femoral head trauma. The evolution of minimally invasive hip surgery, however, has led to re-exploration and adaptation of the anterior approach for total hip replacement.

Several techniques have been described using the anterior interval between the tensor fascia muscle and the sartorious muscle. This interval provides excellent exposure of the acetabulum and anterior column. The distinction between the different anterior techniques is in reference to femoral preparation. One technique, known as the Zimmer two-incision approach, involves a second incision for femoral preparation. The other technique entails preparing and implanting the femoral stem through a single-incision anterior approach. This technique was originally described by Judet in France using the Judet table and has been modified in its current form by several surgeons using tables that allow extreme extension and rotation of the leg. This chapter describes the modification of Matta, which uses the PROfx table (Orthopedic Systems, Inc. [OSI], Union City, Calif.) with rigid traction that allows predictable delivery of the femur into the wound for safe femoral preparation.

It is important to distinguish between the anterior approach and the anterolateral and modified lateral approaches (Hardinge). All of these incisions require an anterior capsulotomy with anterior dislocation of the hip. However, the anterior approach is the only true internervous and intermuscular dissection. The anterolateral and the modified lateral approaches are not internervous and require extensive splitting of the gluteus medius–vastus lateralis muscle complex, or at least partial detachment of the abductor mechanism. These approaches violate the superior gluteal neuromuscular interval. This increases the risk of postoperative limp, which historically has been associated with the anterolateral approach.

INDICATIONS

The anterior approach is appropriate for routine primary total hip replacement but is ideally indicated for the patient at high risk for dislocation. The anterior approach preserves the posterior capsule and external rotator muscles, which protects against dislocation. Classic risk factors for dislocation include neuromuscular disease, alcoholism, Parkinson's disease, and epilepsy. An additional advantage is the ease of augmenting visualization of component positions with fluoroscopic control. Fluoroscopy allows real-time intraoperative assessment and adjustment of implant position, and it assists in the biomechanical reconstruction of offset and hip length. In contrast to the Zimmer two-incision technique, the single-incision anterior approach allows for either cemented or cementless fixation of either the acetabular or the femoral component. Operating with the patient in the supine position permits easy and reliable assessment of leg lengths.

There are disadvantages to surgeons unfamiliar with the supine position and the Smith-Peterson approach. Implant positioning can be disorienting with the patient in the supine position. Early on, there can be confusion regarding identification of appropriate muscular intervals. Visualization of the posterior column is less complete. Straight reaming of the femoral canal is difficult, and the approach works best with broach-only stem systems.

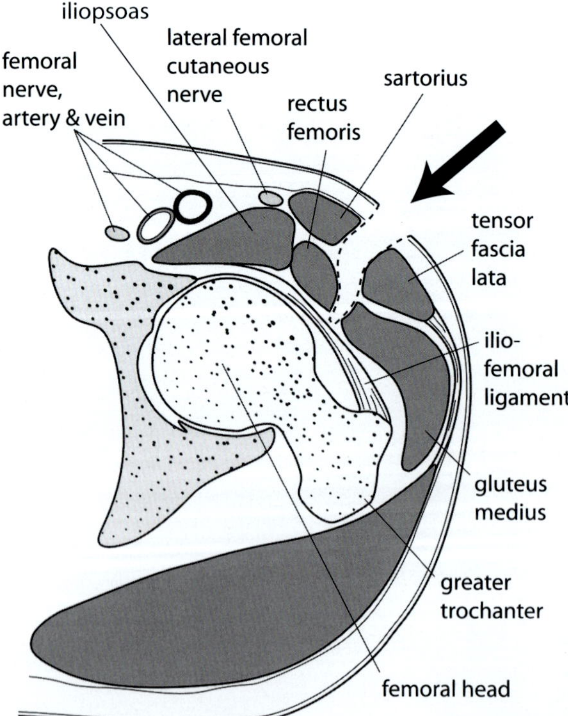

Figure 8–1 *The internervous and intermuscular Smith-Peterson interval (arrow). Note the location of the femoral nerve neurovascular bundle and the lateral femoral cutaneous nerve medial to the sartorius and iliopsoas muscles.*

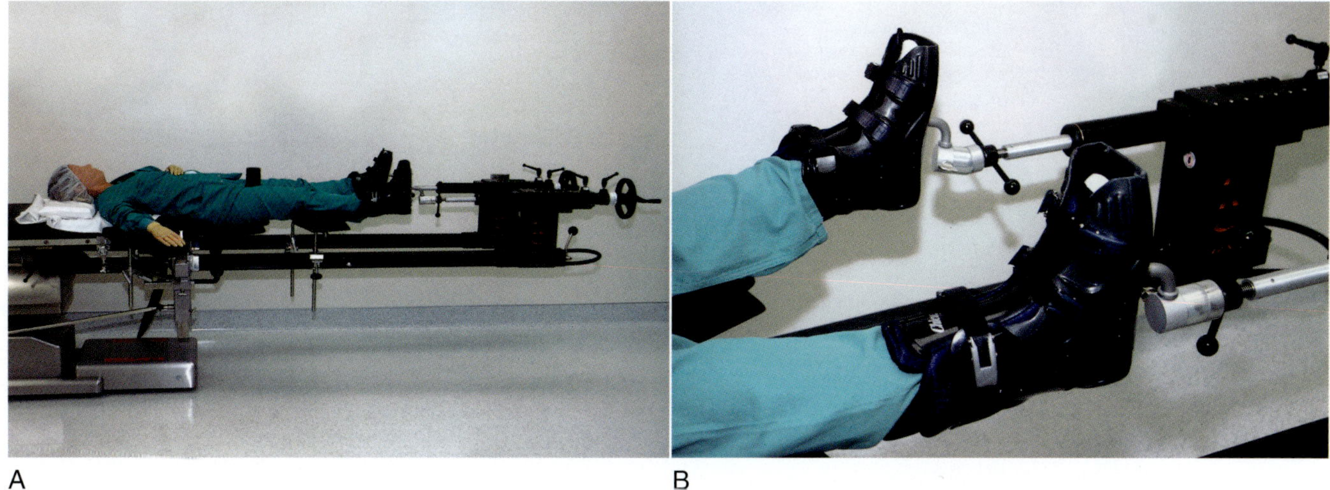

Figure 8–2   **A,** *The OSI PROfx table.* **B,** *Close-up of the traction boot system attached to the leg spars.*

IMPLANTS AND INSTRUMENTATION

Although acetabular exposure was always predictable, the anterior approach had been largely abandoned over past decades because of difficulty with femoral exposure and preparation. The development and use of segmented tables, such as the PROfx, has solved the problem of femoral preparation for the stem. The table provides stable leg control and the leverage necessary for controlled dislocation (Fig. 8–2).

A broach-only system is preferable for the femur. The broach handle needs to be modified specifically for the procedure (Fig. 8–3). Systems that use femoral reaming are not recommended because of the difficulty in obtaining the angle necessary for easy diaphyseal reaming.

Fluoroscopy is not critical to the procedure. Operations using this anterior approach have been done in France for decades without fluoroscopic control. However, during the learning phase, it is recommended that fluoroscopy be used to aid in implant positioning and assessment of hip biomechanics.

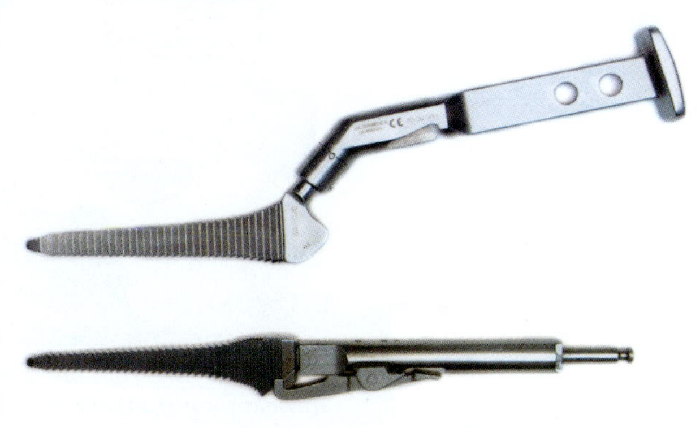

Figure 8–3 *A comparison of the standard* (bottom) *and modified Zweymüller broach handle* (top). *Note the modified broach insertion handle, which is angled off the plane of the femoral shaft. This allows direct access to the femoral canal through a single incision.*

OPERATIVE TECHNIQUE

Positioning and Incision

The patient is placed supine on the PROfx table with the arms extended 90 degrees to the body. Sequential compression devices are placed on the bilateral lower extremities for intraoperative deep venous thrombosis prophylaxis (Fig. 8–4). Both feet are securely fixed in the traction boots, with the legs extended and slightly internally rotated 10 degrees (Fig. 8–5). The leg is pre-

pared to allow exposure from proximal to the iliac crest to just proximal to the patella (Fig. 8–6). Palpable landmarks are important for accurate positioning of the incision. The anterior superior iliac spine and iliac crest should be easily palpable in any patient, regardless of his or her size.

The incision starts approximately 2 fingerbreadths posterior and lateral and 1 fingerbreadth distal to the anterior superior iliac spine. It continues for approximately 10 cm anterolaterally to just proximal to the anterior border of the greater trochanter (Fig. 8–7). The incision should run directly superficial to the fibers of the tensor fascia lata muscle (Fig. 8–8). In thinner or muscular patients it may even be possible to visualize or palpate the tensor fascia lata muscle. The approach

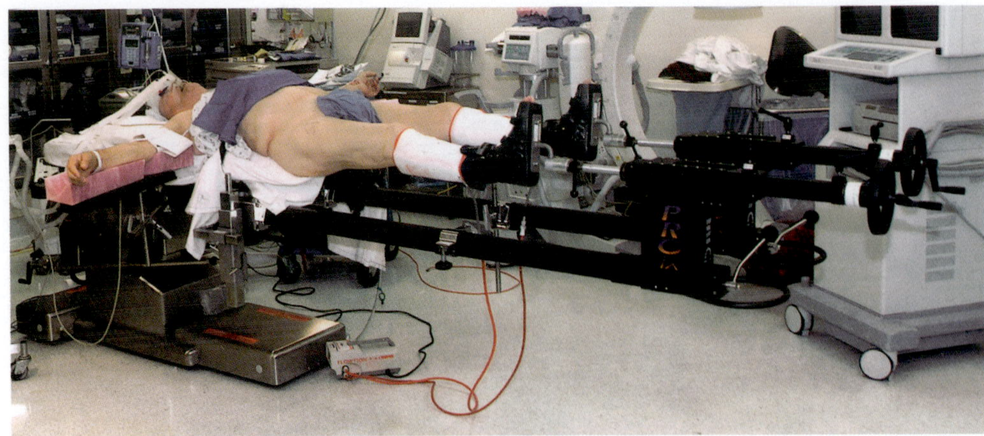

Figure 8–4 The patient is positioned supine on the PROfx table. Arms are extended 90 degrees to the body and the legs are in the neutral position.

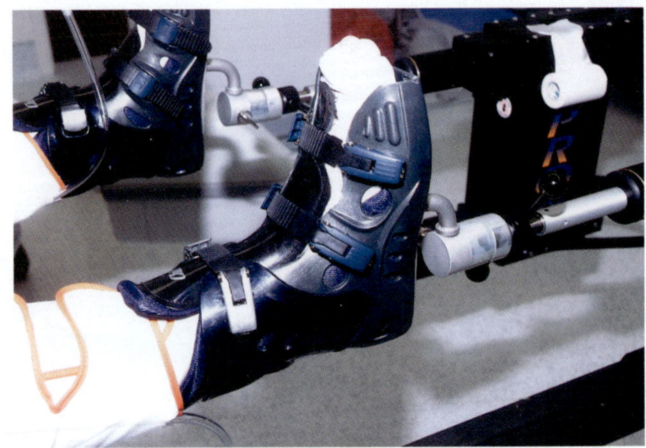

Figure 8–5 Traction boots with sequential compression devices for intraoperative deep venous thrombosis prophylaxis.

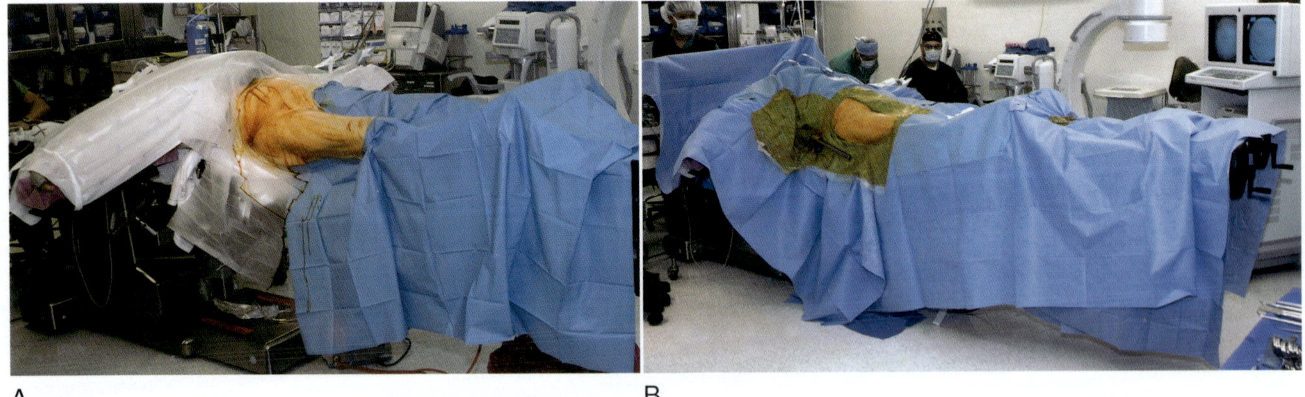

A

B

Figure 8–6 **A,** The patient is prepared and draped with the first layer of drapes. **B,** Final layer of drapes. The iliac crest and the distal femur are exposed.

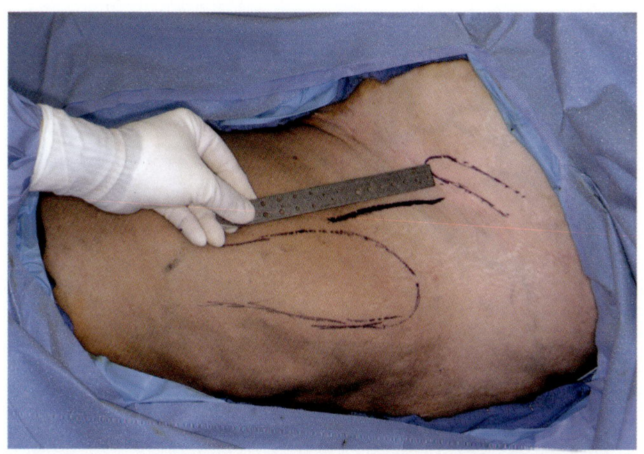

Figure 8–7 *Incision landmarks based on the anterior superior iliac spine and greater trochanter. Approximately 8 to 10 cm in length, the incision runs obliquely over the tensor muscle.*

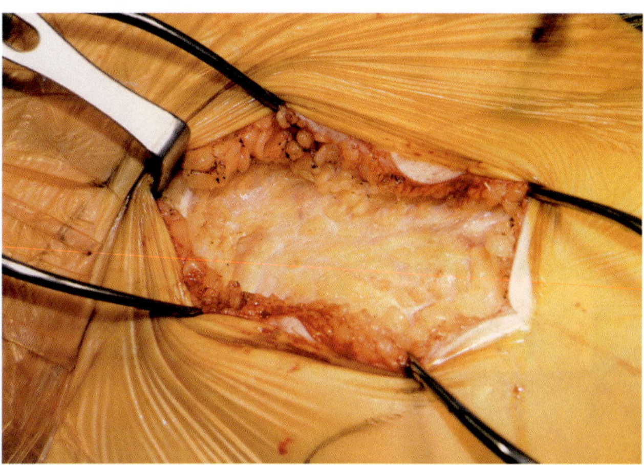

Figure 8–9 *Superficial dissection down to the level of the subcutaneous fat.*

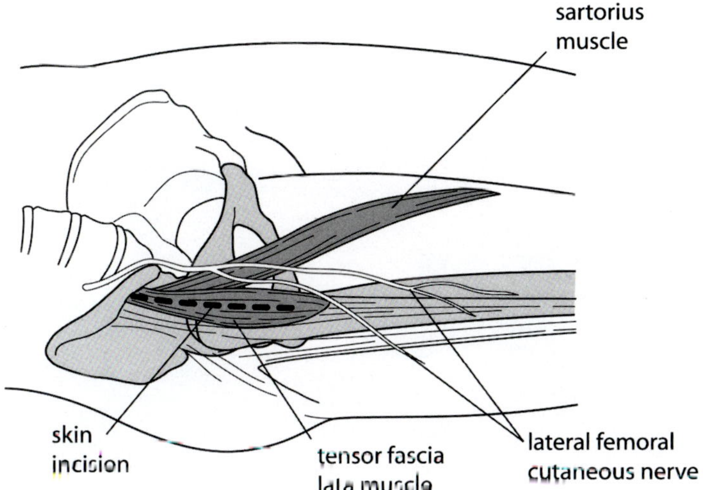

Figure 8–8 *Location of the skin incision with the location of the lateral femoral cutaneous nerve medial to the incision.*

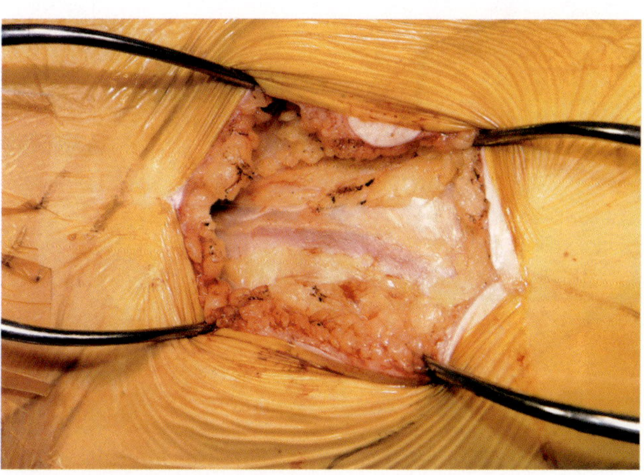

Figure 8–10 *Dissection down to the level of the fascia directly overlying the tensor fascia lata muscle.*

is slightly more lateral than the original Smith-Peterson interval to protect against injury to the lateral femoral cutaneous nerve. The nerve usually tracks medial to the incision (see Figs. 8–1 and 8–8).

Exposure

Dissection is carried through the subcutaneous fat (Fig. 8–9) to the deep fascia overlying the tensor fascia lata (Fig. 8–10). Once the fascia is identified and opened, the muscle fibers of the tensor fascia lata are easily visualized to run in-line with the incision (Fig. 8–11). The exposure of the tensor provides a safe window for superficial dissection by avoiding the lateral femoral cutaneous nerve (see Fig. 8–8). The fascial sleeve is elevated medially with two Allis clamps (Fig. 8–12). Blunt

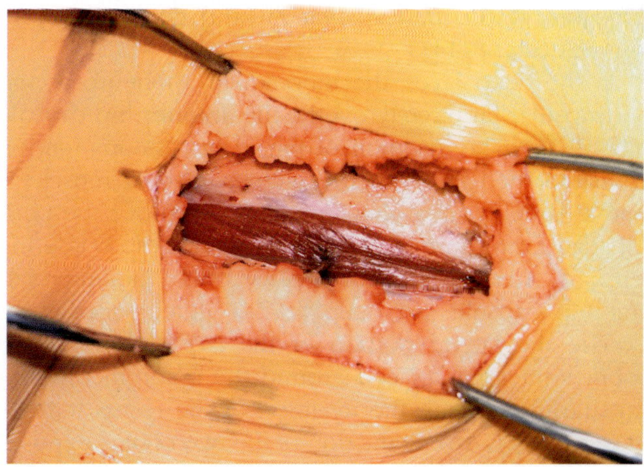

Figure 8–11 *Splitting of the fascia in line with the fibers of the tensor fascia lata muscle. Oblique fibers of the muscle are visible below.*

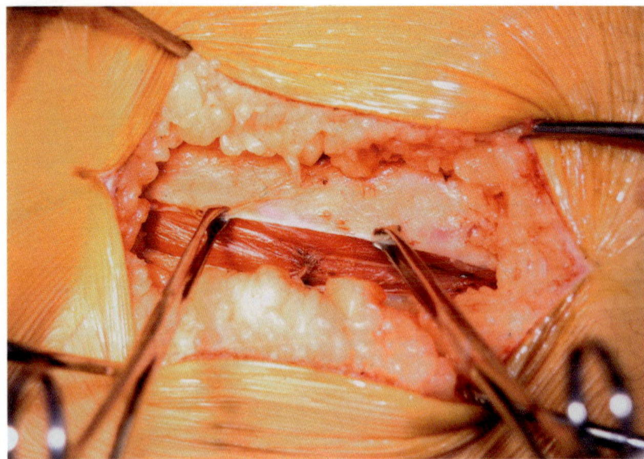

Figure 8–12 *Defining the interval between the medial border of the tensor and the fascia of the sartorius. Two Allis clamps retract the fascia medially.*

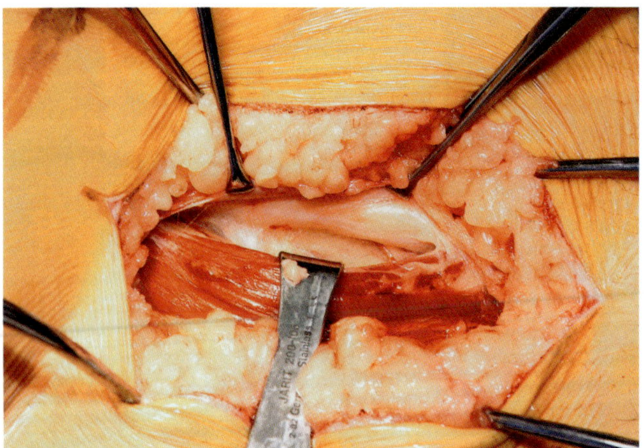

Figure 8–13 *Blunt dissection of the tensor laterally and the sartorius medially down to the level of the pericapsular fat.*

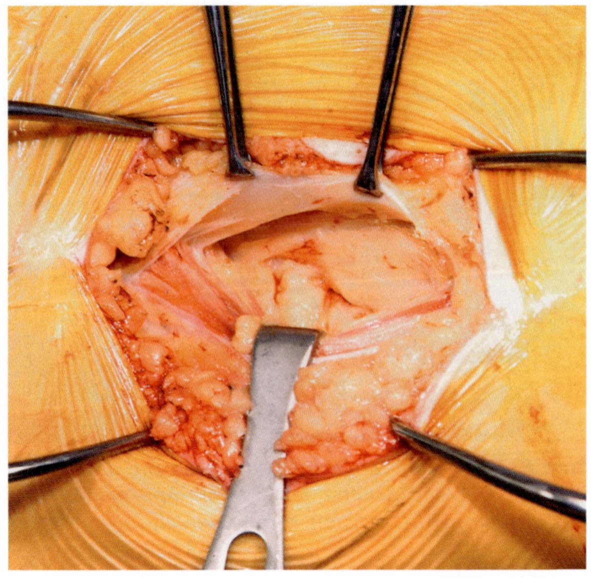

Figure 8–14 *Pericapsular fat overlying the hip capsule.*

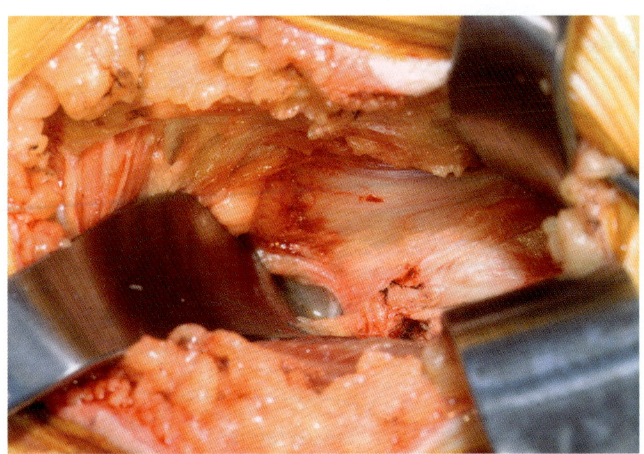

Figure 8–15 *The innominate aponeurosis overlying the anterior hip capsule.*

dissection between the medial border of the tensor fascia lata fibers and the fascia of the lateral border of the sartorius muscle (Fig. 8–13) provides immediate exposure of the pericapsular fat and deeper layer of muscles (Fig. 8–14).

At the deep layer, the innominate aponeurosis and pericapsular fat directly overlie the anterior hip capsule (Fig. 8–15). The insertion of the rectus femoris tendon is visible medially, and the gluteus medius muscle is visible laterally. A rongeur is used to remove the pericapsular fat to improve visualization of these bordering tendons. A cobra retractor is placed over the anterolateral hip capsule just deep to the gluteus medius to expose the lateral portion of the capsule. A second cobra retractor is placed around the anteromedial hip capsule underneath the insertion of the rectus femoris muscle (Fig. 8–16). Retraction of the two cobras exposes the entire length of the anterior hip capsule.

Gentle retraction of the cobras also exposes the ascending branches of the lateral femoral circumflex artery. The vessels cross horizontally at the apex of the incision (Fig. 8–17; see Fig. 8–16A) and can be safely coagulated or ligated.

The femoral head is visualized deep to the capsule with gentle internal or external rotation of the leg through the leg spar. The surgeon can choose to do either an anterior capsulectomy or capsulotomy. Capsulectomy involves excision of a trapezoidal window anteriorly. I prefer an H-shaped capsulotomy that extends in-line with the femoral neck (Fig. 8–18). The two perpendiculars of the "H" run parallel to the acetabular rim and the greater trochanter. The two capsular sleeves are tagged for later closure. With capsulotomy, the hip capsule can be repaired at the conclusion of the operation to increase anterior stability.

Once the capsulotomy has been completed, retractors are placed inside the capsule and around the

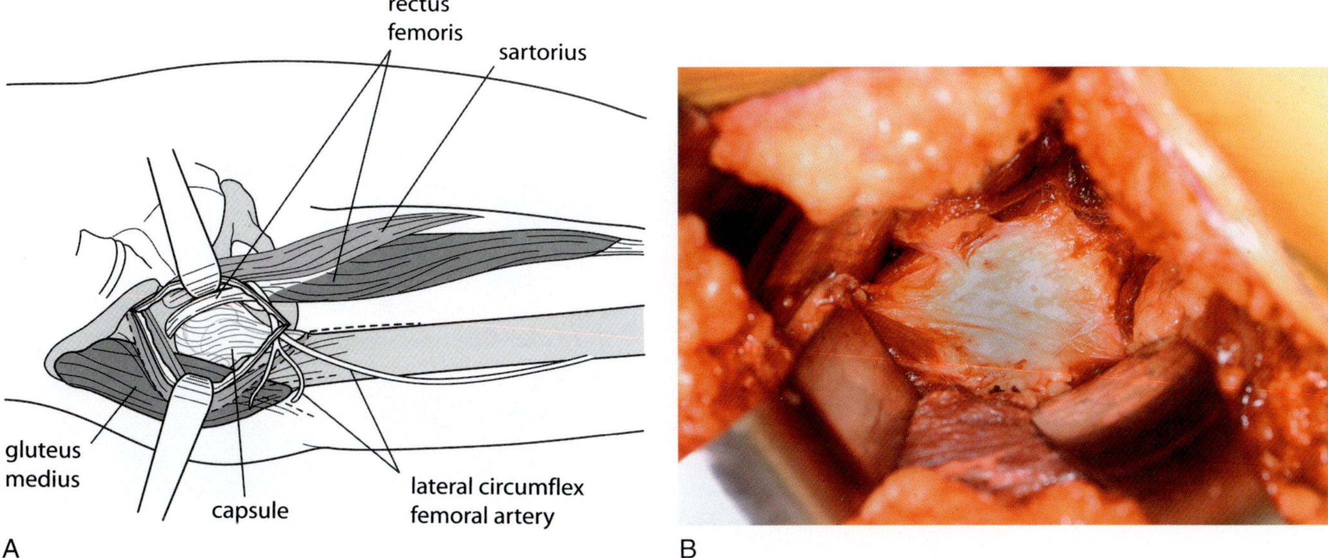

Figure 8–16   **A,** *The hip capsule, below. Note the indirect head of the rectus femoris medially and the gluteus medius laterally.* **B,** *The anterior hip capsule is exposed. Cobra retractors are placed superiorly and inferiorly.*

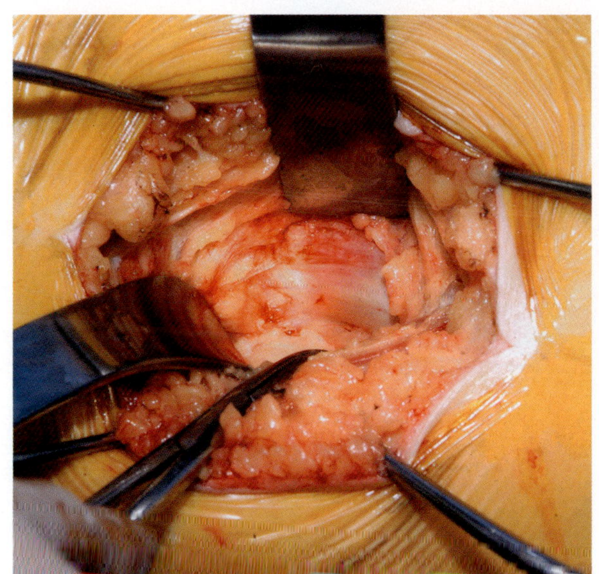

Figure 8–17   *Identification of the lateral femoral circumflex vessels at the apex of the distal end of the incision. These vessels should be coagulated or ligated.*

femoral neck superiorly and inferiorly. The labrum can be identified along the anterior rim and removed. In stiff joints with osteophytes seen on preoperative radiography, an osteotome can be used to remove the anterolateral border of osteophytes to open up the acetabulum. Gentle traction of the leg using the table opens up the joint space 2 to 3 mm (Fig. 8–19). Into this space, an osteotome is inserted to cut the ligamentum teres and intervening soft tissue (Fig. 8–20). The osteotome can then be used in conjunction with the table to lever out the femoral head. Release of

the traction and external rotation of the leg to 90 degrees completes the surgical dislocation anteriorly (Fig. 8–21). To increase mobilization of the femur with external rotation, a small, straight Homans retractor may be placed along the medial border of the femoral neck to aid in medial capsular release with a Bovie electrocautery. In excessively stiff hips or in hips with protrusio acetabuli, the femoral head can be removed in situ without intervening dislocation by a provisional osteotomy of the femoral neck (Fig. 8–22). Fluoroscopic guidance can be used to identify the neck cut level.

Femoral Osteotomy

The femoral osteotomy can be done in one of several ways, at the surgeon's discretion. As mentioned previously, the neck can be cut with the head in situ before dislocation. Alternatively, the neck can be cut with the hip dislocated and externally rotated 90 degrees. In this position, the head and neck point directly anterior and out of the wound into the field. The center of the femoral head and lesser trochanter are easily visualized in this position to aid in neck resection measurements. This is the technique originally described by Judet, but it may be disorienting for surgeons initially. I recommend a secondary reduction of the femoral head back into the acetabulum after the dislocation step. An accurate level of neck resection can be determined by measuring from the center of the femoral head distally (Fig. 8–23). The correct level can be confirmed using a final fluoroscopic check. This additional dislocation and subsequent reduction step is recommended before osteotomy because it seems to improve femoral

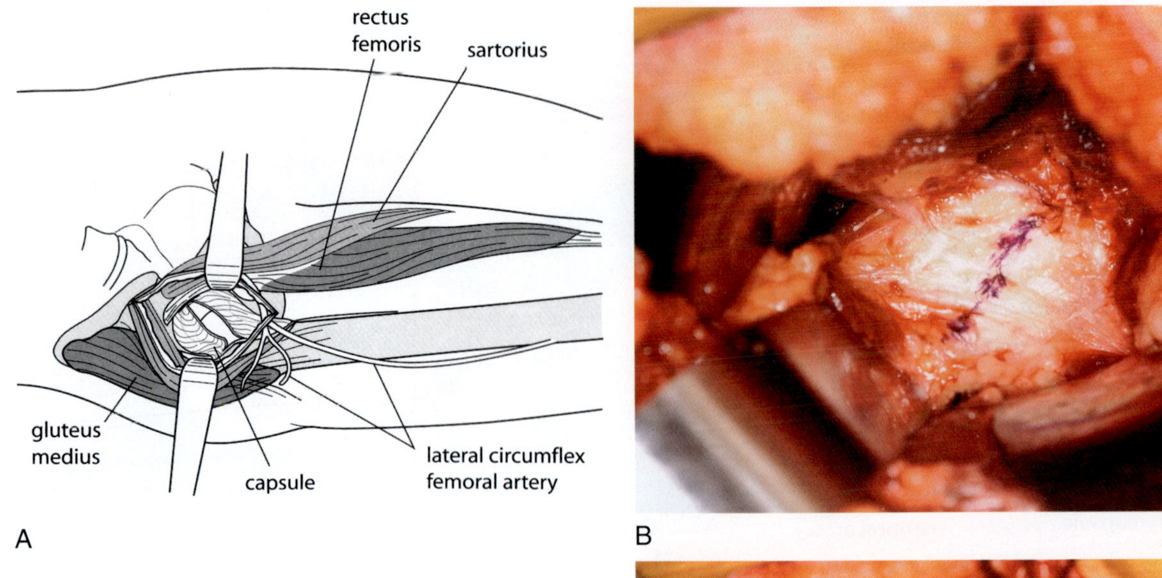

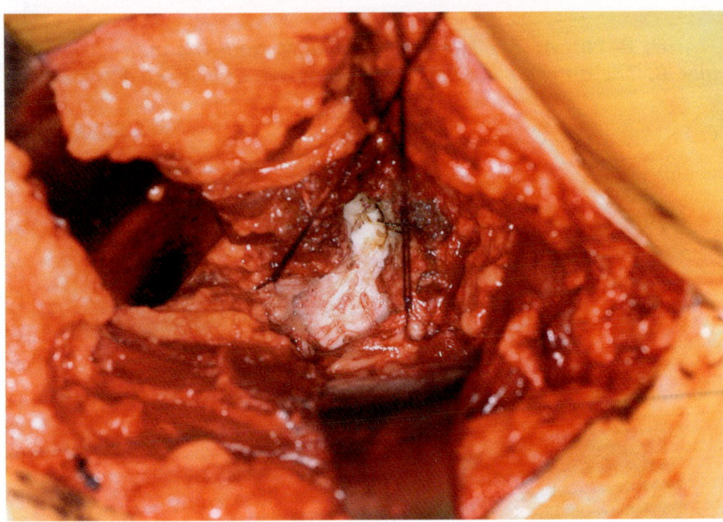

Figure 8–18 **A,** *The anterior capsulotomy.* **B,** *Pen mark outlining the direction of the intended anterior capsulotomy.* **C,** *Capsulotomy has been made and the leaves of the capsule have been tagged for later closure. Note the femoral head below.*

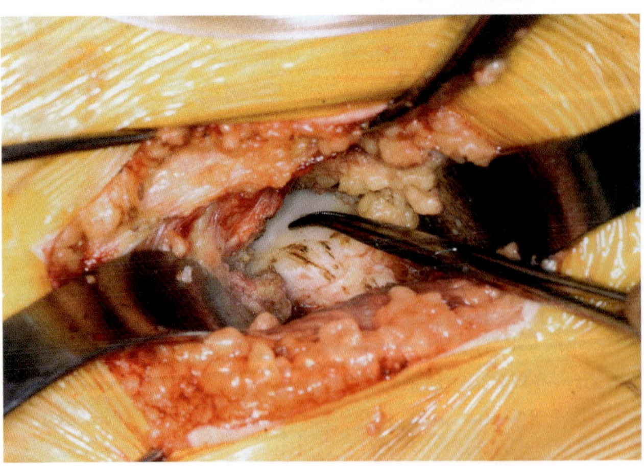

Figure 8–19 *The femoral head is identified with retractors placed around the inferior and superior femoral neck.*

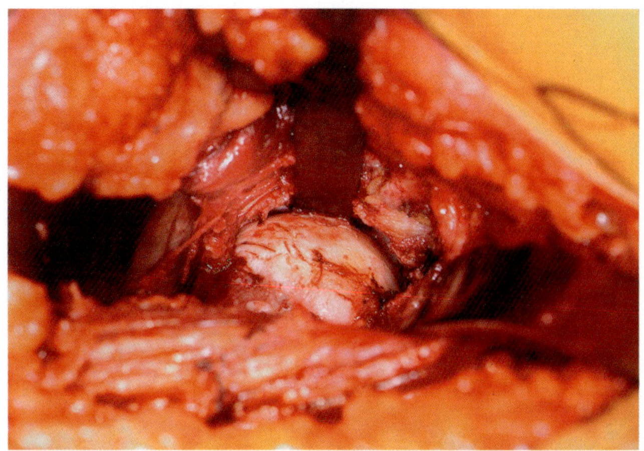

Figure 8–20 *An osteotome is placed between the femoral head and acetabulum. This cuts the ligamentum teres to facilitate dislocation.*

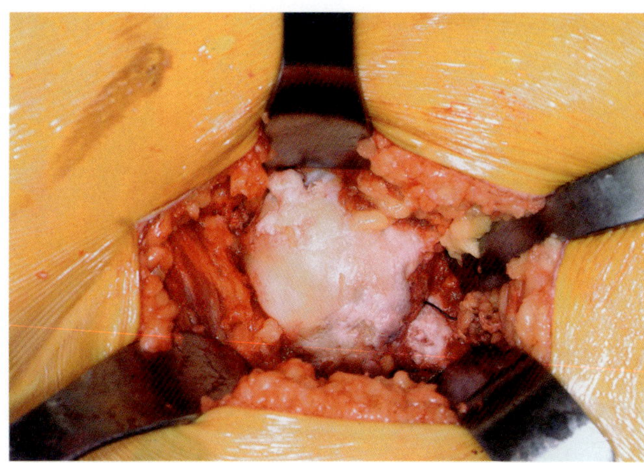

Figure 8–21 *Head dislocated anteriorly.*

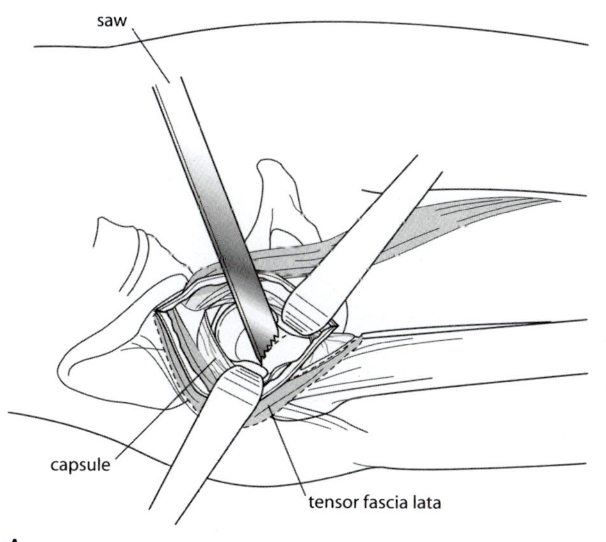

A

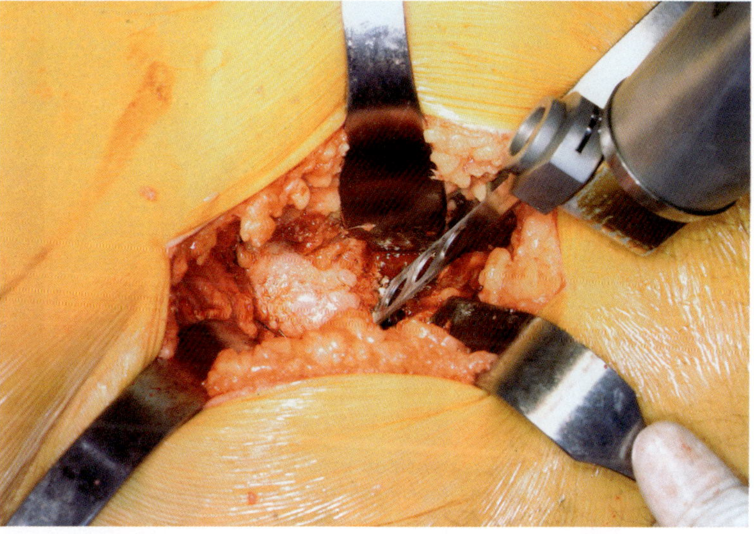

B

Figure 8–22 *A, In situ cutting of the femoral neck. Retractor around the femoral neck protects the tensor laterally and the rectus medially. B, In situ cutting of the femoral head. Intraoperative view.*

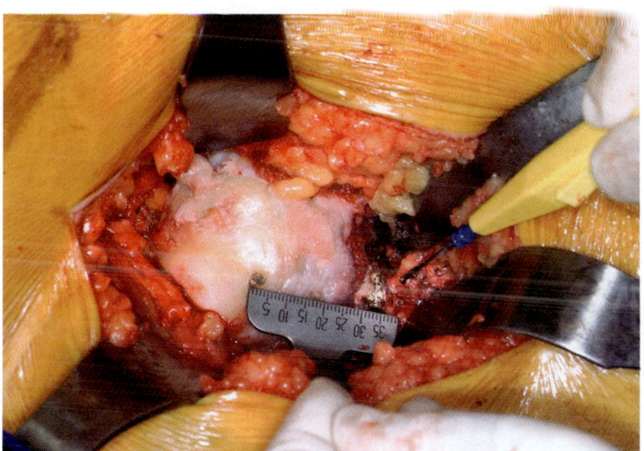

Figure 8–23 *Measurement of the osteotomy. A ruler measures the distance distally from the center of the femoral head.*

and inclination, which is important for later portions of the procedure.

After osteotomy is completed, the head is drilled and stabilized with a corkscrew (Fig. 8–24). The femoral head is then removed from the wound (Fig. 8–25).

Acetabular Exposure and Preparation

The acetabulum can now be exposed and prepared. Using the table, the femur is rotated externally approximately 30 degrees to displace the femoral neck out of the field (Fig. 8–26). A large, bent Homans retractor is placed anteriorly between the rectus and the anterior ilium to provide exposure of the anterior column. A cobra retractor is placed posteriorly between the capsule

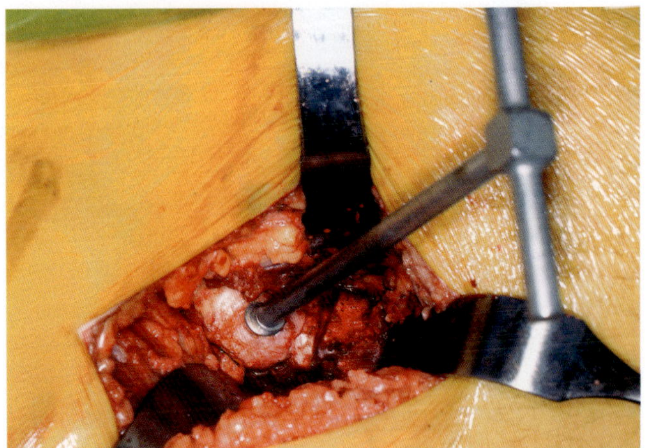

Figure 8–24 *After osteotomy is complete, the head is drilled and then tapped with a corkscrew.*

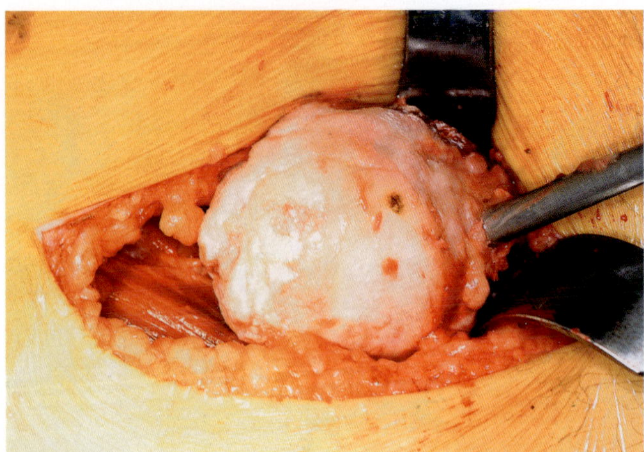

Figure 8–25 *A corkscrew is used to remove the femoral head out of the wound.*

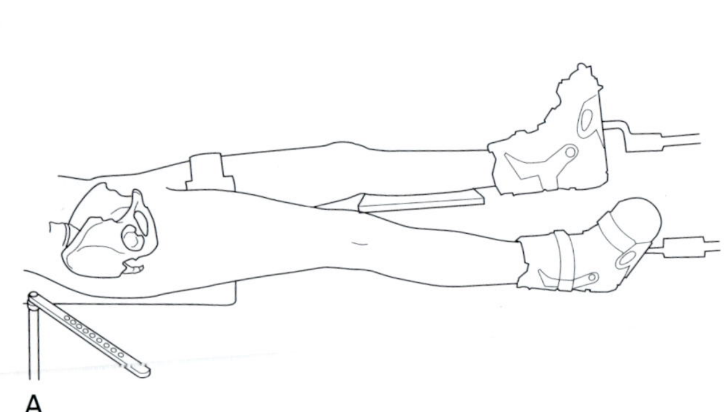

A

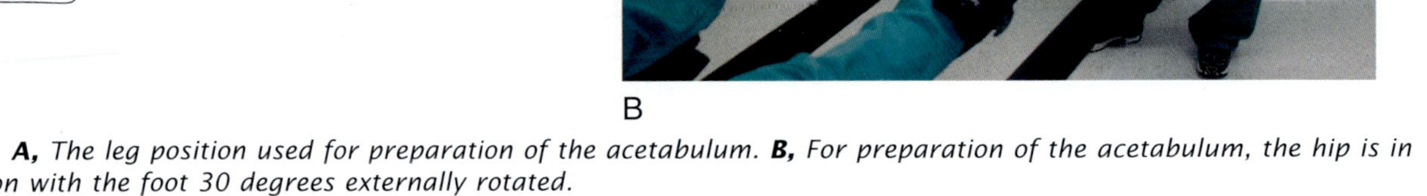

B

Figure 8–26 *A, The leg position used for preparation of the acetabulum. B, For preparation of the acetabulum, the hip is in neutral position with the foot 30 degrees externally rotated.*

and the labrum onto the ischium. This not only retracts the posterior capsule but also displaces the femur posteriorly for acetabular exposure. A second cobra retractor may be placed against the tear drop for inferomedial exposure (Fig. 8–27). The labrum is debrided.

Acetabular Reaming

Attention is then turned to the acetabulum. Reaming can be done under direct visualization (Fig. 8–28) or under fluoroscopic control (Fig. 8–29), at the discretion of the surgeon. Using fluoroscopy, the surgeon is able to ream under real-time assessment. The reamer should approach but not pass Köhler's line for appropriate medialization (Fig. 8–30). Proper sizing is confirmed by examining the fill of the reamer in the acetabulum under direct vision (Fig. 8–31) or by fluoroscopy. Further information is provided by the increase in torque the surgeon feels as the reamer contacts the anterior and posterior columns. The reamer should pene-

trate through the remaining cartilage and sclerotic bone to expose a uniform surface of bleeding subchondral bone (Fig. 8–32).

Trial Cup Placement

A trial cup is then placed under direct vision or fluoroscopic guidance. The exact amount of anteversion is difficult to quantify. Traditional mechanical alignment guides may be used. Under fluoroscopy, a radiographic ellipse is formed by the separation of the anterior and posterior rims of the shell. With experience, a small opening angle of the ellipse will be shown to correspond to 15 to 20 degrees of radiographic anteversion (Fig. 8–33). The stability of the trial is then tested by pulling firmly on the cup. The real cup is then impacted. Under fluoroscopy, bottoming out of the cup is easily determined for surgeons who choose to use a no-hole cup. Stability is checked by pulling on the impactor (Fig. 8–34).

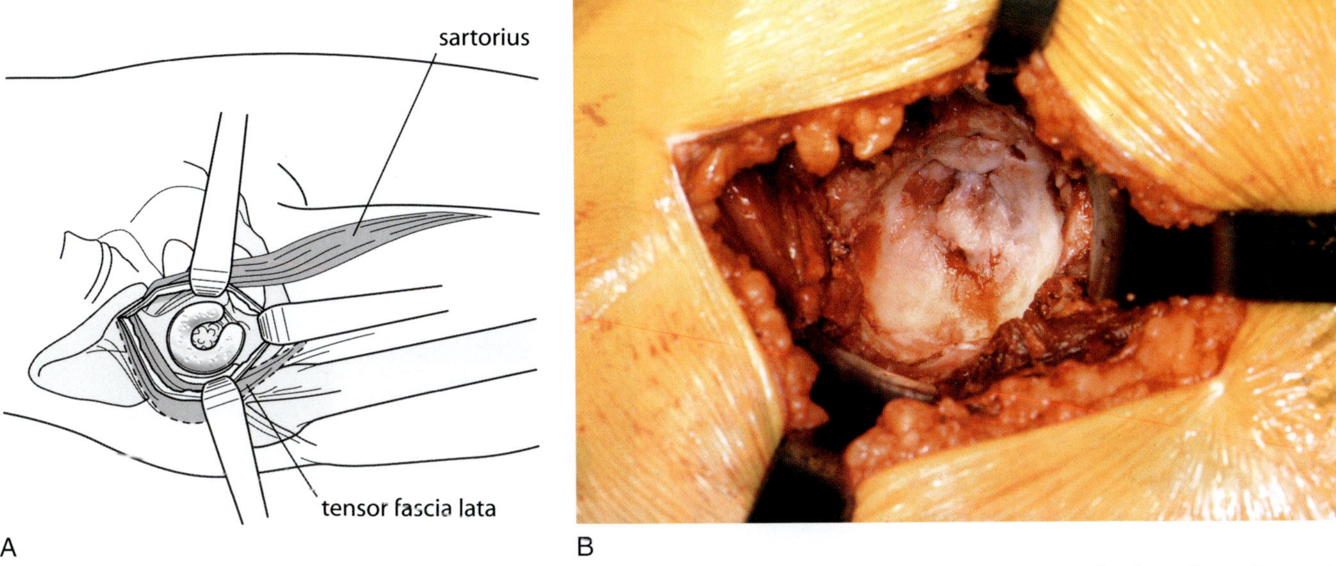

Figure 8–27 **A,** *Retractors are placed anteriorly deep to the rectus, posteriorly along the ischium, and inferiorly in the notch to provide circumferential exposure.* **B,** *Clear circumferential visualization of the acetabulum is obtained.*

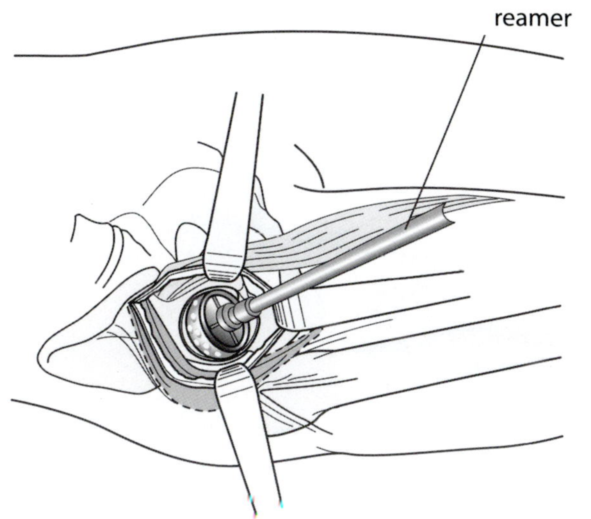

Figure 8–28 *Reamer position with retractors in place.*

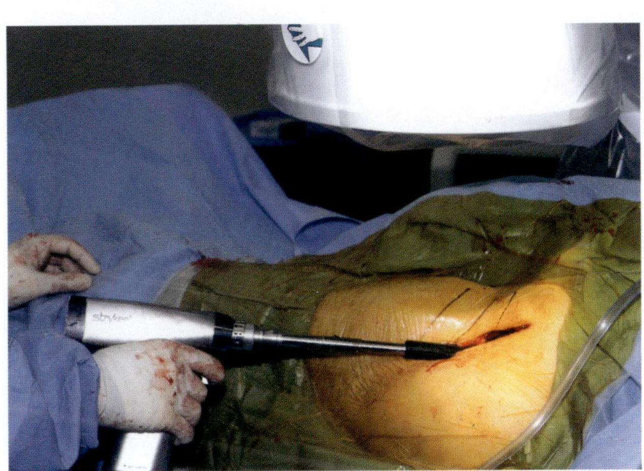

Figure 8–29 *Reaming done under fluoroscopic control.*

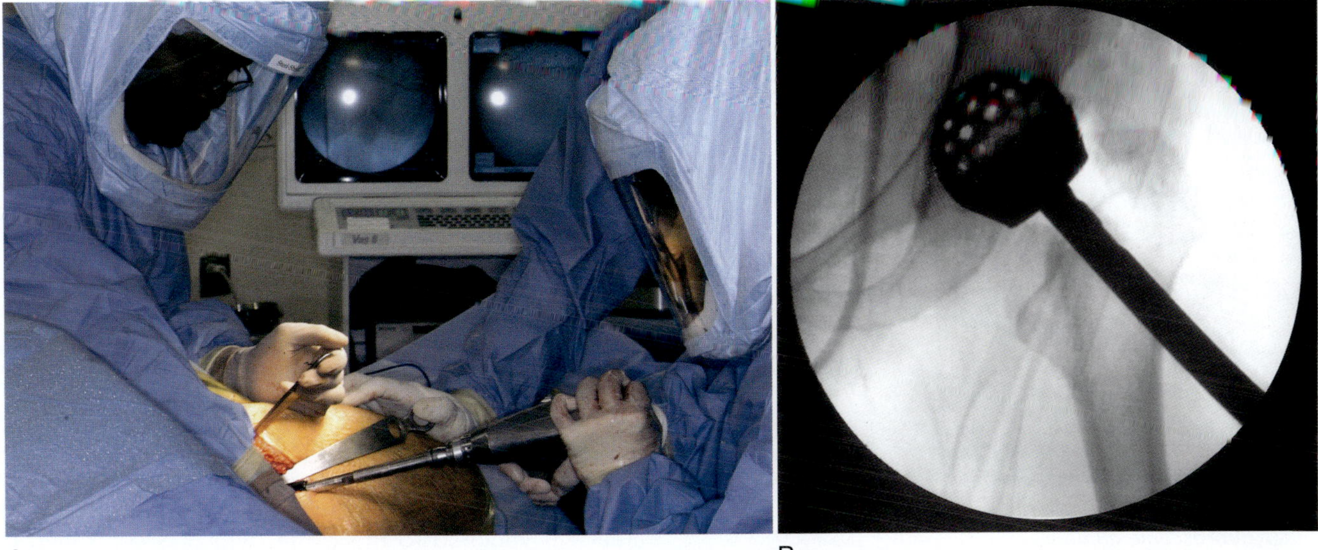

Figure 8–30 *Fluoroscopic images of the reamer. Note the medialization of the reamer to Köhler's line.*

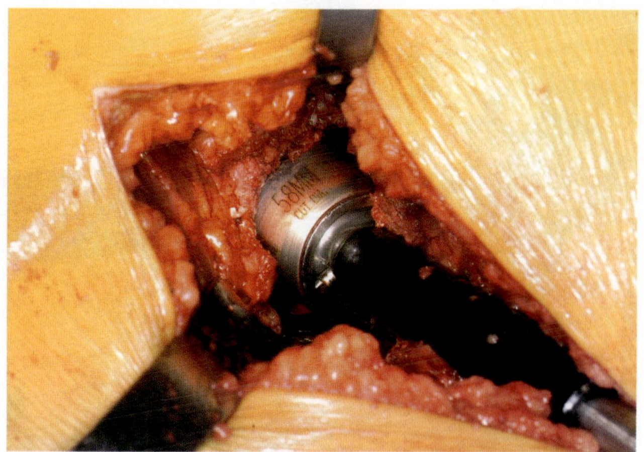

Figure 8–31 *Usual view when reaming the acetabulum under direct visualization.*

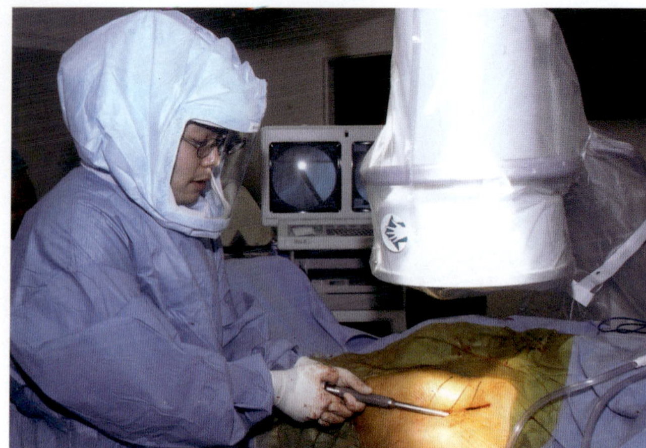

Figure 8–34 *Testing of acetabular stability by the push-pull test.*

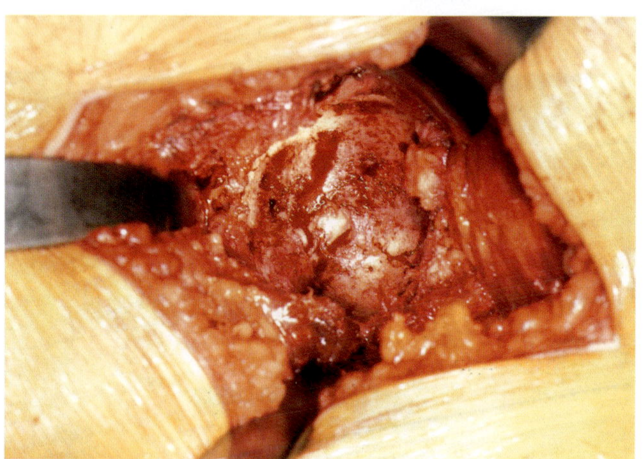

Figure 8–32 *Bleeding subchondral bone of the acetabulum is exposed after final reaming.*

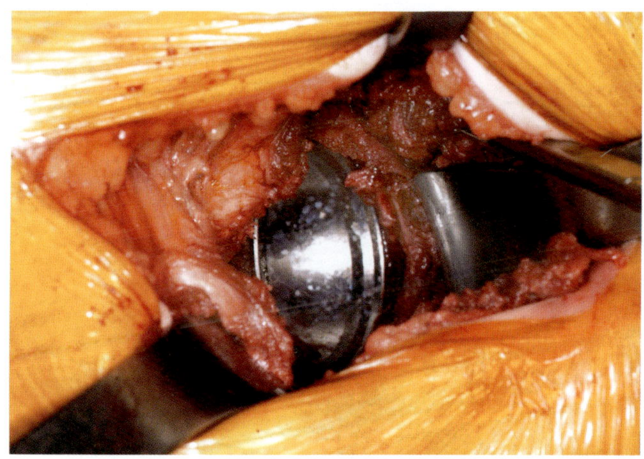

Figure 8–35 *Evaluation of component position in relation to bony landmarks.*

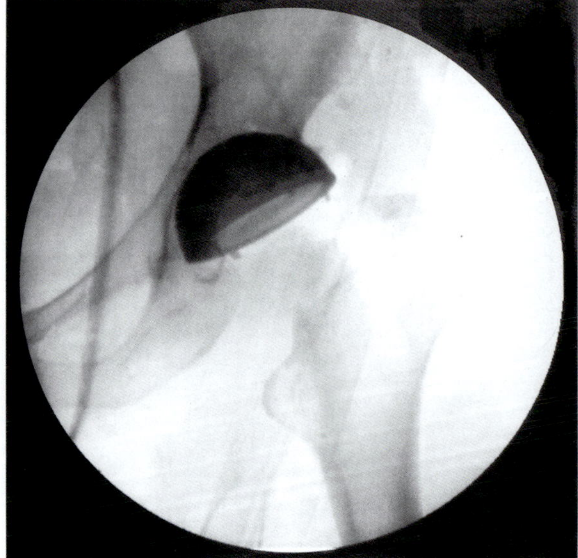

Figure 8–33 *Correct position of the acetabular component under fluoroscopic guidance.*

Retractors are once again placed around the acetabulum to provide circumferential exposure (Fig. 8–35). Stability is finally confirmed by tapping against the edge of the cup with a tamp. If there is any concern regarding stability or if the bone is osteoporotic, two screws can be easily inserted into the superior ilium. Fluoroscopy is not necessary but can be used to evaluate the position of the screws. Osteophytes are debrided (Fig. 8–36), and the real liner is inserted (Fig. 8–37).

Femoral Exposure

Femoral exposure involves extensive use of the PROfx table. First, the hip is internally rotated 10 degrees to expose the vastus tubercle (Fig. 8–38). The large femoral hook is placed through the wound just distal and lateral to the bony ridge of the vastus tubercle (Fig. 8–39). The base of the hook is attached to the adjustable bracket on the PROfx table (Fig. 8–40), and this mechanism is attached to the crank, which is controlled by

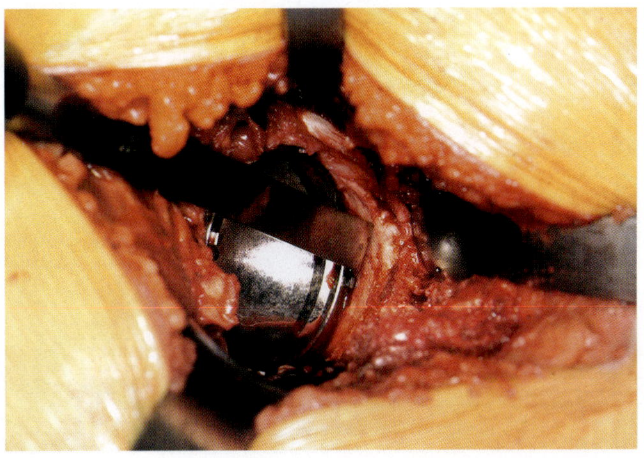

Figure 8–36   *Removal of osteophytes before liner insertion.*

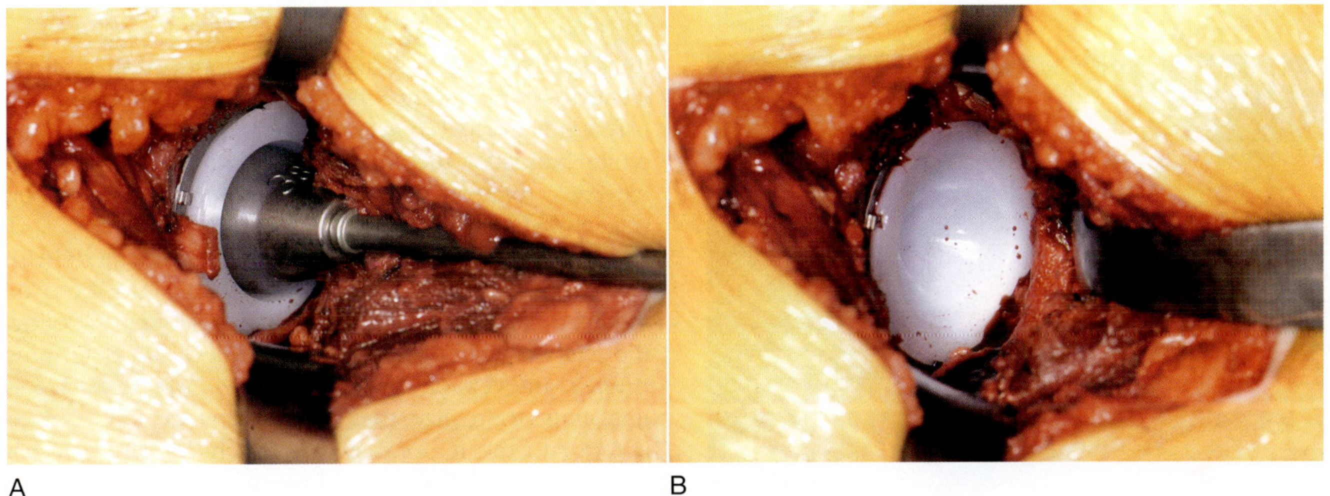

A

B

Figure 8–37   **A,** *Insertion and seating of the liner.* **B,** *The acetabular portion of the procedure is complete.*

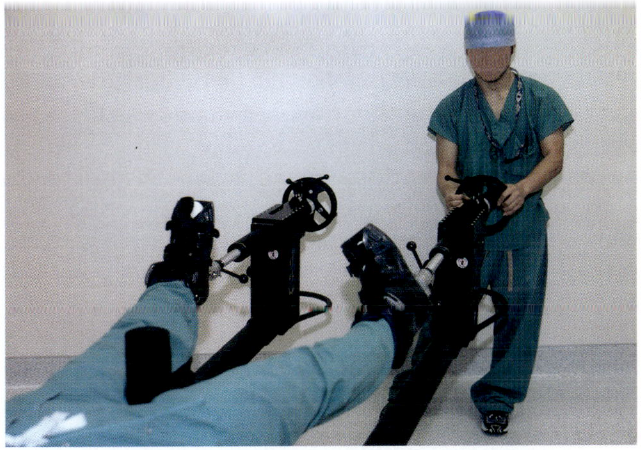

Figure 8–38   *For preparation of the femur, the leg is internally rotated 10 degrees to expose the vastus tubercle.*

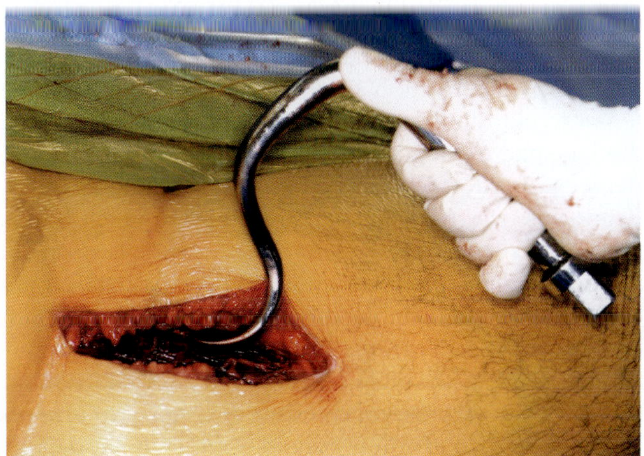

Figure 8–39   *The hook is placed into the wound just distal to the vastus tubercle.*

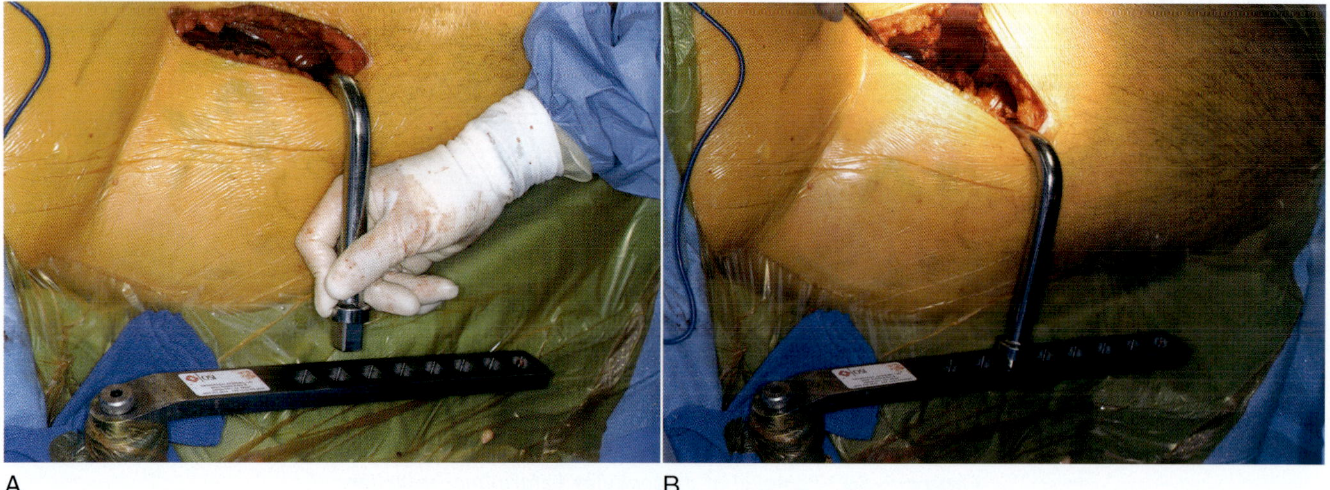

A   B

Figure 8–40   **A,** *The hook is placed around the proximal femur and attached to the sidebar.* **B,** *Final position of the proximal femoral retractor and actual position of the leg spars. Note the amount of hip extension needed to expose the proximal femur.*

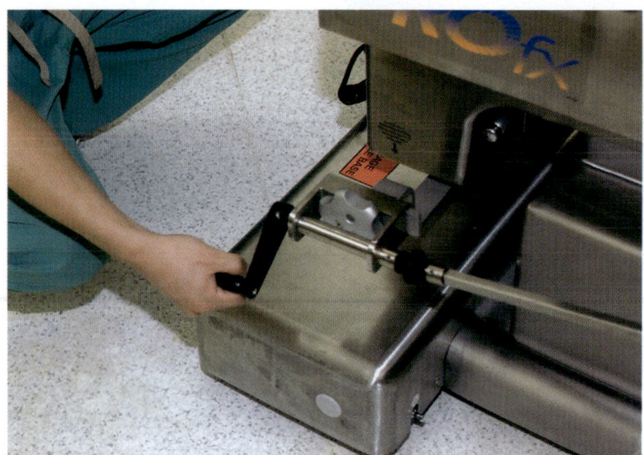

Figure 8–41   *A crank connected to the head of the table allows for superior and inferior control of the femur.*

the anesthesiologist at the head of the table (Fig. 8-41). Rotation of the crank raises or lowers the hook. The hook provides traction superiorly against the proximal femur to elevate the osteotomy out of the wound. Using the leg spar, the leg is then placed into a position of 40 degrees of extension, 10 degrees of adduction, and 90 degrees of external rotation (Fig. 8–42). All traction must be removed from the system to relieve tension on the femoral nerve. Gentle elevation of the proximal femoral hook allows predictable delivery of the femur out of the wound (Fig. 8–43).

This creates an angle of easy entry for the femoral broaches in an anteroposterior direction. If anterior displacement of the hip becomes difficult in patients with a stiff hip, the posterior capsule can be released, maintaining the integrity of the external rotator muscles (Fig. 8–44). This can be done using a Bovie electrocautery along the posterior border of the osteotomy as the hip is gradually externally rotated. The white bands of the tendinous insertions of the short external rotators are visible and can be avoided (Fig. 8–45).

The preparation of the femur is more difficult to learn than that of the acetabulum. The tibia cannot be used to determine the correct rotation of the stem. I follow the cut surface of the posterior neck to determine proper anteversion (see Figs. 8–44 and 8-45). It is important to realize that the femoral neck is bowed anterior to the femoral shaft. To achieve direct access to the intramedullary canal, broach insertion must begin in the posterior third of the neck (Fig. 8–46). I recommend insertion of a Charnley awl or a similar blunt rod to ensure proper direction of the canal (Fig. 8–47). Fluoroscopic control of broaching is another choice (Fig. 8–48).

I use the Zweymüller stem with a modified broach handle. This system is based on serial bone compaction (Fig. 8–49). The rectangular, flat, tapered Zweymüller stem is made of fully grit-blasted titanium and has an excellent track record of durability (Fig. 8–50). To prevent varus insertion, lateral bone in the medial portion of the greater trochanter can be removed safely with a rongeur or an osteotome (Fig. 8–51). The femur is then prepared by sequential broaching, starting with the smallest size (Figs. 8–52 and 8–53). Appropriate sizing of the femur is judged by comparison with preoperative templating and during surgery by failure of the broach to advance with consistent mallet blows. Appropriate position and fill of the broach can be confirmed and adjusted under fluoroscopy (Fig. 8–54).

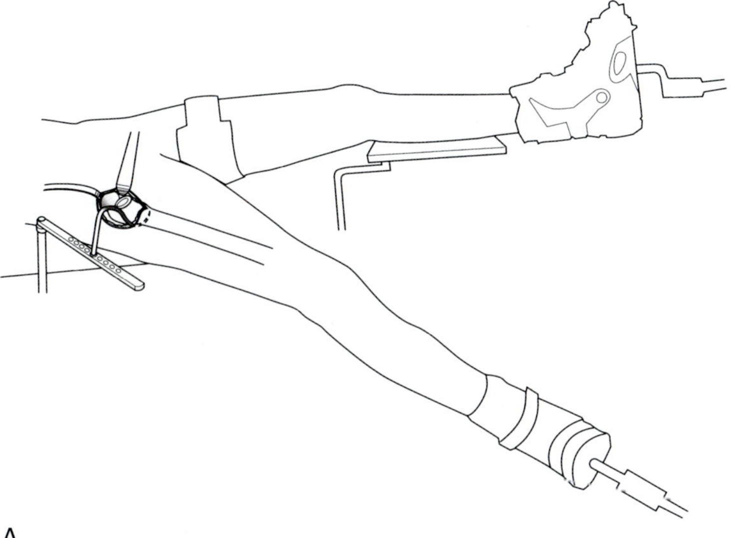

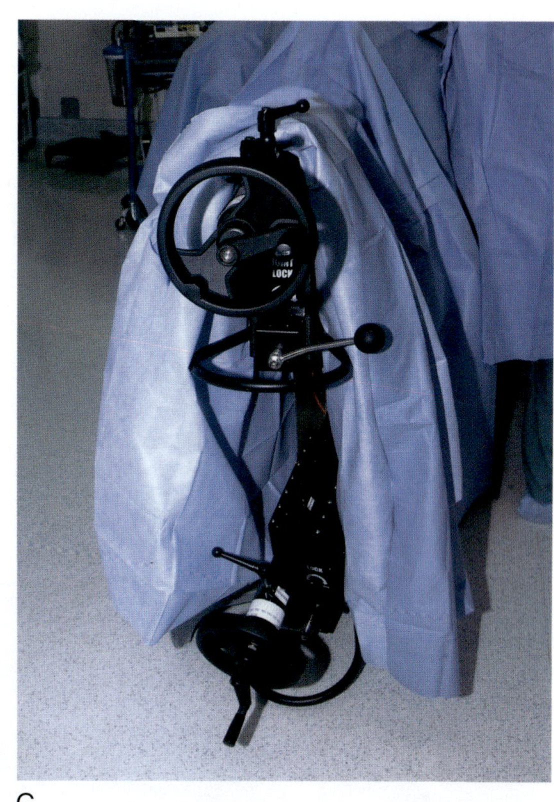

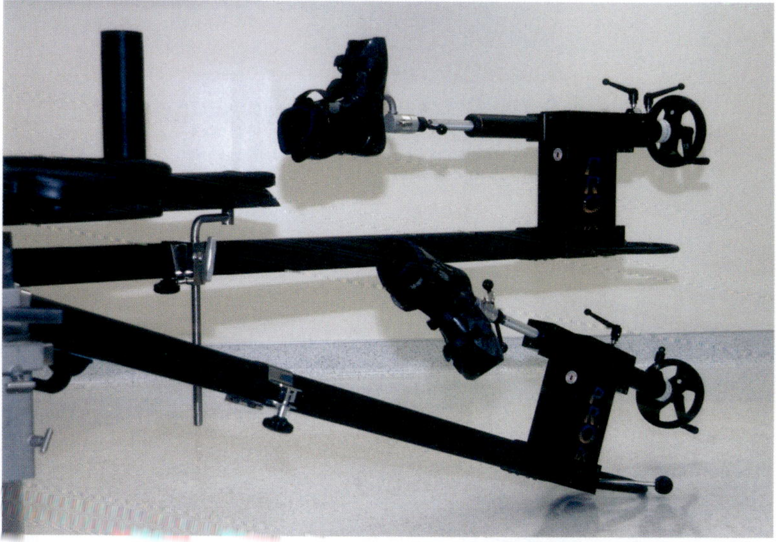

Figure 8–42 **A,** *Correct position of the table for femoral exposure. The hip is extended 40 degrees, externally rotated 90 degrees, and adducted 10 degrees.* **B,** *Intraoperative photo of the correct position of the table for femoral exposure. The hip is extended 40 degrees, externally rotated 90 degrees, and adducted 10 degrees.* **C,** *End-on view of the intraoperative position of the leg spars.*

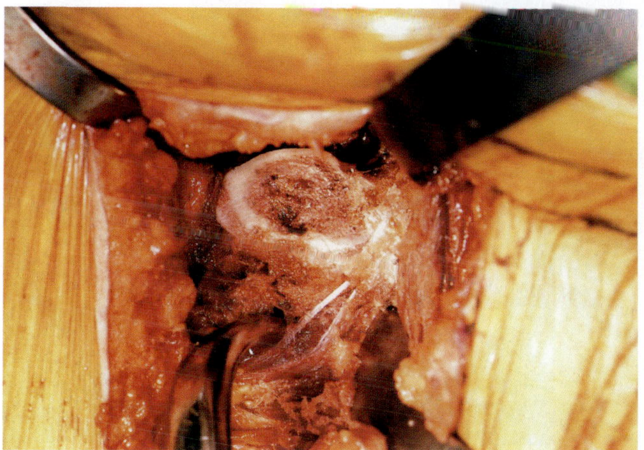

Figure 8–43 *The femur is delivered out of the wound. Note the anterior and posterior cortices of the osteotomy.*

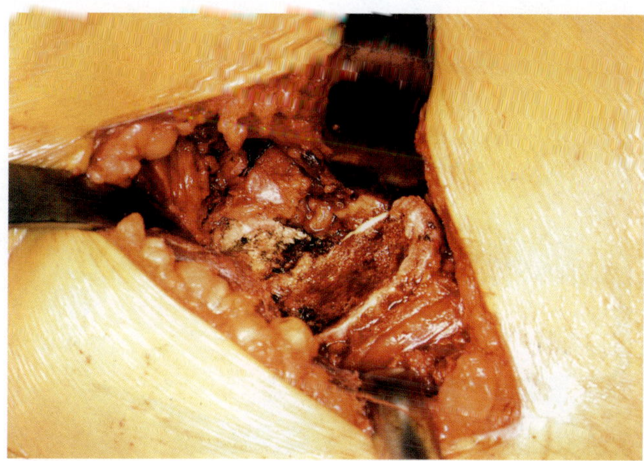

Figure 8–44 *The trochanter is visible proximally. The superior and lateral capsule has been released. External rotators remain attached to the posterior portion of the femur.*

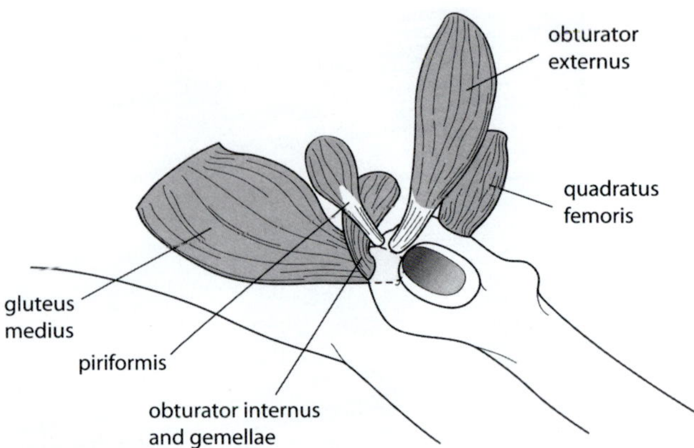

Figure 8–45 *The rotators insert along the posterior trochanter. Note the position of the gluteus medius out of the field posterior to the trochanter.*

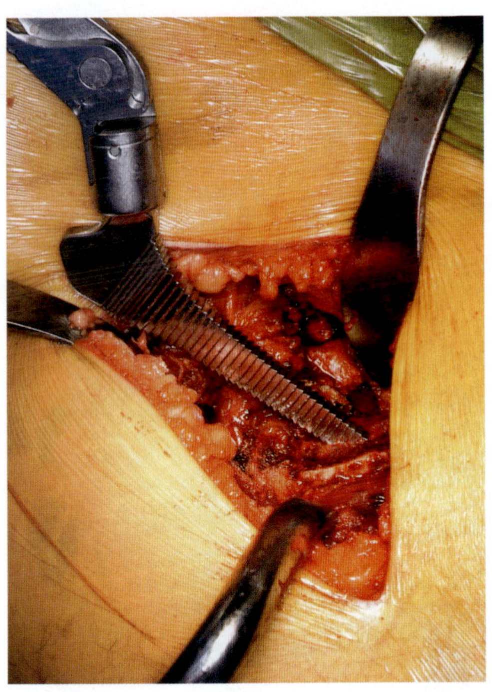

Figure 8–46 *Direct access into the femoral canal with the Zweymüller broach.*

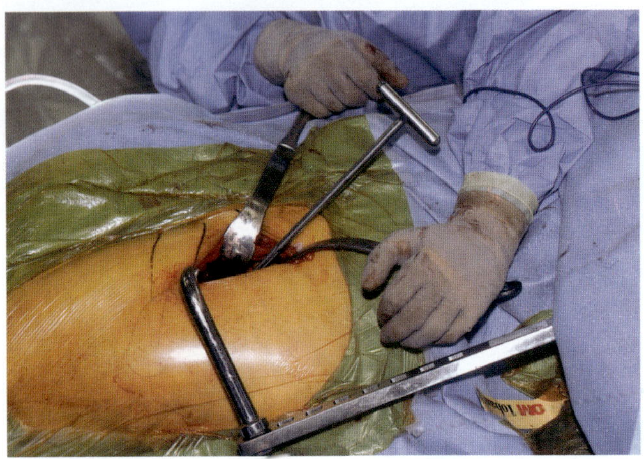

Figure 8–47 *A Charnley awl is used to identify the center of the canal. This minimizes the risk of posterolateral perforation.*

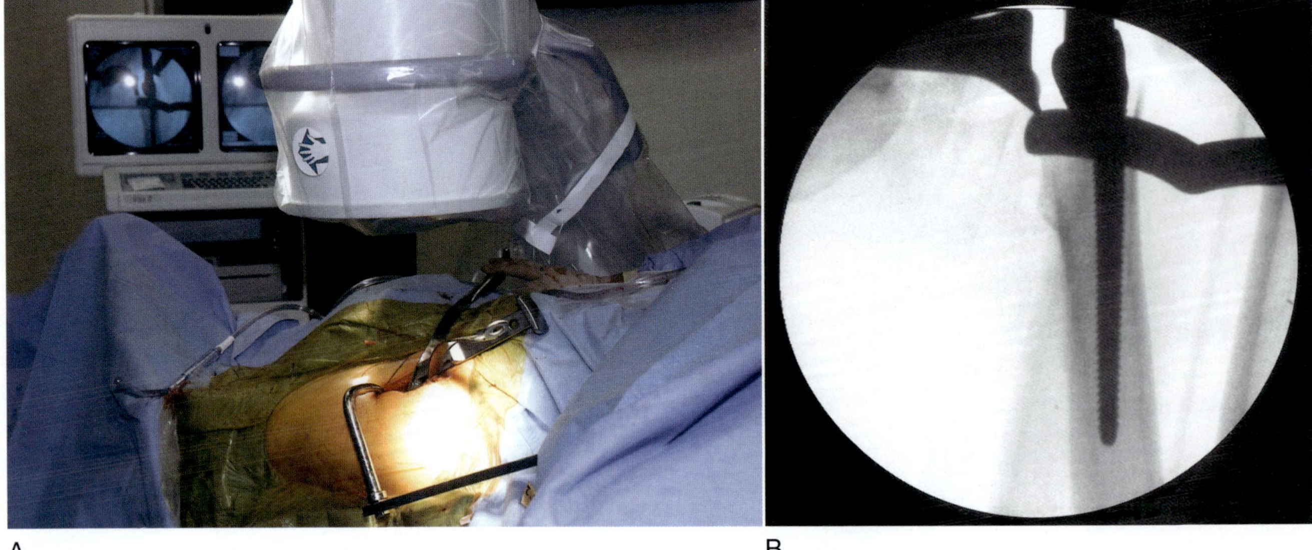

A   B

Figure 8–48 **A,** *Intraoperative check with fluoroscopy to determine that the broach is correctly positioned in an anteroposterior direction.* **B,** *Fluoroscopic image shows that the broach is axial to the femoral shaft.*

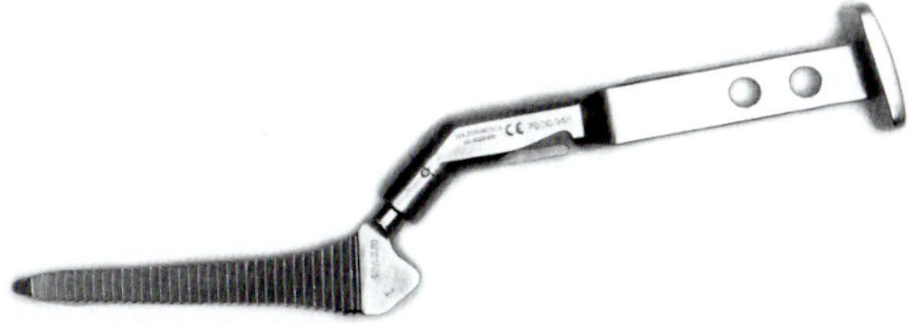

Figure 8–49 *Zweymüller broach with offset impactor handle. Note the ridges in the broach, which allow for bone compaction.*

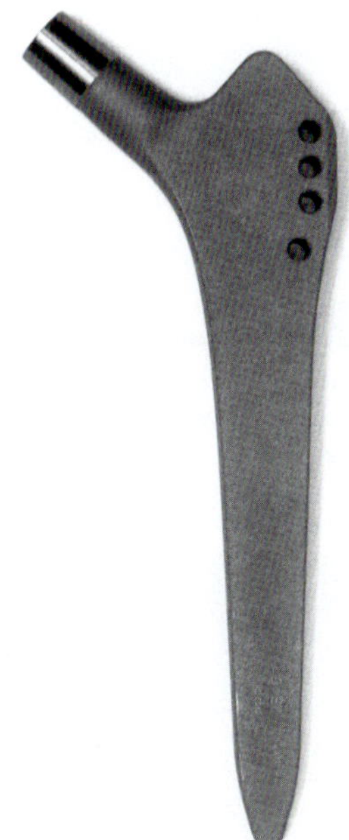

Figure 8–50 *The Zweymüller stem, constructed of grit-blasted titanium. Note the flat rectangular cross section and tapering.*

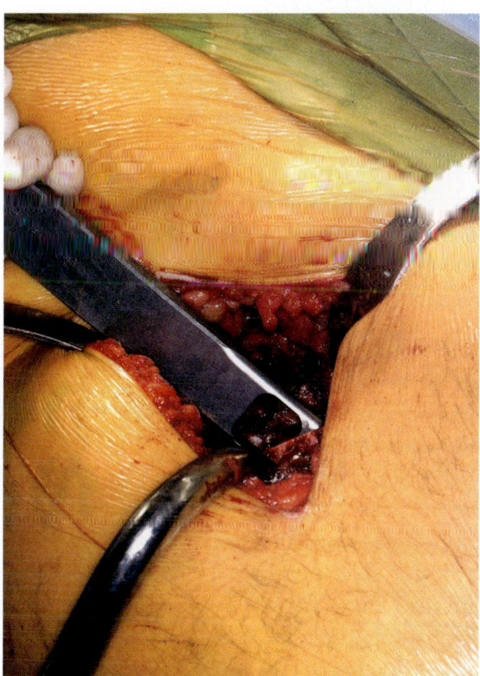

Figure 8–51 *Box osteotome used to clear out the medial portion of the greater trochanter to prevent varus positioning of stem.*

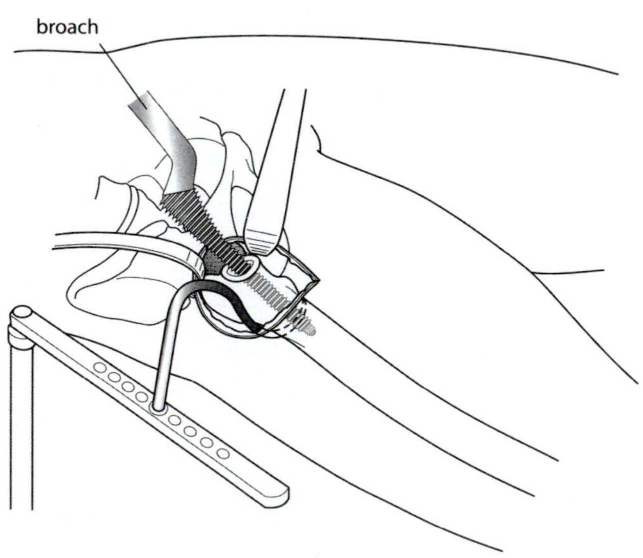

Figure 8–52 *Correct insertion of the broach with retractors in place.*

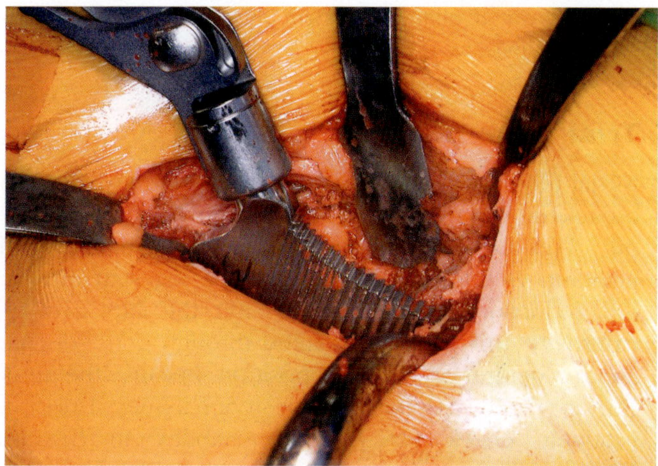

A

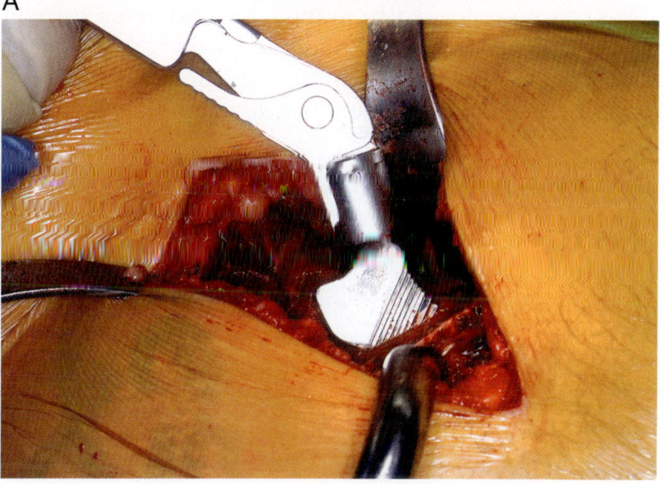

B

Figure 8–53 *A, Serial broaching of the femur in midposition. B, Broach near its final position.*

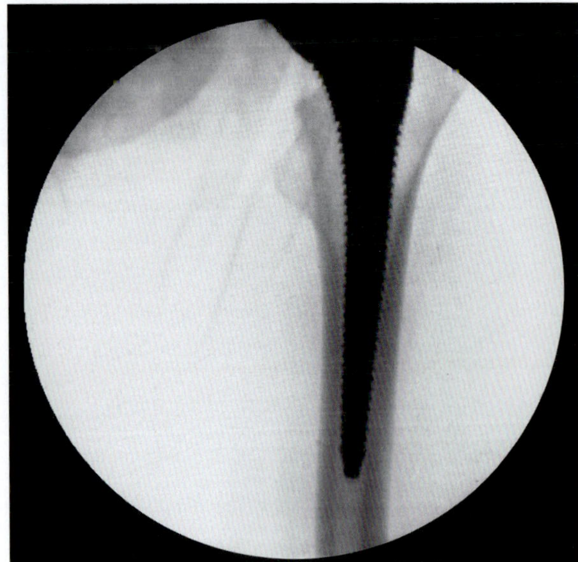

Figure 8–54 *Intraoperative fluoroscopic check confirms correct axial alignment of stem and adequate fill in the femoral canal.*

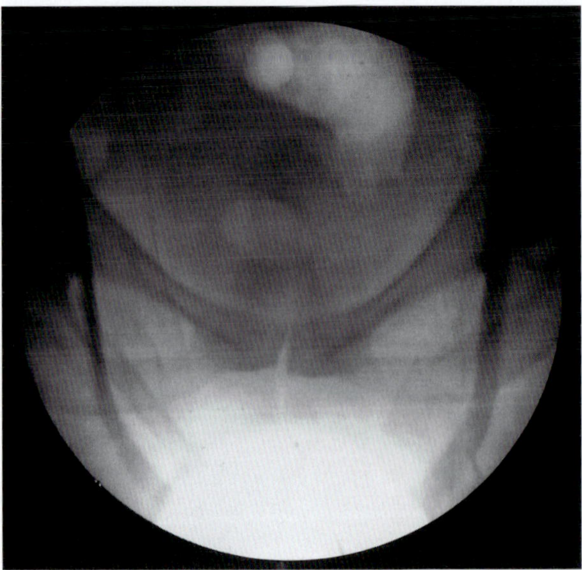

Figure 8–55 *Fluoroscopic view of the obturator foramina to ensure that the pelvis is level. Both foramina should be of equal size and shape.*

Trial Stem Insertion

A trial reduction is performed once the femur has been broached. A trial stem is inserted and the leg is reduced out of its extended, externally rotated, and adducted position. Gentle traction through the leg spar aids in hip reduction. To assess stability, the hip can be externally and internally rotated through a 180-degree arc in a neutral or extended position. Because the anterior approach maintains the posterior tissues, I do not routinely check for posterior stability in flexion. However, if desired, the traction boot on the ipsilateral leg can be unlocked from the table and taken through a full range of motion underneath the drapes by an unscrubbed assistant. After the trial reduction, the leg can be reattached to the table distally.

Leg Length Assessment

Intraoperative assessment of leg length is best done at this time. The image intensifier is used to identify the symphysis pubis and the obturator foramina. If both foramina are of equal size and shape, the pelvis is level (Fig. 8–55). In thin patients, it is also possible to see that the coccyx directly overlies the pubic symphysis. The intensifier is used to image the contralateral hip to visualize the cotyloid notch and ischial tuberosity of the acetabulum, and the greater and lesser trochanters of the femur (Fig. 8–56). This image is saved and printed. An image of the operative hip is taken to ensure that the leg is in an identical position to the contralateral leg, including the same abduction and rotation (Fig. 8–57). The position and size of the lesser trochanter are important in determining the rotation. The image of the operative hip is compared with the

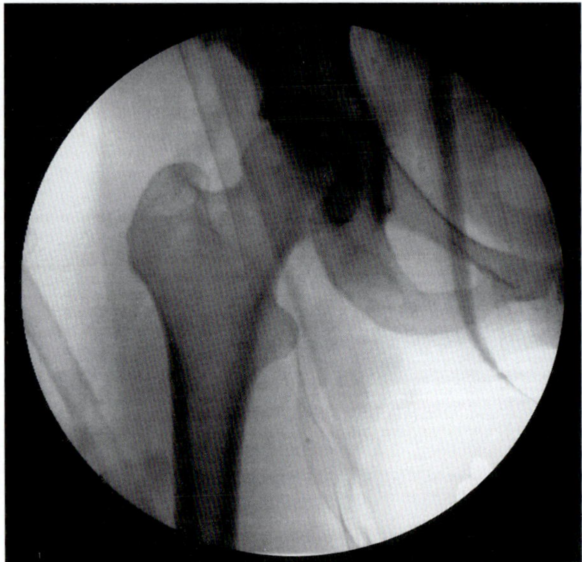

Figure 8–56 *Fluoroscopic view of the contralateral hip used for templating.*

contralateral hip, and leg length and offset can be judged (Fig. 8–58).

Leg length can be modified either through the trial neck and head or by changing the size of the stem. The Zweymüller stem is designed to accept either the size above or the size below the trialed broach. Decreasing the size decreases both the offset and hip length; using the next larger size increases both measurements. If the leg length and canal fill are appropriate but offset needs to be improved, the extended-offset Zweymüller stem can be used instead (Fig. 8–59). Shenton's line can be evaluated as a final check for appropriate restoration of hip biomechanics.

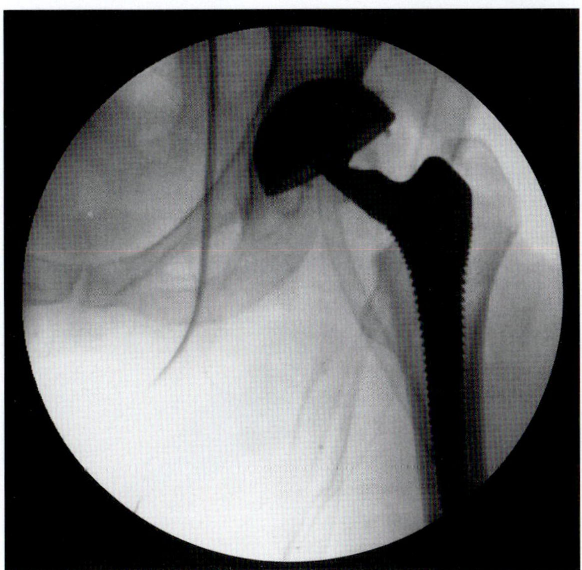

Figure 8–57 *Fluoroscopic view of the trials in place to test leg length and offset.*

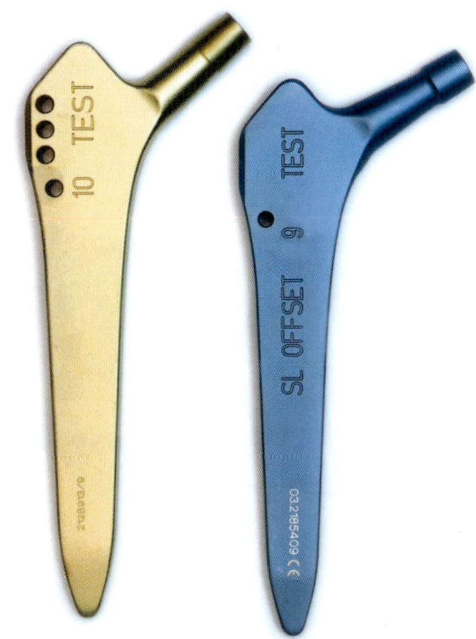

Figure 8–59 *Standard Zweymüller stem* (left) *and extended-offset Zweymüller stem* (right).

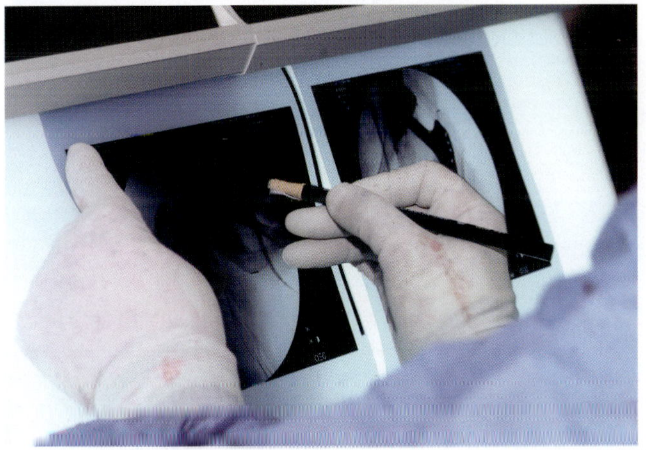

Figure 8–58 *Intraoperative fluoroscopic comparison of the ipsilateral and contralateral hips.*

Stem Insertion

Once the components have been selected, the Zweymüller stem is inserted into the femur (Fig. 8–60). A properly sized Zweymüller stem should advance initially three fourths of its length into the canal (Fig. 8–61). The stem can then be gently impacted until it reaches a stable position (Fig. 8–62); the surgeon will also note a change in the tone of impaction when the stem is fully seated. The trial head can once again be examined fluoroscopically (Fig. 8–63). Once the surgeon is satisfied, the real head is placed (Fig. 8–64) and then reduced. A final fluoroscopic check is made (Fig. 8–65).

Closure

Wound closure is remarkably simple. The capsular tags are used to reapproximate the flaps and the capsule is repaired with 1-0 Vicryl (Fig. 8–66). Fascia over the tensor fascia is closed with running 1-0 Vicryl (Fig. 8–67). Subcutaneous tissue is closed with 2-0 Vicryl and the skin is closed subcuticularly with 3-0 Monocryl and Steri-Strips.

The feet are removed from the traction boots and the leg lengths checked to ensure equality (Fig. 8–68). Postoperative anteroposterior pelvic and frog-leg lateral radiographs of the hip are taken before leaving the operating room (Fig. 8–69).

POSTOPERATIVE REHABILITATION

These patients are not placed on any dislocation precautions, either anterior or posterior, after routine total hip replacement. They do not require elevated toilet seats and are allowed to sleep on their side or back. They are not restricted from putting on their own shoes and socks after surgery. I allow most patients to proceed with full weight bearing as tolerated, although this is subject to individual surgeon preference.

For physical therapy, patients are instructed to walk the day of or the day after surgery. Progress is related to the individual's overall health. In the healthy patient with oligoarticular disease, I quickly advance the patient over the next 24 to 48 hours from a walker to crutches

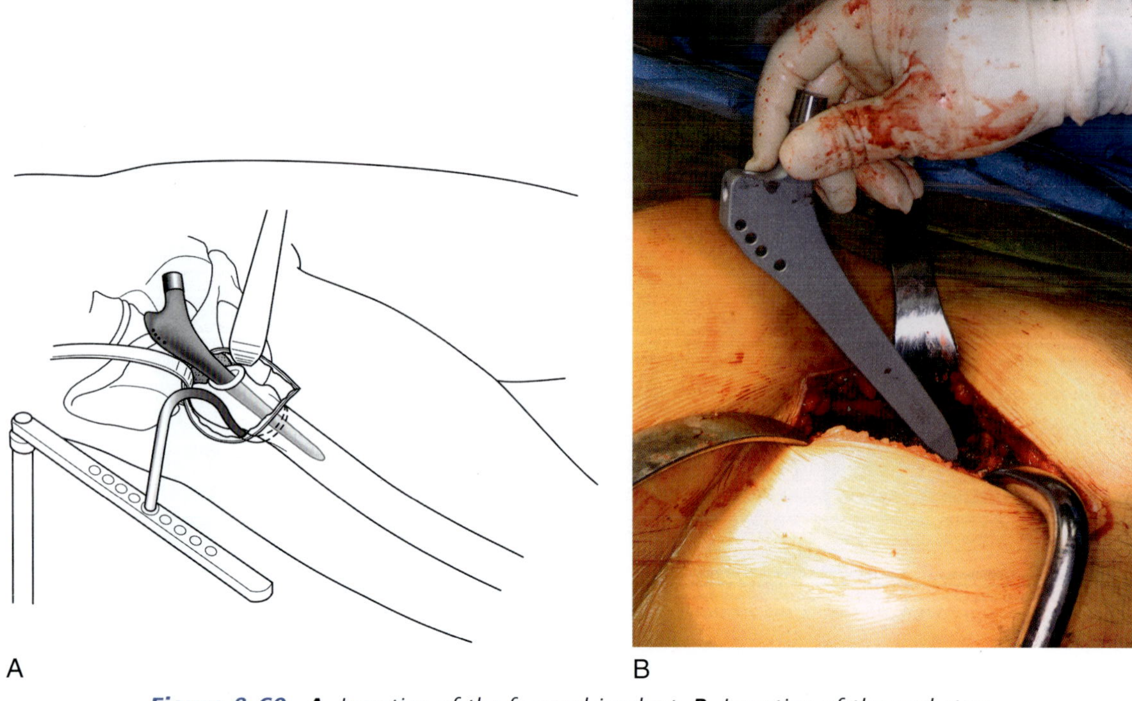

A

B

Figure 8-60 **A,** *Insertion of the femoral implant.* **B,** *Insertion of the real stem.*

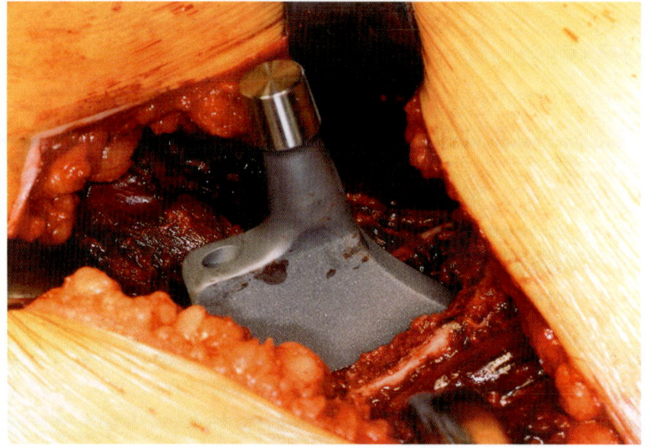

Figure 8-61 *Proper initial position of the real implant when inserted by hand. Approximately one third to one fourth of the femoral stem remains proud.*

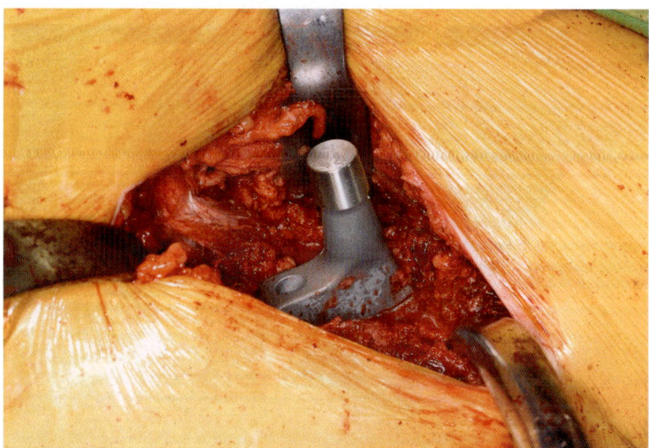

Figure 8-62 *Implant solidly impacted into its final position.*

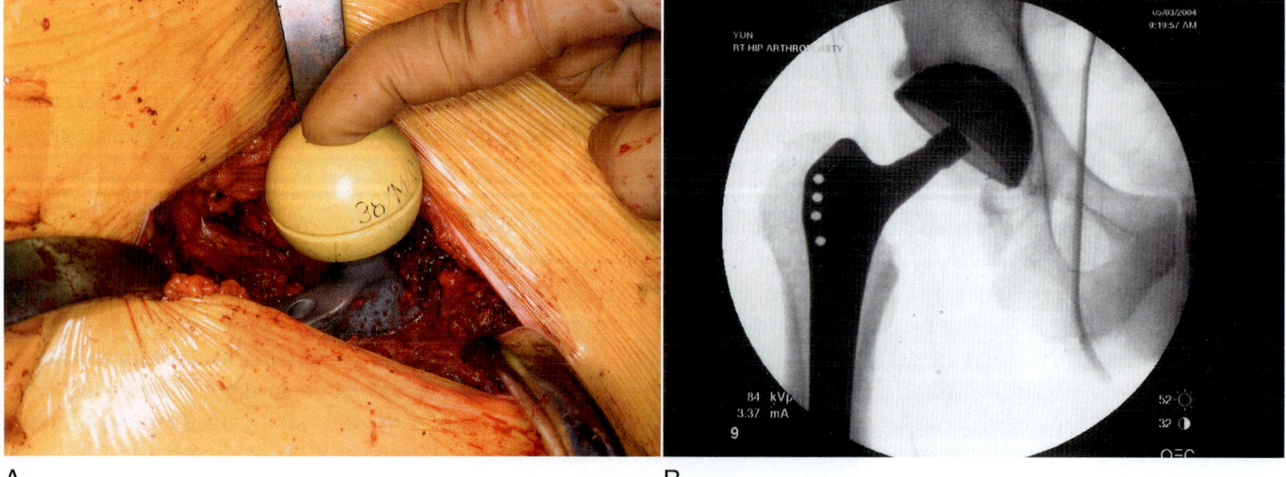

A

B

Figure 8-63 **A,** *Trialing with the trial head.* **B,** *With trials in place, a final fluoroscopic check is performed to confirm correct reconstruction.*

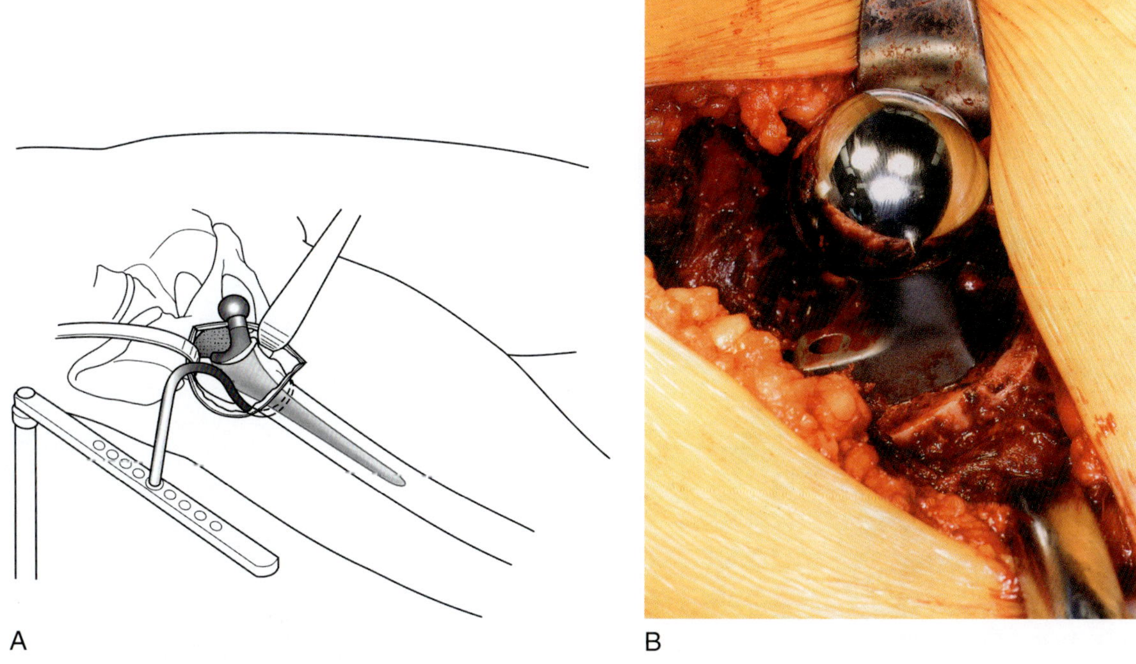

Figure 8-64 **A,** The real implants in place. **B,** The real femoral head is placed.

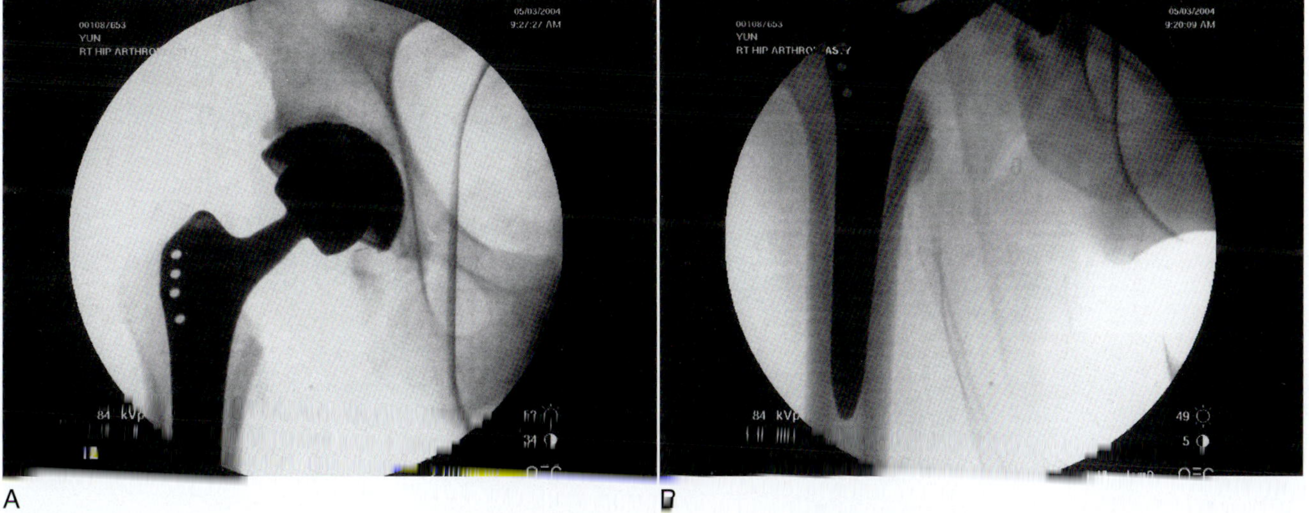

Figure 8-65 **A,** Intraoperative fluoroscopic views of the femoral and acetabular components. **B,** Intraoperative fluoroscopic views of the distal femur to confirm distal fill, proper alignment, and absence of fractures.

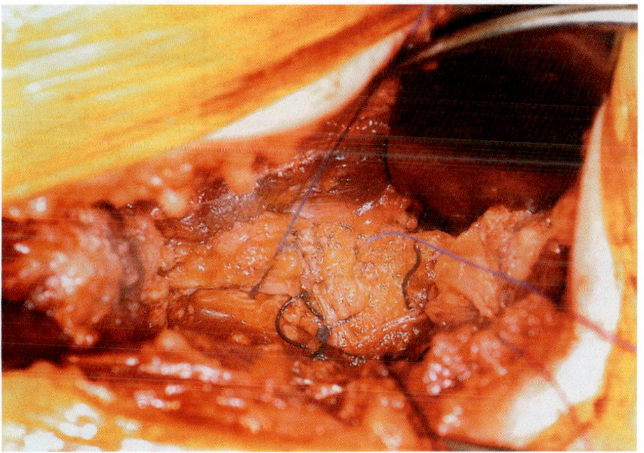

Figure 8-66 Capsular closure, showing obliteration of dead space.

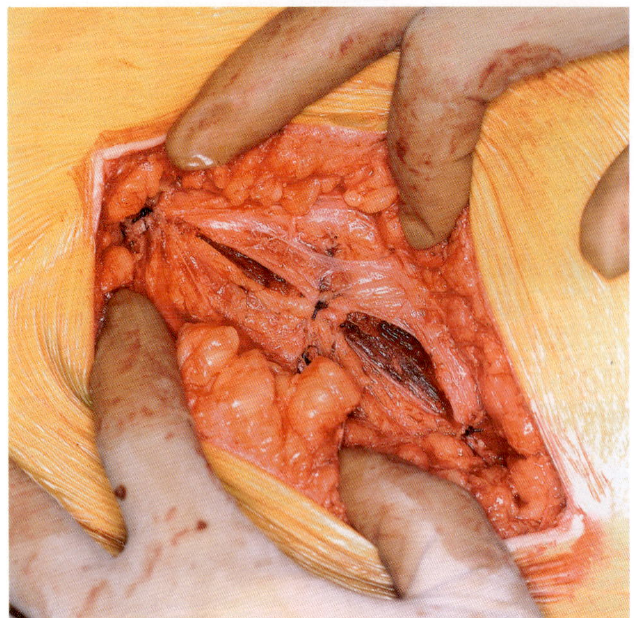

Figure 8–67 *Wound closure of the fascia over the tensor fascia lata.*

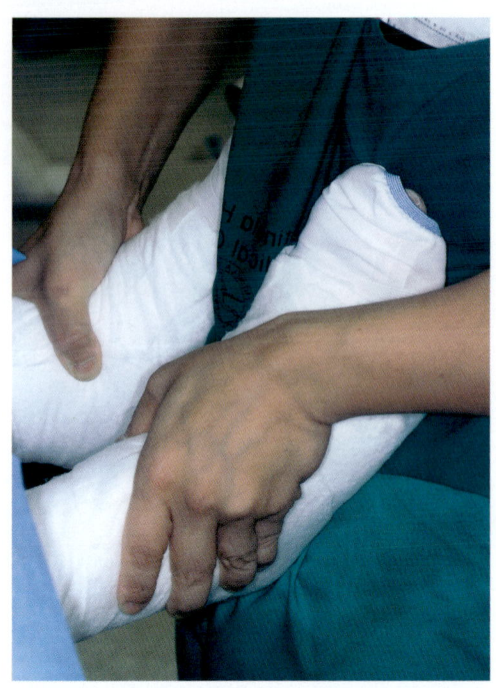

Figure 8–68 *Final intraoperative assessment of leg length.*

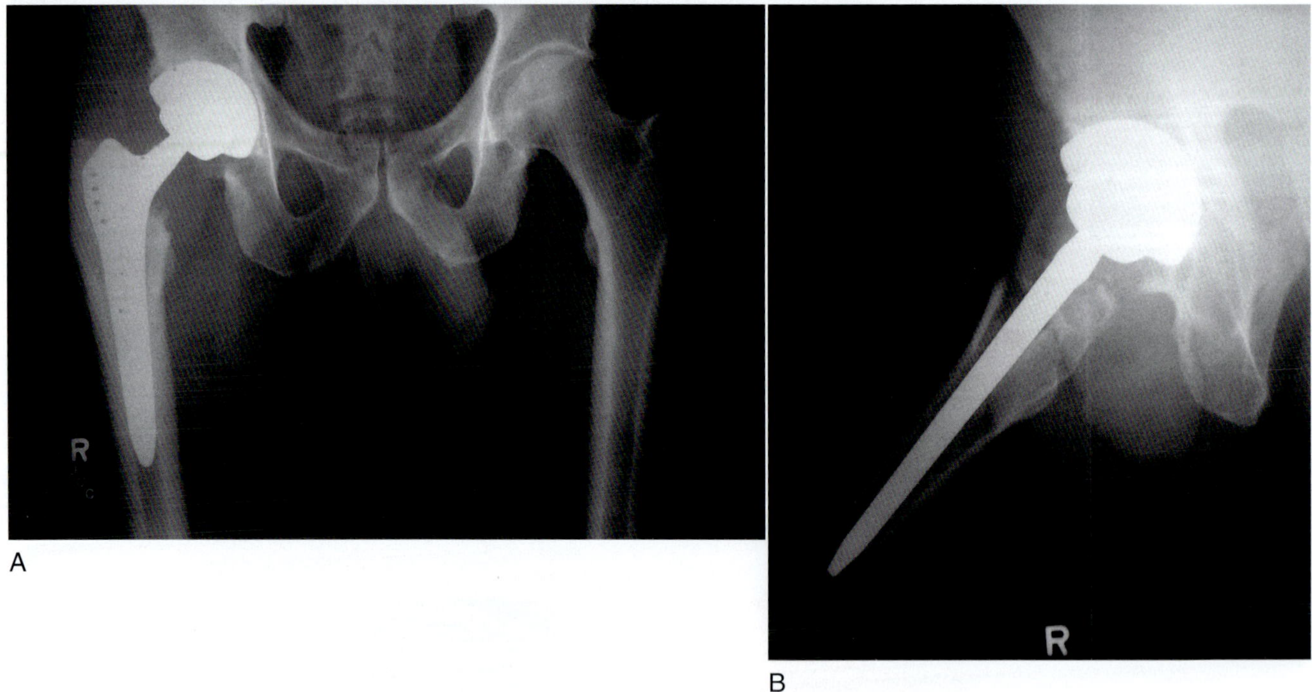

Figure 8–69 **A,** *Postoperative anteroposterior pelvic x-ray of the anterior approach total hip replacement.* **B,** *Posterior Lowenstein lateral x-ray of the anterior approach total hip replacement.*

to a cane. Patients are discharged home on the cane and are instructed to use it for outdoor walking over the next 2 to 3 weeks.

At home, the patient follows a program based on walking with quadriceps and hip abductor strengthening. A physical therapist visits the patient at home two to four times over the next 3 to 4 weeks to ensure timely progress. Formal outpatient physical therapy is rarely necessary in healthy patients.

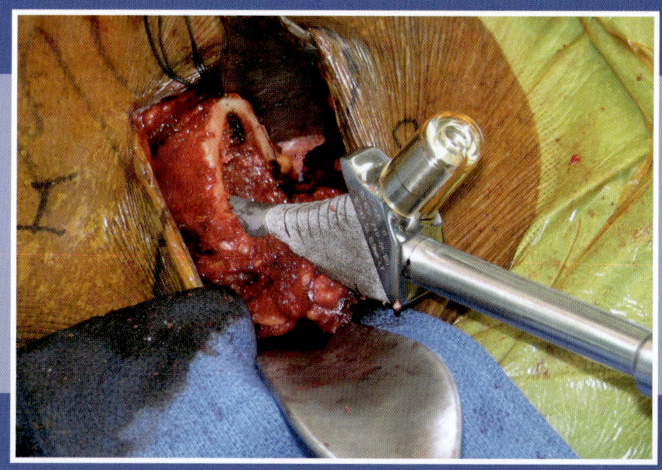

Chapter 9

Anterolateral Approach for Mini-incision Total Hip Replacement*

RICHARD "DICKEY" JONES

*In conjunction with this chapter on the DVD-ROM is the video *"Anterolateral Approach for Total Hip Replacement."*

INDICATIONS

The anterolateral approach to total hip arthroplasty is an alternative to the posterior approach. In the United States, approximately one third of surgeons use the anterolateral approach, with the rest using the posterior approach. Benefits of the anterolateral approach include a lower postoperative dislocation rate and direct access to and visualization of the acetabulum.[1-4] When computer-assisted surgical navigation is not available, the direct access provided by the anterolateral approach can result in more reproducible acetabular positioning.

Mini-incision surgery for total hip arthroplasty is a modification of a well-established and standardized procedure. As the surgeon becomes familiar with minimally invasive total hip arthroplasty, the length of the incision can be gradually shortened. Some authors[5] believe that surgeons need special hands-on training in cadavers or special mentoring before undertaking minimally invasive surgical procedures independently. I believe that because the mini-incision anterolateral approach is simply the same approach done with gradually shorter and shorter incisions, no special training is necessary. The surgeon moves along the learning curve very quickly if the principles outlined in this chapter are followed.

OPERATIVE TECHNIQUE

Positioning and Incision

The patient is positioned in the direct lateral position and the pelvis securely stabilized on the operative table (see Chapter 3). The legs are placed in 30 degrees of flexion at the hip and the knee, in neutral abduction/adduction and rotation. Initially, the surgeon stands on the posterior side and the assistant is on the anterior side of the patient.

The borders of the greater trochanter and vastus tubercle are palpated and marked and the incision is outlined (Fig. 9–1). The initial incision extends from 1 cm proximal to the posterosuperior border of the greater trochanter to 1 cm distal to the anterior distal trochanter at the vastus tubercle ridge. The oblique incision allows better direct access to the acetabulum during acetabular preparation. This incision may vary from 8 to 12 cm in length depending on the size of the patient's greater trochanter. A Cobb elevator can be used to dissect the subcutaneous tissue and fat off the iliotibial band so that the skin moves independently of the fascia, creating a mobile window.

Exposure

The leg is abducted and a Richardson retractor is placed distally to expose the fascia, which is incised in line with the skin incision, continuing to 3 cm proximal to the tip of the greater trochanter (Fig. 9–2). The Richardson retractor is then moved anteriorly to expose the gluteus medius fibers, which are incised from the anterior proximal, in line with the fibers, to the tip of the greater trochanter, and then in an "L" shape distally along the trochanteric ridge to elevate and separate the medius from the underlying minimus (Fig. 9–3). The gluteus medius flap is tagged with interlocking Kessler sutures (#5 Ticron) for reattachment during closure to the retained cuff of tendon along the trochanteric border.

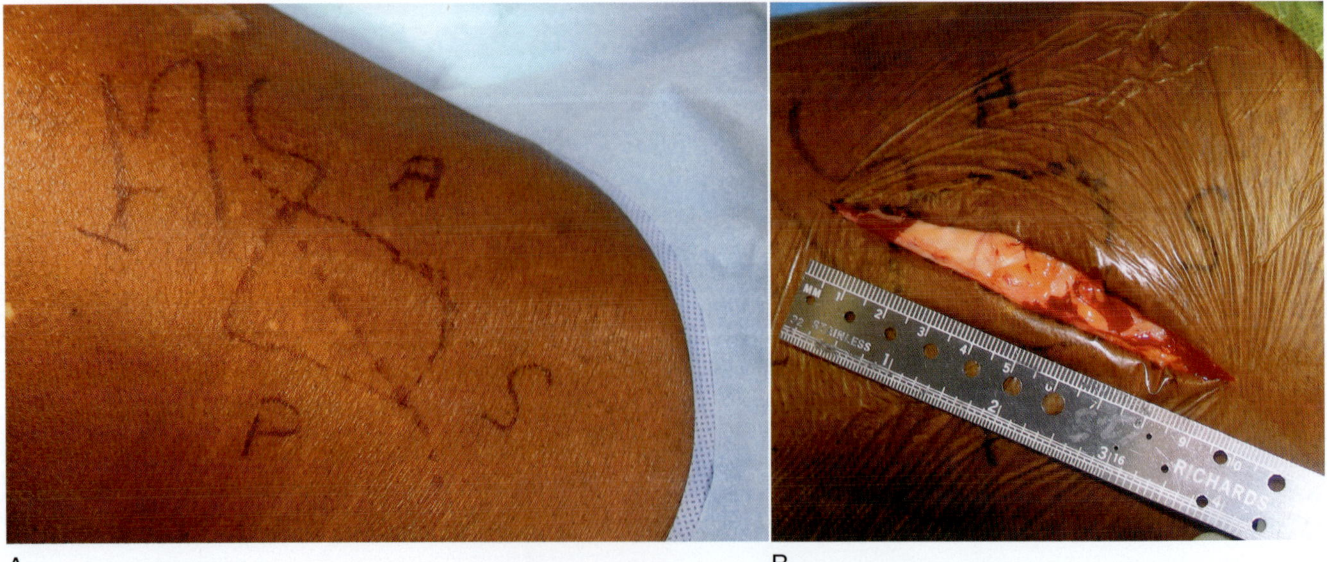

A   B

Figure 9–1   **A,** The greater trochanter is outlined by the rectangle on the skin. Superior, inferior, anterior, and posterior borders are noted. The dotted line is the oblique incision extending from 1 cm proximal to the superoposterior aspect of the greater trochanter to 1 cm distal to the anteroinferior aspect of the greater trochanter. **B,** The 8-cm skin incision is measured with the ruler.

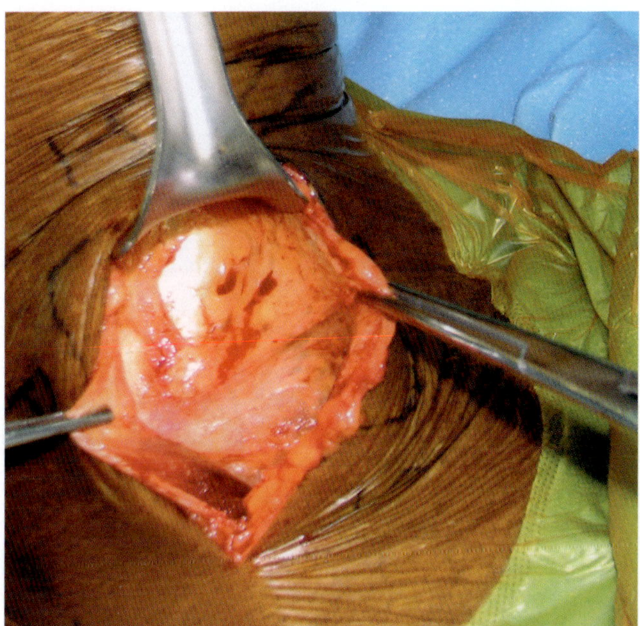

Figure 9–2 *Subcutaneous fat has been elevated and freed from the iliotibial band. The leg is abducted and a Richardson retractor is placed in the distal limb of the skin incision. The iliotibial band will be incised in line with the femur and the skin incision.*

The Richardson retractor is moved under the gluteus medius to retract the anterior two thirds of the medius anteriorly. A blunt cobra retractor is placed under the remaining posterior fibers of the gluteus medius to expose the entire gluteus minimus (Fig. 9–4). The gluteus minimus is incised as a single flap with its underlying capsule from the superior acetabulum over the superior neck, along the trochanteric ridge and distal into the vastus lateralis muscle (Fig. 9–5). The insertion of the minimus is 1 cm medial to that of the medius and it must be repaired to that anatomic position to prevent postoperative limp (Fig. 9–6). The exposure is extended on the medial inferior neck to the lesser trochanter. A Cobb elevator between the inferior femoral neck and capsule can facilitate exposure.

The minimus/capsule flap is tagged with an interlocking Kessler suture (#5 Ticron) for reattachment during closure to the anatomic insertion using a Hewson suture passer and 3.2-mm drill holes through the greater trochanter (Fig. 9–7).

A Meyerding retractor is placed under the minimus capsular flap, retracting it anteriorly (Fig. 9–8). The capsule/labrum is elevated from the superior acetabulum from the posterior acetabulum to the anterior column. A lighted anterior retractor or a blunt cobra retractor is placed between the anterior acetabulum and the iliopsoas tendon (Fig. 9–9).

A special superior acetabular retractor is inserted along the superior acetabular border to gain full vision

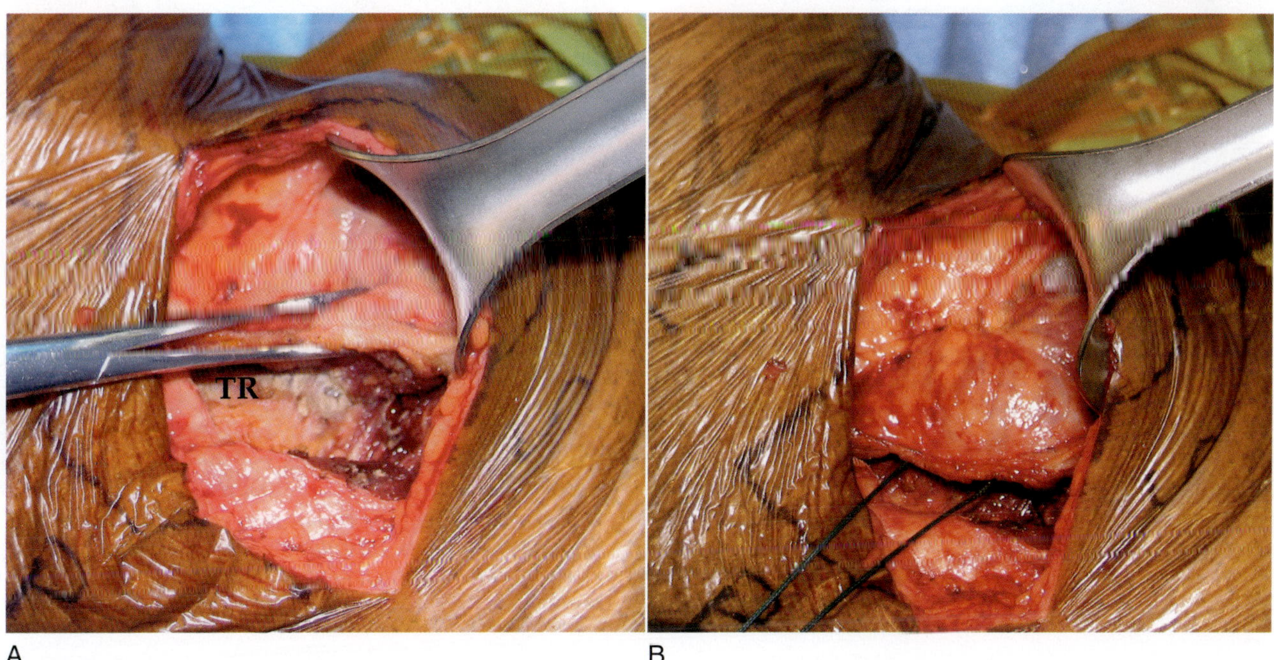

Figure 9–3 **A,** *A Richardson retractor elevates subcutaneous tissue and exposes the anterior two thirds of the gluteus medius muscle (held in clamp). The gluteus medius muscle has been incised from proximal (right) to the greater trochanteric tip and along the trochanteric ridge (TR) to elevate it from the underlying gluteus minimus.* **B,** *The Richardson retractor stays anterior and superior, and #5 Ticron interlocking sutures are placed into the gluteus medius, tagging the muscle for later reattachment to the trochanteric ridge.*

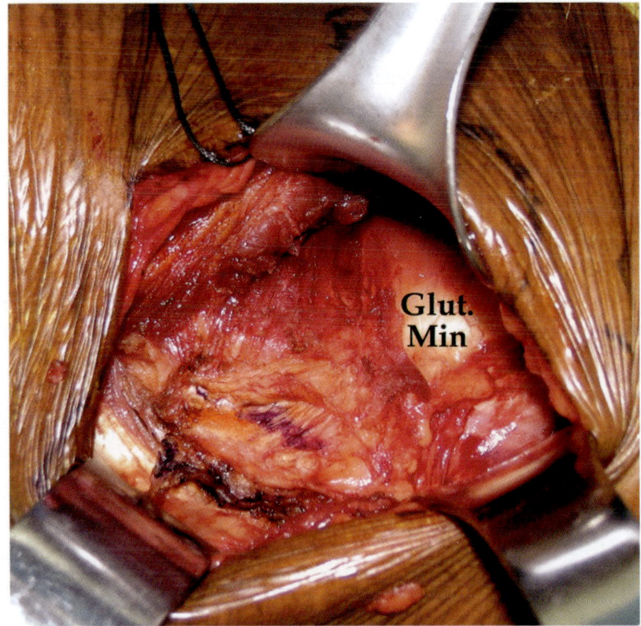

Figure 9–4   *The anterior Richardson retractor (top) retracts the tagged gluteus medius muscle to expose the gluteus minimus (Glut Min). A cobra retractor (bottom right) is placed under the posterior fibers of the remaining one third of the gluteus medius to complete the exposure of the gluteus minimus.*

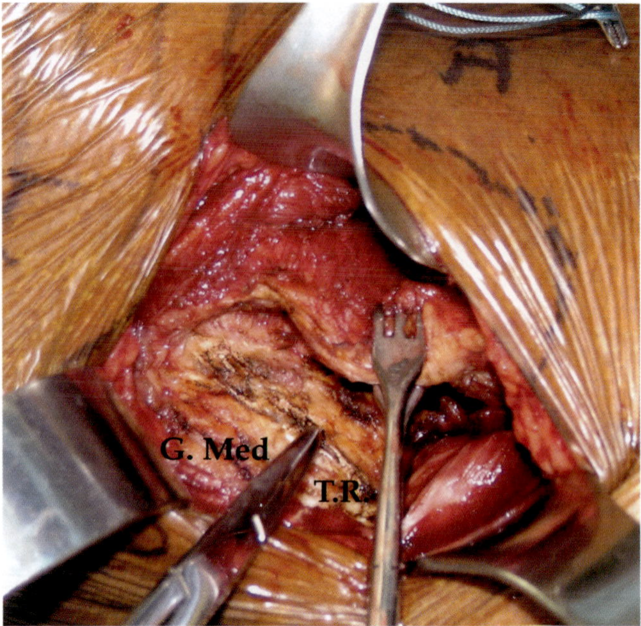

Figure 9–6   *The superior Richardson retractor continues to retract the gluteus medius muscle. A Leahy clamp is placed on the gluteus minimus and capsule flap. The needle holder marks the gluteus minimus insertion into the trochanter, which is 1 cm medial to the gluteus medius (G. Med) insertion on the trochanteric ridge (TR).*

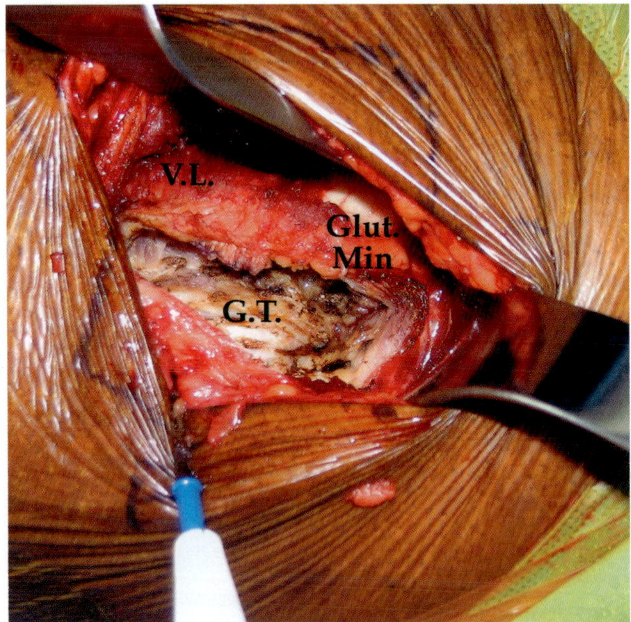

Figure 9–5   *An "L"-shaped incision is made in the gluteus minimus muscle (Glut Min) and capsule from the superior aspect of the femoral neck on the right down along the gluteus minimus insertion into the trochanter (GT), and dissection is continued distally into the contiguous vastus lateralis muscle (VL).*

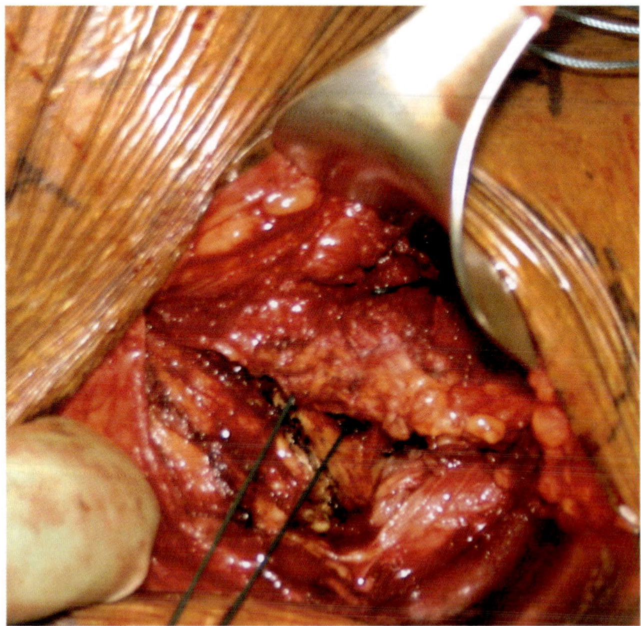

Figure 9–7   *Again, the Richardson retractor is anterior and the gluteus minimus capsular flap has been tagged with #5 Ticron for later reattachment to the trochanter by drill holes.*

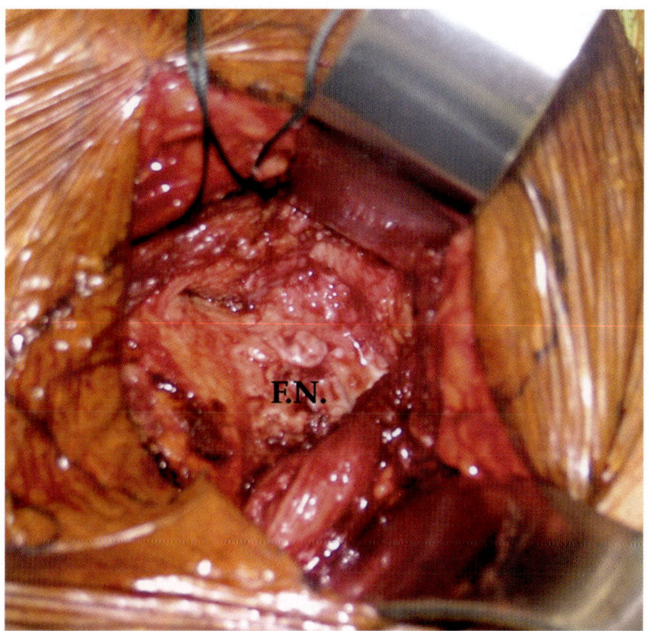

Figure 9–8 *A Meyerding retractor is placed anterior, retracting the gluteus minimus capsular flap anteriorly and exposing the femoral neck (FN).*

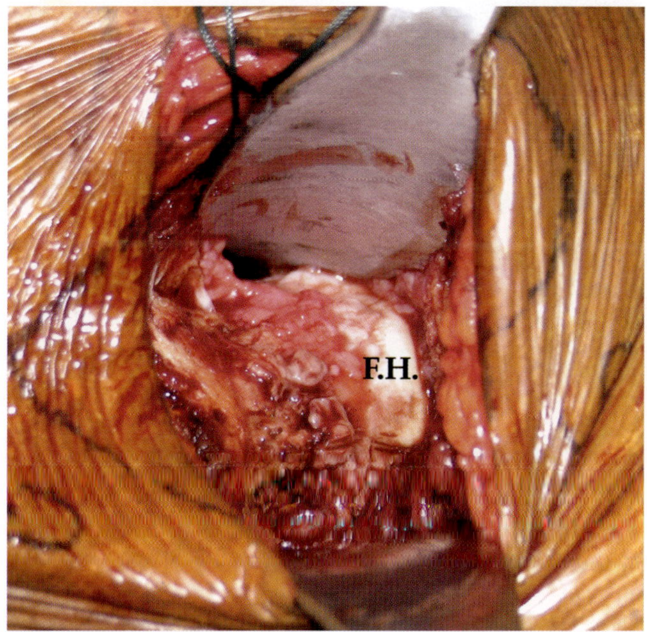

Figure 9–9 *A blunt anterior retractor of the cobra type is placed between the anterior acetabulum and the iliopsoas tendon, further exposing the inferior half of the femoral head (FH; right).*

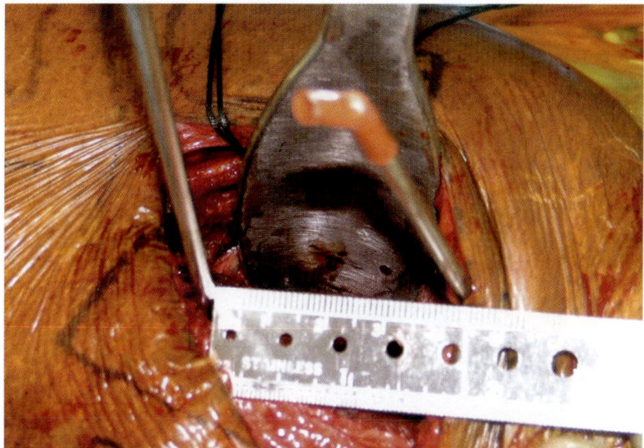

Figure 9–10 *Two Steinmann pins have been placed in the superior acetabular wing and in the greater trochanter. The distance between the two is measured to help obtain appropriate leg lengths after the procedure. Electrocautery marks are made at the sites of the two pins so they can be replaced after final reduction and leg lengths rechecked.*

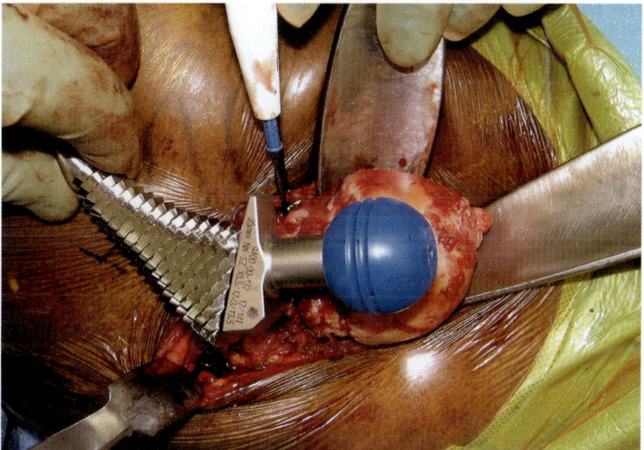

Figure 9–11 *The trial component is superimposed over the femoral head and the site of the neck osteotomy is marked with the trial component. A second check for the level of the femoral neck osteotomy is done by measuring up from the lesser trochanter to the distance determined by the preoperative x-ray templating exercise depicted in Figure 9–10.*

of the acetabulum. Alternatively, one or two Steinmann pins can be placed on the superior acetabulum for retraction and exposure. A 3.2-mm drill bit is drilled into the greater trochanter parallel to the superior acetabular retractor (or Steinmann pin), and the distance between the two is measured to assess preoperative and postoperative leg lengths (Fig. 9–10). The measuring points used on the bone should be marked by methylene blue for identification after the reconstruction.

Osteotomy

The leg is flexed, abducted, and externally rotated to dislocate the femoral head. If necessary, a bone hook can be used to lift the head out of the acetabulum. The flexed, abducted, and externally rotated position delivers the femoral head and neck into the wound. The osteotomy level can be measured with a trial femoral component (Fig. 9–11), or from the preoperatively

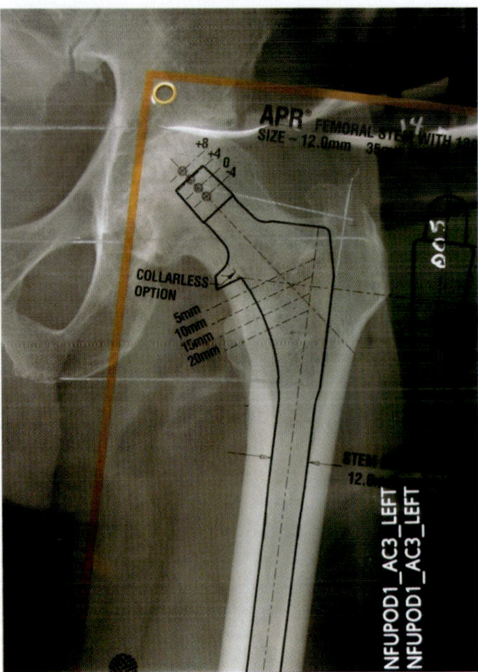

Figure 9–12 *The APR femoral stem x-ray template is superimposed over the hip x-ray. Templating should be done for a neutral or zero head. In this example, the femoral neck osteotomy site is 10 mm above the proximal portion of the lesser trochanter and correlates closely with the clinical determinations made with the component trial, as shown in Figure 9–11.*

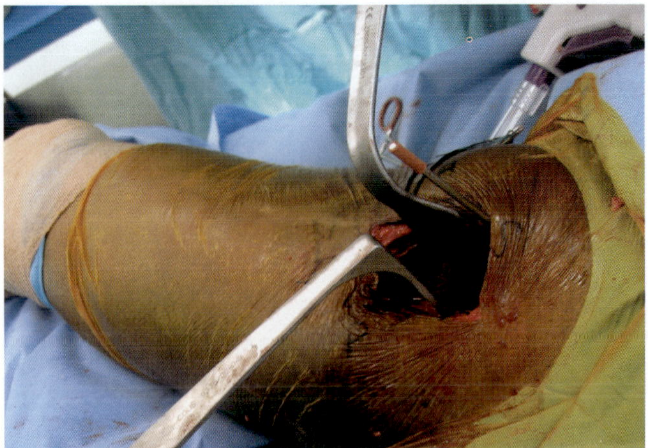

Figure 9–13 *The leg is placed on the table in 30 degrees of external rotation on top of the contralateral leg. The posterior retractor has been placed so that it straddles the ischium behind the posterior column. With the anterior cobra retractor and posterior retractor in place, the acetabulum can be directly visualized. The Steinmann pin is just proximal to the anterior retractor.*

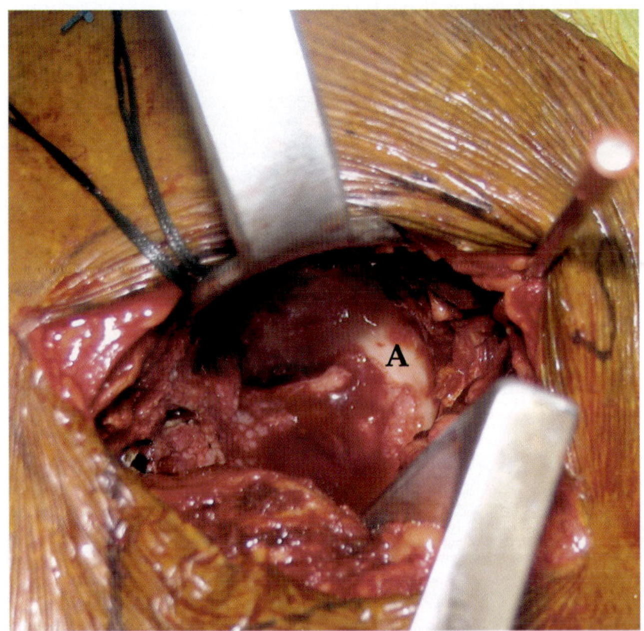

Figure 9–14 *The anterior retractor (top) remains in place between the anterior acetabular rim and the iliopsoas tendon. The posterior retractor below moves the femur posteriorly and allows direct visualization of the acetabulum (A). Acetabular reaming is directed toward the sciatic notch, which is a reliable anatomic landmark and yields an anteversion angle of 20 degrees for the acetabulum. The acetabulum is medialized to the cortical bone of the cotyloid notch (the quadrilateral plate). The Steinmann pin is superior.*

templated position above the lesser trochanter (Fig. 9–12).

The femoral neck osteotomy is completed, the head is removed, and the leg is placed on the table in 30 degrees of external rotation on top of the contralateral lower leg.

A bone hook can be used to elevate the proximal femur for palpation of the ischium, and a posterior retractor is placed either directly onto the ischium or straddling the ischium behind the posterior column of the acetabulum (Fig. 9–13). The "mobile skin window" is readily retracted to expose the acetabulum (Fig. 9–14).

Acetabular Preparation and Implantation

The surgeon should move to the anterior side of the table for acetabular preparation because there is much better visualization of the acetabulum in this position. Reaming is done, with the medial end point being the cortical bone of the cotyloid notch (quadrilateral plate). The reamer is directed toward the sciatic notch, which can be plated by a finger. A Steinmann pin is used as a visual guide for the direction of reaming. Figure 9–15 shows the reamer handle pointing toward the sciatic

notch with a Steinmann pin as a guide. Figure 9–16 shows a close-up view of the reamer preparing the acetabular bone.

A trial acetabular component is inserted to judge the fit and position of the acetabulum. The inclination rec-

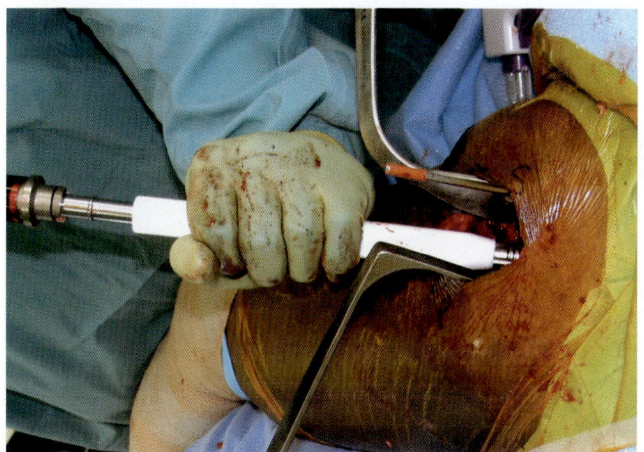

Figure 9–15 *Long view of the reamer handle pointing toward the sciatic notch. The rubber-tipped Steinmann pin confirms correct anteversion position.*

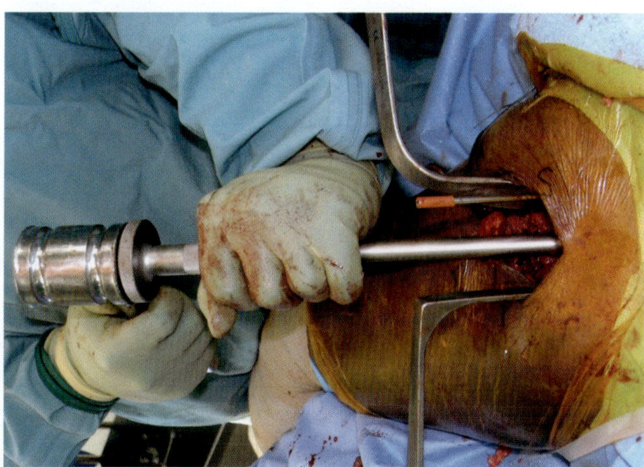

Figure 9–17 *The trial and the actual acetabular component are impacted into the acetabulum by pointing the long holder toward the sciatic notch.*

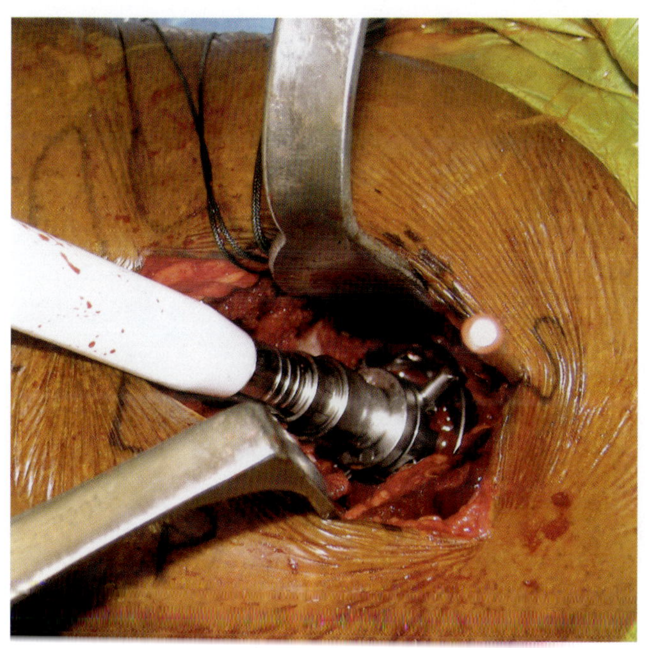

Figure 9–16 *Anteversion on the acetabular reamer is determined by aiming directly at the sciatic notch, which can be palpated by a finger. The rubber-tipped Steinmann pin to the right of the anterior retractor and above the reamer is a visual guide for the sciatic notch. The Steinmann pin also retracts tissue at the superior acetabular brim. This view shows the ease of access to the acetabulum for preparation of the acetabular bone.*

ommended for the acetabulum is 40 to 45 degrees. The anteversion is determined by aiming the center of the socket to the sciatic notch (Fig. 9–17). The average acetabular anteversion with this technique is 20 degrees. The trial component is then removed and the actual acetabular component is impacted into the same accepted position and tested for stability by levering on the impactor handle. Slurry is placed into the bony

acetabulum before impaction of the component (Fig. 9–18). Screw fixation is used if needed for immediate stabilization of the cup. Using screw fixation is technically easy. The insert is then implanted into the metal shell. If a hood is needed for extra stability, it should be placed in the anterolateral position of the acetabular shell with the apex of the hood in line with the anterior superior iliac spine (Fig. 9–19).

Femoral Preparation and Implantation

Femoral preparation begins with the surgeon moving to the posterior side of the table. The superior acetabular retractor and posterior acetabular retractors are removed, but the anterior acetabular retractor remains in place. The leg is flexed, abducted, and externally rotated with a femoral neck elevator retractor positioned between the greater trochanter and posterior fascia for exposure during femoral reaming and broaching. This retractor must be positioned with the leg in the neutral position on the table (to prevent entrapment of the sciatic nerve; Fig. 9–20). After this retractor is positioned, the leg is moved to the flexed, abducted, and externally rotated position (Fig. 9–21).

Reaming (Fig. 9–22) and broaching (Fig. 9–23) can then be performed under direct visualization. The final broach is used as a trial, and a head/neck attachment is placed onto the broach and then reduced into the hip. The superior acetabular retractor and the drill bit in the trochanter are replaced and leg lengths are measured (see Fig. 9–10). The measuring points on the posterior acetabulum and the greater trochanter had been marked with the cautery or methylene blue, so the identical pin positions are known. The final choice for head length can be made by testing stability with the trial reduction. The drill bit and superior acetabular

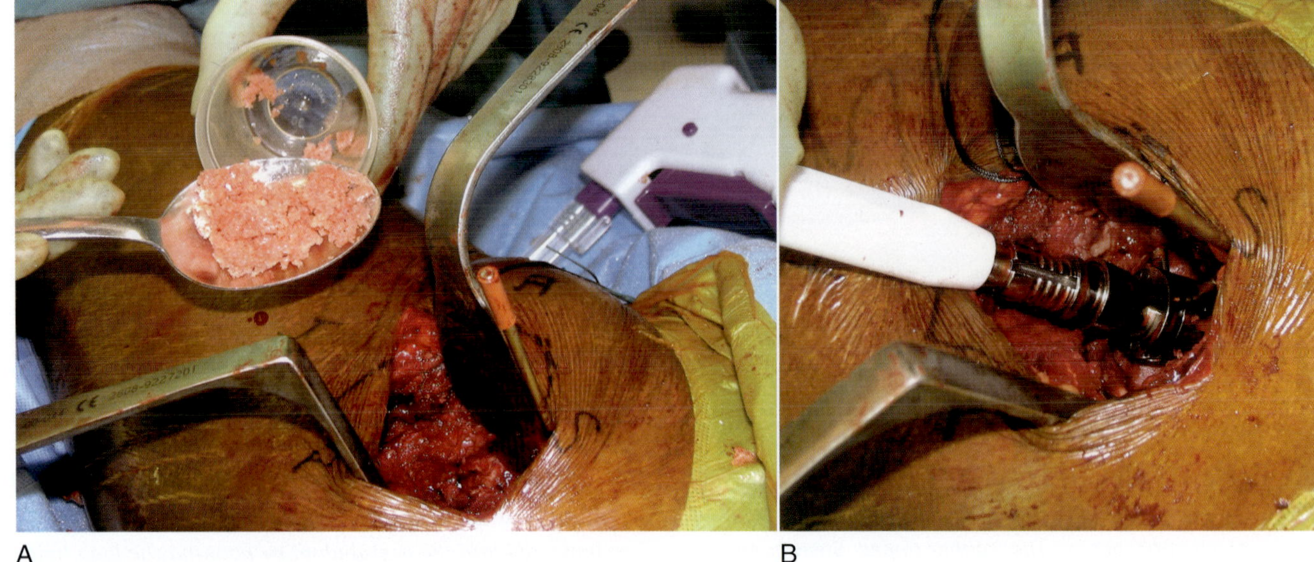

Figure 9–18 **A,** *Cancellous bone reamings removed from the femoral head and defatted in a lap sponge are placed into the prepared acetabulum.* **B,** *The reamings are impacted into the acetabular bed with either a smooth acetabular reamer or a regular acetabular reamer in reverse. This reamer is directed toward the sciatic notch.*

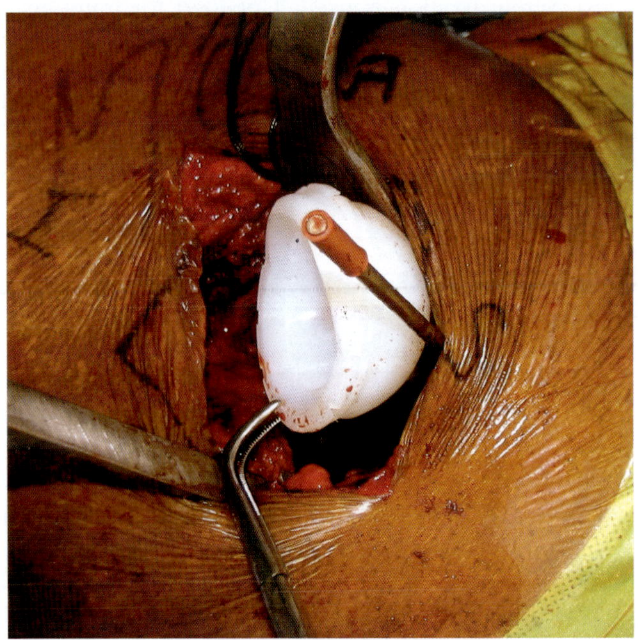

Figure 9–19 *A 10-degree hooded acetabular polyethylene component is placed with the hood directed anterior and lateral at the 10 to 11 o'clock position for the left hip and at the 1 to 2 o'clock position for the right hip.*

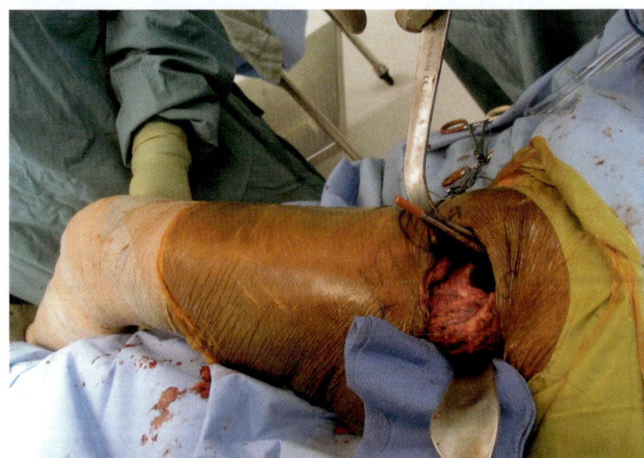

Figure 9–20 *To protect the sciatic nerve, the femoral neck elevator is placed behind the greater trochanter with the leg still on the table in neutral position (bottom right of wound). The retractor is on the blue towel.*

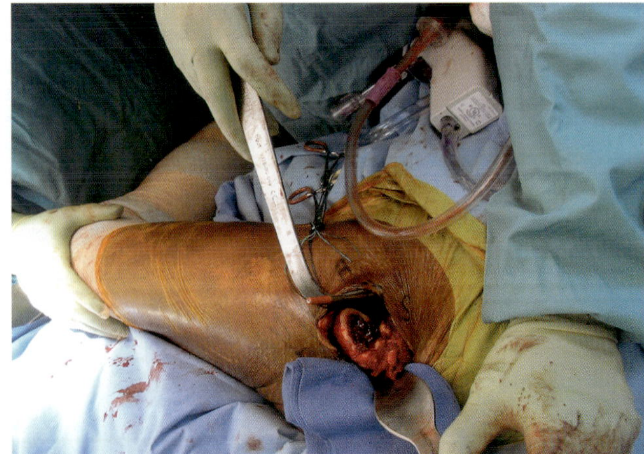

Figure 9–21 *The leg is moved to a flexed, adducted, and externally rotated position by the assistant. This provides direct access to the femoral neck in the center of the wound.*

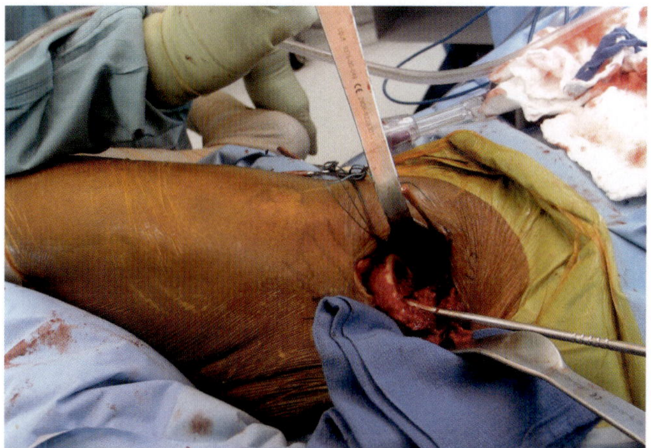

Figure 9–22 *Femoral reaming is done with direct visualization of the proximal femoral neck.*

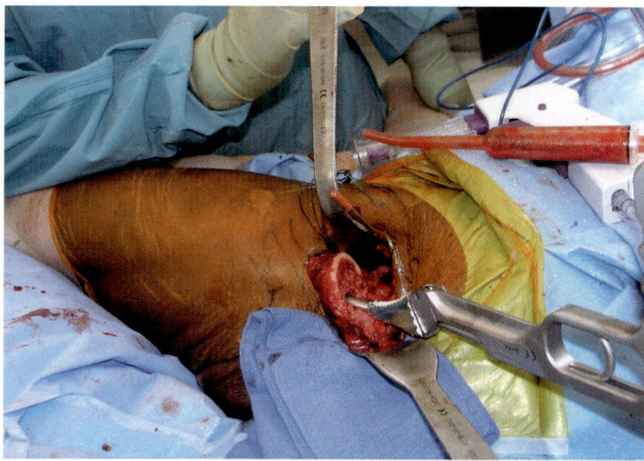

Figure 9–23 *Femoral broaching is then accomplished after reaming to appropriate size. Note that a single assistant holds the operative leg in the flexed, adducted, and externally rotated position and also holds the anterior retractor, which remains in place to aid visualization. Long handles on the retractors allow this.*

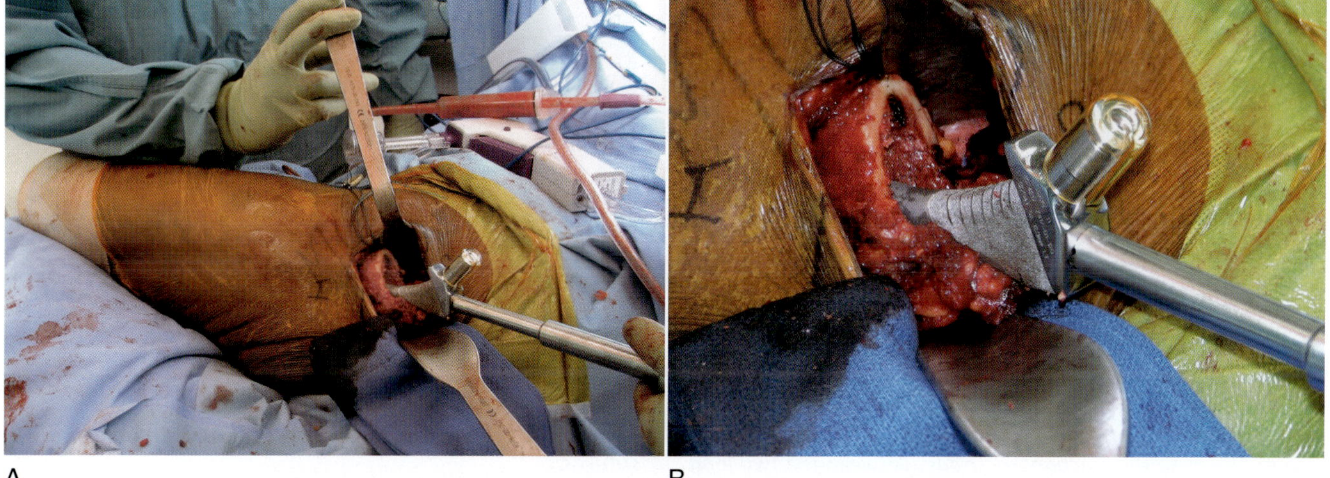

A   B

Figure 9–24 **A,** *The correct size of femoral component is impacted. The collar should be in intimate contact with the calcar for maximum initial stability.* **B,** *Close-up of femoral stem insertion.*

exterior and removed. The proximal femur is again delivered into the wound and the leg is placed in a neutral position for positioning of the posterior retractor (to protect the sciatic nerve; see Fig. 9–20). The femoral trial is removed and the actual femoral stem is implanted to the same level of femoral neck cut as was the broach (Fig. 9–24).

Closure

All retractors are removed from the wound and pulsatile lavage irrigation is done. The gluteus minimus/capsular flap is reattached through drill holes to its anatomic position (Fig. 9–25). The gluteus medius is reattached

to the undermost edge with the previously placed #1 Ticron suture (Fig. 9–26). The subcutaneous tissue is closed with 2-0 Vicryl suture. A running subcuticular skin suture is done with #2-0 Monocryl, which produces an excellent cosmetic result (Fig. 9–27).

CONCLUSION

Mini-incision surgery for total hip arthroplasty using the anterolateral approach is an excellent option because the smaller incision reduces the length of muscle that must be incised, divided, or released to provide femoral and acetabular access for component implantation.

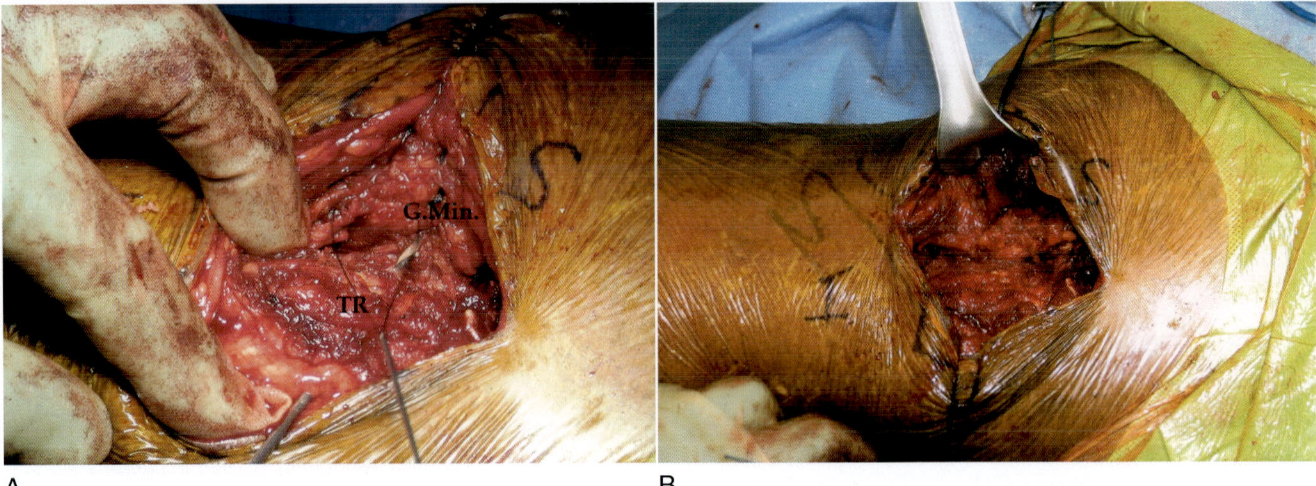

Figure 9–25 **A,** *The gluteus minimus/capsular flap (G Min) is reattached to its position 1 cm medial to the trochanteric ridge (TR) through drill holes using a Hewson suture passer. Reattachment is performed with the leg in the abducted position on folded sheets, or on a Mayo stand.* **B,** *The gluteus minimus flap has been reattached.*

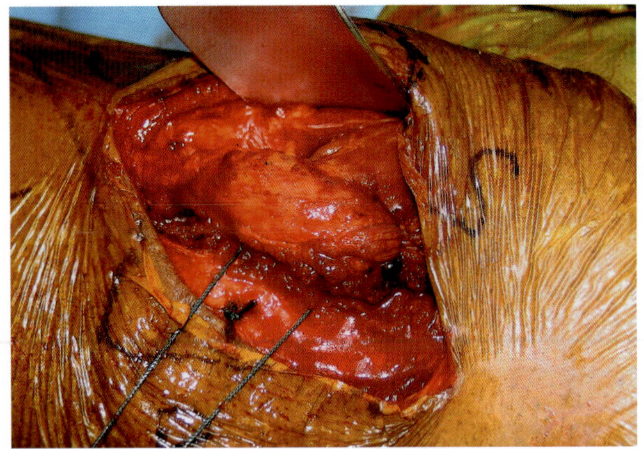

Figure 9–26 *The gluteus medius is then reattached with direct sutures to the trochanteric ridge. Between the two long sutures visible at the bottom is the already tied drill hole reattachment of the gluteus minimus/capsular flap.*

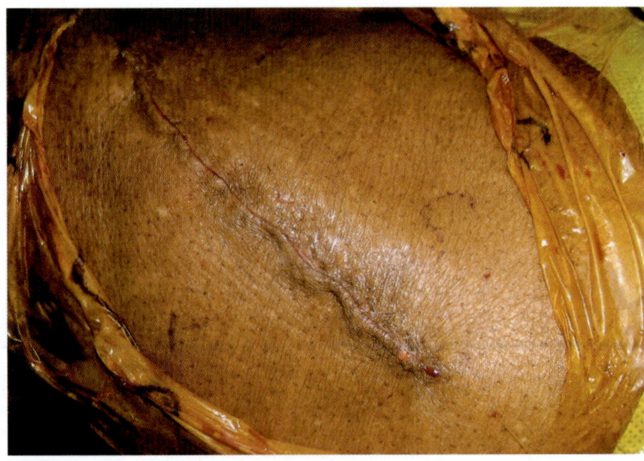

Figure 9–27 *Final closure of the incision with subcuticular sutures.*

Instrumentation designed for this exposure facilitates the efficiency of the operation. This instrumentation, combined with a single assistant manipulating the leg, allows easy performance of the operation without the need for a larger incision. However, the approach is also readily extensible if more exposure is needed, and there should be no hesitation to extend the incision if needed for safe performance of the hip reconstruction.

References

1. Barber TC, Roger DJ, Goodman SB, Schurman DJ: Early outcome of total hip arthroplasty using the direct lateral vs. the posterior surgical approach. Orthopaedics 19:873-875, 1996.
2. Hardinge TR: The direct lateral approach to the hip. J Bone Joint Surg Br 64:17-19, 1982.
3. Hedlundh U, Hybbinette CH, Fredin H: Influence of surgical approach on dislocations after Charnley hip arthroplasty. J Arthroplasty 10:609-614, 1995.
4. Mulliken BD, Rorabeck CH, Bourne RB, Nayak N: A modified direct lateral approach in total hip arthroplasty: a comprehensive review. J Arthroplasty 13:737-747, 1988.
5. Mears DC: Development of a two incision minimally invasive total hip replacement. J Bone Joint Surg Am 85:223-224, 2003.

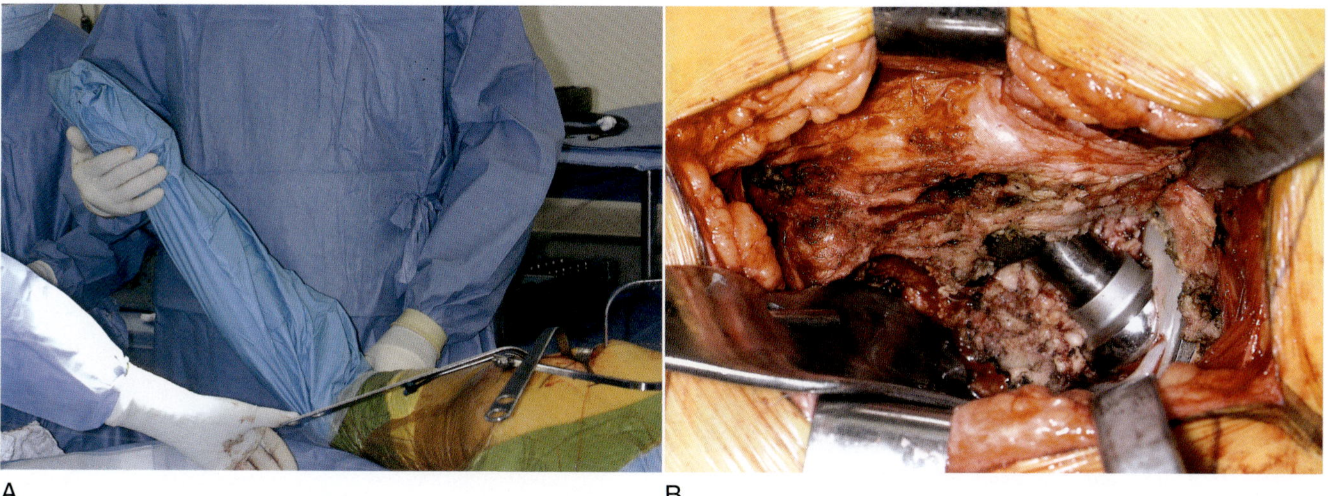

A　　　　　　　　　　　　　　　　　　　　　　　B

Figure 10–6 **A,** *The leg is continually internally rotated with support against the knee, so that the knee stays on top of the lower leg and is pushed posterior to relax the posterior tissues.* **B,** *The scar that was overlying the superior and posterosuperior cup has been removed, leaving the superoanterior and inferior scar tissue.*

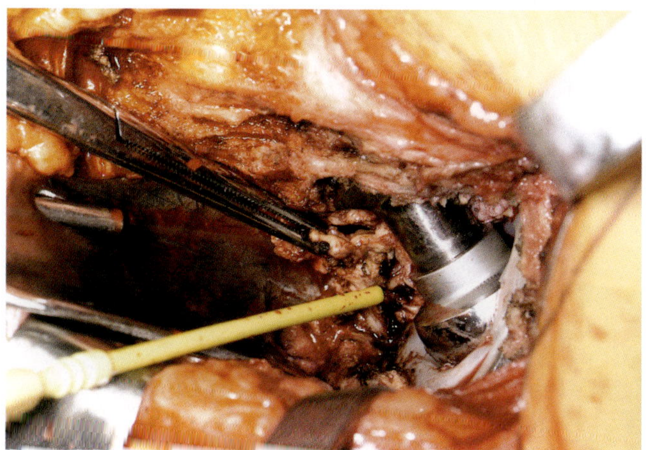

Figure 10–7 Scar tissue in the anteroinferior quadrant is removed with a Bovie electrocautery.

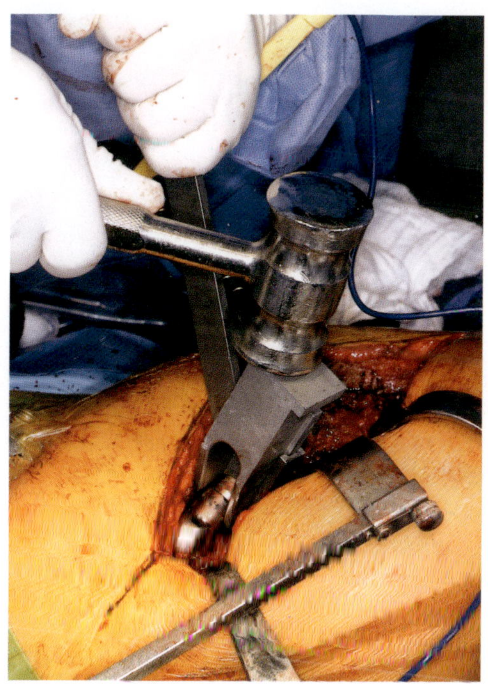

Figure 10–8 *The metal femoral head is wedged off the stem taper.*

which can be used with any brand of prosthetic hip, wedges the femoral head off the tapered neck (Fig. 10–8). Once the femoral head has been removed, there is access to the anterior femoral neck and to the scar tissue between the medial acetabulum and the anterior femoral neck. A retractor is placed around the lesser trochanter to retract the posterior flap. The patient's leg is placed on top of the lower leg in the middle of the table and is maximally internally rotated in this position (do not internally rotate the leg when it is over the side of the table) (Fig. 10–9).

The scar tissue anterior to the metal neck must be incised off the anterior femur and anterior greater trochanter to allow the femur to be retracted anterior to the acetabulum. The scar can be incised with a Bovie electrocautery if there is adequate access; if not, an osteotome is the best tool to cut this tissue and release it. A sharp osteotome is placed along the anterior neck and, with the help of a mallet, is used to cut through the tissue (Fig. 10–10). The osteotome can also cut through the tissue attached to the anterior greater trochanter, thus creating an anterior flap of tissue from the anterior femoral neck along the anterior greater trochanter.

When the anterior femur has been freed of scar tissue, the femoral neck usually points up and away

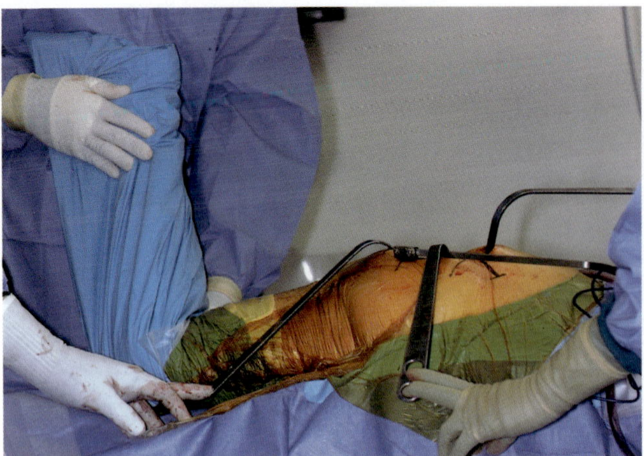

Figure 10–9 *The leg has been advanced to a 90-degree internally rotated position but remains on top of the lower leg.*

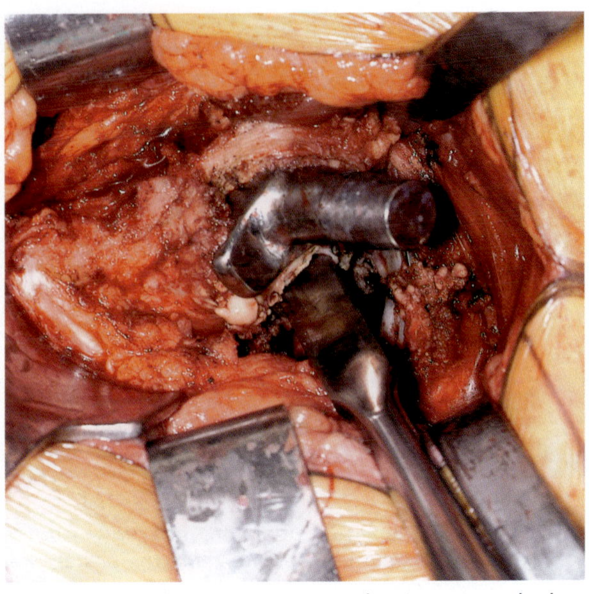

Figure 10–10   *The osteotome cuts the tissue attached to the anterior femoral neck.*

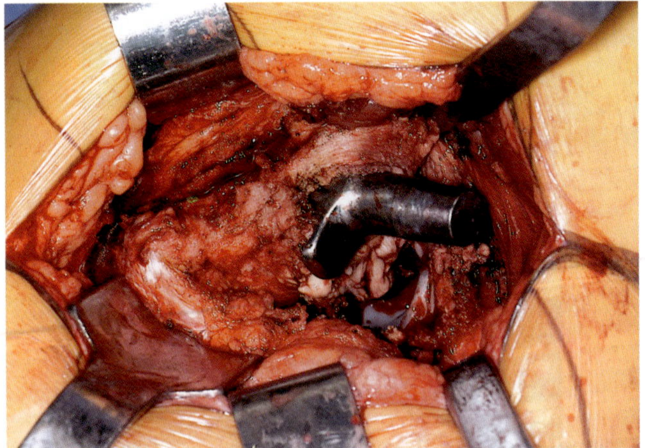

Figure 10–11   *The metal femoral neck is pointing up and out of the wound.*

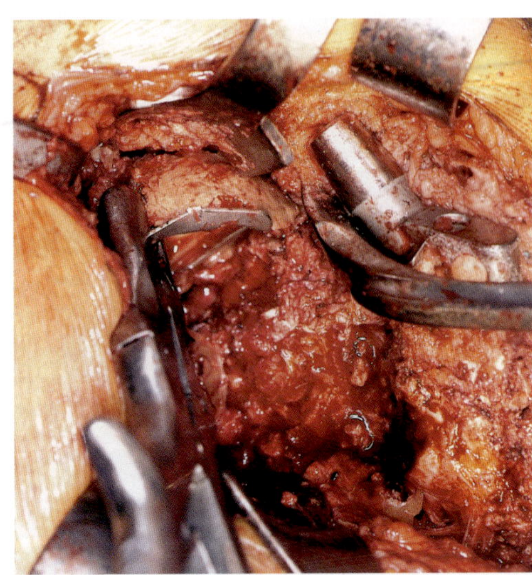

Figure 10–12   *The snake retractor is retracting the femoral component anteriorly against the femoral neck, but not against the taper of the neck. A metal ring is removed from the acetabulum with a rongeur.*

from the wound and rises out of the wound (Fig. 10–11). When this occurs, the femur is free enough for the snake retractor to be inserted. The snake is placed onto the ilium and malleted into position. It should retract against the base of the femoral neck and not against the modular articulating surface (Fig. 10–12). It is preferable not to scratch the articulating surface of the taper; the surface can be covered with a gauze or lap sponge if doing so will not block the view of the acetabulum. As the snake retracts the femur anteriorly, the leg is rotated from internal to external rotation and laid flat on the table (Fig. 10–13). Laying the leg flat on the table retracts the femur anterior of the acetabulum, allowing visualization of the entire acetabulum.

Anterior scar tissue must be excised along the anterior edge of the acetabulum (Fig. 10–14), preferably with a Bovie electrocautery. Additionally, an incision is made in the scar tissue inferomedially to provide an opening to place the tip of a #7 retractor against the cortical bone of the cotyloid notch, so that its paddle can be seated on the ischium and retract the posterior tissue (Fig. 10–15). The exposure of the acetabulum is now complete.

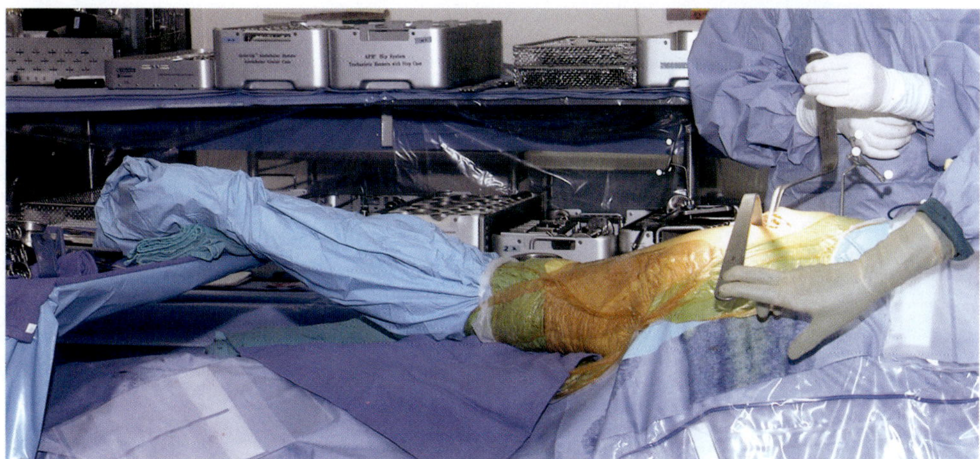

Figure 10–13 The leg is moved from internal rotation to lying flat on the table or with the foot lying on the Mayo stand.

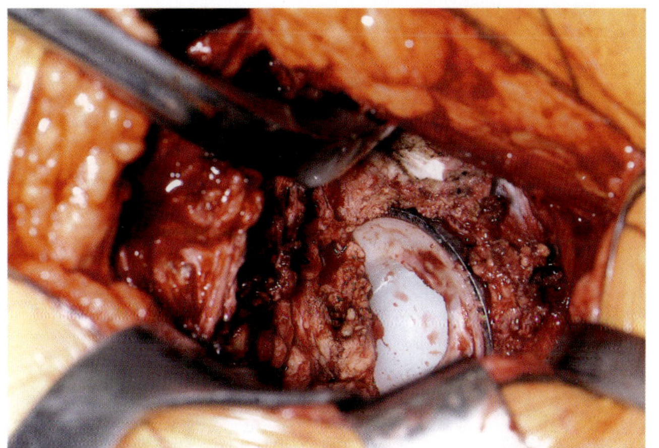

Figure 10–14 Hip capsular scar tissue, which needs to be excised to completely expose the acetabular component, is present along the anterior and anteroinferior cup.

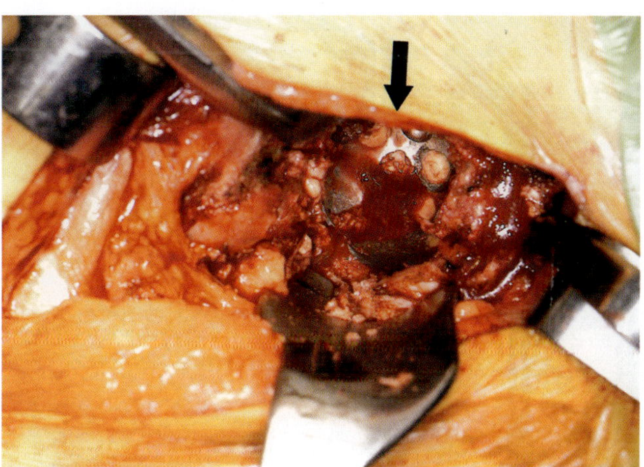

Figure 10–15 The arrow points toward the acetabular cup. At the bottom of the wound, the #7 retractor is seen, with its tip against the cotyloid notch and the paddle sitting on the ischium.

Femoral Exposure with the Posterior Approach

In revisions that include the femur, the femoral component should be removed before exposure of the acetabulum. Doing so simplifies the exposure of the acetabulum and the anterior retraction of the femur. Whether the femoral bone is prepared for a new femoral stem before exposure of the acetabulum is up to the surgeon. I usually prepare the femur before exposing the acetabulum simply because I find it more efficient.

After the hip is dislocated and the metal femoral head is removed, the scar tissue around the proximal femur can be excised with a Bovie electrocautery and a rongeur. The osteolytic tissue is easily peeled away from the femur with a rongeur. Often, any remaining femoral neck is necrotic from the osteolytic tissue and simply peels away as well (Fig. 10–16). If the proximal femoral neck is not necrotic, I usually remove it with a saw. Removing the femoral neck to the level of the lesser trochanter provides good exposure of the most proximal femoral stem and simplifies the work of removing it. Almost all revision prostheses are designed to work without bony femoral neck support, so removing the femoral neck has no effect on the revision stem implantation or fixation (Fig. 10–17).

Access to the scar tissue on the anterior side of the femur can sometimes be difficult to obtain. Again, an osteotome can be used to cut through this tissue and release it (Fig. 10–18). It is important that all the soft tissue and bone around the proximal portion of the femoral stem be removed; this essentially eliminates the chance of fracturing the femur when removing the femoral stem. If the femoral stem is grossly loose and can be pulled out, this is advantageous for the surgeon,

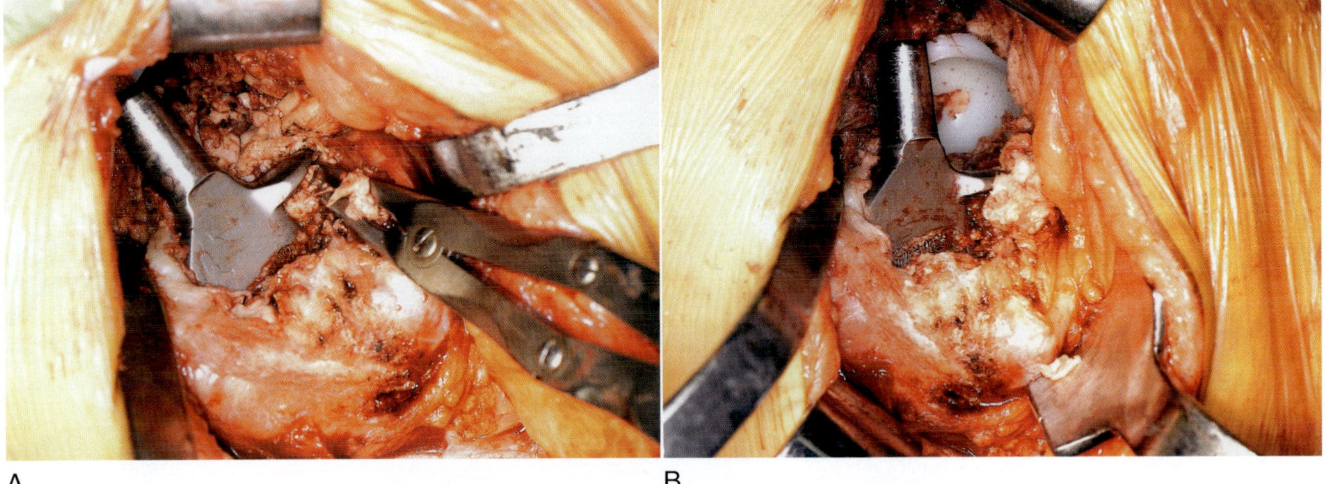

Figure 10–16 **A,** *Necrotic tissue, including necrotic bone around the neck, is removed with a rongeur.* **B,** *The proximal porous coating is exposed after removal of the necrotic tissue.*

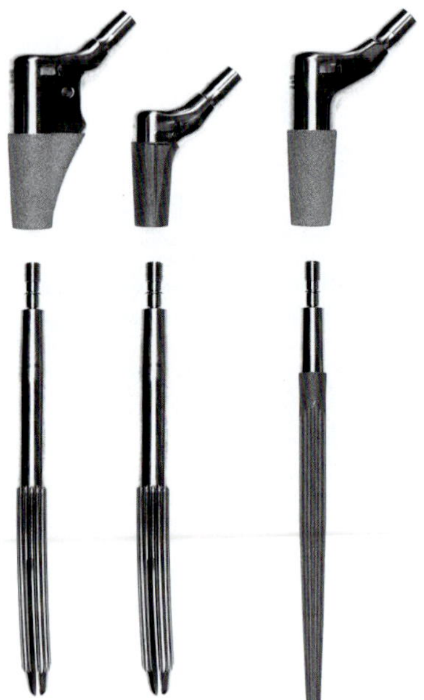

Figure 10–17 *Revision implants provide a proximal neck length that does not require any support from the femoral bone. The Zimmer modular revision (ZMR) stem pictured has a proximal segment that functions irrespective of bone support.*

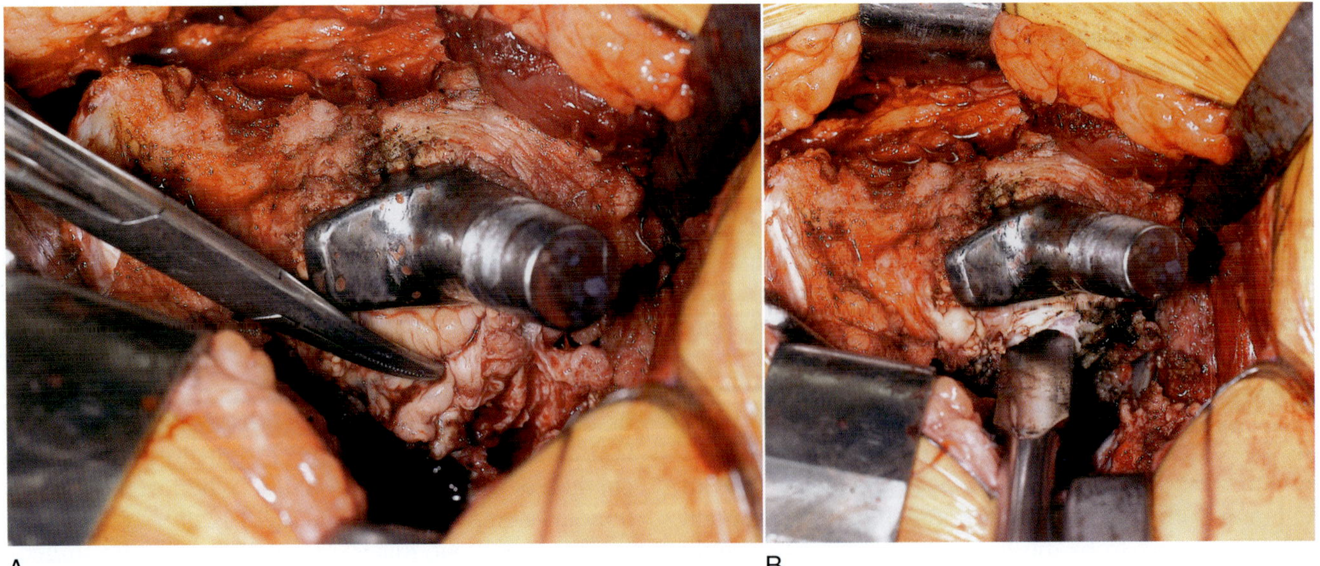

Figure 10–18 **A,** *Anterior scar tissue is attached between the anterior acetabulum and the anterior femoral neck.* **B,** *An osteotome is the most effective tool to cut through and strip this tissue.*

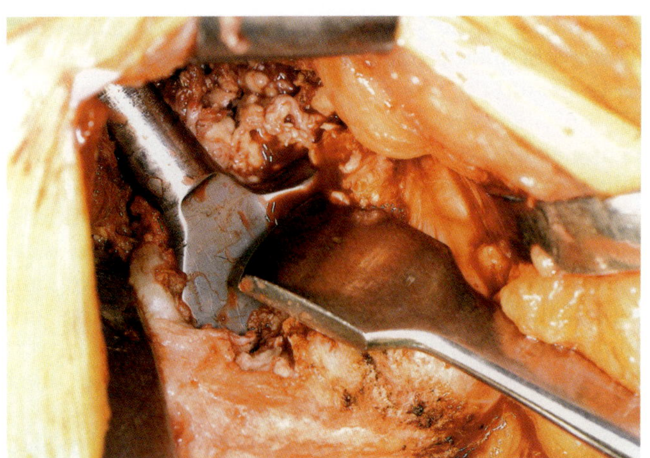

Figure 10–19 *The entire lateral prosthesis is cleared of tissue (and cement, if present) so that it can be extracted (with a periosteal elevator) without endangering the greater trochanter.*

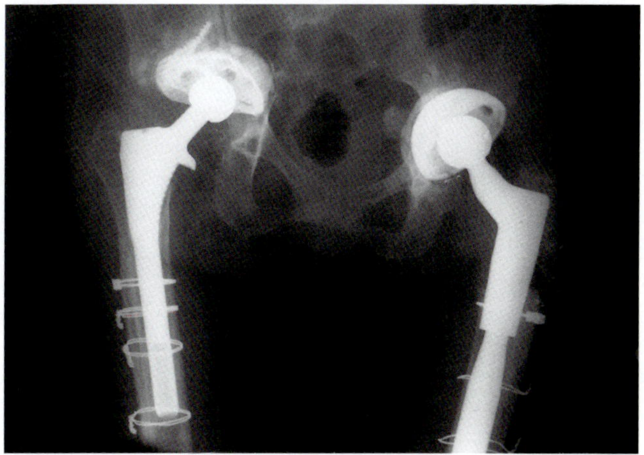

Figure 10–20 *The difficulty of reattaching the greater trochanter is illustrated in the left hip of this patient in this x-ray. The greater trochanter is not united to the remainder of the femur and just sits against the implant because any wires used would have to be against the metal of the implant.*

but this is generally not the case. Usually, tissue has grown into gaps around the femur, or the stem has sunk to a position where it is wedged into the femur and needs the tissue and bone cleared away before it can be safely removed.

Cementless Stem Removal. It is critical that the bone or cement along the lateral side of the proximal prosthesis (the trochanteric bed) be entirely eliminated so that the prosthesis can be removed without fracturing the trochanter (Fig. 10–19). As the prosthesis is extracted from the femoral canal, it always moves laterally. Therefore, if the bone or cement is not removed from the lateral side of the femur, it will create stresses at the base of the greater trochanter and cause fracture. This complication can result in less than optimal clinical results for the patient. Sometimes, achieving healing of this type of fractured trochanter is nearly impossible—the trochanteric bone has thinned from osteolysis, and there is no metaphyseal bone around which trochanteric reattachment cables or wires can be placed to provide secure fixation of the trochanter (Fig. 10–20). There are trochanteric fixation devices that attach to the diaphysis and have a hook that pulls on the trochanter, but the use of such devices increases the time and complexity of the operation. Thus, the importance of meticulously clearing the lateral side of the prosthesis before its extraction cannot be overstated.

If the surgeon decides that the lateral side of the prosthesis cannot be easily cleared, or the prosthesis has sunk so low in the femur that extraction endangers the trochanter, a controlled removal of the trochanter with an extended slide should be performed (see later). The extended slide enables the trochanter and lateral femur to be repaired, with an excellent chance for

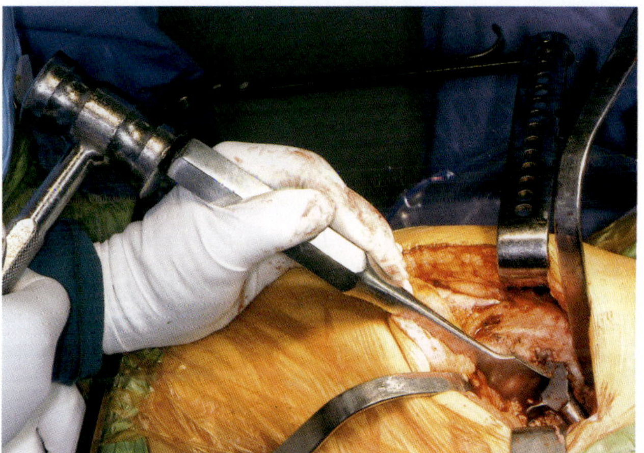

Figure 10–21 *An elevator is used to mallet an implant in an axial direction out of the femur.*

healing. In a revision situation, it is better to have a controlled removal of the greater trochanter than a fractured trochanter.

The implant can be removed from the femoral canal with an extraction device. If no extraction device is available and the implant has a collar, a periosteal elevator can be placed under the collar and used as a lever to drive the implant out of the femur (Fig. 10–21). If there is no collar, a carbide bit from the Anspach power burr set can be used to make a divot in the implant; a tool is then placed in the divot to drive the implant out of the femur proximally. Sometimes, making a divot requires the creation of a window on the anterolateral side of the femur below the greater trochanter (Fig. 10–22).

Other options for removing the implant include the use of the extended slide or a femoral window (Fig.

10–23). A femoral window can be made for any length along the anterolateral side of the femur below the greater trochanter. The advantage of the window is that it keeps the trochanter intact proximally, obviating concern about its healing. The disadvantage is that a fracture of the diaphysis can occur at the distal end of

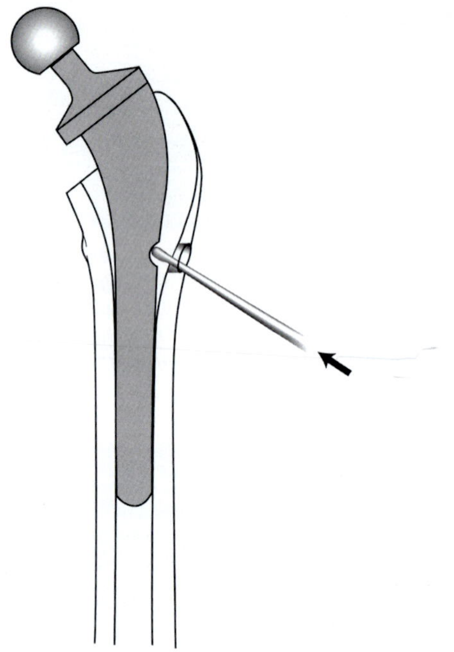

Figure 10–22 *A small window can be made in the femur just distal to the trochanter using a power burr. A carbide bit makes a divot in the metal of the implant, and a tool is then used to mallet the implant proximally. If necessary, sequential divots can be made in the metal as the implant is advanced. The arrow points in the direction of the mallet force.*

the window if the surgeon does not guard against this. To prevent such a fracture, the surgeon should place a cable around the femur at the distal end of the window; this provides strong hoop stresses to the femur, protecting against extension of a corner of the window distally into the femur, most commonly manifesting as a spiral fracture. When the work through the window is completed, the window should be replaced and wires placed over it to support the femur before reaming and implantation of the femoral stem. If reaming and implantation are done with the window still removed, the femur will be further weakened and at a much higher risk for fracture.

A window can be used instead of an extended slide when the lateral side of the prosthesis can easily be freed from the trochanteric bed and the proximal lateral femur. An extended slide should be done if there is strong bony fixation of a cementless prosthesis, because the implant cannot be extracted in the presence of this lateral fixation.

Cemented Implant Removal. With cemented implants, a window is commonly used to remove distal cement or a cement plug after the proximal cement has been removed from the proximal end of the femur.

Once a cemented stem has been removed from the femur, it is necessary to remove the cement retained in the femoral canal. The proximal cement is removed with osteotomes specially designed for this purpose (Fig. 10–24). The distal cement, particularly the distal plug, is difficult to remove. I use a cement drill made by LINK (Hamburg, Germany). A hole is drilled through the cement and gradually enlarged; then, using a hook

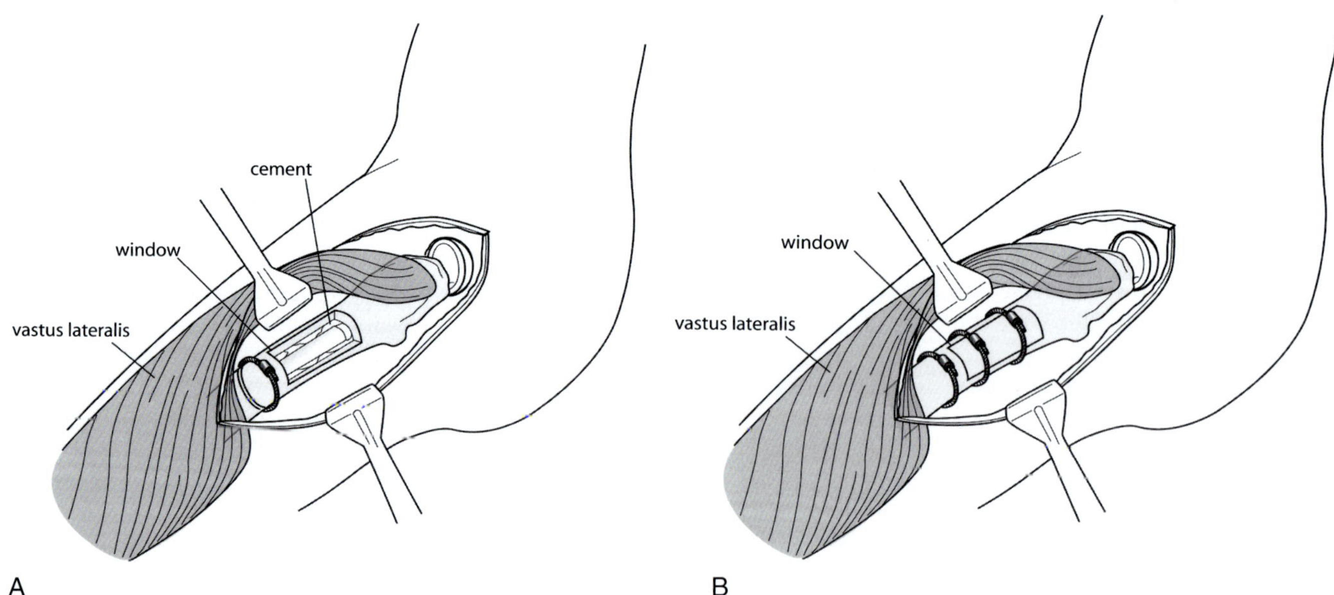

Figure 10–23 *A, A femoral window is made on the anterolateral bone. Initially, holes can be made with a drill or a pointed burr to facilitate the saw cut of the window. The saw cuts are made obliquely so that the cut window will be stable when it is reduced back into position. B, The window has been replaced and is secured with two wires.*

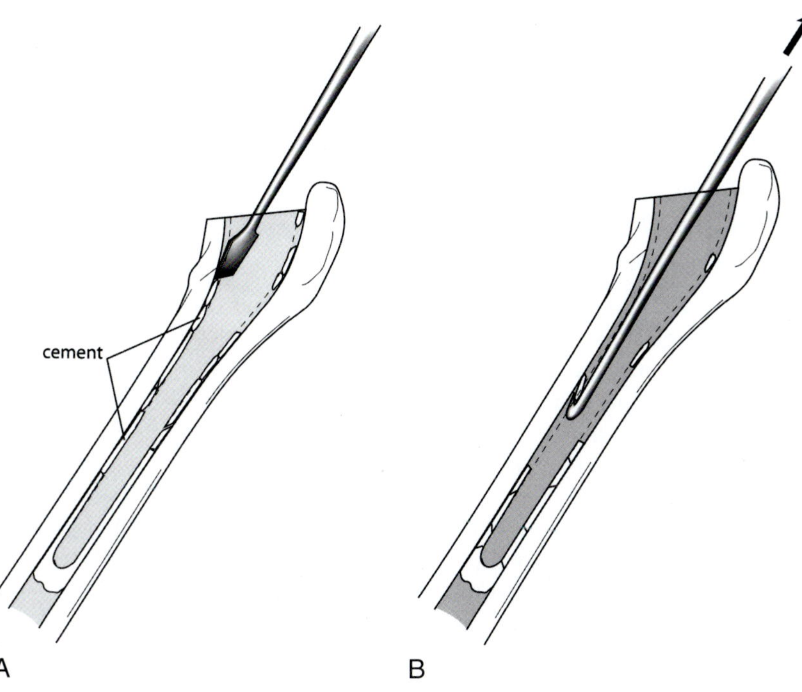

Figure 10–24 **A,** A cement osteotome is used at the interface of the cement and bone. **B,** A backhoe-type tool is used to hook the cement fragments off the femoral wall and out of the wound.

A

B

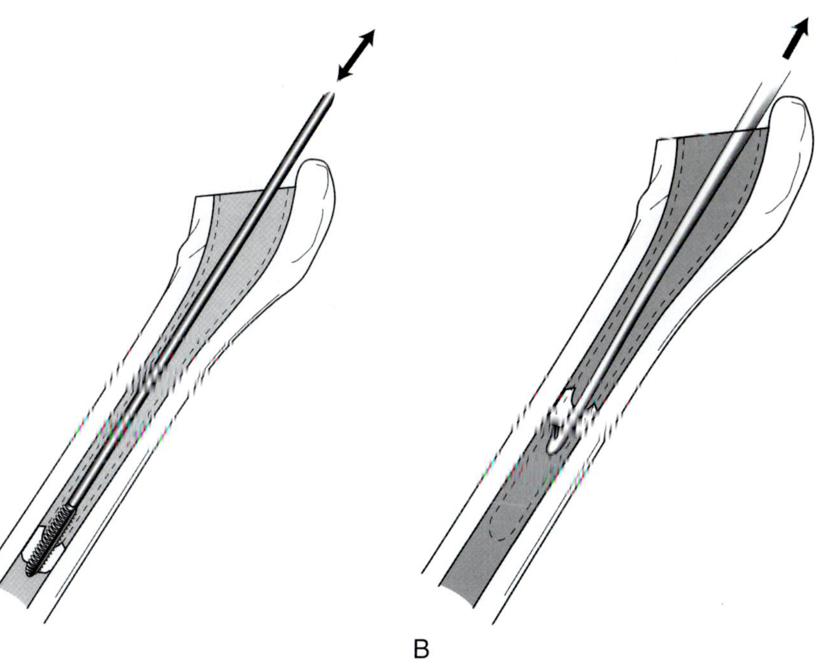

Figure 10–25 **A,** A power drill is used to drill a hole through the center of a cement plug. A short plug is shown, but this can be done for either short or long cement plugs. **B,** The backhoe-type tool is passed through the drill hole and used to hook the fragments, which can then be malleted free from the femoral bone and removed proximally.

A

B

or backhoe-type tool, the distal cement is removed and pulled out the proximal end of the femur (Fig. 10–25). Care must be taken not to drill the drill out the side of the femur rather than through the distal cement. If this occurs, and the hole in the femur is enlarged in error, the femur will have to be exposed by elevation of the vastus lateralis over the defect site. If I make this type of defect in the femur, I usually enlarge it into a window and remove the cement through it; then I replace the window, secure it with a wire, and finish preparing the femur. However, most often the drill passes through the cement column and remains inside the intramedullary canal, providing an efficient means of cement removal.

Once the cementless implant, or the cement and stem, have been removed from the femur, the femur is prepared with reamers and broaches for the new femoral stem. This preparation should be individualized according to the prosthesis system selected. However, no matter what type of cementless stem is used, the reamer should obtain contact over 7 cm of the femoral diaphysis to allow stable rotational fixation of the stem. (See Stem Implantation, later.)

Anterior Slide and Anterior Extended Slide

The extended slide technique must be learned and used by any surgeon who plans to perform revision hip replacement surgery. The anterior slide and anterior extended slide are valuable techniques that significantly improve the versatility of exposure for revision hip replacement (*see "Simple Techniques for Revision Total Hip Replacement"*).

This technique was initially described by Wagner and then popularized in the United States by Engh.[3] Paprosky published his results with this technique and showed that the healing of the extended slide is nearly always complete.[4] My experience with the extended slide is that it provides excellent exposure for revision surgery and is necessary when implants are well fixed in the femoral canal. A well-fixed bone-ingrown or cemented implant is best removed from the femur with the extended slide, extending the femoral bone elevation as far distally as necessary to the level of the isthmus. For the fixation of a new revision implant, it is critical that at least 7 cm of the isthmus be retained, so the distal end of an extended slide should be planned with this in mind. If the prosthesis remains fixed distal to this level, and it is bone ingrown, the prosthesis should be cut and the trephine technique (see under Femoral Preparation, later) (*see "Simple Techniques for Revision Total Hip Replacement"*) used to remove the more distal stem. If there is retained cement distal to this level of the isthmus, the cement should be removed with drill, burrs, and hooks, as described earlier. Maintenance of an intact femur from the level of the isthmus distally provides a much more stable result and more predictable fixation for the new implant.

The slide technique requires that the vastus lateralis be elevated sufficiently to allow a transverse cut of the femur. With only an anterior slide of the trochanter, the cut is made at the level of the vastus tubercle, and the vastus lateralis and gluteus medius are left attached to the greater trochanter fragment. Most commonly, a section of the lateral femur should remain attached to the trochanter fragment so that a single piece of bone (i.e., the greater trochanter and 5 to 7 cm of lateral femur) are elevated. Retaining 5 to 7 cm of lateral femur makes it easier to reattach the entire bony fragment with two cables around the diaphyseal lateral bone. Because there is often no metaphyseal bone to put a wire around for reattachment to the greater trochanter, the lateral

extension provides a surface around which fixation cables or wires can be placed.

When the slide is extended to the isthmus, the vastus lateralis is elevated distally (Fig. 10–26). The femur is cut on the lateral posterior side to the level selected for the transverse cut. The femur is then cut transversely to allow a lateral segment that is approximately 2 to 3 cm wide to be elevated. The vastus lateralis should remain attached both to the fragment proximal to the level of the transverse cut and to the femur distal to the transverse cut. If there is any concern about the strength of the femur distal to the extended slide, a cable should be placed around the femoral shaft distal to the transverse cut (see Fig. 10–23).

If there is a cemented implant in the femur, the extended slide can usually be cut on the anterior side by simply sawing across the cement column. This allows elevation of the extended slide femoral fragment and access to all the retained cement, which can be removed. Distal cement is removed with the drill, burr, and hook technique.

With a cementless implant, the large size of the implant probably will not allow the saw to cut across the femur for elevation of the fragment, necessitating the use of an osteotome to separate the anterior femoral bone. An initial saw cut is made in as much of the anterior bone as possible, and the remainder of the anterior cut is extended proximally with an osteotome (see Fig. 10–26). Once the anterior cortex has been cut with the osteotome, the osteotome is placed into the posterior cut, and the fragment is levered off the cementless

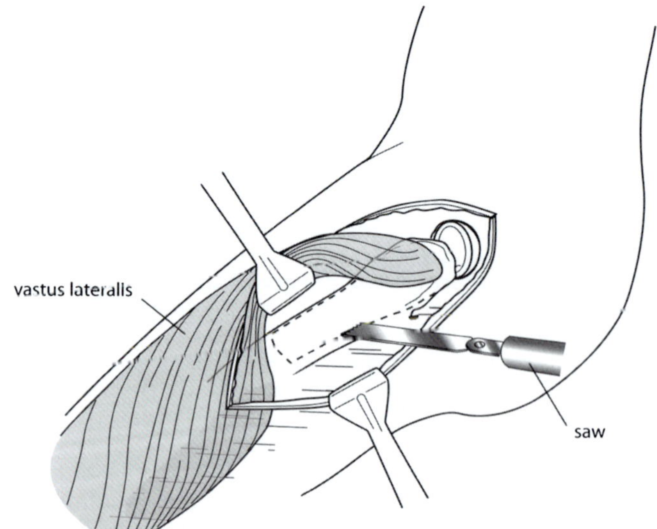

Figure 10–26 *The vastus lateralis is retracted anteriorly to expose the femoral bone just enough to create the extended slide. The slide is created by sawing the femoral bone from the greater trochanter distally to just above the isthmus and then transversely for 2 to 3 cm, depending on the size of the femur. The saw can be used to open as much of the anterior bone as possible, but an osteotome will be needed to complete the anterior cut of the femoral bone.*

implant. It is critical that if this fragment is attached to the trochanteric bed and the proximal lateral femur it be separated with a high-speed burr with a pointed attachment. If this is not done, the anterior elevation of the extended slide fragment can cause fracture of the trochanter from the diaphyseal segment or fragmentation of the trochanter. Either of these complications can result in postoperative weakness of the gluteus medius because of poor trochanteric bone stability.

A bone-ingrown implant can be removed once the extended slide fragment is elevated. Again, a pointed burr may be necessary to fragment bony fixation in the femoral canal. A good technique for detaching bone fixation from the medial side of the prosthesis is to pass a Gigli wire along the medial implant for the length of the slide. If the implant is fixed distal to the slide, the implant must be cut with a carbide bit from the Anspach set, and a trephine used to loosen the distal fragment.

Closure of Extended Slide. When the new prosthesis has been implanted into the femur, the extended slide is closed by reducing it and securing its reduction with wires (Fig. 10–27). If the vastus lateralis remained intact with the majority of the proximal fragment, usually only a distal wire is necessary. Repair of the vastus lateralis muscle and restoration of leg length with the revision arthroplasty keep the fragment reduced. If the vastus lateralis was elevated off the proximal fragment, two or three wires are necessary to maintain its secured, reduction position until bone healing occurs. Thus, the number of wires used is dependent on the amount of vastus lateralis muscle attached to the proximal fragment.

One technique that can be used to advance the trochanter and increase the tension on the gluteus medius muscle is to cut some of the distal end of the proximal segment (Fig. 10–28). Shortening the proximal segment and then reducing it against the cut edge of the distal segment advances the trochanter and muscle. The amount of bone removed from the distal end is generally only 1 to 2 cm, because that is the most that can be advanced and maintain contact between the cut surfaces. This advancement of the trochanter is not required in many hips, but it may be necessary when the tension of the gluteus medius needs to be increased to provide better muscle function and better stability of the hip joint. A second reason to advance the greater trochanter is to avoid its impingement on the pelvis during range of motion of the hip after reconstruction. In some cases, the implants, when reduced, change the offset of the hip such that impingement on the bone occurs, which can be avoided intraoperatively by advancing the trochanter.

Exposure for Revision with Trochanteric Nonunion

Some hips have a trochanteric nonunion from a previous hip replacement operation (Fig. 10–29). Most commonly, the greater trochanter has been a nonunited

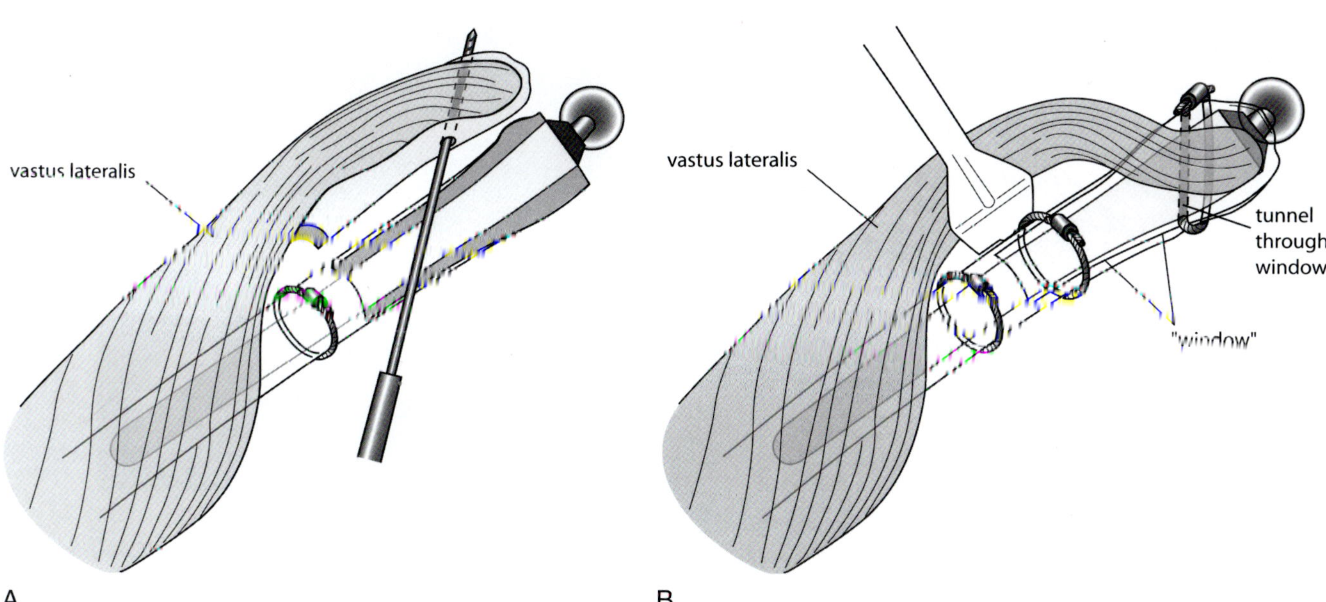

Figure 10–27 **A,** *A drill hole is passed through the greater trochanter for the most proximal wire used to close the extended slide fragment of the femoral bone. A cable distal to the extended slide is seen in position to prevent a fracture from either corner of the end of the slide.* **B,** *The extended slide is reduced to the femur and held with a proximal and distal wire or cable. The prophylactic cable is seen distal to the end of the slide.*

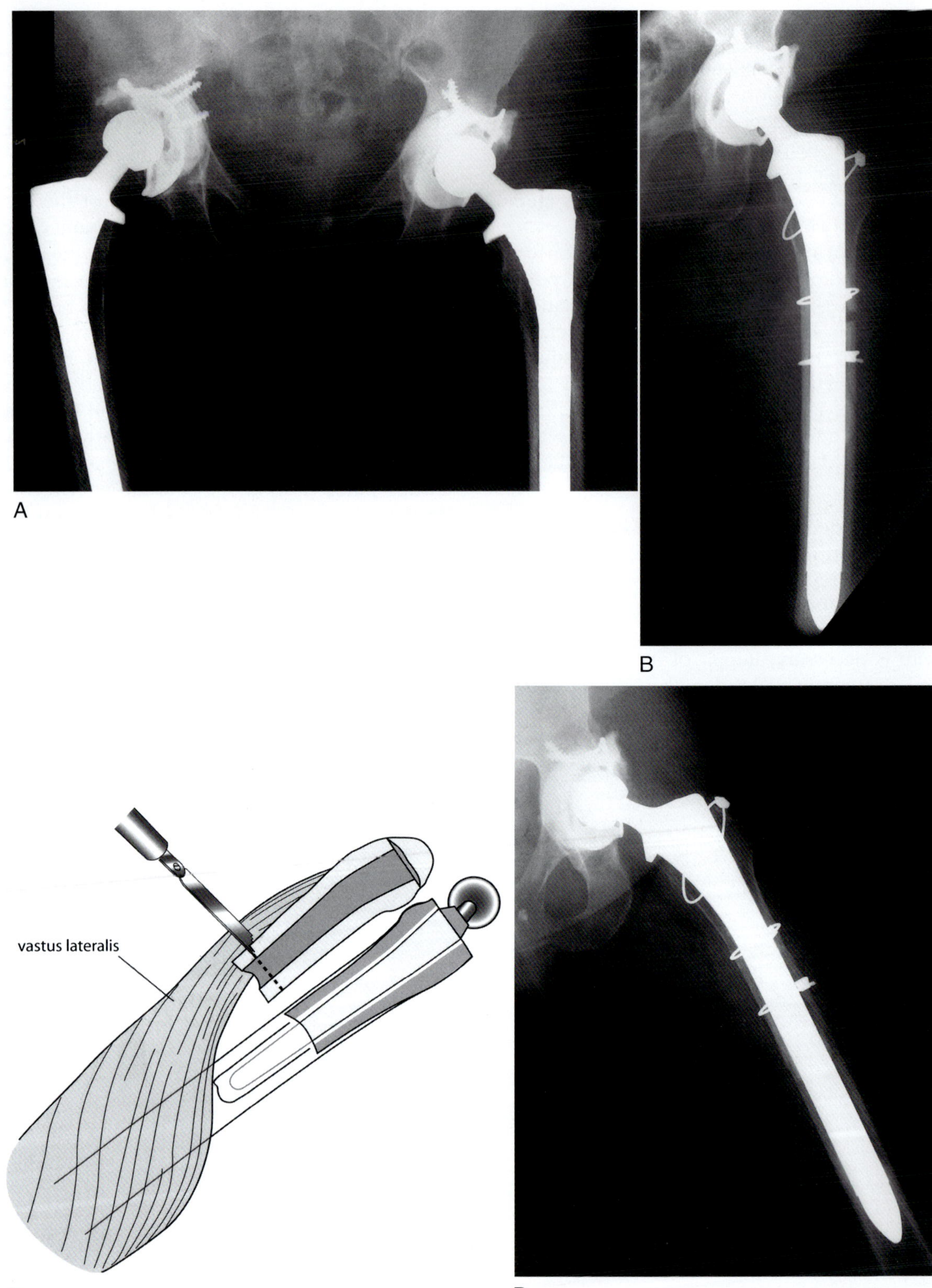

Figure 10–28   **A,** Preoperative x-ray. The left hip of this patient had a femoral stem revision because of pain from the chemicals of the recalled Sulzer cup. The acetabulum had already been revised. The stem was not loose and was cut with a trephine to remove the distal stem (see Fig. 10–49). **B,** The extended slide has been repaired, and the distal 2 cm of the proximal slide was removed to advance the greater trochanter. There is a gap between the proximal and distal fragments. The stem used for revision was the AML Solution (DePuy, Warsaw, Ind.). **C,** It is possible to remove 1 or 2 cm from the distal end of the slide with a saw and then reduce the slide into position and close it, as shown in Figure 10–27A and B. **D,** The 1-year postoperative x-ray shows that the initial gap between the proximal slide and the femoral diaphysis has healed and is filled with bone. There is bone-ingrowth fixation of the stem, as demonstrated by the spot weld at the distal coating and the proximal osteopenia.

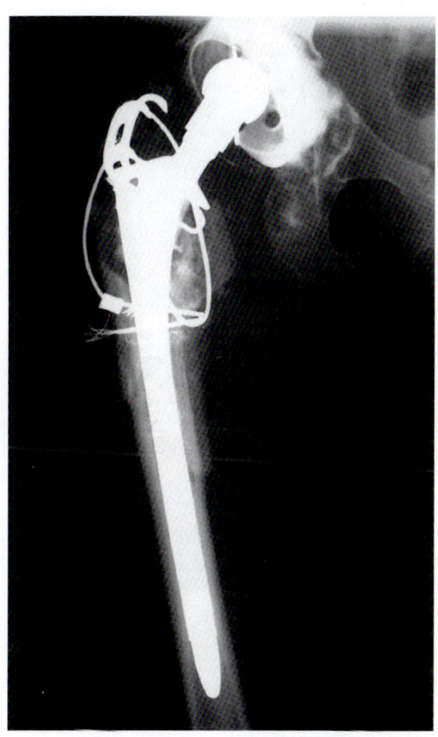

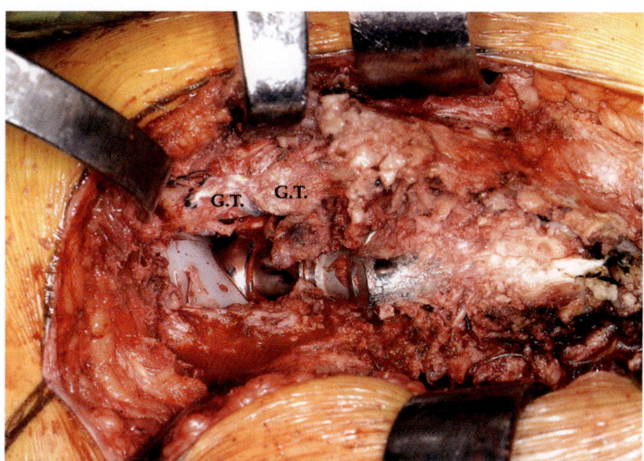

Figure 10–30   *The greater trochanter fragment is identified by the two labels, GT. The position of this greater trochanter bone, particularly with it being scarred, creates difficulty in exposing the acetabulum while retaining the femoral component.*

Figure 10–29   *The trochanter has migrated proximally, and the fragment is below the trochanteric hook. The cables broke because they could not resist the proximal migration of this now nonunited trochanteric bone fragment. The patient had a revision because of a loose and migrated acetabular construct. The removal of this greater trochanter fragment is illustrated in Figures 10–30 to 10–34.*

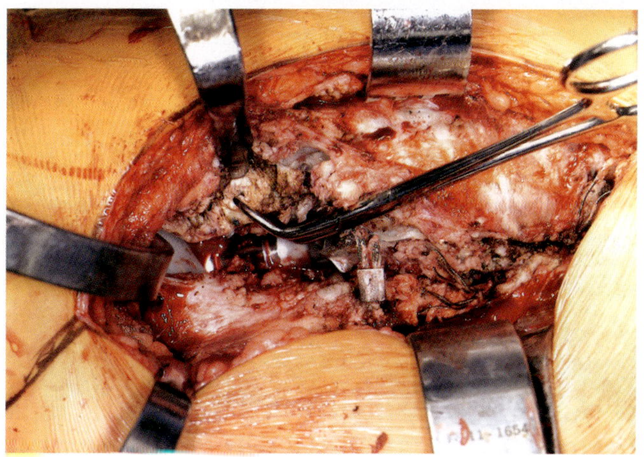

Figure 10–31   *Soft tissue has been removed over the top of the greater trochanter bone.*

bone fragment for years. The nonunited fragment is usually encased in scar tissue and retracted proximally, so that the chance of successful reattachment of the greater trochanter to the femoral bone is near zero. Often the greater trochanter bone is necrotic (which is probably one of the reasons that reattachment always fails). Leaving a nonunited trochanter fragment would create a click, or a sense of motion or "slipping," that is noticeable to the patient, leading to the baseless fear that subluxation of the hip is occurring. The best choice is to excise the greater trochanter fragment. This excision should be done carefully so that there is no disruption of the gluteus medius–vastus lateralis sling. The patient's function may be even better after the fragment is removed because there is better tension in the gluteus medius muscle. The removal of the greater trochanter also makes it much easier to expose the hip for the revision.

After the exposure of the hip joint, the greater trochanter fragment is identified (Fig. 10–30). Any soft tissue that is occluding visualization of the bone should be removed (Fig. 10–31). This work is done while the hip is still reduced so that the metal femoral head and neck do not obstruct access to the greater trochanter bone. Using a high-speed power burr is the simplest and fastest way to begin removing this bone (Fig. 10–32). Once the fragment is reduced in size and thinned, it can be more easily separated from the muscle attachment, using a sharp osteotome at the bone-muscle interface (Fig. 10–33). The osteotome can also isolate the remaining bone that was not destroyed with the burr. This bone is removed with a rongeur and further use of the high-speed burr (Fig. 10–34). When the trochanteric bone is entirely removed, there is easy access to the entire proximal femur and hip joint. The vastus lateralis–gluteus maximus sling remains intact and is retracted anteriorly (Fig. 10–35). For acetabular preparation, the femoral component is retracted anteriorly, easily accomplished in the absence of the greater

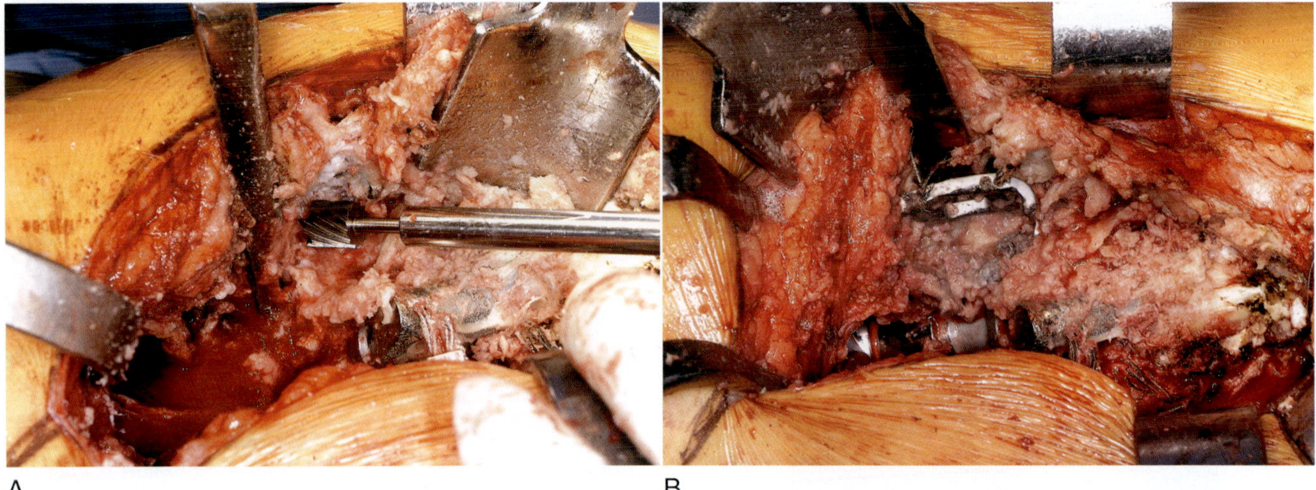

A   B

Figure 10–32 **A,** *A power burr is used to destroy the greater trochanter bone while preserving the gluteus medius–vastus lateralis muscle sling.* **B,** *The greater trochanter bone has been mostly removed, and the trochanteric hook from the cable system has been exposed and can easily be removed (see x-ray in Fig. 10–29).*

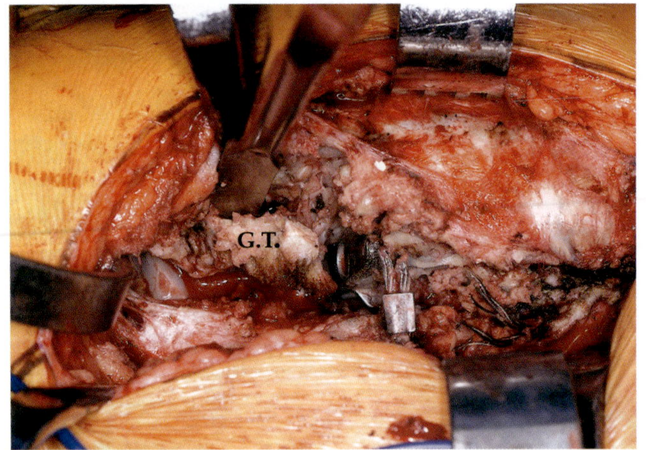

Figure 10–33 *The remaining greater trochanter fragment (GT) can be separated from its attached soft tissue with a sharp osteotome.*

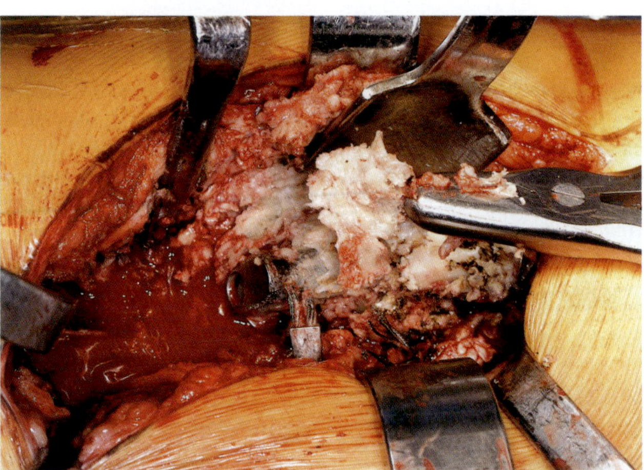

Figure 10–34 *When the remaining bony fragment has been separated from its soft tissue, it can be completely removed with a rongeur.*

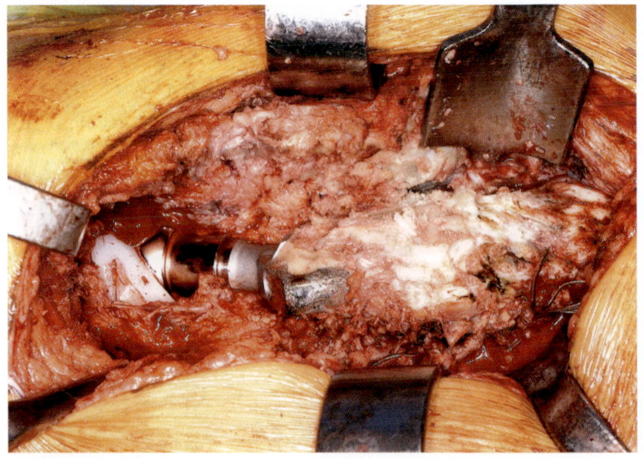

Figure 10–35 *The bone has been entirely removed, and there is an intact gluteus medius–vastus lateralis muscle sling along the anterior hip. The vastus lateralis has been elevated from the femoral bone to further mobilize the femur.*

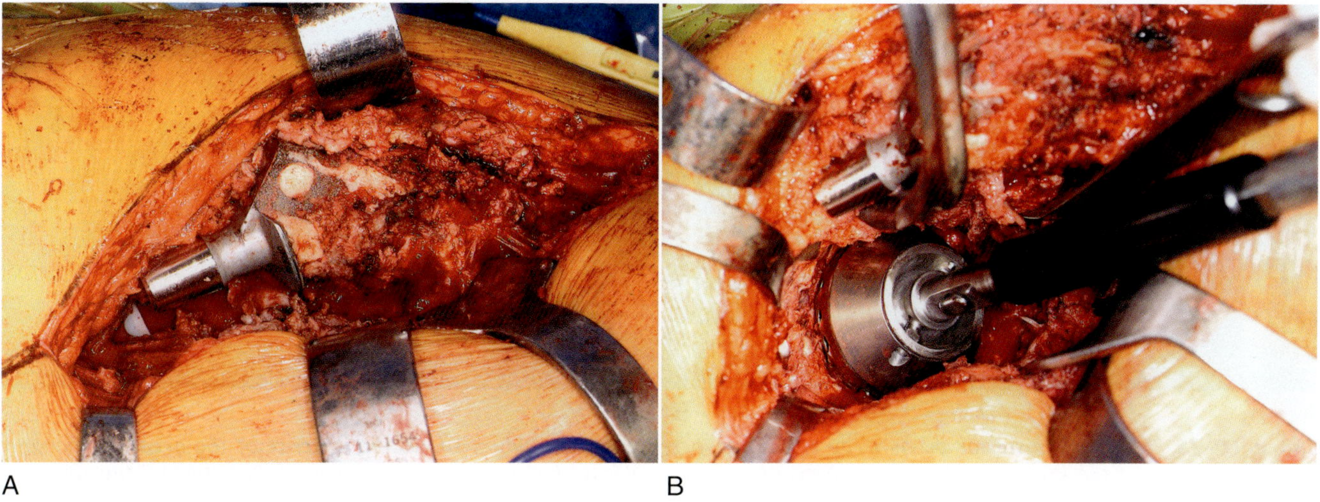

A   B

Figure 10–36 **A,** *The femoral component is mobilized and has been dislocated with the femoral head removed. All necrotic tissue has been excised from around the proximal femur, and the muscle sleeve is anterior.* **B,** *The femur can now be easily retracted anteriorly to allow acetabular preparation.*

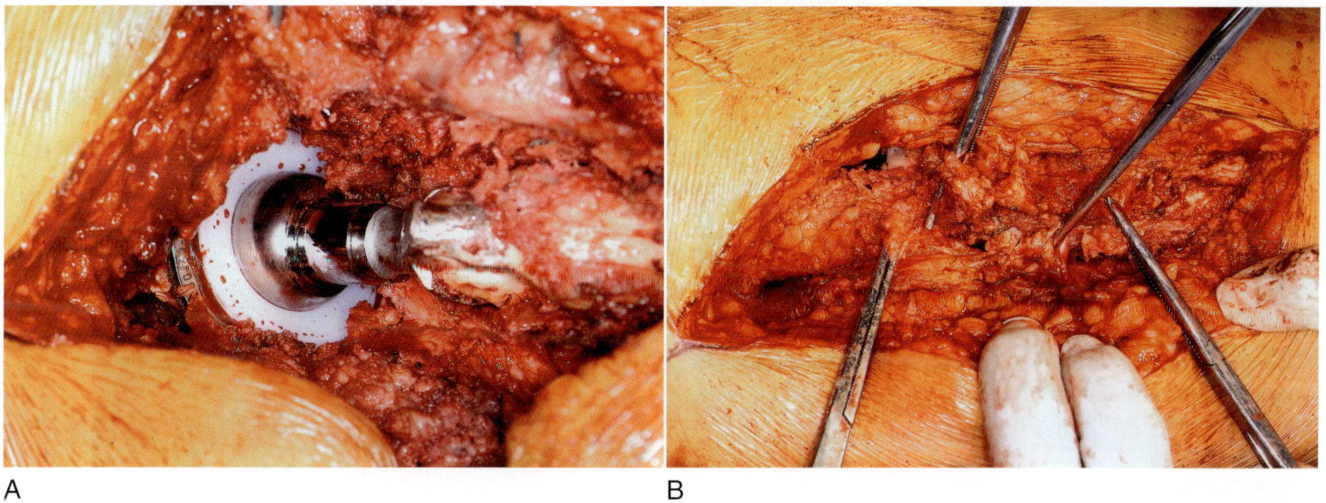

A   B

Figure 10–37 **A,** *The hip has been reconstructed, and the posterior muscle flap can be closed to the anterior muscle flap. The anterior muscle flap is seen lying against the anterior femoral neck. The mobility of the hip tissues can be compared with that in Figure 10–30, which was before removal of the greater trochanter fragment.* **B,** *The posterior and anterior flaps have been approximated with Kocher clamps, illustrating the excellent closure that can be obtained by eliminating dead space.*

trochanter bone (Fig. 10–36). When the reconstruction of the acetabulum or femur is complete, the hip is reduced and the posterior capsule and muscle are repaired to the anterior muscle flap to eliminate dead space around the hip and restore tension to the muscle sling (Fig. 10–37). The postoperative x-ray should verify elimination of the greater trochanter fragment (Fig. 10–38).

Loss of the trochanter affects walking capability. Figure 10–39 is a preoperative x-ray showing a nonunited, proximally migrated greater trochanter. The postoperative x-ray shows the absence of the trochanter fragment and shows a constrained liner that has been cemented into the acetabular shell (Fig. 10–40). Walking one gait cycle of heel-strike through toe-off produces a minimal lurch (Figs. 10–41 to 10–43) that will increase as the muscle fatigues, generally after about one-and-a-half blocks of walking. Thus, these patients do not have the same endurance as people with normal hip anatomy. However, patients with trochanter nonunion who have the trochanter fragment removed have a compromised but satisfactory gait that is better, in my opinion, than the gait of patients with retained fragments.

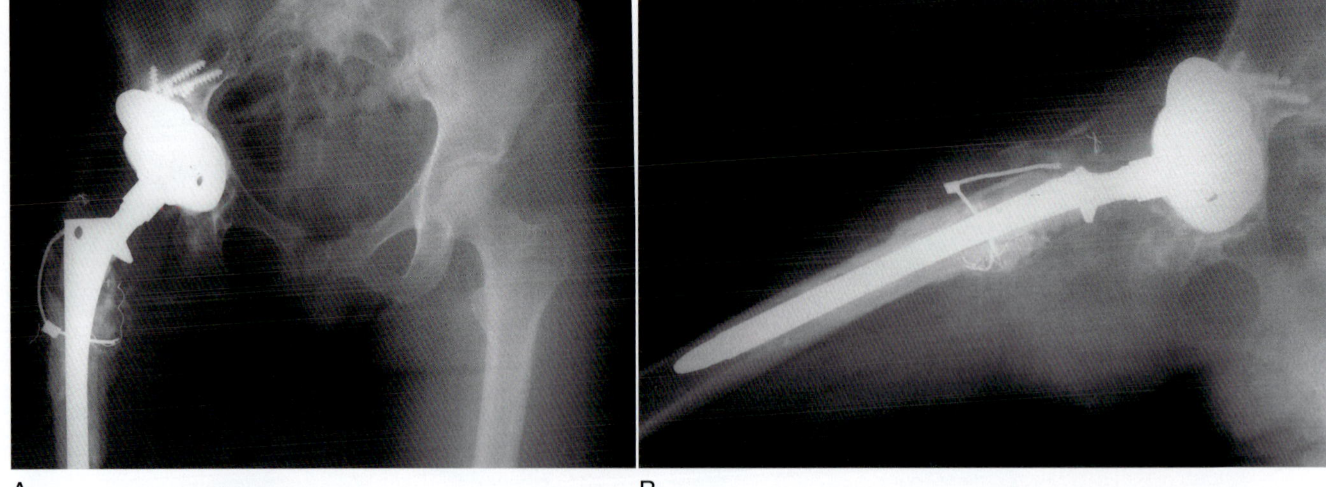

A

B

Figure 10–38 **A,** Anteroposterior pelvic x-ray of the reconstructed acetabulum shows the absence of the greater trochanter fragment. Not all of the broken cable was removed because it could not be visualized in the wound. **B,** Lateral x-ray shows the absence of the greater trochanter fragment.

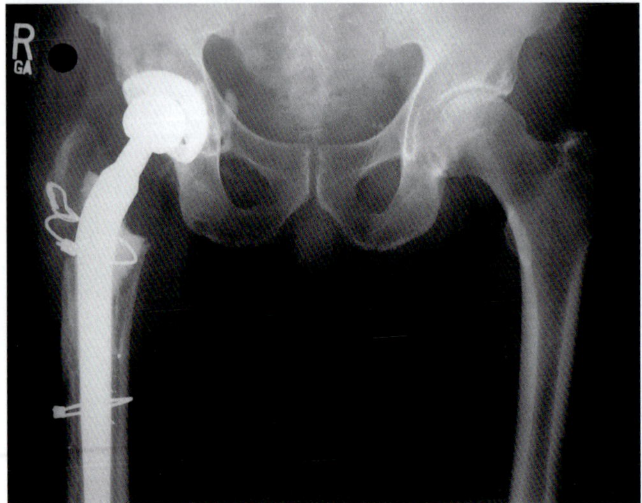

Figure 10–39 Preoperative x-ray of a patient with a non-united trochanter and dislocation.

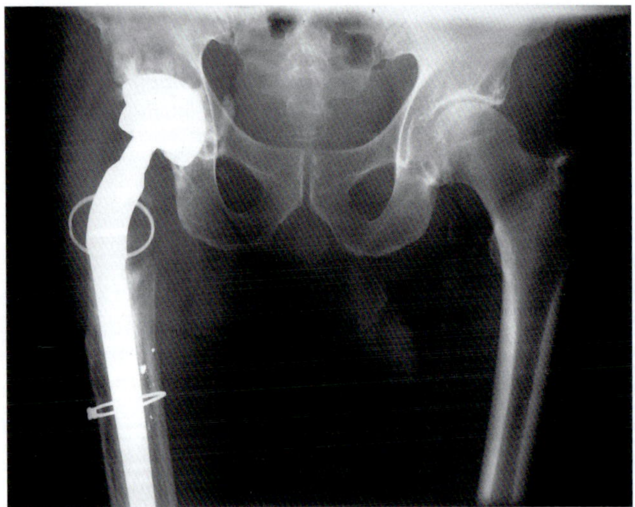

Figure 10–40 Postoperative x-ray shows that a constrained liner has been implanted to give mechanical stability to this hip, which had compromised soft tissue balance. The greater trochanter fragment has been removed. The metal ring from the constrained liner has disengaged and migrated distally around the proximal femoral stem. The femoral head is still constrained by the plastic.

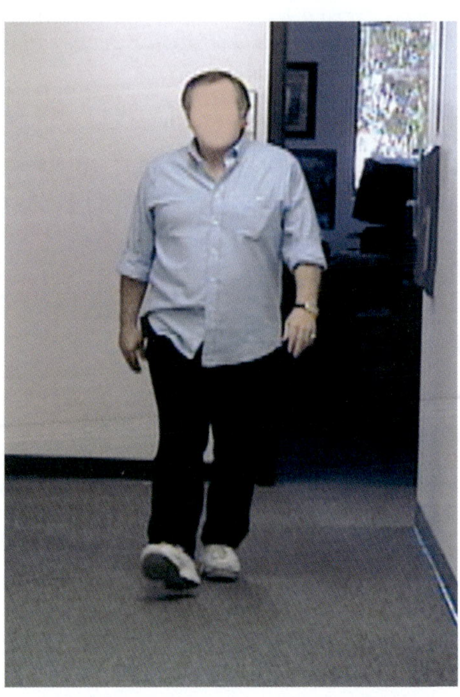

Figure 10–41 The patient whose x-rays are shown in Figures 10–39 and 10–40 walks a gait cycle. Observe the level of the right shoulder, which best demonstrates the amount of abductor lurch. This photograph was taken just before heel-strike and shows only a slight depression of the right shoulder.

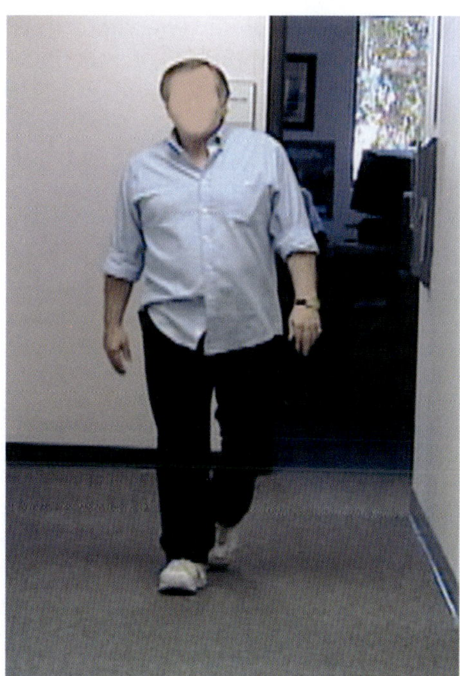

Figure 10–42 When the patient is fully loaded on the right leg, there is accentuation of the lurch, but it is not profound.

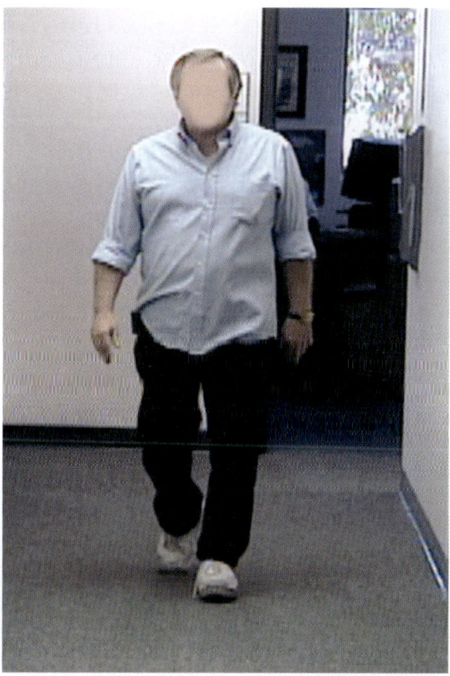

Figure 10–43 As the patient toes off, the shoulders are almost level. Observe that the right forearm is also swinging through during this gait cycle, which means that the patient is not holding it still to guard the right side.

Muscle Preservation

One of the most important features of successful revision surgery is retention of the muscle function of the hip and leg. In my experience, the most common cause

of pain after revision surgery is failure of good muscle function. The worst case is total loss of muscle function, as may occur with the gluteus medius muscle. The proximity of the superior gluteal nerve to the superior acetabulum is one cause of profound loss of gluteus medius function after revision surgery (see Fig. 10–2). Because so many acetabular components migrate superiorly, the nerve may be quite close to the work being done to reconstruct the acetabulum. Certainly, if a #7 bone graft or plates and screws are used on the ilium, the nerve is at risk. It is absolutely incumbent on the surgeon to ensure that all work is done subperiosteal to the gluteus medius.

I learned the importance of muscle function from Dr. Jacqueline Perry, an orthopedic kinesiologist with whom I worked at Rancho Los Amigos Hospital in Downey, California. Gait studies we performed made it apparent that we could have a great postoperative x-ray but a patient with a poor clinical result. Most often this occurred because of severe functional disability caused by muscles that did not work properly or fatigued rapidly. Patients with poor muscle function also had more aching at night because of muscle fatigue. I realized that it was often easier to get satisfactory implant position and fixation than to retain muscle function.

It is important for the surgeon to understand the patient's preoperative muscle function so that realistic postoperative expectations can be estimated. Before revision, the hip has often been shortened by proximal migration of the acetabulum or sinking of the femoral component. A hip that is shortened for longer than 3 months has lost at least 50% of the conditioning of the gluteus medius muscle, and it can take a year after surgery for this muscle function to approach "normal" on gait analysis studies. Even after primary total hip replacements, achieving normal function of the gluteus medius can take as long as 1 year. If there is profound preoperative weakness of the gluteus medius muscle (or the abductor complex, consisting of the gluteus medius and upper gluteus maximus muscles), the patient should be told to expect to have a permanent limp and limited endurance capability.

The muscles that are most commonly injured during revision surgery are the gluteus medius, gluteus maximus, and vastus lateralis muscles. The gluteus medius can be injured by too aggressive splitting of that muscle with a posterior approach. The gluteus minimus muscle can be injured by aggressive or incorrect muscle splitting with an anterior approach. Rough retraction can also injure these muscles, more so than their controlled cutting.

Muscles that have been incised more than twice become more sensitive to injury and more atrophied than would be expected based on the objective damage done to them. Therefore, in complex revisions or in patients with multiple revisions, it is wise to use an extended slide exposure rather than a direct anterior or direct posterior exposure. The extended slide exposure protects the muscles because the bone is cut instead. Bone repairs itself well no matter how many times it is cut, whereas muscles are more sensitive to frequent injury. Therefore, the extended slide approach may be chosen for muscle protection and not just because of the ease of femoral preparation.

Muscle Preservation Techniques

Gluteus Medius. Protection of the gluteus medius requires knowledge of its innervation. The gluteus medius is innervated by the superior gluteal nerve, which is present within the muscle 5 cm above the tip of the greater trochanter *when the hip is in its normal position.* Sometimes with revision surgery the trochanter is elevated, and the tip of the greater trochanter is itself 5 cm above its normal position. Therefore, when planning revision surgery, the position of the nerve should be calculated preoperatively based on the normal position of the tip of the trochanter (Fig. 10–44). If it is necessary to attach implants or bone graft to the ilium, protection of this nerve is paramount. Damage to this nerve results in a totally neurologically dead gluteus medius, resulting in a permanent, profound limp and pain for the patient.

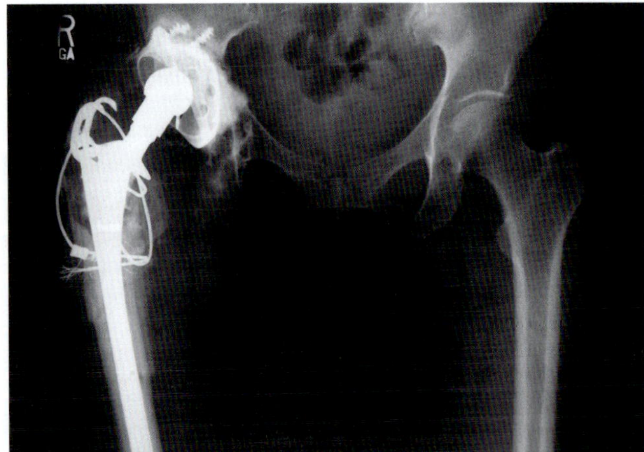

Figure 10–44 *This acetabular construct has migrated superiorly, as evidenced in this x-ray by the zone 3 space and the broken screws. This proximal migration means that the superior edge of the acetabulum is at the level of the inferior gluteal nerve (compared to the level of the ilium of the left hip, where the nerve would be present just above the superior subchondral bone). When an acetabular component has migrated this far proximally, it may cause irreparable damage to the nerve. Thus, if the patient has a profound limp preoperatively, he or she must be advised that the limp will be present postoperatively.*

Gluteus Maximus. The gluteus maximus muscle is the second most important abductor of the hip (after the gluteus medius) and is most commonly injured by aggressive proximal splitting. This technique causes damage to the inferior gluteal nerve, which innervates the superior head of the gluteus maximus. This can leave a patient with a permanent lurch, even if the gluteus medius muscle functions. This combination results in poor endurance of the abductor complex, causing a limp and fatigue and pain after only one-and-a-half blocks of walking. There is no reason to take a finger and split the entire gluteus maximus (which endangers the nerve); instead, it should be split in line with its fibers using the coagulation Bovie. If the Bovie electrocautery is used, the nerve will be stimulated (and contract) before it is totally injured, and the surgeon can stop. The extent of separation of this muscle should be limited to only that necessary for adequate exposure of the acetabulum (Fig. 10–45); it is not necessary to split this muscle proximally for its entirety.

Vastus Lateralis (*see "Simple Techniques for Revision Total Hip Replacement"*). The best way to expose the femoral shaft is by doing as little damage as possible to the vastus lateralis muscle. This means elevating the vastus lateralis posteriorly from the interosseous membrane toward the anterior femur, using a periosteal elevator. As this muscle is peeled from the interosseous membrane anteriorly, the perforating vessels can be visualized and independently clamped, cut, and cauterized, thus decreasing hemorrhage in the wound and into the muscle (Fig. 10–46). The sacrifice of these vessels is necessary to enable muscle retraction anteriorly, so it is beneficial to do so in a controlled manner that minimizes the amount of devascularized muscle and the amount of hemorrhage into the muscle, which further damages muscle fibers. The periosteal elevator exposes the vessel on the posterior side of the muscle. The vessel is ligated with two clamps and cut between the clamps. The two cut ends are cauterized to prevent them from bleeding, and the muscle is then retracted anterior to the femur to expose the femoral shaft. This technique can be used for the entire length of the femur. The first vessels are usually encountered about 7 cm below the lesser trochanter. When work with the femur is completed, the vastus lateralis should be repaired by sutures to its bed at the interosseous membrane. I make an incision through the fascia of the vastus lateralis muscle just anterior to the interosseous membrane to permit this suture repair. This leaves a bit of the muscle still attached to the interosseous membrane. By the time the work on the femur is completed, any necrotic muscle will be evident—dark and purplish in color, with a ragged appearance compared with the normal muscle color and texture—and a large rongeur can be used to peel away all the dead fibers. This sig-

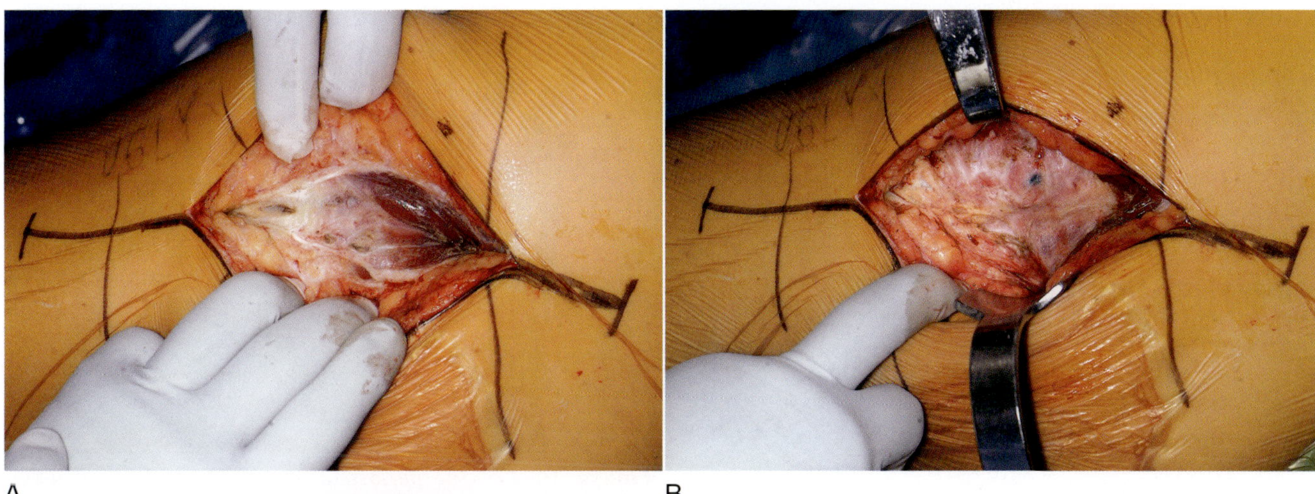

A

B

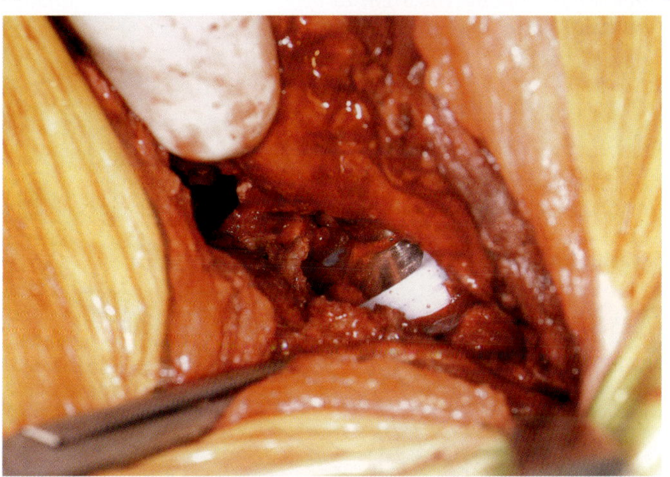

C

Figure 10–45 **A,** The iliotibial band has been divided distally, and the gluteus maximus muscle proximally. The good quality of this muscle can be ascertained by its color and texture. The muscle has been divided gently with a Bovie electrocautery and has not been divided any further than necessary for exposure. **B,** At the right edge of the wound, the division of the gluteus maximus muscle can be seen. The muscle is being retracted anteriorly and posteriorly to expose the posterior hip. The blue dot locates the greater trochanter. **C,** The posterior hip structures have been incised, and the superior margin of the gluteus maximus can be seen just below the subcutaneous fat. Division of the gluteus maximus has been carried just superior to the superior edge of the acetabulum, because that is all that is needed for exposure.

Figure 10–46 The vastus lateralis muscle is peeled off the interosseous membrane using a periosteal elevator to expose the perforating arteries. The perforating arteries are clamped and then divided with the coagulation Bovie electrocautery. The cut ends are also coagulated. This allows anterior retraction of the muscle without much blood loss and with minimal muscle trauma and necrosis. (See "Simple Techniques for Revision Total Hip Replacement" *for a dynamic demonstration of this technique.*)

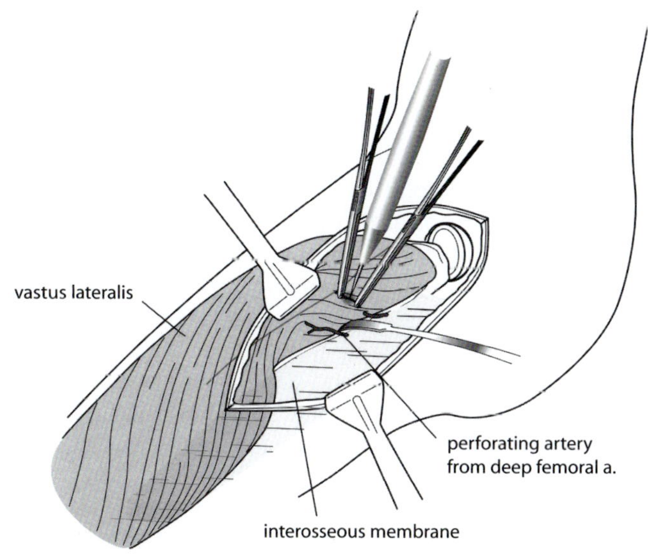

nificantly reduces the risk of infection and drainage from this tissue. This technique optimizes the postoperative function of the vastus lateralis muscle by preventing injury to the maximum amount of muscle possible.

FEMORAL PREPARATION

Removal of Implant

The initial steps for removal of the implant were delineated earlier in the exposure section. The proximal end of the femur must be cleared of all soft tissue and necrotic bone, as described. If the femoral neck bone is not necrotic, I remove it with a saw to nearly the level of the lesser trochanter to expose the most proximal implant. For some porous coated implants, this provides enough exposure for the bone fixation to the coating to be loosened using a high-speed drill with a pointed burr, allowing the implant to be extracted from the femur. Even if the burr does not destroy enough fixation to allow implant removal, it clears the lateral side of the prosthesis in the trochanteric bed and proximal lateral femur so that a window or extended slide can be used safely without the risk of fracturing the trochanter. The use of very thin, flexible osteotomes to break up the bone fixation in the proximal femur has been advocated, but I do not subscribe to that technique. When mature, the bone fixation has the structure of strong cortical bone; therefore, I believe that the power burr is a more efficient and safer tool for removing this fixation.

When the full extent of the power burr has been reached and the implant is still fixed, the remainder of the implant must be exposed by techniques previously described. Exposure of the femoral bone is necessary, and elevation of the vastus lateralis should be done with the muscle-saving technique. An extended slide or window can then be used to finish disrupting the fixation to allow removal of the implant proximally.

Usually the implant has an extraction device that allows it to be delivered out of the femur. If there is no extraction device, a bone tamp or periosteal elevator can be used under the collar, if present, allowing the stem to be malleted out of the femoral canal (Fig. 10–47). Another option is to make a divot in the metal with a carbide metal-cutting burr and then use a tool in the divot to pound the implant proximally (see Fig. 10–22).

If the implant is a bone-ingrown stem with fixation in the diaphysis beyond the level of the isthmus, the implant may have to be cut and the proximal and distal halves removed separately. This technique was initially developed for the AML stem (Anatomic Medullary Locking, Depuy, Warsaw, Ind.). The proximal femoral stem is exposed with an extended slide. At the distal

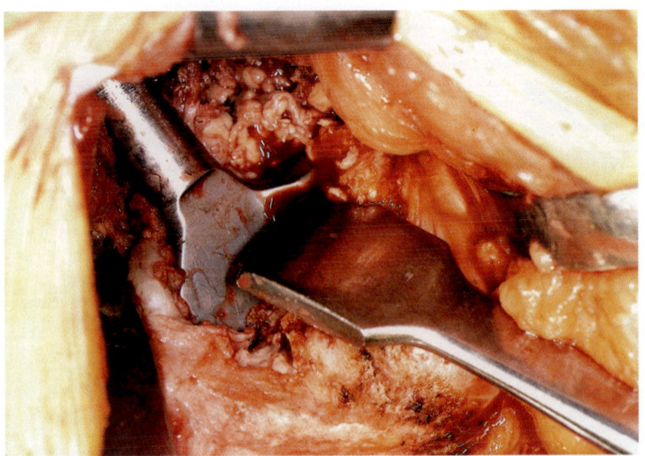

Figure 10–47 *The periosteal elevator is positioned under the collar to allow the stem to be malleted out of the canal in an axial direction.*

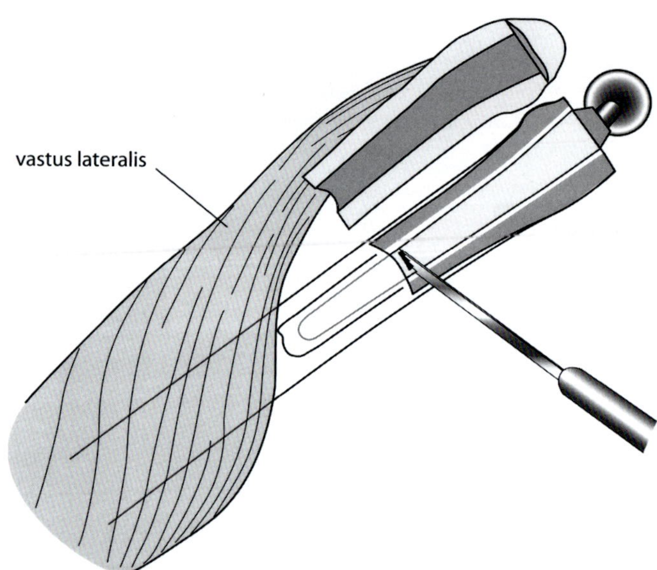

Figure 10–48 *The metal carbide burr divides the femoral stem at the distal end of the extended slide.*

end of the extended slide (which should be at the proximal end of the isthmus), the stem is divided with a carbide metal-cutting burr (Fig. 10–48; *see "Simple Techniques for Revision Total Hip Replacement"*).

The proximal stem is removed. The fixation that remains between the distal circular stem and the femur is disrupted with a trephine cutting tool (Fig. 10–49). At the interface between the metal and the bone, the trephine is introduced and drilled distally (Fig. 10–50). Appropriate-sized trephines should be selected, and because they can become dull, it is important to have at least two of each size available.

Once the trephine has disrupted the fixation interface between the metal and the bone, the distal metal

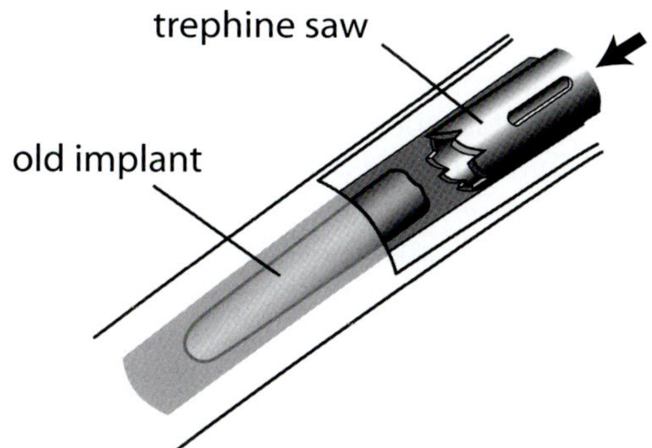

Figure 10–49 *The trephine cutting tool is positioned to cut at the interface between the distal femoral stem and the bone.*

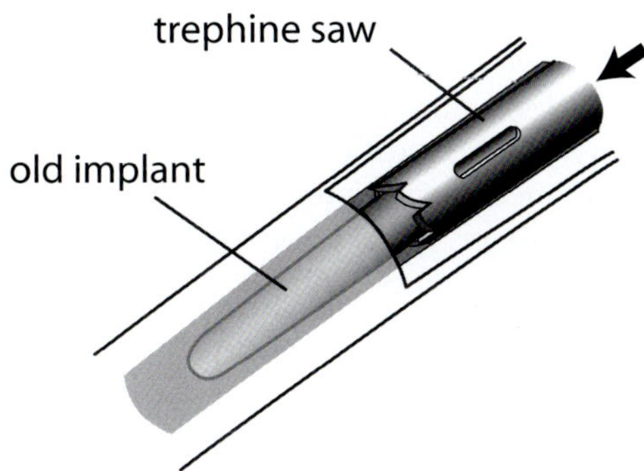

Figure 10–50 *The trephine is drilled at the interface to disrupt it, so that the femoral stem can be lifted out of the femur.*

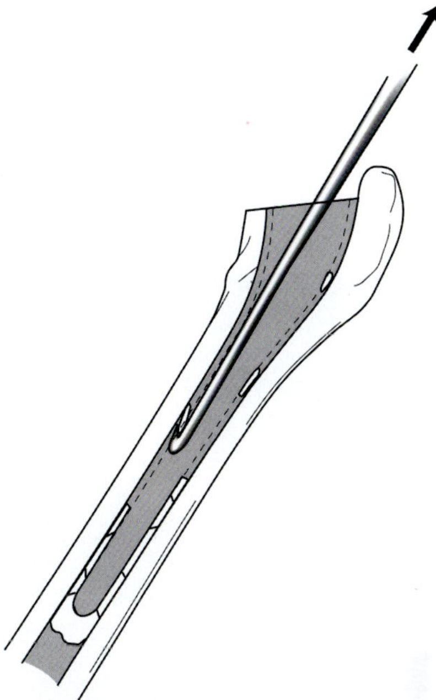

Figure 10–51 *The cement column is fragmented by the osteome, and the fragments can be removed from the canal by gripping them and lifting them out or by using a backhoe-type tool to retract them proximally.*

rod of the stem can be easily removed. The bone is then prepared by reaming the isthmus and the distal femur for the new implant. The extended slide is repaired once the new implant is in place (see Fig. 10–27).

Removal of Cement

Whenever possible, cement should be removed from the proximal end of the femur without violating the intact structural tube of the femur. This is not possible when there are long cement "tails" or when the cement is still rigidly interdigitated into the femoral bone. In these cases, an extended slide is the best technique for cement removal.

Cement removal begins by meticulous cleaning of the proximal opening of the femur. All fibrous tissue from around the edge of the cortical bone of the neck should be removed. If the cortical bone of the neck is gone due to necrosis, the osteolytic bone and tissue should also be removed (see Fig. 10–16). The goal of this cleaning technique is to expose the interface between the cement and the bone so that the cement osteotomes can be used most effectively.

When the interface between the bone and cement is clear, the cement column is initially separated from the bone by using a straight osteotome at that interface. The proximal cement fragments into pieces of variable size (Fig. 10–51), depending on how well fixed the cement was to the bone (very small pieces when well fixed). If the x-rays show a continuous radiolucent line around the cement column for its entire length, it is possible that the cement will come out of the femur with the femoral stem (Fig. 10–52). Sometimes this loose cement column does not come out with the stem simply because wedges of cement are blocking its extraction. In that situation, removing the proximal metaphyseal and diaphyseal cement with the osteotome can permit the entire distal cement column to be removed with its cement plug.

When the cement column cannot be removed in large segments, the surgeon must patiently remove the metaphyseal and upper diaphyseal cement with osteotomes. At first, the visibility of the interface between the cement and the bone is good, but as the cement column gets deeper into the diaphysis, and as the bow of the diaphyseal bone comes into play, the distinction between bone and cement is not so easy to see. When this occurs, the surgeon has to decide whether to use a cement removal system or make a femoral window (already described) to remove the cement.

To remove the distal cement, I prefer using the drills and burrs of the LINK cement removal system. Once the central hole has been made through the cement plug, backhoe-type tools are used to extract the cement from the walls of the femur (see Fig. 10–25). Once the walls are free of cement, the femur can be prepared for the new implant.

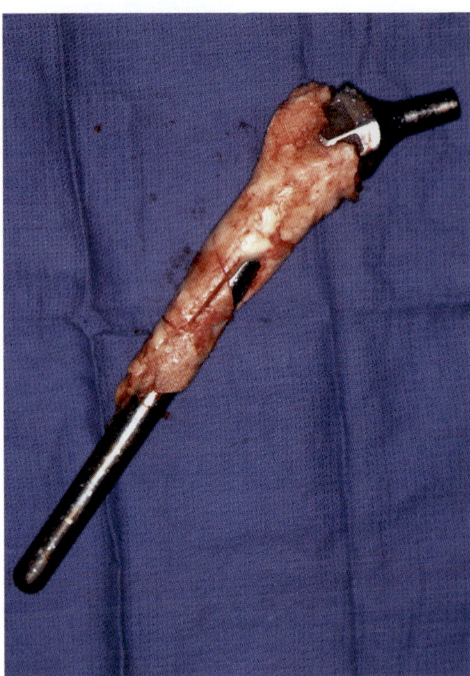

Figure 10–52 *A femoral stem with the cement attached. This can happen when there is a complete cement-bone interface seen on the x-ray.*

Removal of Neocortex

When a bone-ingrown or cemented implant is removed, there is an interface between the fixation surface and the original femoral cortex. This is termed a *neocortex*, because it forms as a cortical layer around the fixation surface of the stem and often has cancellous trabeculae that radiate from the neocortex to provide attachment to the original cortex (Figs. 10–53 and 10–54).

The neocortex, which can be easily visualized when looking into the femur after removal of an implant (Fig. 10–55), should be disrupted, and the fixation surface for the new implant should be prepared to the original cortex. If the new implant is to be cementless and bone ingrown, removal of the neocortex allows proper sizing; retention of the neocortex can result in a painful and ultimately loose implant. With cemented implants, failure to remove the neocortex results in poor fixation and a rapidly loosening implant. If the neocortex cannot be completely removed, it should at least be grooved so that some mechanical interlock occurs with the new implant. The inner surface of the neocortex is very smooth, and there is no way that cement can interdigitate with it.

Removal of Fibrous Tissue

Fibrous tissue forms in a femoral canal containing a loose implant (Fig. 10–56). After removal of a loose noncemented implant, it is imperative that all the fibrous tissue be removed so that the host cortical bone is available for fixation to the new implant. Although

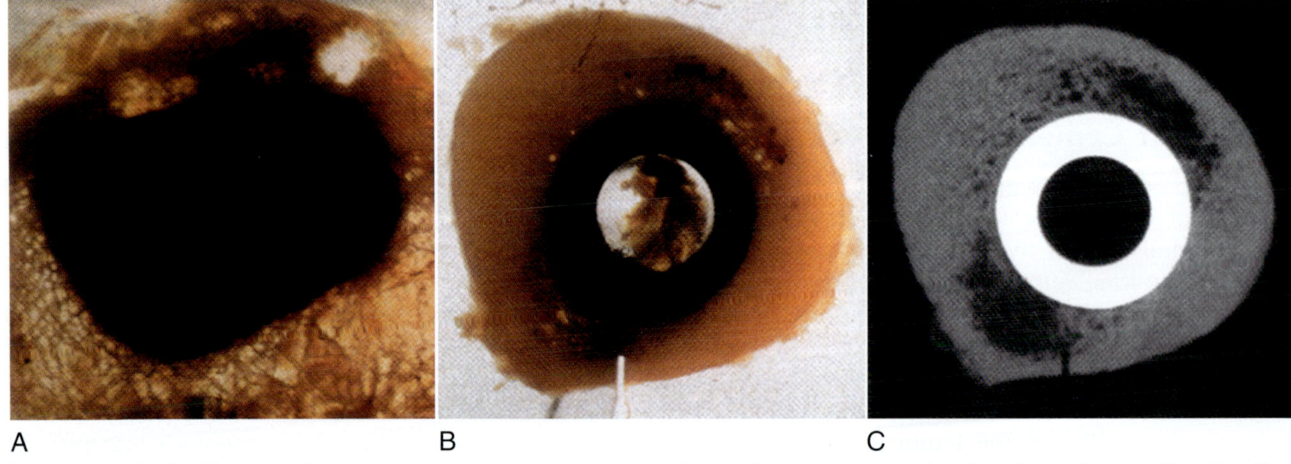

A   B   C

Figure 10–53 **A,** *Histology from an autopsy implant retrieval shows that new cortex that has formed immediately adjacent to the femoral stem and is separate from the original femoral cortex. The level of the femur is just above the lesser trochanter. The new cortex is the dark brown layer adjacent to the black metal of the stem. Cancellous bone radiates from the cortex surrounding the black stem to the original metaphyseal cortex.* **B,** *Autopsy implant retrieval of the distal end of a femoral stem that was fully grit-blasted to achieve bone attachment. There is intimate contact between the stem and the cortical bone of the femur.* **C,** *Microradiograph of the histology section in Figure 10–53B. The white circle is the stem. Between the 7 and 12 o'clock positions (left side of the stem) is a layer of cortical bone attached to the stem. Cancellous bone radiates from that layer of cortical bone and attaches the neocortex to the original cortex.*

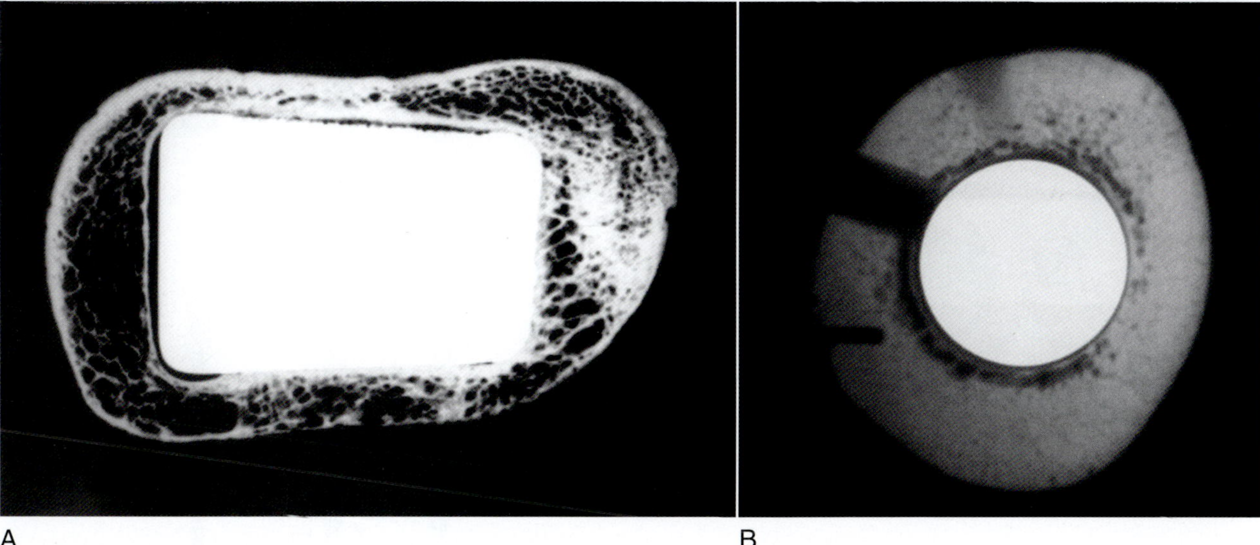

A   B

Figure 10–54 **A,** *Microradiograph of the histology section in Figure 10–53A. The neocortex is seen surrounding the white metal stem. On the left side (lateral stem), where there was only smooth metal, there is no attachment of the bone to the stem, but there is neocortex. The neocortex and cortical bone are connected by cancellous trabeculae.* **B,** *Microradiograph of a different stem that is smooth (not grit-blasted) in the diaphysis of the femur. The neocortex around the smooth stem is evident, with cancellous trabeculae from the neocortex to the diaphyseal cortical bone. Sections have been taken from this autopsy retrieval specimen for study.*

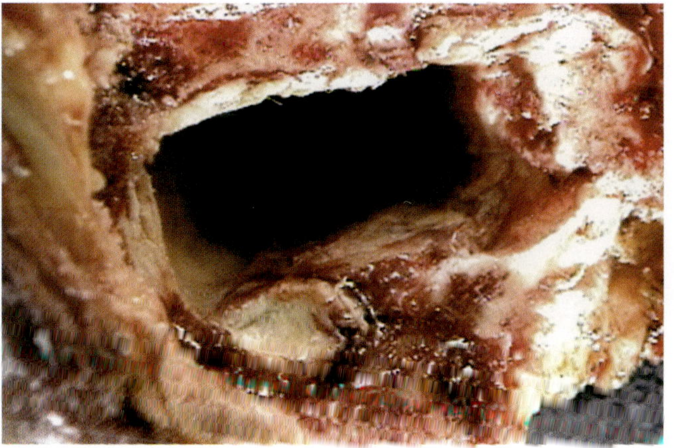

Figure 10–55 *Intraoperative view of neocortex that remains after removal of the stem. This cortex will have to be removed using a high-speed burr or osteotome to allow implantation of the new stem against the femoral cortex. The neocortex takes the shape of the implant used (the implant removed in this case was rectangular, so the neocortex formed adjacent to the implant in that shape).*

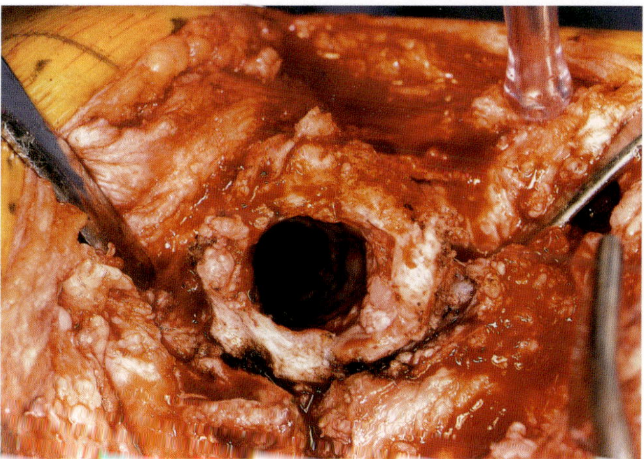

Figure 10–56 *The endosteal surface of the femoral canal is lined with fibrous tissue after a loose femoral component has been removed.*

the fibrous tissue can be removed using curettes, I prefer a high-speed burr. By lightly moving the burr along the endosteal surface in a clockwise manner (so that the entire surface is debrided), the surgeon can easily loosen fibrous tissue from the bone and remove the tissue from the femur. To confirm that the femoral canals are clear, a backhoe or long curette is moved around the circumference of bone, again in a clockwise fashion, to ensure that all the fibrous tissue has been removed (Fig. 10–57).

Reaming

Almost all revision implants allow distal fixation, such as the Zimmer modular revision (ZMR) stem (Warsaw, Ind.) (Fig. 10–58). The canal is reamed to determine the correct size of the stem (Fig. 10–59). Soft tissue protectors can be used to prevent injury during reaming (Fig. 10–60). The ZMR stem is tapered and fully coated

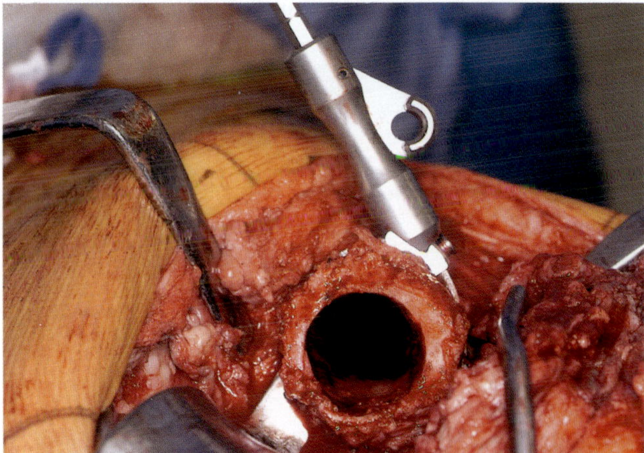

Figure 10–57 *Appearance of the femoral canal once the fibrous tissue has been removed (compare with Fig. 10–56).*

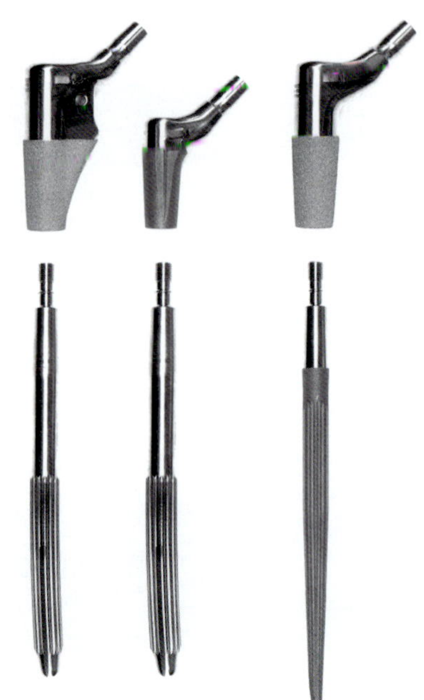

Figure 10–58 *Zimmer modular revision (ZMR) stems.*

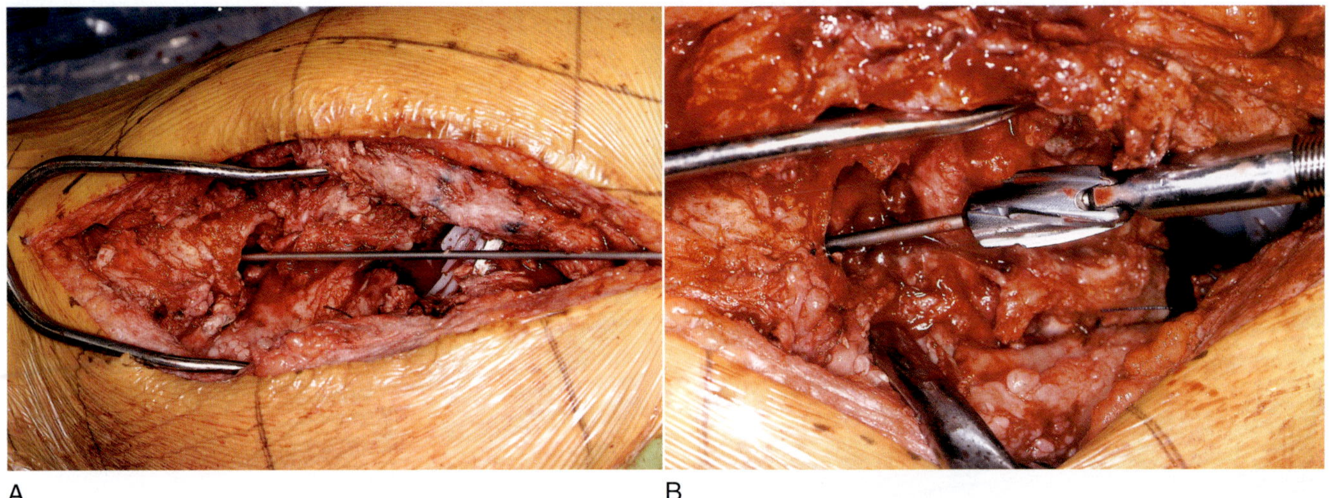

A B

Figure 10–59 *A, The guidewire for the flexible reamer has been placed into the femoral canal. Observe the amount of missing proximal femur, as demonstrated by the position of the acetabular cup. B, The flexible reamer is passed, using the guidewire to keep it centralized in the femoral canal.*

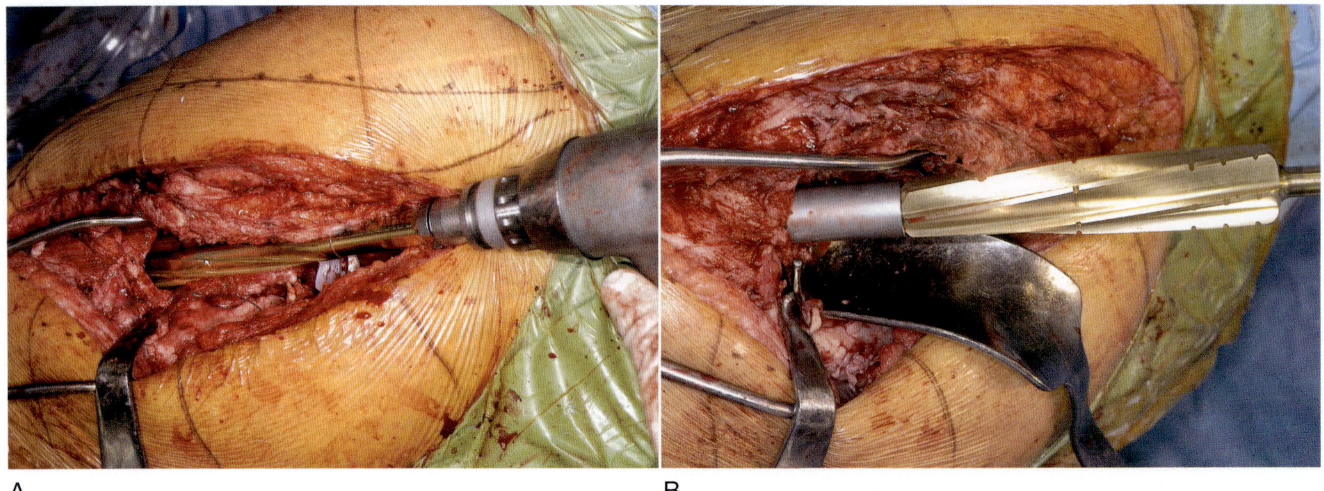

A B

Figure 10–60 *A, The reamer is used to prepare the femur for the ZMR stem. B, Sleeves can be used to protect the soft tissues from injury when the reamer is activated.*

so that it will achieve fixation over a long distance of the diaphysis. This tapering reduces the stiffness of the stem and permits its length to be implanted without violation of the anterior cortex. The isthmus must be preserved for satisfactory initial rotational stability of almost all revision stems, including the ZMR. There should be solid contact with the reamer over 7 cm of diaphysis for satisfactory stability. Implantation of the stem provides a long surface for excellent permanent bone ingrowth fixation (Fig. 10–61). The modularity of the stem allows its proximal segment to be correctly positioned for anteversion and offset (Fig. 10–62).

Durable results have been achieved with revision stems that have fixation in the diaphysis. There are different brands of stems, all with the same principle of distal fixation; some of these are monoblock, and some are modular. My choice for a revision implant is one that can provide diaphyseal fixation.

Stem Implantation

Once the femur has been prepared by reaming and broaching, the final stem implantation is delayed until after acetabular reconstruction. As stated earlier, I prepare the femur before the acetabulum partly because it is my habit and partly because, with the initial exposure for revision surgery, decisions regarding femoral exposure (e.g., extended slide or window) must be made for removal of the implanted femoral stem. It is most efficient for me to complete the femoral preparation before returning to the acetabulum. If the femoral component is grossly loose and can be manually extracted from the femur, the order of preparing the femur and the acetabulum is of no consequence. In fact, in that situation it might be more efficient to do the acetabular exposure and reconstruction first, because removing the soft tissue around the acetabulum would also help mobilize the proximal femur.

Regardless of whether the femoral or acetabular preparation is completed first, the final implantation of the femur is the last step of the revision. This should be a simple matter of malleting the implant into place, because once the femoral preparation is complete, the implantation of a distally fixed stem is straightforward. The only complication that could occur is related to incorrect sizing of the implant. If the implant is too small and loose, the surgeon must exchange the small stem for one of the correct size, despite the cost of the implant. If the stem is too big and a longitudinal

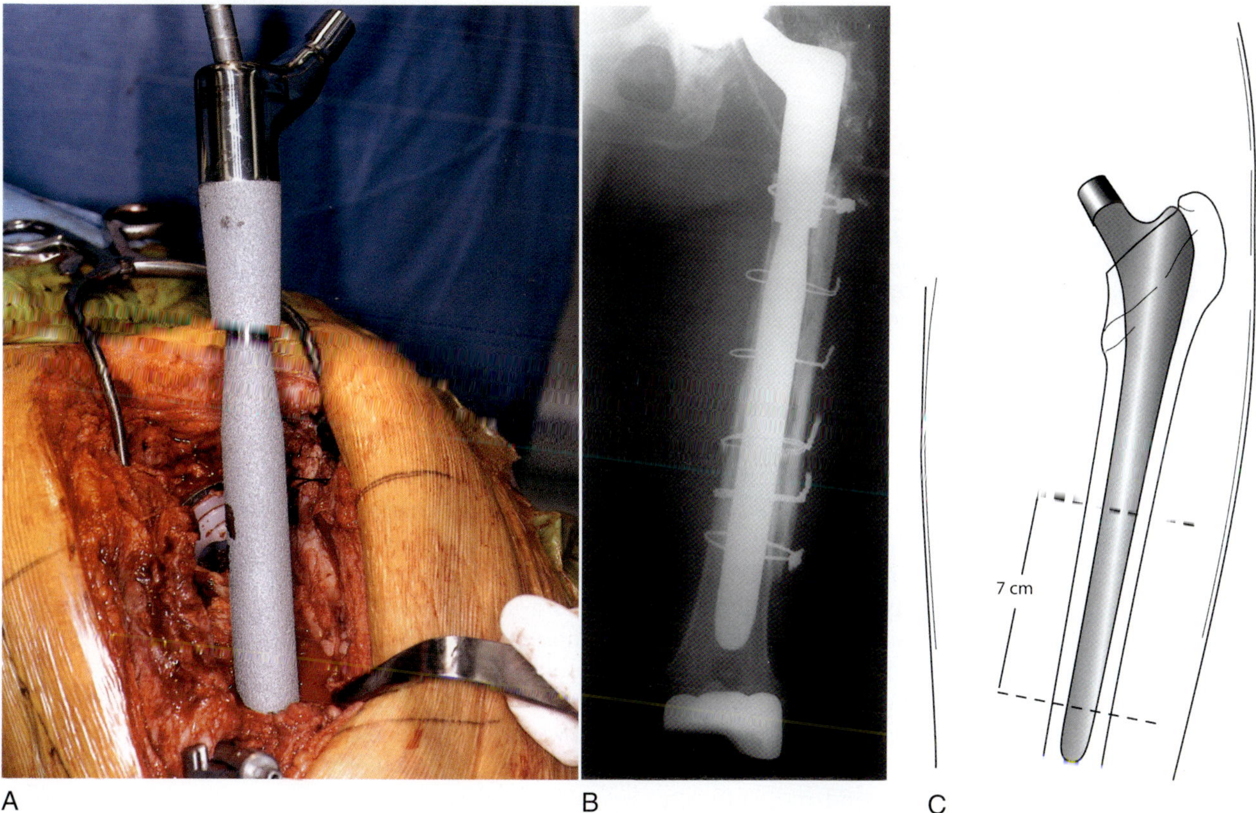

ABC

Figure 10–61 *A, The long fixation surface of the porous ZMR stem. B, The position of the ZMR stem in the femur as seen on x-ray, showing an area of contact that is at least 7 cm long. C, Diagram illustrating that the grip of a revision stem should be at least 7 cm through the isthmus.*

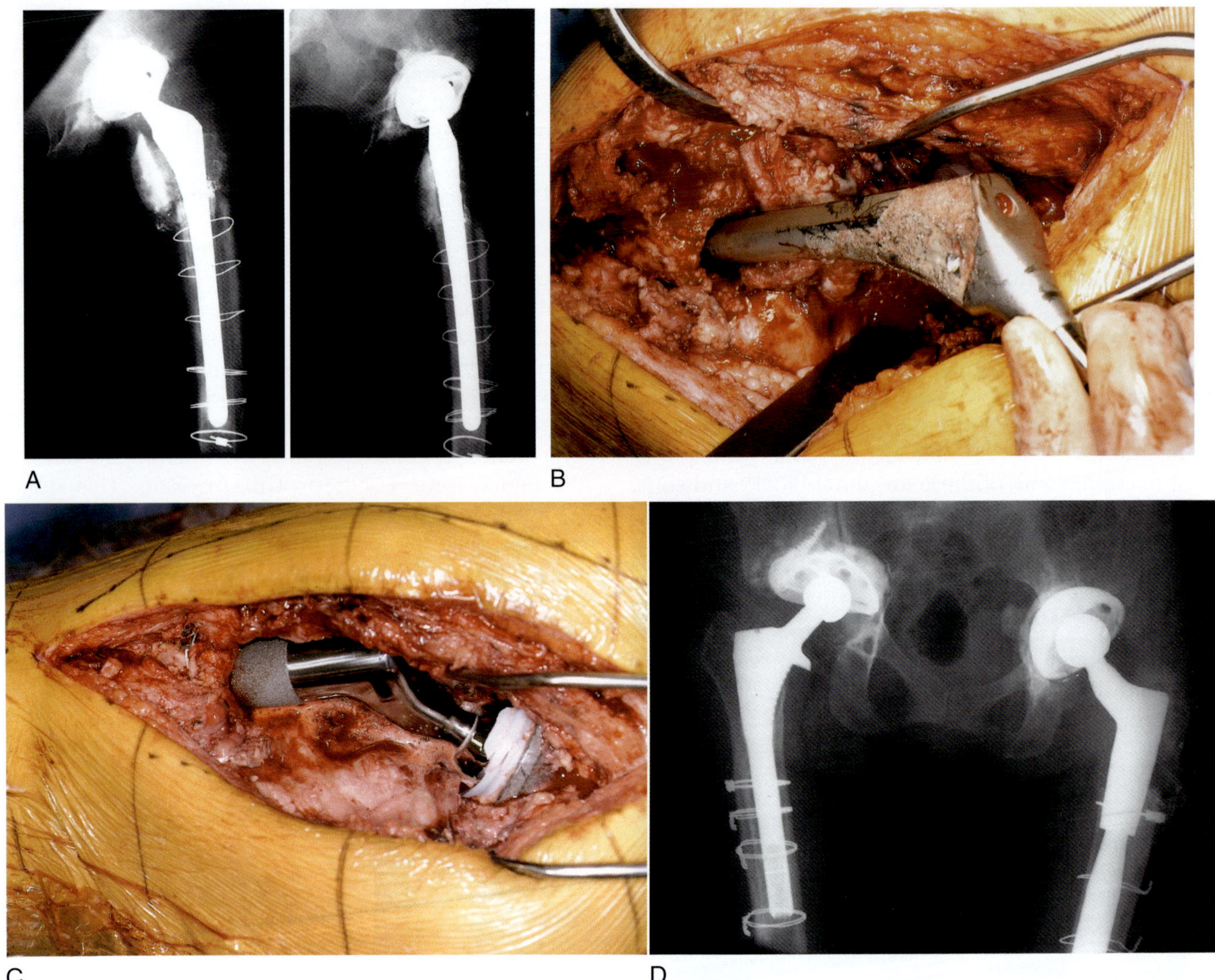

Figure 10–62 *A, Preoperative x-rays of a loose stem, with necrosis of the proximal femoral bone. B, This loose femoral stem could simply be lifted out of the distal femur because the necrotic proximal femoral bone was the only bone to which there could have been any fixation. C, The revision stem can replace the lost proximal femoral bone because of its strength and geometry. The absence of any structures to which the greater trochanter could be reattached is evident. D, X-ray of the implantation of the revision stem. The greater trochanter fragment was left in place in this patient, but it could have been excised (see Figs. 10–30 to 10–34) at the discretion of the surgeon. Usually, I would have excised the fragment, for reasons explained in the text.*

diaphyseal fracture occurs, usually the only treatment necessary is to wire the femur so that it has hoop stress support during healing. If the fracture is complex, such as a long spiral fracture, it must be repaired before completion of the operation. This may require the placement of a plate, bone strut grafts and wires, or wires or cables around the femur (Fig. 10–63).

If a fracture occurs, the surgeon must decide whether to treat the fracture with the stem in place or to remove the stem, repair the fracture, and reimplant the revision stem. Most commonly, the simplest and most efficient technique is to leave the revision stem in place and treat the fracture. The treatment is no different from any other fracture treatment, except that the presence of the

stem can obstruct screw fixation of the plate to the bone. In this situation, a unicortical screw can be used, or the surgeon can use plates that allow cable fixation. In my experience, however, cable fixation seems to have a significant failure rate, so unless the surgeon is confident that the plate fixation is adequate, a cast should be used in addition to the plate. The plate selected should be of the correct length to allow at least four screws to be used above or below the extent of the fracture, particularly if the screws are unicortical.

When bone struts and wires are used to secure a fracture, it is most common to use two bone struts—one medial and one anterolateral. This technique is not difficult and simply requires selection of the correct

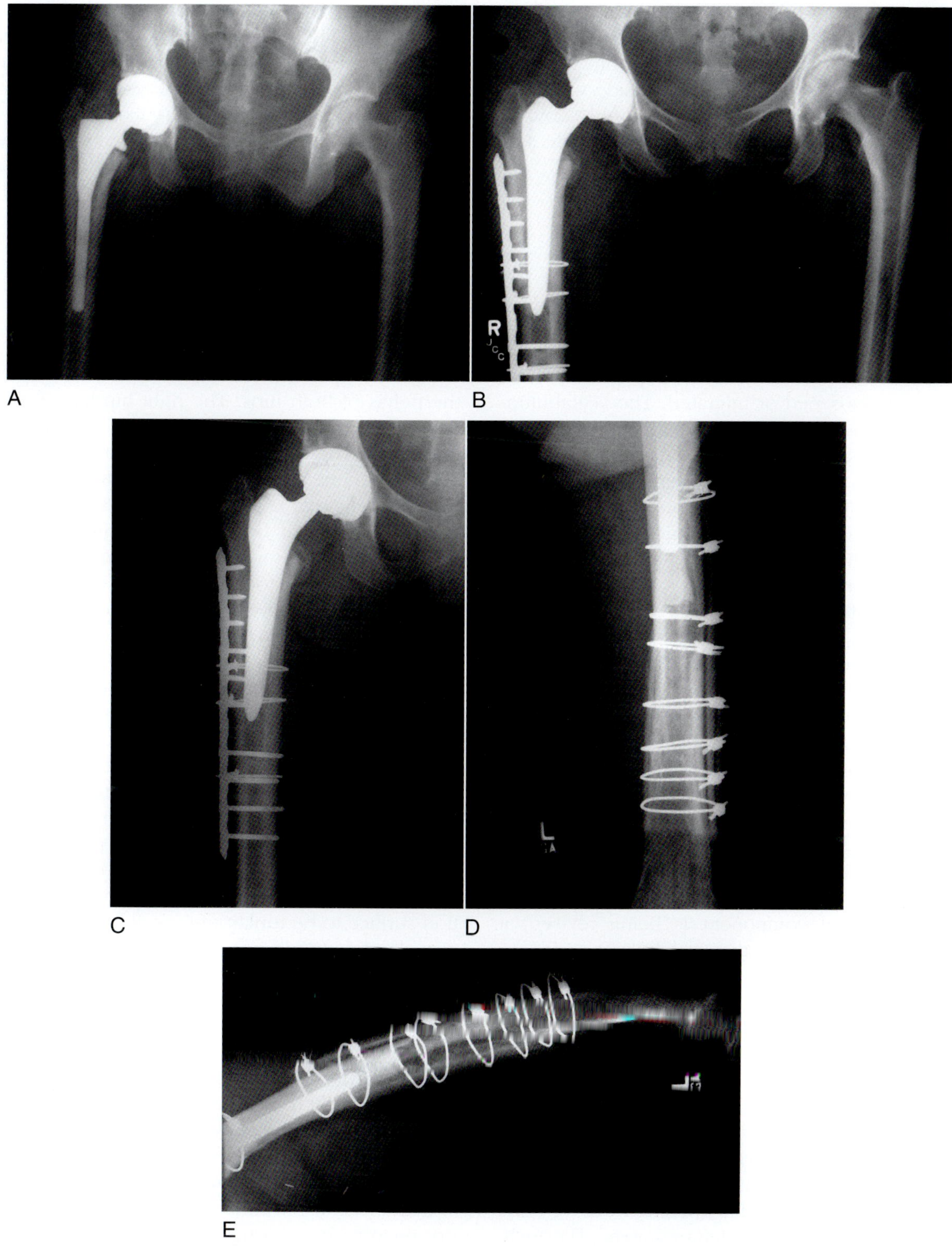

Figure 10–63 **A,** *An intraoperative fracture occurred during implantation of this stem. A split in the greater trochanter is evident on this x-ray, and the distal extension of the fracture is seen laterally, just above the tip of the stem.* **B,** *A plate was initially placed to stabilize the fracture, and cables and unicortical screws were used proximally. The bone healed, but the implant was loose. A second operation was performed to replace the APR stem with the Alloclassic stem, which had a better fit and could be placed without removal of the plate. This x-ray was taken 1 year after placement of the plate and 6 months after revision of the stem. The patient had no pain and no limp.* **C,** *Anteroposterior x-ray shows the entire length of hip plate used to repair the femur, with screw fixation used distally and unicortical screws with two wires used proximally. The healed femur fracture can be seen between the two wires.* **D,** *Anteroposterior x-ray of the femoral shaft showing a bone plate attached to the femur with cables. There is an intact medial and lateral cortex in this femur, demonstrating repair of a fracture at the distal end of the cement column.* **E,** *Lateral x-ray of the same femur showing the anterior bone plate and the attachment with cables. There is healing of the femoral fracture.*

length of bone graft and then great care by the surgeon to ensure that the cable or wire passed posteriorly around the femur is directly adjacent to bone, so that there is no risk of including the artery inside the wire. The length of the bone strut selected should allow at least two cables or wires to secure the bone above and below the extent of the fracture.

ACETABULAR PREPARATION

Revision of the acetabulum is probably the most creative operation in total joint replacement. The acetabular bone can have several different geometries once it has had an acetabular component in place and that component has loosened or migrated. The acetabulum is always larger than it was with the primary operation, which means that a larger acetabular metal shell will be needed and that screws will almost certainly be needed for initial security of that shell. Jumbo-sized acetabular hemispheric cups (generally defined as cups that are 65 to 81 mm in diameter) are available for large cavitary defects. With today's materials, it is critical to use the largest head possible with these jumbo cups. Even a 44-mm femoral head in an 81-mm cup is likely to cause impingement of the metal femoral neck against the edge of the cup, but when smaller cup sizes are combined with the largest femoral head possible, impingement can usually be avoided. The only reason to use a large acetabular component with a 28- or 32-mm femoral head is the presence of a fixed monoblock head on a retained femoral component.

Revision of the acetabulum can be performed in isolation, with retention of the femoral component, or it can be combined with revision of the femoral component. If the femoral component is being revised, it should be removed before the acetabular revision to simplify exposure of the acetabulum. If the femoral component is being retained, the acetabular revision must be performed so that the retained femoral component does not impede the satisfactory reconstruction of the acetabulum.

One of the most common revisions performed is for osteolysis of the pelvis or wear of the plastic insert of the hip replacement. This revision requires exchange of the plastic insert and femoral head and sometimes revision of the acetabular cup. This operation can be done without interference from the femoral stem. The technique for an isolated acetabular revision should be understood by all joint surgeons, and any surgeon who practices total joint replacement should be able to perform one capably. This section presents a case report of an isolated revision of the acetabulum, detailing the technical methods necessary to expose the acetabular component by retracting the femoral component anteriorly. After the technique for removing scar tissue around the acetabulum is described in the case report, the remainder of the section focuses on techniques to simplify the removal and reimplantation of the acetabular component. These techniques concentrate on straightforward acetabular revisions. Experienced surgeons interested in the techniques required for complex acetabular revisions with severe segmental defects or acetabular discontinuity are directed to the writings of Wayne Paprosky (Rush Presbyterian Hospital, Chicago, Ill.) and Alan Gross (Toronto).

Case Report of Isolated Acetabular Revision

The patient pictured in Figure 10–64 has osteolysis in the pelvis of both hips. The right hip has already been operated on, with a new femoral head and plastic insert implanted. The left hip is going to have the same operation. It is generally my practice not to use a bone graft for the acetabular defects in these patients.

If an acetabular bone graft is going to be done, a window must be made in the ilium, and the fibrous membrane needs to be removed from the cavitary defect so that the bone graft has a chance to unite to the host bone. (The extent of bone cavity is always greater than anticipated from the x-ray and usually extends more posteriorly than expected.) This technique was performed for the patient pictured in Figure 10–65. Because the graft material used was hydroxyapatite granules, the site of bone graft is easily seen. In my opinion, there is no chance that this bone graft will heal to the cup, and I do not expect the bone graft to incorporate into the cavity. The only possible benefit of this bone graft would be to strengthen the bone supporting the cup; however, if the cup had enough fixation surface to be functioning well for the patient, there was clearly enough bone support. If the fixation of the cup, or the bone support of the cup, were not sufficient to withstand the forces to which it was subjected, it would have become loose, in which case this would have been discovered at surgery and a revision of the cup could have been done. Thus, the bone graft offers no great benefit to the longevity of the hip replacement. I believe that no bone graft can prevent future loss of fixation of the cup. Therefore, I do these operations without a window and without bone grafting.

The incision for an isolated acetabular revision does not need to be as long as the traditional conventional incision. Therefore, an old incision does not need to be opened in its entirety to perform this operation (Fig. 10–66). The incision is made with the leg lying on top of the contralateral leg, with the hip and knee both flexed about 30 to 40 degrees. This relaxes the tissues at the hip sufficiently to allow incision of the skin, fascia, and gluteus maximus muscles. A small Homans retractor can be used to retract the anterior flap of the

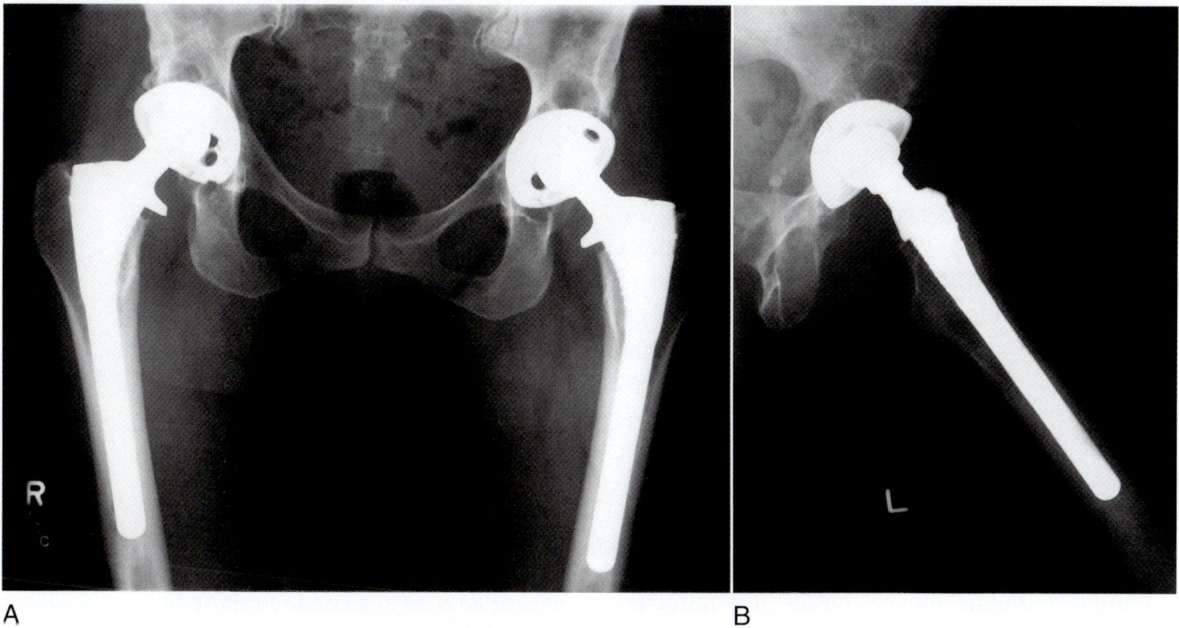

A   B

Figure 10–64 **A,** This x-ray shows osteolysis of both hips, with severe wear in both cups. The right hip was operated on first; the operation on the left hip is illustrated in subsequent figures. **B,** Lateral x-ray of the left hip shows the osteolysis superiorly as well as medioposteriorly.

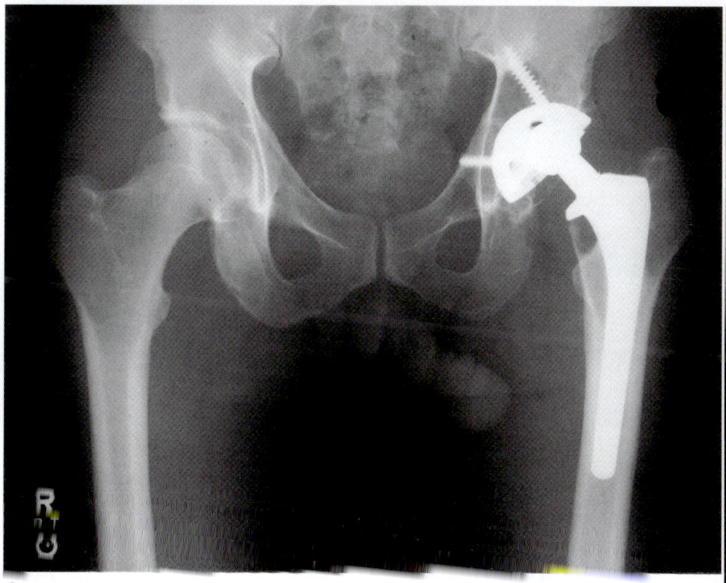

A

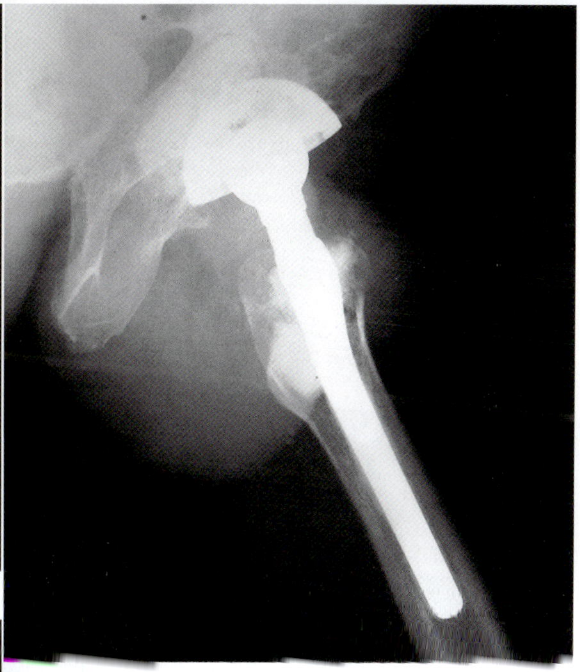

C

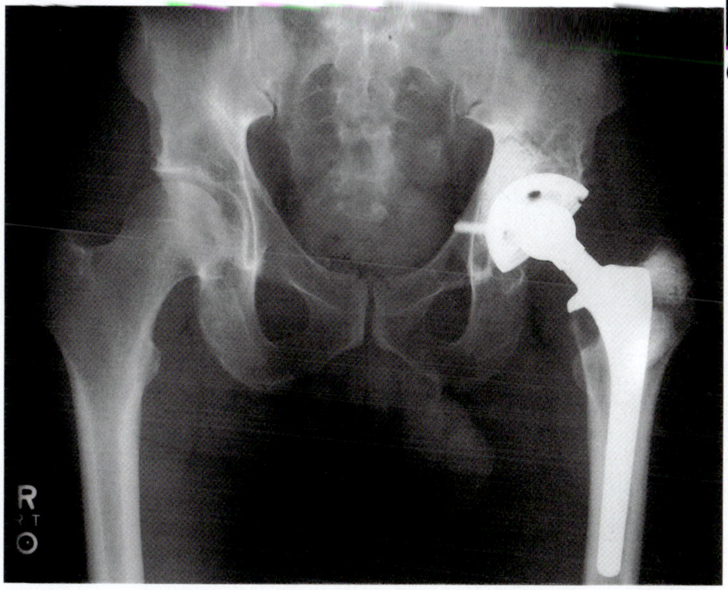

B

Figure 10–65 **A,** Severe osteolysis is seen around the acetabulum, with severe wear of the plastic in the cup. When there is a large superomedial defect, such as that seen on this x-ray, it means that there is significant posterior extension of the osteolysis. There is also osteolysis in the trochanter and medial femur. **B,** Postoperatively, hydroxyapatite granules were used to bone graft these defects. These granules allow easy visualization of the extent of the grafted defects in both the acetabulum and the femur. The medial femoral lytic defect was not grafted. The components were rigidly fixed and therefore were not changed. **C,** Postoperative lateral x-ray shows the acetabular and femoral defects that were packed with graft material. The extent of the medioposterior acetabular defect can be seen.

wound, allowing the surgeon to use his or her hand to retract the lower edge of the wound, giving exposure for division of the tissues down to the hip (Fig. 10–67). The fascia of the tensor fascia lata muscle is opened distally, and this is extended into the gluteus maximus muscle proximally (Fig. 10–68). When these tissues are opened, divided, and retracted, the posterior hip is visualized, with the scarred structures from the index operation being attached to the posterior greater trochanter. The leg is internally rotated 30 to 40 degrees (Fig. 10–69); this rotates the trochanter anteriorly and away from the sciatic nerve and gives better access to the posterior greater trochanter so that a flap of posterior tissue can be incised off it and the femur. A posterior flap is incised from the level of the gluteus maximus tendon into the gluteus minimus muscle below the retracted

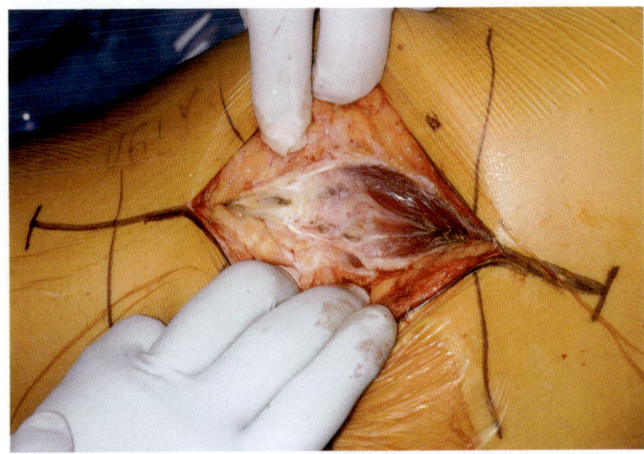

Figure 10–68 *The tensor fascia and gluteus maximus muscle have been incised to expose the greater trochanter.*

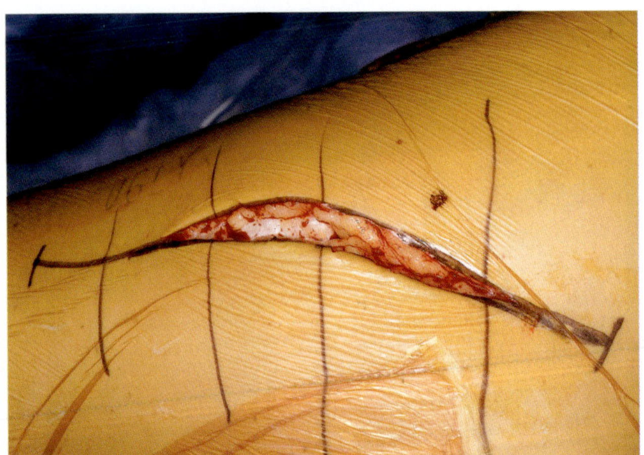

Figure 10–66 *For isolated acetabular revision, the entire previous long incision need not be used.*

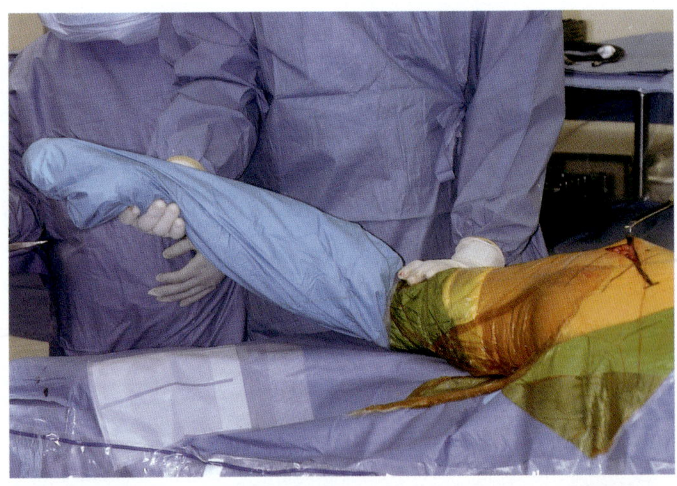

A

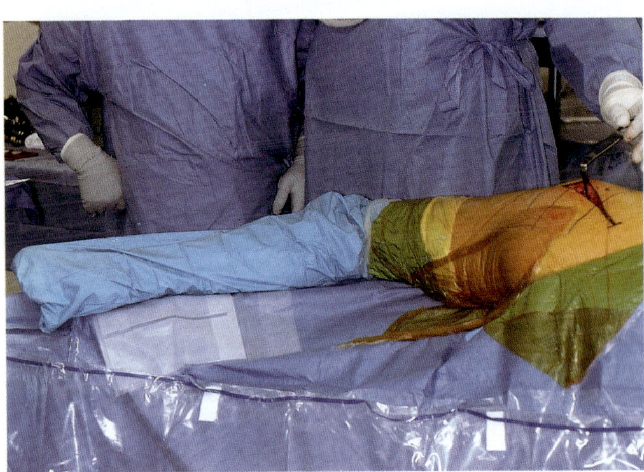

Figure 10–67 *The anterior flap is retracted to allow easier dissection of the posterior structures.*

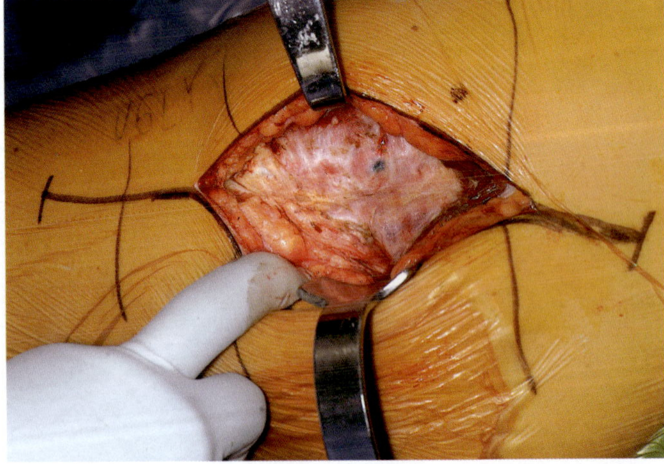

B

Figure 10–69 **A,** *The leg is internally rotated with the knee kept in the center of the table to provide easier access to the posterior structures and to retract the trochanter anteriorly away from the sciatic nerve.* **B,** *With the leg held in this position, the trochanter is rotated anteriorly (blue dot), and the scar can be easily incised off the greater trochanter.*

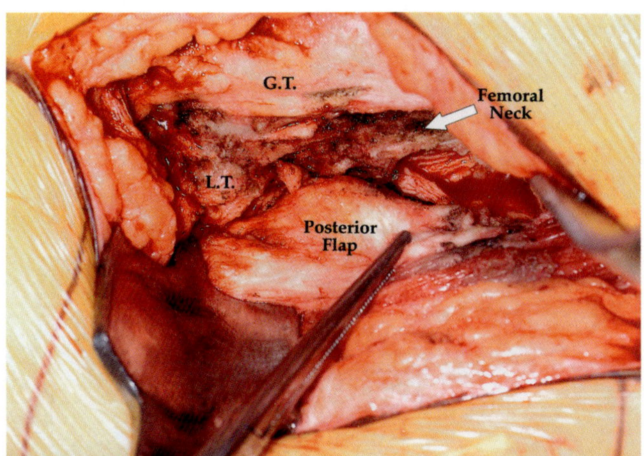

Figure 10–70 *The posterior flap is created from the lesser trochanter (LT) to the superior edge of the acetabulum. This posterior flap can be repaired at the end of the operation. GT, greater trochanter.*

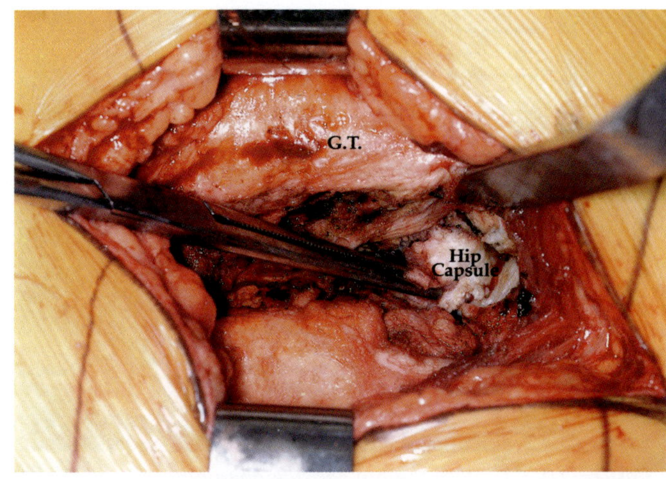

A

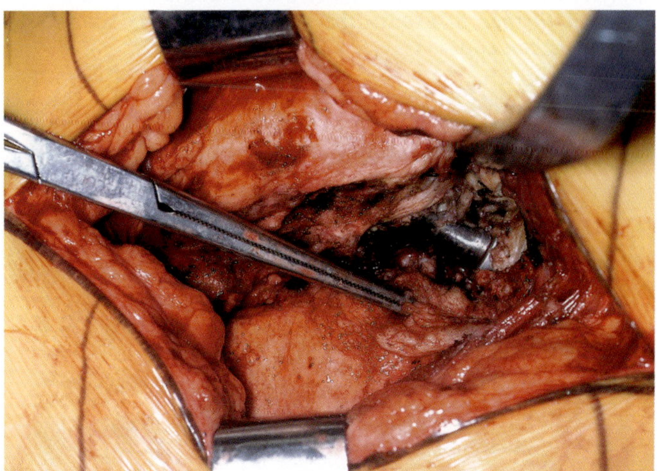

B

Figure 10–71 *A, Beneath the posterior flap is a scarred hip capsule over the hip replacement. B, The hip capsule is incised to create a posterior flap that can be closed at the completion of the operation. This flap is held by a Kocher clamp, and the hip replacement is exposed. Scar is present along the superoposterior and superior cup. GT, greater trochanter.*

gluteus medius tendon (Fig. 10–70). This posterior flap can be retracted en masse to expose the femoral neck and the scar of the hip capsule, and it will be used to provide closure of the posterior hip at the end of the operation. The hip capsule is then incised to create a posterior flap of hip capsule that can also be closed at the completion of the operation (Fig. 10–71).

The scar within the hip is then excised in quadrants. Retractors are placed to protect tissue and expose the scar to be excised. First, the posterosuperior quadrant scar is excised, clearing the edge of the superior and superoposterior acetabular component (Fig. 10–72). After this tissue has been incised, the leg is internally rotated further (Fig. 10–73). The posterior and posteroinferior scar tissue is removed next (Fig. 10–74). The leg is continually internally rotated without dislocation of the hip during excision of this tissue. When it has reached maximal internal rotation tension, the anteroinferior scar is usually visible and can be excised (Fig. 10–75). Following excision of the anteroinferior capsule, the hip is dislocated, the leg is brought to a 90 degree flexed position at the knee, and the femoral head is removed (Fig. 10–76). Once the femoral head is removed, the femoral neck begins to point out of the wound (Fig. 10–77). The tighter the anterior scar or capsule, the less the metal neck points out of the wound; the more relaxed the anterior scar, the higher the metal neck points out of the wound and the easier it is to retract the femur anterior to the acetabulum (Fig. 10–78). This anterior retraction must be accomplished for final exposure of the acetabulum.

The point of the snake retractor is malleted into the ilium to secure the leverage needed to retract the femur with the femoral component anteriorly. This cannot be done until the anterior scar or capsule is relaxed. If the

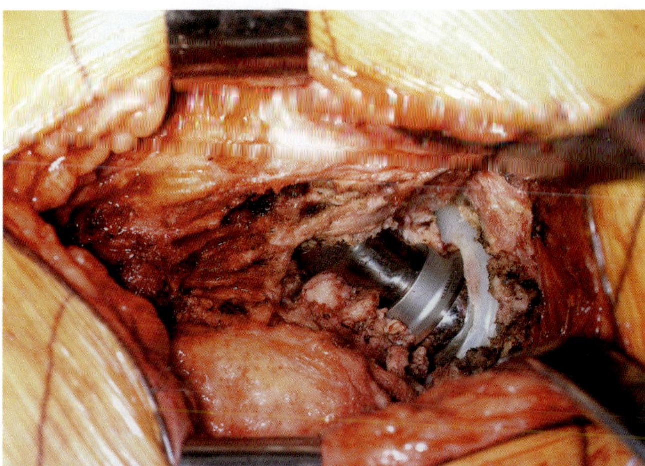

Figure 10–72 *The posterosuperior and superior scar has been excised, exposing the plastic of the cup. Impingement was present at the 1 to 2 o'clock positions, as seen by the deformation and discoloration of the plastic.*

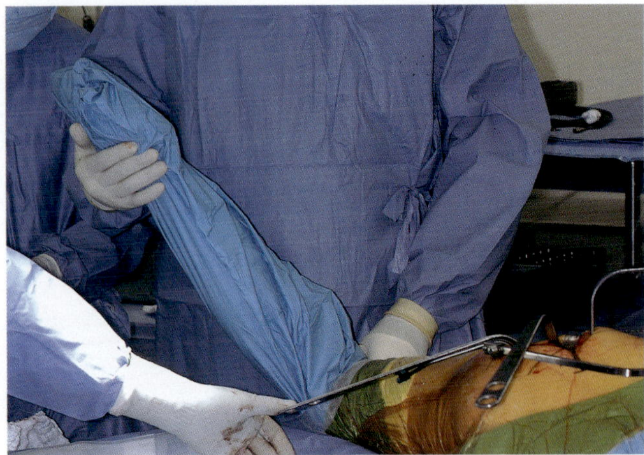

Figure 10–73 *With the hip capsule open and the scar tissue partially excised, the hip is more mobile and can be internally rotated further to expose the remainder of the scar tissue overlying the cup.*

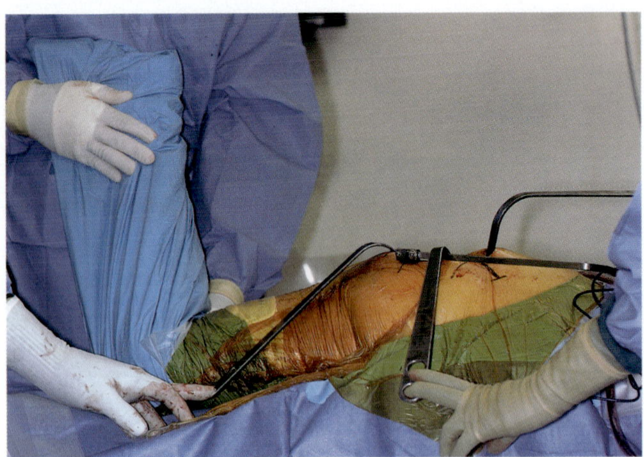

Figure 10–76 *The leg has been brought to 90 degrees internal rotation and still rests on the lower leg.*

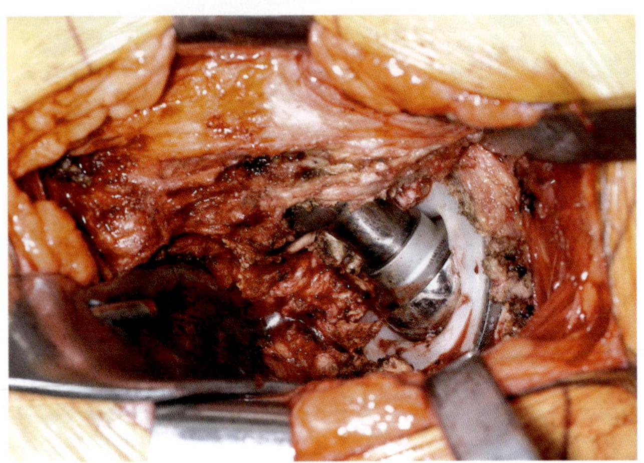

Figure 10–74 *With the leg in the position shown in Figure 10–73, the inferoposterior and inferior hip capsular scar is excised.*

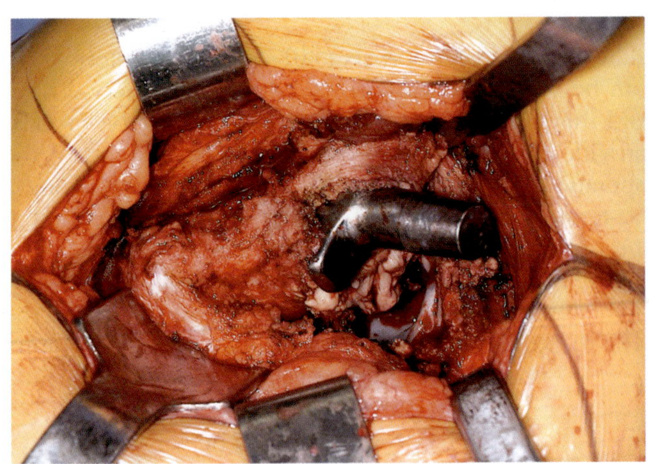

Figure 10–77 *The metal femoral neck is pointing out of the wound, indicating that the anterior capsule is not tethering it deep in the wound.*

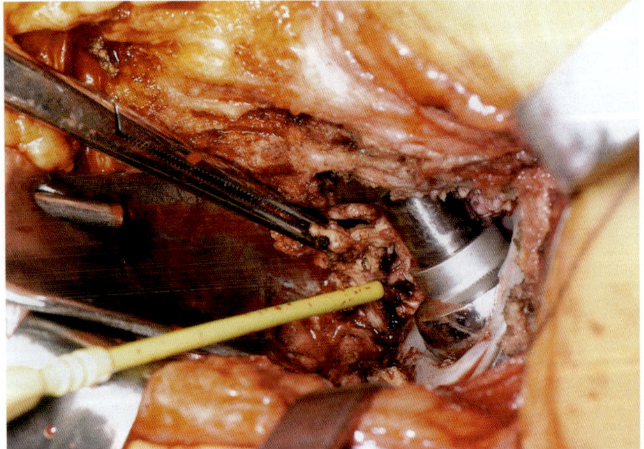

Figure 10–75 *The anteroinferior hip capsular scar is excised as it is held by a Kocher clamp.*

scar is tight and access to it is difficult, I internally rotate the leg maximally, placing a retractor around the lesser trochanter and incising as much as 50% to 60% of the iliopsoas tendon off the lesser trochanter. This maneuver provides access to the anterior femoral neck. A Bovie electrocautery can be used to incise the tissue along the anterior femoral neck, but this may not be sufficient to loosen it. The best technique to incise the tissue along the anterior neck, and thereby loosen the tether of the femur to the anterior acetabulum, is the use of an osteotome (Fig. 10–79). A sharp osteotome will cut this tissue and has the leverage to cut along the entire anterior neck without the surgeon's needing visible access. Secondly, the osteotome can be used to

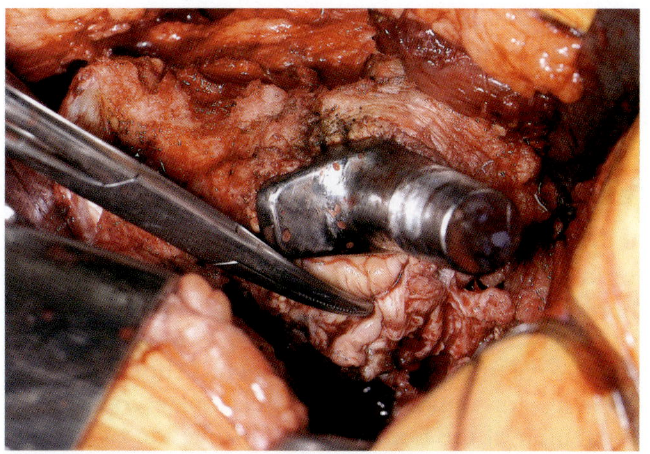

Figure 10–78 *The anterior scar is easily visualized. It extends between the anterior and medial acetabulum and the anterior femur.*

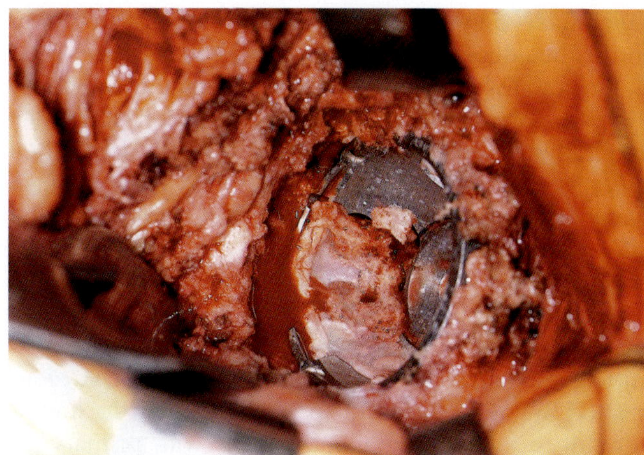

Figure 10–80 *The femur is retracted anterior to the acetabulum, providing complete exposure of the acetabulum.*

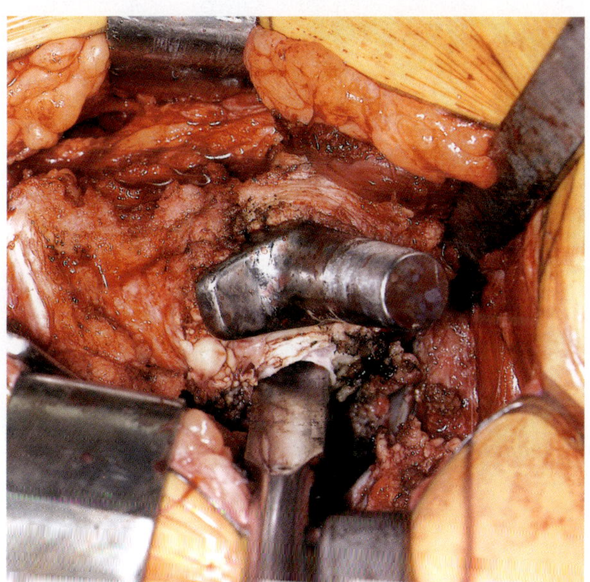

Figure 10–79 *An osteotome is used to cut the anterior capsule and strip it from the femoral neck.*

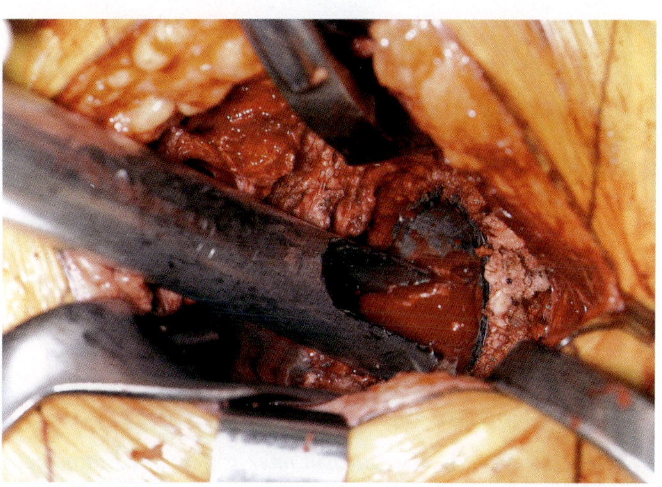

Figure 10–81 *A metal tool is used to hit the edge of the acetabular cup to ensure that it is solidly fixed. If there is no motion of the cup and the tool makes a ringing sound, the cup is solidly fixed.*

peel tissue off the anterior neck once it has cut through the initial scar. A Bovie electrocautery does not have the length or strength of the osteotome to be able to accomplish what can be done with this tool.

Once the anterior scar has been incised, the femur can be retracted completely anterior to the acetabulum with the snake retractor. This retractor should be held against the bottom of the metal femoral neck and not on the articulating taper (Fig. 10–80). The anterior and inferior scar needs to be excised to completely expose the acetabular component, and this can now be easily accomplished. The plastic insert is removed by the drill and screw technique (see under Removal of Implants, later). When scar tissue is removed, the stability of the acetabular component can be tested by hitting a tool against the metal edge of the shell and determining whether there is any motion of the acetabular component (Fig. 10–81). A solidly fixed acetabular component also has a unique sound, almost like a ringing.

Once it has been determined that the metal acetabular component is securely fixed, preparation for a new plastic insert can be done. If the new plastic insert will simply be mechanically locked into the metal shell, only the scar tissue inside the acetabulum and at the edges of the acetabulum needs to be cleared. If the new insert will be cemented into the acetabular shell, the cementing technique described later (see under Cementation of the Liner into the Metal Shell, later) is performed. In this patient, a new Durasul acetabular liner (Zimmer, Warsaw, Ind.) was implanted (Fig. 10–82). After successful acetabular implantation and impaction of a new femoral head onto the metal femoral taper, the reduction is done, and a complete range of motion is performed to ensure that there is no impingement and good stability. Closure is then accomplished. Initially, the hip capsule is brought to the cut edge of the gluteus minimus, just as with primary hip replacement (Fig. 10–83). The posterior flap is then closed to the posterior trochanter, and the fascia and muscle layer are closed on top of that. The postoperative radiograph of this operation is shown in Figure 10–84.

Techniques for Acetabular Revision

The previous case report described the organized excision of scar tissue around the acetabulum by quadrants. This section begins with the assumption that this scar tissue has already been removed, with or without retention of the femoral component. The techniques necessary for removal of the acetabular component, preparation of the bone, and reimplantation of cavitary defects are discussed here.

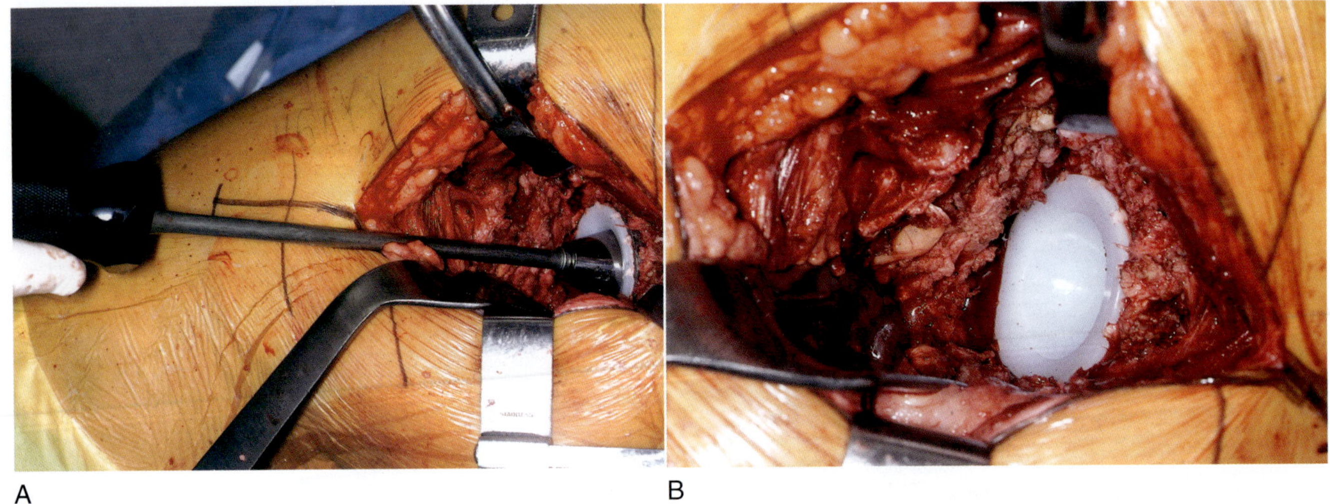

A   B

Figure 10–82 **A,** *The Durasul liner is cemented into the metal shell. Pressure is kept on the liner until the cement is hard.* **B,** *All excess cement has been removed, except that present in the interdigitations of the plastic, which aids in fixation.*

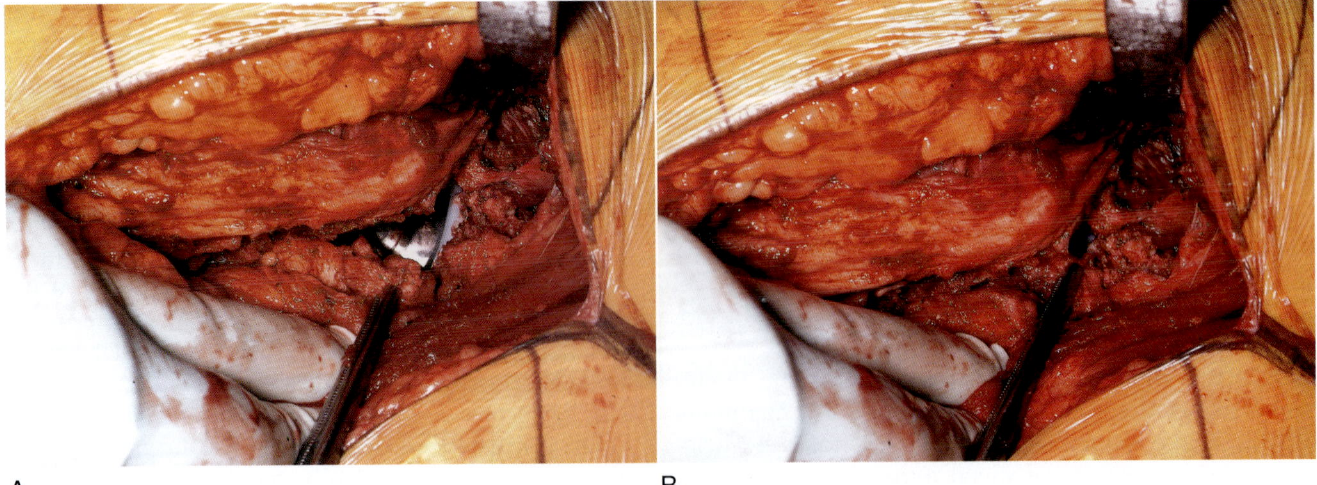

A   B

Figure 10–83 **A,** *The preserved posterior capsular flap is held by a Kocher clamp and will be brought anteriorly, up to the edge of the gluteus minimus muscle.* **B,** *Closure of the posterior capsule, which will be sutured to the anterior gluteus minimus muscle.*

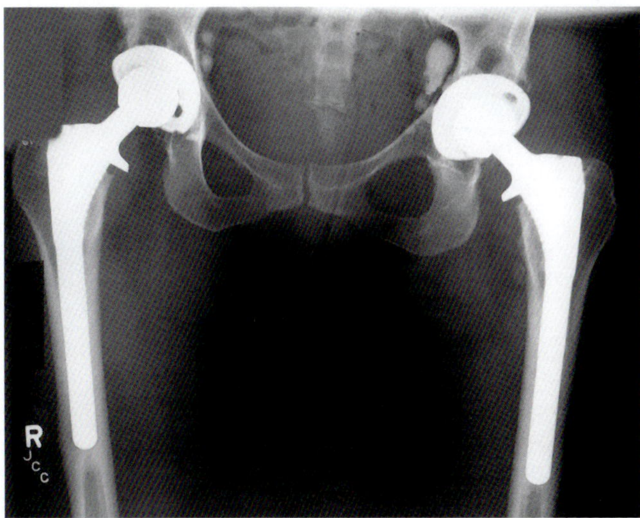

Figure 10–84 *Postoperative radiograph shows that the Durasul liner has been cemented into place, and cement has extruded into the pelvis through bony defects. Both hips have been reconstructed, with some cement extrusion into the pelvis in the right hip as well.*

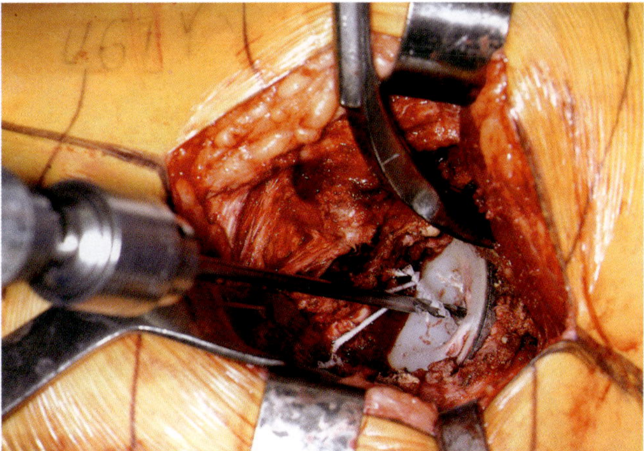

Figure 10–86 *The drill is inserted through the plastic until it hits the metal shell. This creates a spiral plastic fragment that must be removed from the wound.*

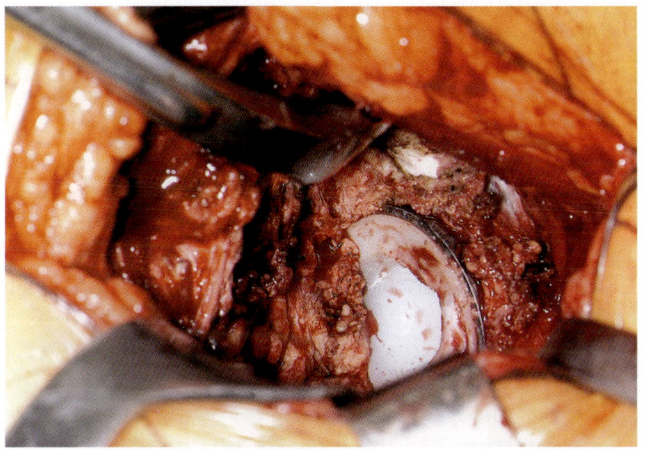

Figure 10–85 *Hip capsular scar overlying the anterior acetabulum must be removed.*

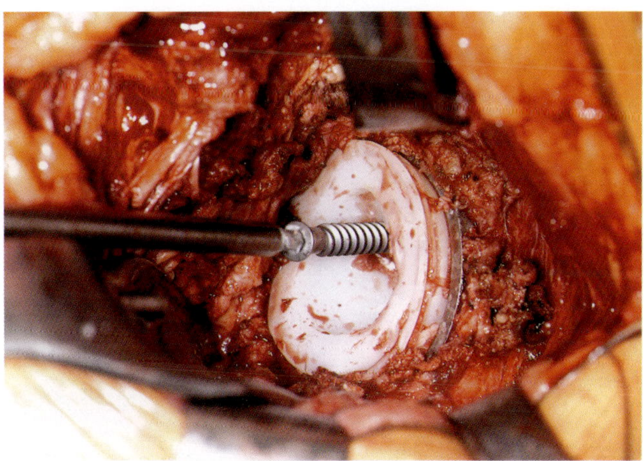

Figure 10–87 *The screw is inserted until the locking mechanism disengages and the plastic begins to disengage from the metal shell.*

Removal of Implants

Once the femur has been retracted anterior to the acetabulum, any remaining scar tissue that overlies the modular plastic insert of bone-ingrown implants or the plastic edge of a cemented acetabular component should be excised (Fig. 10–85). When the edges of the plastic have been exposed, the insert can be removed from the metal shell by the drill and screw technique. In this technique, a 4.5-mm drill is used to drill through the plastic to the metal shell. It is important that the drill bit hits metal and does not enter one of the screw holes in the metal shell. This ensures that when the screw is inserted, its tip will also hit the metal shell, and

with continued torque on the screw, the pressure backs out the plastic component. Drilling of the plastic produces spiral plastic debris, which should be lifted out of the wound with a tonsil clamp (Fig. 10–86). A 6.5 mm screw is inserted into the hole, and with most conventional plastics, this one screw causes the locking mechanism to disengage and the plastic to disassemble from the metal shell (Fig. 10–87). With some of the newer locking mechanisms (such as the Converge cup with a Durasul or Metasul liner), more than one screw is necessary to disassemble the plastic. With Durasul, two screws are often necessary, and these are usually crossed so that the levering-out pressure is exerted at a nearly 90 degree angle (which is almost always successful). With metal-on-metal inserts, the drill must be directed through the periphery of the plastic at an almost vertical angle to disengage the locking

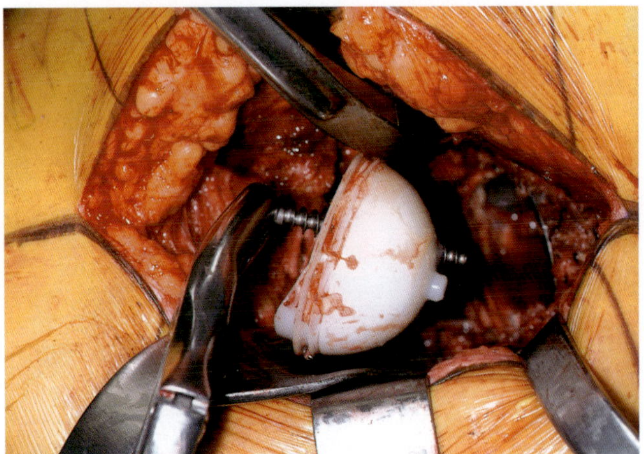

Figure 10–88   *The disengaged plastic is lifted out of the wound by grabbing the screw with a rongeur and twisting the plastic free.*

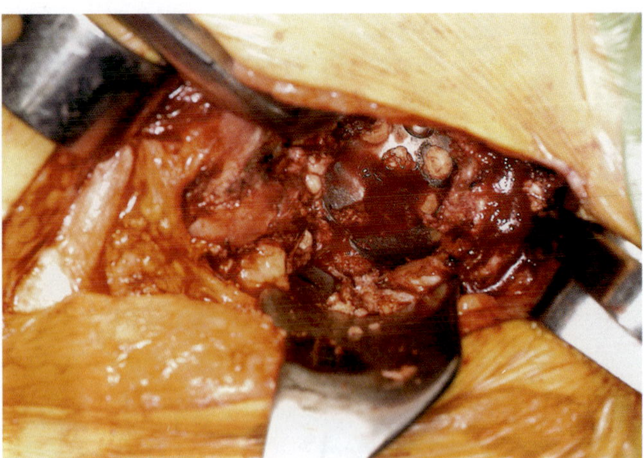

Figure 10–90   *After removal of the plastic, the scar tissue along the edges of and inside the acetabular shell must be removed for implantation of a new plastic insert.*

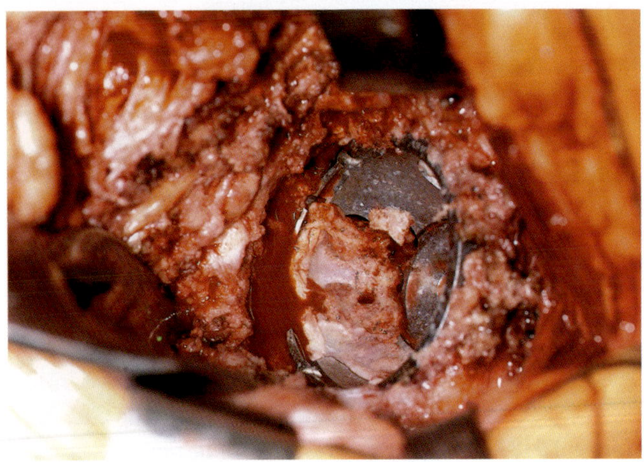

Figure 10–89   *A fibrous membrane is often present inside the acetabular shell and must be removed. The easiest way to do this is with a high-speed burr.*

mechanism. With Metasul, it is usually necessary to direct two screws vertically at the plastic-metal interface to disengage the liner. When the plastic has been disengaged from the metal shell, it is easily lifted out of the wound by grabbing the screw head with a rongeur and twisting the plastic free of the metal shell (Fig. 10–88).

In nearly all first- and second-generation conventional polyethylene inserts, there was a gap between the metal shell and the plastic that allowed the latter to be seated into the former so that the locking mechanism could engage. The gap resulted in a fibrous membrane inside the metal acetabular shell (Fig. 10–89). This fibrous tissue had to be removed to gain access to the screw heads and to free any fibrous tethering of the

acetabular shell to the underlying bone. This was generally accomplished with a high-speed burr, a curette, and a rongeur. Most current implants have a much tighter fit between the plastic and the metal shell, which eliminates any sizable gaps.

To remove the metal shell, its edges must be exposed so that osteotomes can be inserted at the interface of metal and bone. Further, all screw holes must be exposed to ensure that all screws have been removed (Fig. 10–90). Removal of scar tissue inside and on the periphery of the metal shell is most easily done with a high-speed burr; alternatively, osteotomes, rongeurs, or scalpel excision can be used. A high-speed burr easily and quickly identifies the metal-bone interface as it "chews up" the scar tissue overlying the cup (Fig. 10–91). Once the entire periphery of the cup is exposed, the cup can be removed by inserting osteotomes between the edge of the cup and the bone (or cement) to fragment the fixation (Fig. 10–92). Zimmer has a device called the Cup Out, with different osteotome blade sizes, that circumferentially fragments the fixation between the metal shell and bone (Fig. 10–93). Occasionally, use of this tool alone releases the cup, but sometimes it is necessary to use long, curved osteotomes to completely disengage the cup from the bone. It is critical that the bone attachment be separated at the dome of the cup and in zone 3 (at the cortical bone of the cotyloid notch). Often, the bone in zones 1 and 2 is easily accessible and is separated with the cup and removed, taking with it bone from the medial floor of the bony acetabulum and leaving a precarious rim and a large medial segmental defect. The Cup Out tool helps prevent this because it permits circumferential cutting of the bone. Long, curved osteotomes also help achieve circumferential fragmentation of the fixation. Thus, the surgeon must use

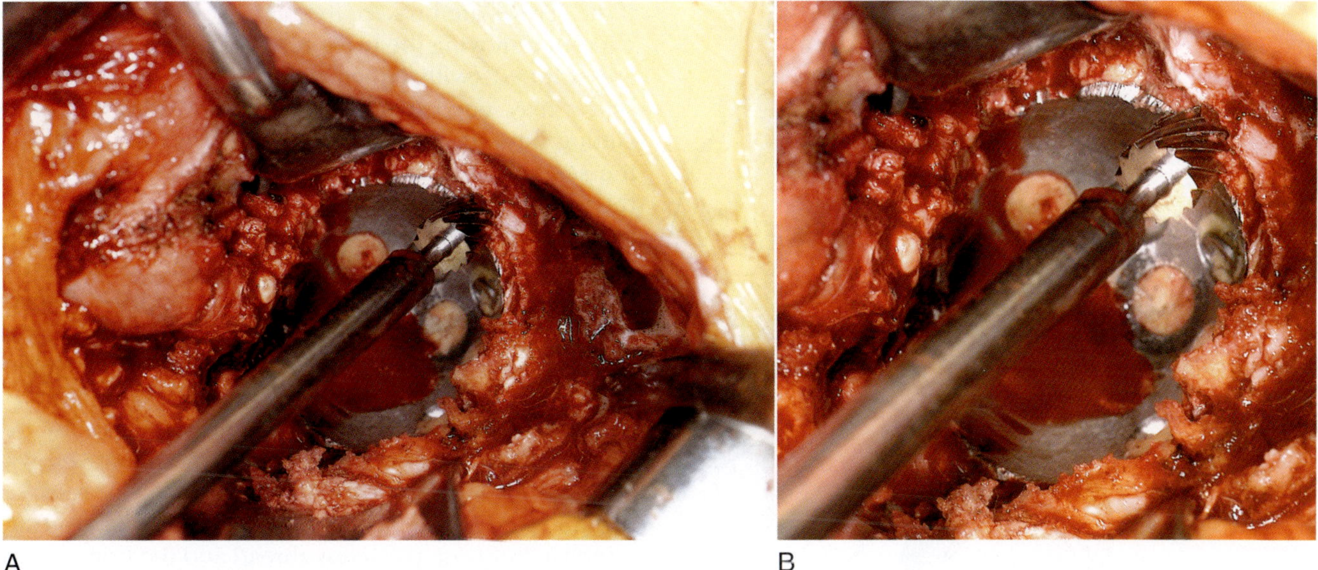

A   B

Figure 10–91 **A,** *A power burr is used to remove the scar from the metal edges of the acetabular shell to prepare for the locking or cementation of a new plastic insert.* **B,** *Close-up view of the burr clearing the edge of the acetabular shell.*

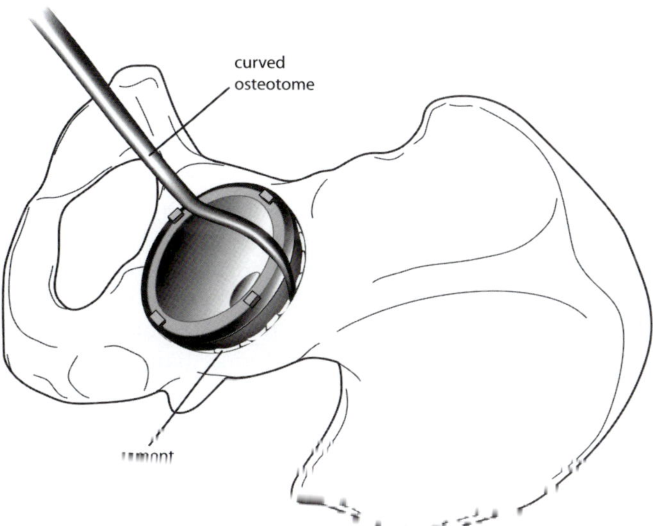

Figure 10–92 *A cemented osteotome is inserted at the interface of the metal shell and bone (or shell and cement) to fragment the fixation and allow the cup to be removed.*

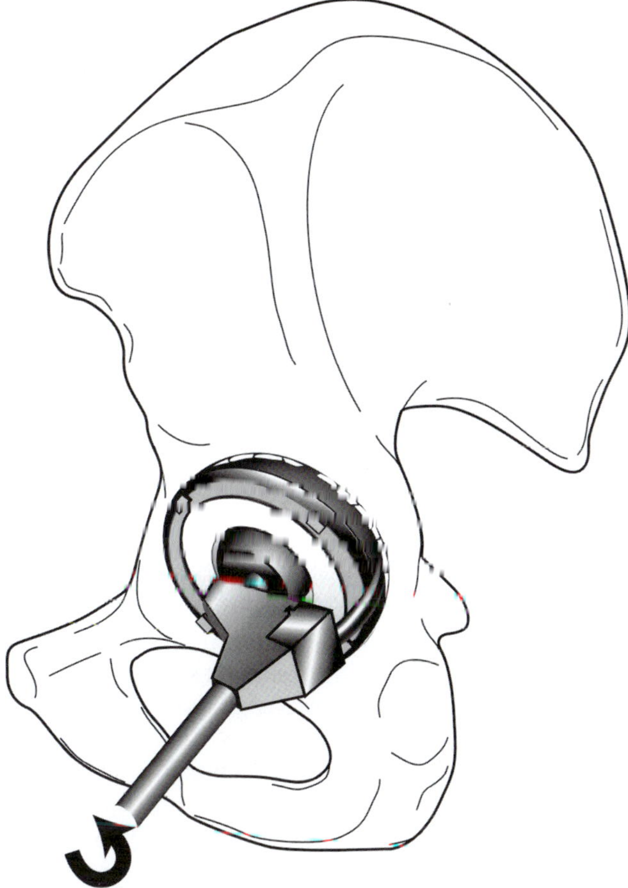

Figure 10–93 *The Cup Out tool is stabilized with a femoral head that fits the plastic left in place. There is a correct size of tool for each cup size. Once the tool is stabilized, curved blades are fitted at the interface of the cup and bone. There are two links of blades, so the surgeon should start with a short blade and progress to a long blade. This allows circumferential fragmentation of the fixation, which minimizes the risk of retained bone when the cup is removed.*

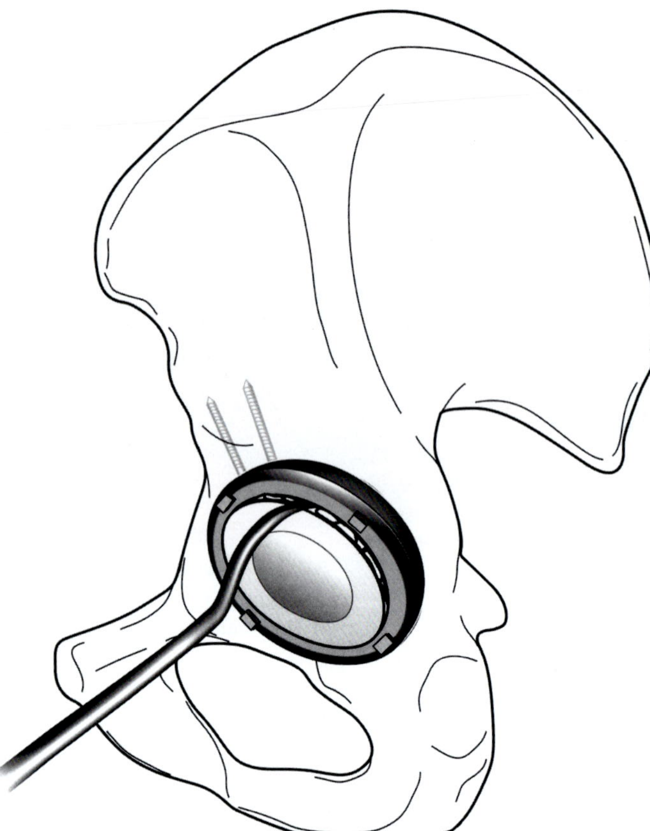

Figure 10–94 *An osteotome is used to separate the cemented plastic insert from the metal shell or ring.*

a cutting tool in the zone 3 area to fragment that bone before twisting the cup free from the acetabular bone.

Removal of an acetabular component consisting of a ring or a cage or that has a polyethylene monoblock in the metal shell can be done with the following technique. The construct is usually loose, so removal is simpler than a fixed cup removal, described previously. Because there are usually screws through the metal ring, the cemented polyethylene must be separated from the ring before the ring itself is removed (Fig. 10–94). The sequence for this technique is similar to that described for the metal hemispheric bone-ingrowth cup. The fibrous tissue overlying the plastic of the acetabular construct is removed with a high-speed burr (Fig. 10–95), and the interface between the cemented polyethylene cup and the metal cage is identified. An osteotome is inserted into the cement-metal interface to extract the polyethylene from the metal cage (Fig. 10–96; see also Fig. 10–94). Once the polyethylene has been removed from the construct, the metal shell can be removed. Initially, exposure of any screws through the metal ring must be done as described for a metal cup. A high-speed burr is used to remove cement or fibrous tissue over the screw heads, and then the screws are removed.

If the screws are broken, the metal ring can be removed without removing the broken screws. If the screw heads are stripped (with either a metal shell or a ring), the screw may need to be destroyed by using a carbide cutting bit with a high-speed burr. After destruction of the screw head, the cup or ring can be removed from the acetabular bone, and the remaining threads of the screw can be removed separately. When the metal ring has been uncoupled from the underlying acetabular bone by releasing the screw fixation and the cement-bone interface, it can be twisted out of the acetabular bone by gripping it with a rongeur in a twisting fashion and lifting it out of the wound (Fig. 10–97).

If screw threads remain in the acetabular bony bed and are firmly fixed in bone, they can be removed with a screw-out tool set. They can also be easily removed using a high-speed pencil-point burr, which creates an interface between the screw thread and the bone, allowing the screw to be simply twisted out. This is my preferred technique. Because I am already using the high-speed burr for clearance of the periphery of the acetabulum, it is a simple matter to change the bit, loosen the screw thread, and remove it from the bone.

Once the implant from the failed acetabular construct has been removed, the remaining bone—and its geometry—should be assessed by the surgeon. Most commonly, there is a cavitary defect of varying size (Fig. 10–98). If the defect's shape is nearly hemispheric, the simplest reconstruction is to use a hemispheric revision acetabular component, including jumbo cups. The implantation of this cup is similar to that of a primary acetabular component once the bone of the acetabulum has been prepared. If the acetabulum has an oblong shape (greater superoinferior than mediolateral diameter), a decision must be made whether to fill in the superior defect and use a cup that restores the center of rotation to nearly normal or to place a cup more superiorly, use a very long femoral neck head segment, and restore length in this fashion. I almost always choose the former option, and this is the technique described here.

Preparation of Acetabular Bone

Any fibrous tissue overlying the remaining acetabular bone must be removed. There can be no bone fixation to a new bone-ingrowth component or bony union between the graft and host if there is intervening fibrous tissue. The easiest way to loosen the fibrous tissue is to pass a high-speed burr lightly across all the acetabular bone (Fig. 10–99). I do this by quadrants (as described earlier) to have an organized pattern of fibrous tissue destruction.

When the thickest and greatest volume of fibrous tissue has been removed with the high-speed burr, a reamer can be used to capture any remaining fibrous

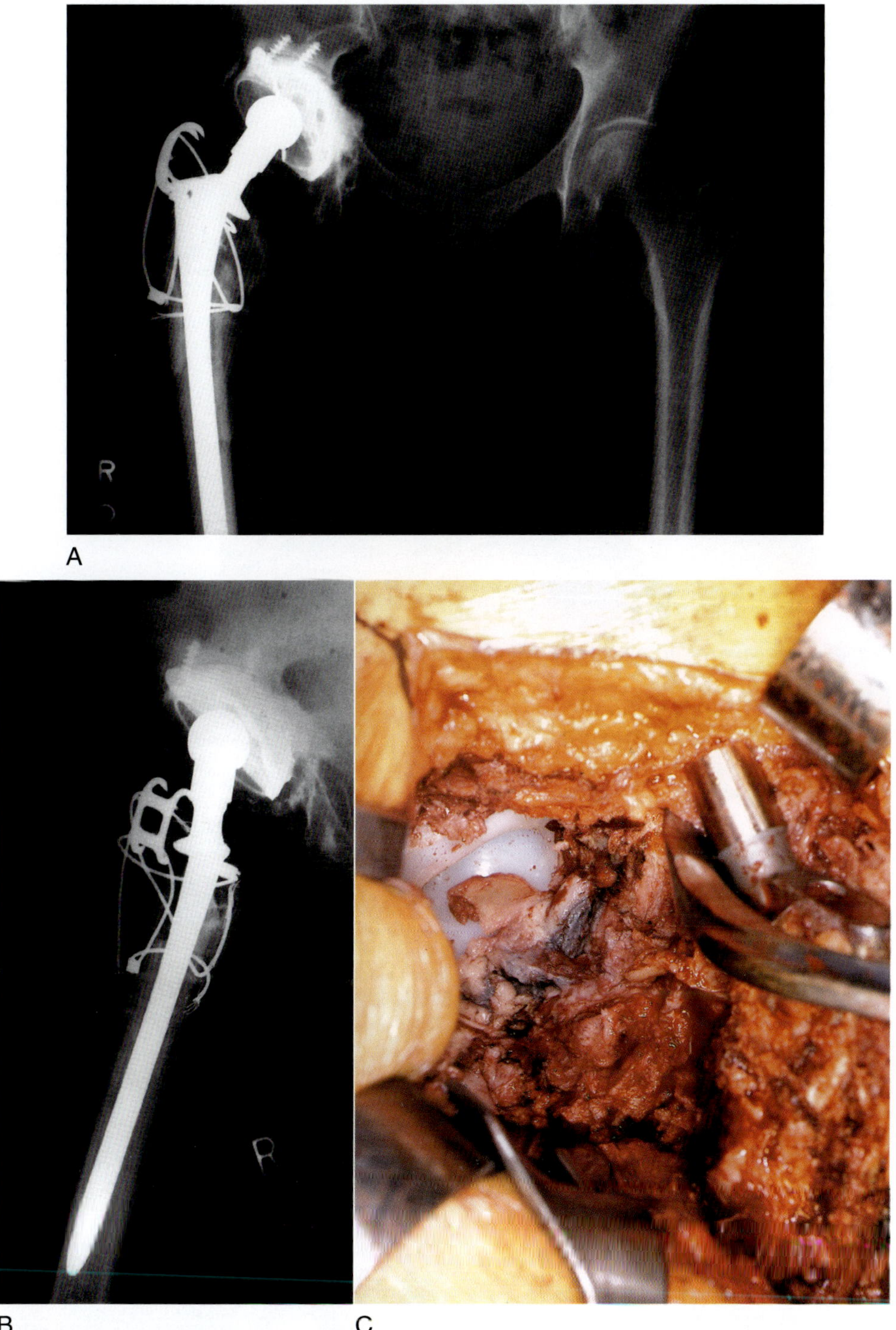

Figure 10–95 **A,** *Acetabular construct of a metal Muller ring with a plastic insert cemented into it. In this x-ray, demarcation between the cement and the bone is seen in zone 1, and the construct is loose.* **B,** *Lateral x-ray shows the gap in zone 3, indicative of migration of the construct.* **C,** *Fibrous tissue is seen overlying the plastic after the femur has been retracted anteriorly.*

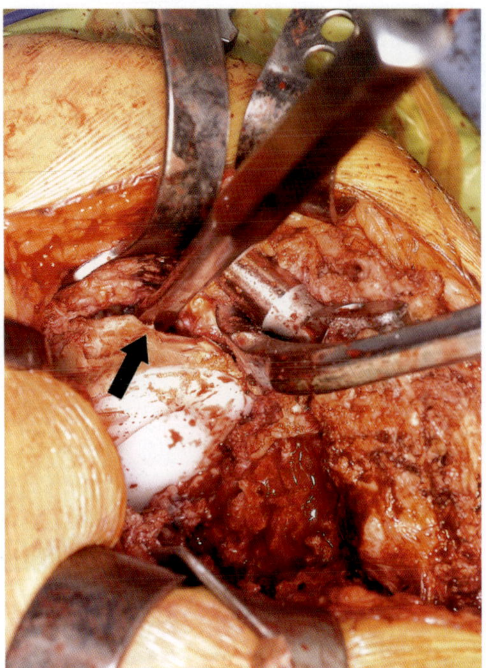

Figure 10–96 *Intraoperative view of an osteotome being used at the cement-bone interface to loosen the cemented fixation* (arrow).

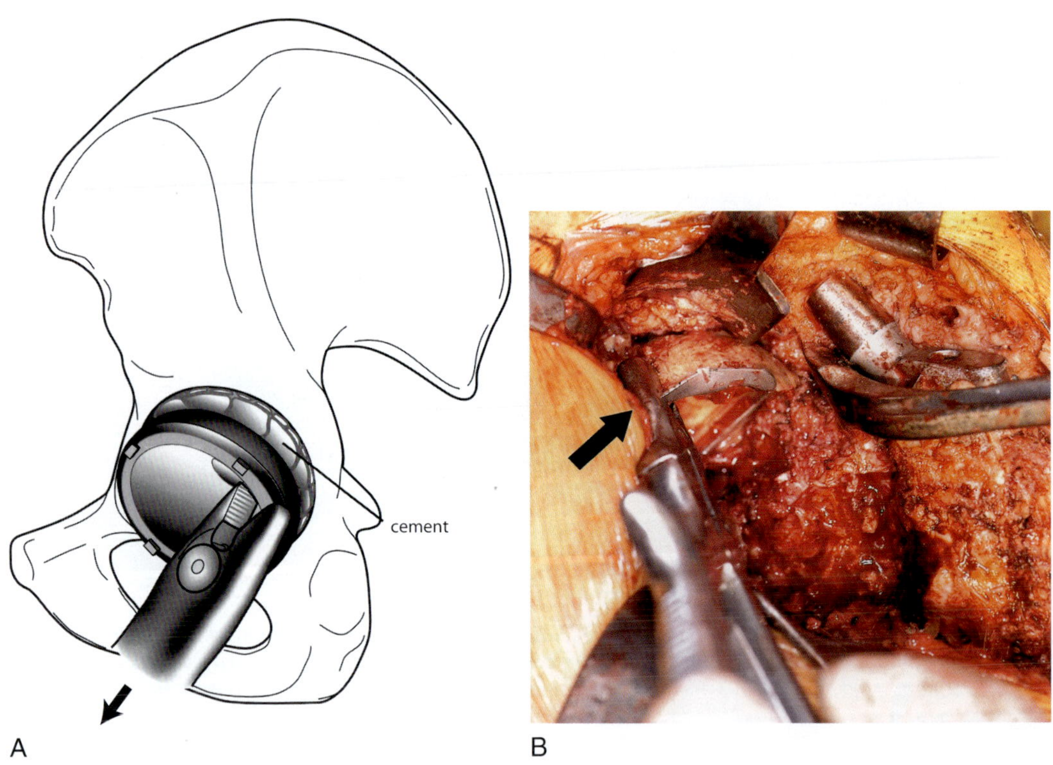

Figure 10–97 **A,** *Illustration of a rongeur rotating the metal cup out of the cement bed after fragmentation of the cement.* **B,** *Intraoperative view of a rongeur rotating the metal ring and cement out of the acetabular bed* (arrow) *after the fixation was loosened by an osteotome.*

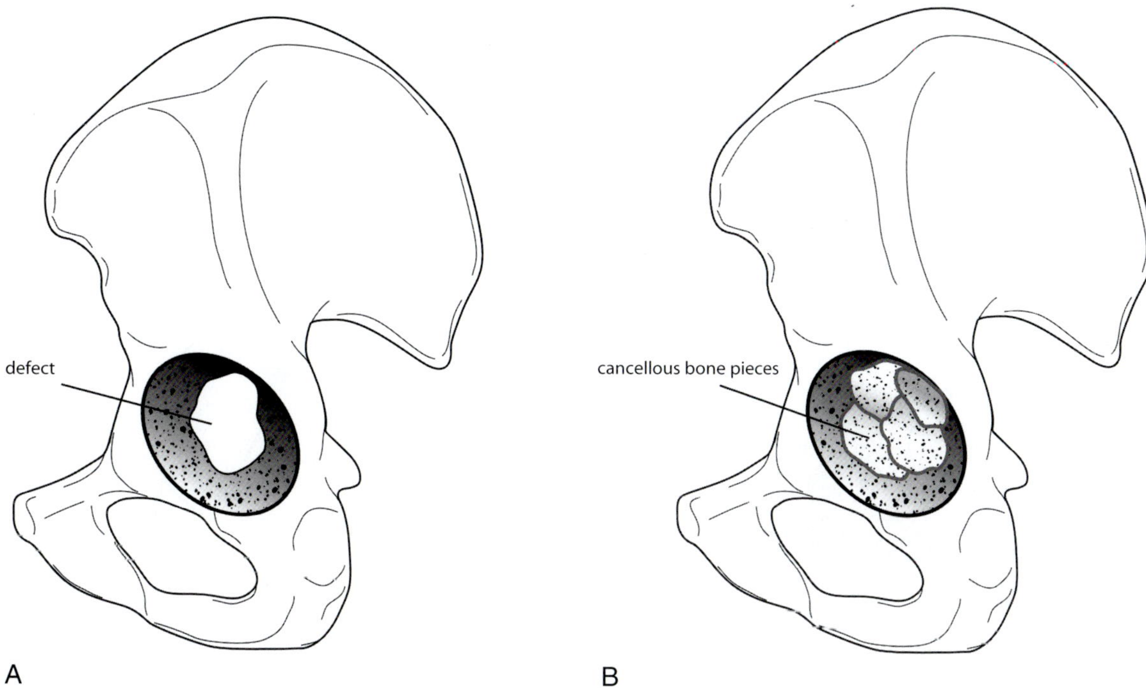

Figure 10–98 **A,** *Illustration of a cavitary defect medially, with intact peripheral walls. With this type of defect, a hemispheric cup can always be used with success.* **B,** *The cavitary defect can be packed with cancellous bone allograft to fill it in. The allograft probably will not heal in the center, but it can unite to the edges of the defect and provide more solid support to the dome of the cup. It is not absolutely necessary to use bone graft.*

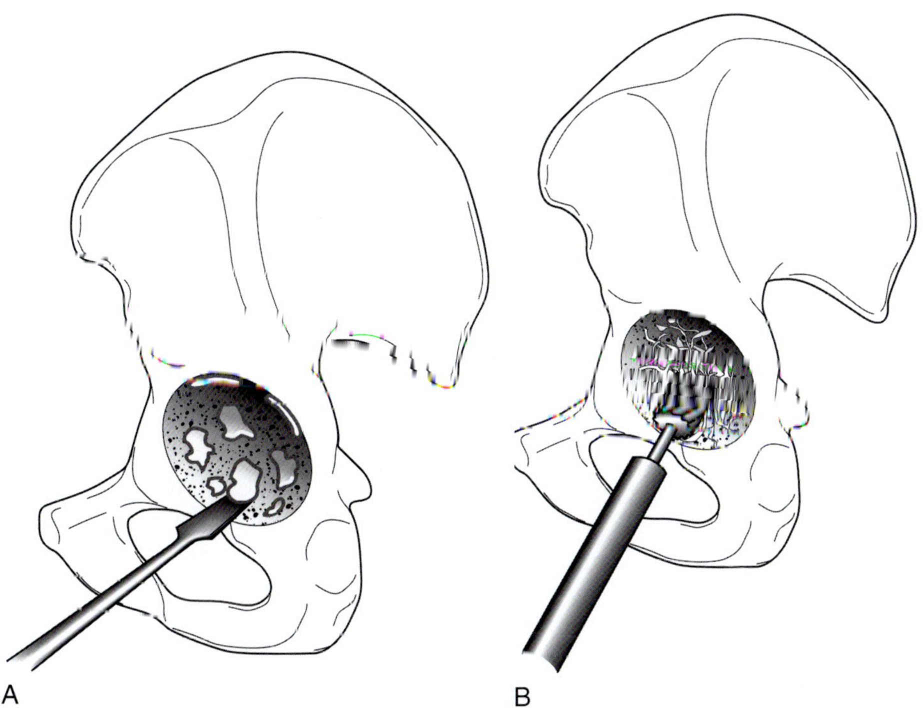

Figure 10–99 **A,** *All loose cement fragments or necrotic bone should be removed from the acetabulum with an osteotome.* **B,** *A high-speed burr is the best tool to remove, or at least loosen, the fibrous tissue attached to the acetabular bony bed. When there is a thick acetabular membrane (as is sometimes present with loose cemented polyethylene cups), a curette can be used to remove the bulk of the fibrous tissue, and the high-speed burr can be used to remove the remaining fragments, leaving a clean bony surface for ingrowth to a porous cup.*

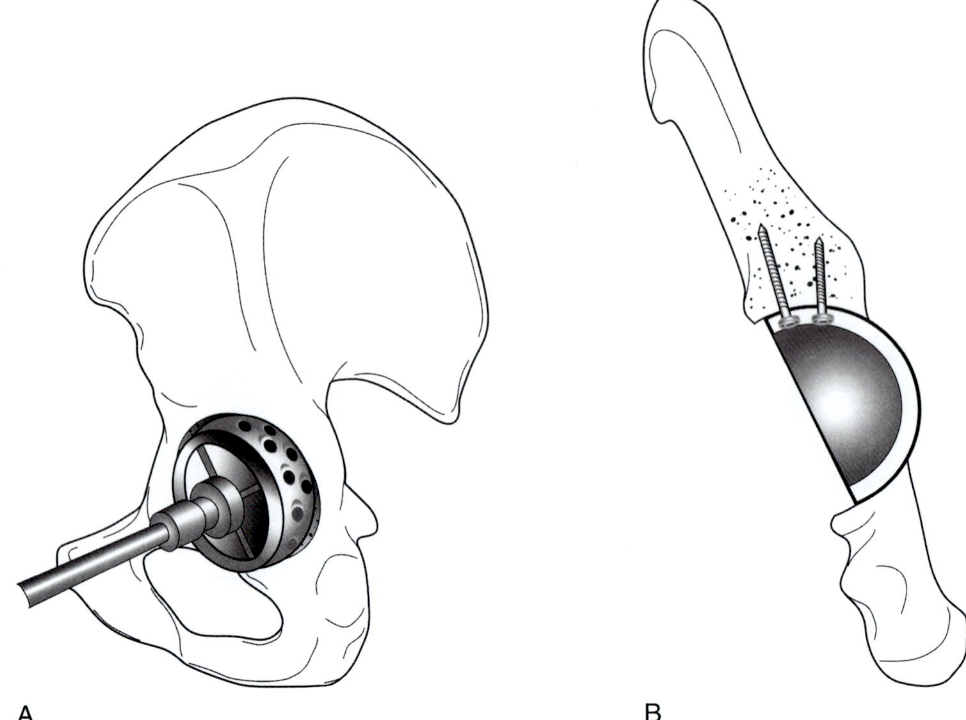

A   B

Figure 10–100 **A,** *If the reamer can reach the entire periphery of the acetabulum, a hemispheric cup (sometimes a jumbo cup) should be used for the reconstruction.* **B,** *The periphery of the acetabulum may be expanded by migration of the previous cup, so the size of the acetabular cup needed to reach the periphery may result in the dome of the acetabulum protruding into the pelvis. This is acceptable. The dome will simply be against iliacus muscle. Achieving a stable fit against the periphery is more important than the dome's protrusion. Screws should be used to augment the press-fit fixation of this cup.*

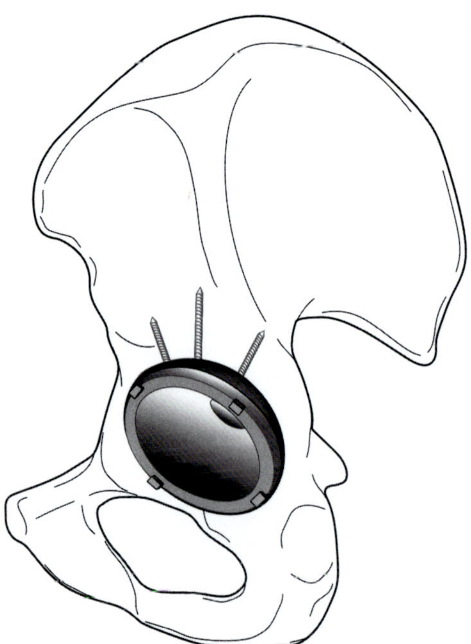

Figure 10–101 *A revision cup should have the same criteria as a primary cup. The anterosuperior edge should be flush with bone, but the anterior surface of the cup may be proud to bone if there is significant bone loss. If this is the case, the iliopsoas tendon should be recessed or released from the lesser trochanter if that was not done during the exposure. The posterosuperior edge of the cup always has uncovered metal.*

fragments and to begin shaping the acetabular bone into a cavity that can accept a new acetabular construct. At this point, the surgeon decides, with the use of the reamer, whether a hemispheric cup can be used. If a reamer can reach the circumferential periphery of the acetabular bone, a hemispheric cup can be implanted (Fig. 10–100). There is often exposed metal from a reimplanted hemispheric cup because the bone geometry does not allow complete coverage. As with a primary cup, the greatest area of uncovered cup will be posterosuperior (Fig. 10–101). With a revision cup, it is essential that the anterosuperior corner of the cup be covered and that the cup not be lateralized. These principles are the same as for a primary implant and can be reviewed in Chapter 5. I now use screws with every hemispheric cup revision reimplantation, although I have done many without screws and have described that method.[5] This no-screw technique can be used with absolutely solid press-fit fixation. However, the bone of the revision acetabulum is not of the same quality as with a primary arthroplasty, and the risk of motion or migration of the acetabular component is much higher. I believe that at least two screws should be used to augment the initial fixation of the revision cup, based on my personal experience with loss of fixation of revision cups implanted without screws.

During revision surgery, use of the computer for absolute knowledge of inclination and anteversion is of great benefit because it is difficult to orient the acetabular component with the same facility as that which can be achieved during a primary operation. In primary acetabular reconstruction there are bony landmarks that are easy to identify, and the acetabulum has a shape that can be controlled by the surgeon. A revision operation involves disruption of some of the bony landmarks, and for the most part, the shape of the acetabulum is out of the surgeon's control. Therefore, it is more difficult to get secure fixation of the cup position, particularly when screws are added. It is necessary in some revision operations to accept a less than ideal acetabular component. If the surgeon knows that the exact position of the acetabulum is less than ideal, a hooded liner can be used to provide further mechanical protection against dislocation. One of the main reasons that dislocation is more of a problem in revision surgery is the limited control the surgeon has over acetabular position. The computer allows greater control and provides information on the final acetabular position, which can then be compensated for as necessary by the acetabular liner.

Reconstruction of the Oblong Acetabular Defect

The bone preparation of an oblong acetabular defect is the same as that for a hemispheric defect. Fibrous tissue is removed, and the reamer is used to shape the acetabulum to accept the new construct. If a bone graft is planned, the distal femur is commonly used, which provides enough bulk to fill the superior defect. This is commonly shaped as a Paprosky type 7 graft, which allows the cortical wing of the graft that lies against the ilium to be fixed with transiliac screws (Fig. 10–102). If the graft fits very securely into the superior defect and the graft can be secured with screws into the ilium, the iliac wing does not have to be used. Not using the iliac wing provides some protection against nerve damage affecting the gluteus medius. If the bone graft is needed to fill the majority of the acetabular defect, the cup should be cemented into the bone graft (Fig. 10–103). If the graft covers the superior half of the acetabular component, but the inferior half can be placed against good host bone, I cement only the portion of the cup that is in contact with the bone graft and allow the remaining porous coating of the cup to have surface contact with the host bone, permitting bone-ingrowth

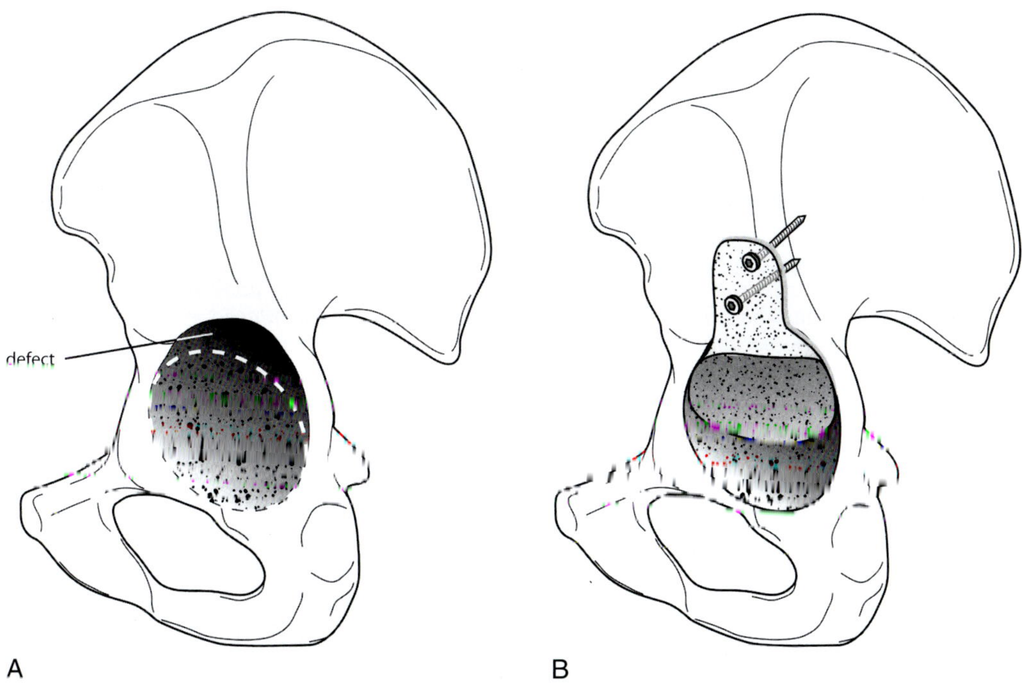

Figure 10 102   **A,** *The anteroposterior diameter of the acetabulum is much less than the superorinferior diameter. This means that there will be a superior defect that cannot be compensated for with a hemispheric cup, even a jumbo cup. In this situation, the defect must be filled with bone graft or metal.* **B,** *The defect has been filled with a distal femoral allograft shaped into a type 7 graft, so that an iliac extension of the graft fills the acetabular defect. The iliac extension allows the graft to be fixed with transiliac screws. This is advantageous because it is not always possible to get good fixation with screws through the acetabular portion of the graft. Also, the screws in the acetabular portion of the graft may interfere with the positioning of the cup.*

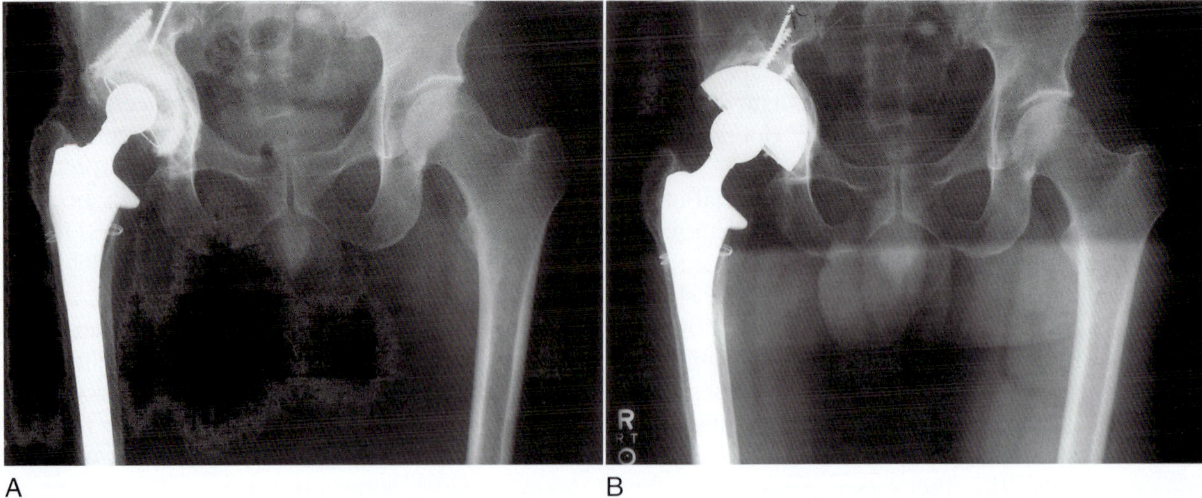

Figure 10–103 **A,** Ten-year postoperative x-ray of a cemented cup in an acetabulum that was reconstructed with a superior bone graft. **B,** The revision of this loose cemented cup was done with a jumbo hemispheric cup with a porous coating. A protrusio liner was used to reestablish leg length and offset.

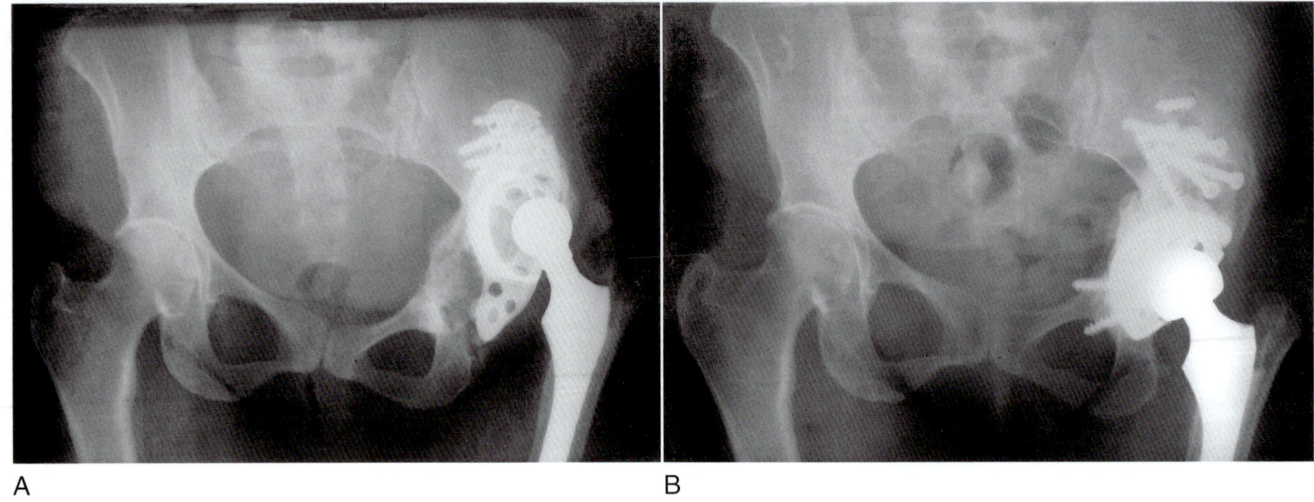

Figure 10–104 **A,** The Burch-Schneider cage has migrated, and the revision will leave a large superior defect. **B,** The superior defect is reconstructed with an allograft shaped into the type 7 graft. There was good host bone in the acetabulum, but fixation could not be achieved between the superior cup and the graft, so cement was placed in between them to provide immediate fixation. This will reduce the micromotion of the acetabular cup and promote bone fixation into the remainder of the cup. This is similar to the principle I use when cementing a cup against a metal wedge.

fixation into that portion of the cup (Fig. 10–104). This is not unlike the technique currently used for trabecular metal wedges (described later).

The reamer can be used to shape and size the superior defect so that it has a hemispheric surface (Fig. 10–105). If a bone graft is planned, a reverse reamer can be used on the bone graft to match the size of the reamed hole in the acetabular bone (Fig. 10–106). This results in a large surface area of graft-to-bone contact, permits some press-fit of the graft into the bone, and simplifies screw fixation through the graft into the host bone. A high-speed burr can initiate the shaping of this graft; it removes graft bone efficiently and with less stress on the fixation of the graft compared with a

reamer. The final hemispheric shape is formed with a hemispheric reamer.

Trabecular Metal Wedges and Cup

The trabecular metal implant has replaced the bone graft in my practice. I have more confidence in the durability of the metal wedge than in that of a cadaver bone graft. The cadaver bone graft can unite to the host bone in areas where it has cortical contact, but the graft will never be entirely converted to host bone and will always be subject to migration (see Fig. 10–103).

Use of the metal wedge requires the same acetabular preparation: fibrous tissue is removed, and the superior defect is reamed. A trial wedge of the appropriate size is then inserted as a template for fit and surface contact with the host bone (Fig. 10–107). With this trial wedge in place, the correct size of hemispheric cup is fitted into the acetabular bed, approximating the correct level of center of rotation. The metal wedge selected should allow the anteroposterior fit of the hemispheric cup, its purpose being to supplant the missing superior peripheral bone contact (Fig. 10–108).

Once an implant of the correct size has been selected, the metal wedge is implanted into the superior defect and secured with screws (Fig. 10–109). The acetabular bone is well prepared so that bony fixation from the acetabular bone to the hemispheric cup can occur. Cement is placed at the interface between the cup and the wedge. The cement provides some fixation at the interface and reduces fretting motion between the wedge and cup (Fig. 10–110). The noncemented trabecular metal cup is then implanted in the desired anteversion and inclination. The cup does not have to be perfectly flush with the trabecular metal interface; the cement prevents motion between the two imprecisely aligned surfaces (Fig. 10–111). The cup must have the correct inclination and anteversion to provide good mating of the acetabulum and femur and good stability through the range of motion of the hip replacement (Fig. 10–112). Screw holes in the trabecular metal cup allow additional screw fixation, if necessary. I recommend the placement of two screws for the same reasons mentioned earlier. The liner is cemented into the trabecular metal cup (Fig. 10–113). There is a good surface for interdigitation of the cement, making this a very safe, reproducible, and predictably durable construct. The rim of the plastic fits flush against the metal of the shell, which is one of the highest criteria for durability (Fig. 10–114).

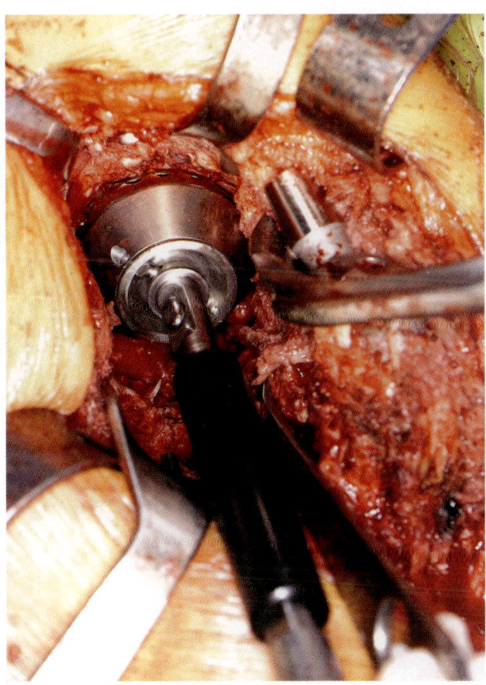

Figure 10–105   *The reamer is used to shape the superior defect so that the bone graft can be mated to its size and provide a large surface area of contact between graft and host.*

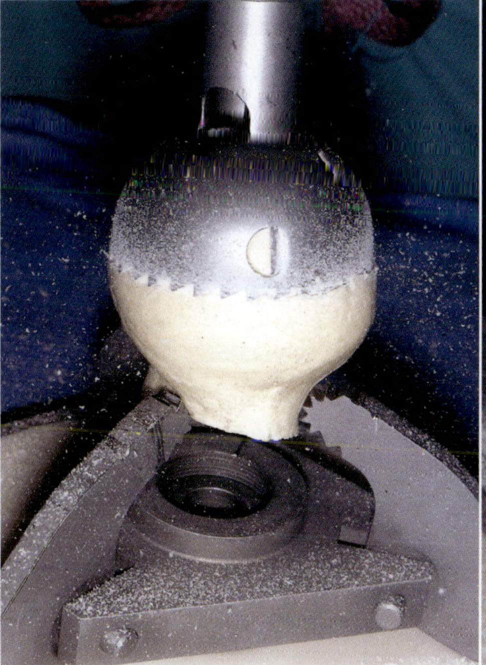
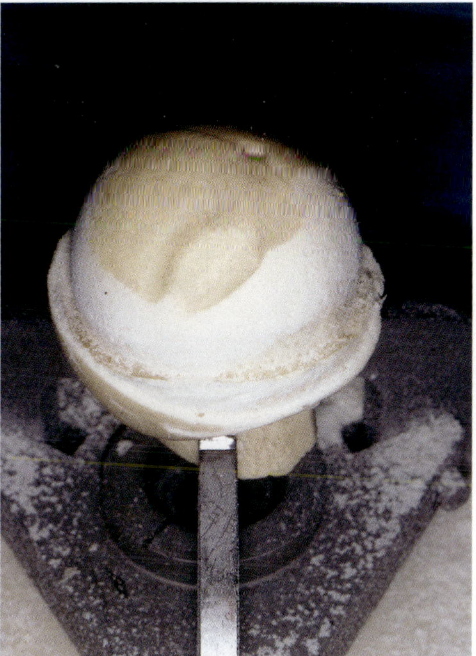

Figure 10–106 A, *A reverse reamer is used on the femoral bone graft to match the size determined by the reamer in the acetabulum (see Fig. 10–105). Matching the size of the graft to the acetabular defect results in a congruent surface area of contact between the two.* **B,** *The femoral head has been reamed to match the size of the acetabular defect. There is always a rim of bone remaining that must be removed with a rongeur or a high-speed burr.*

A

B

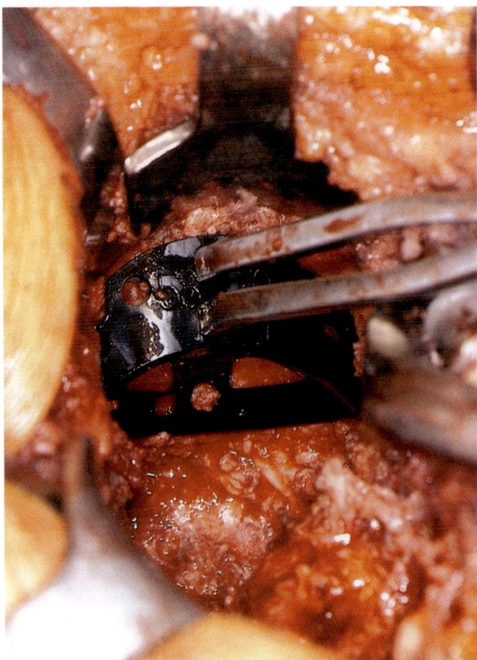

Figure 10–107   *Trial wedges from the trabecular metal set are used to determine the best fit. The wedge size used should be the same as the reamed size.*

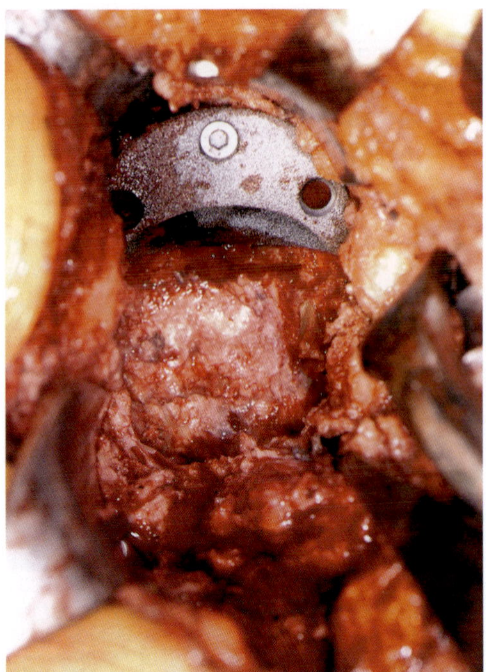

Figure 10–109   *The metal wedge is fitted into the superior defect and secured to the ilium with the greatest number of screws possible.*

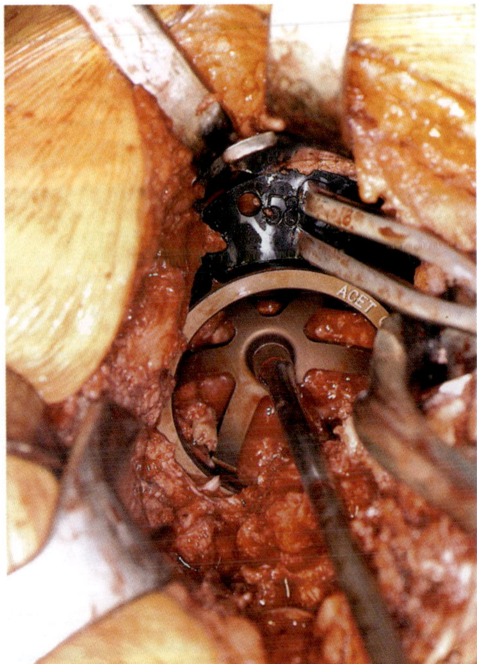

Figure 10–108   *The trial metal wedge is held in place, and the trial template for the acetabular shell is fitted to determine the size needed for a press-fit. This fit should be the same as if there were an intact periphery of the acetabulum; therefore, the anteroposterior fit should match the superoinferior fit. There does not have to be a congruent match between the edge of the wedge and the edge of the cup; the cup can be anteverted and inclined to the correct position.*

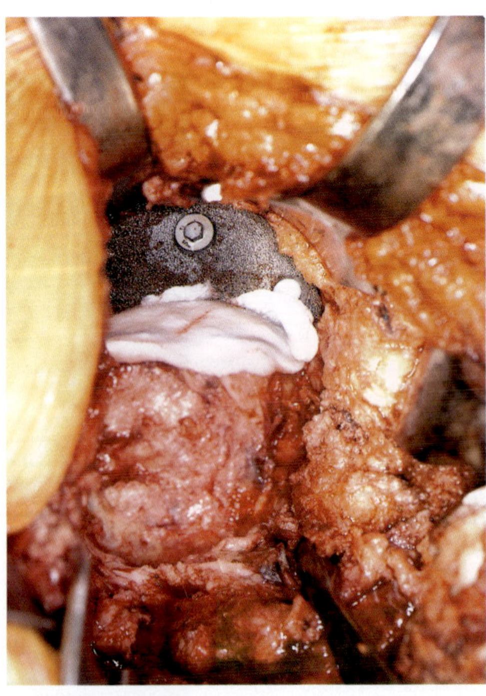

Figure 10–110   *Cement is placed on the caudal surface of the wedge, which will be the interface between the wedge and the cup.*

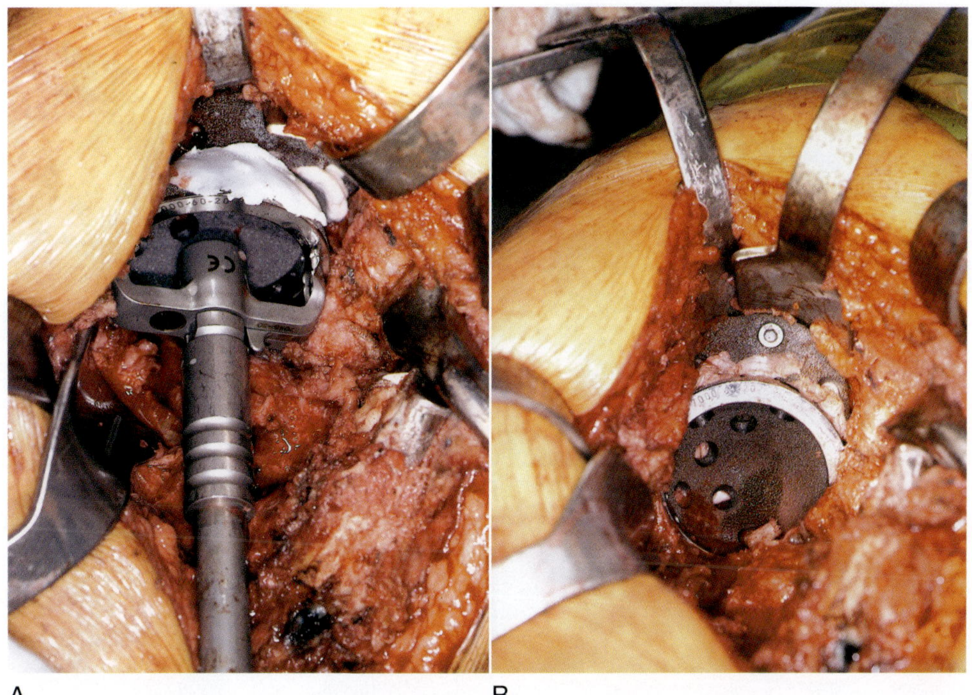

A　　　　　　　　　　　　　B

Figure 10–111　**A,** *The cup is implanted as it would be into an intact acetabulum. The cement on the cup's superior surface will interface with the undersurface of the wedge. The acetabular inserter tool gives the surgeon good control while manipulating the cup into the correct position. Cement extruding from the interfacing surfaces should be cleaned as completely as possible, but this is difficult to do from porous surfaces.* **B,** *The cup is implanted and has a good press-fit between the bone inferiorly and the wedge superiorly. The cement is fixed, and there is extruded cement at the interface between the wedge and the cup. It is best to remove this with an osteotome or even a high-speed burr, because this cement could fragment and, over time, act as a third body at the articulation surface.*

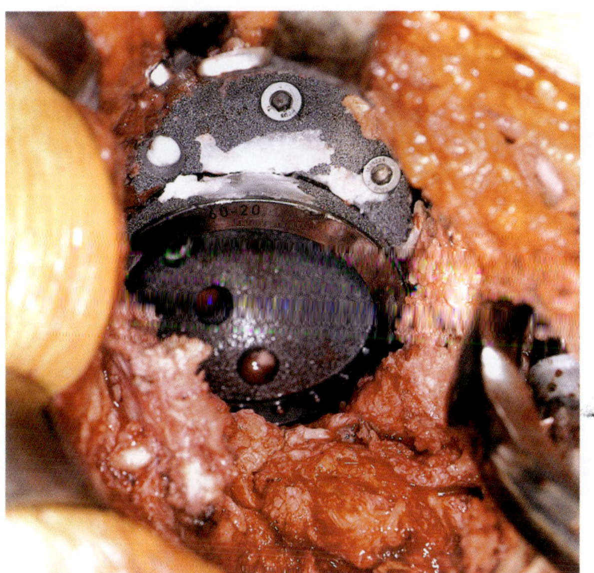

Figure 10–112　*The cup does not have to mate perfectly with the wedge. The correct inclination and anteversion of the cup are more important than the match between the edges of the wedge and the cup.*

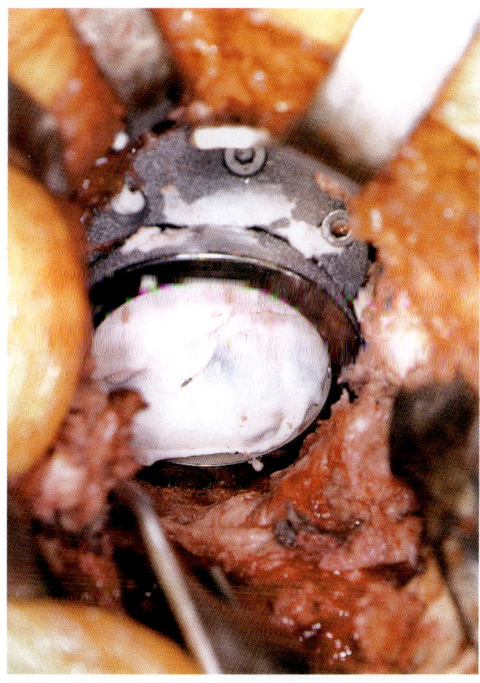

Figure 10–113　*The liner is cemented into the cup.*

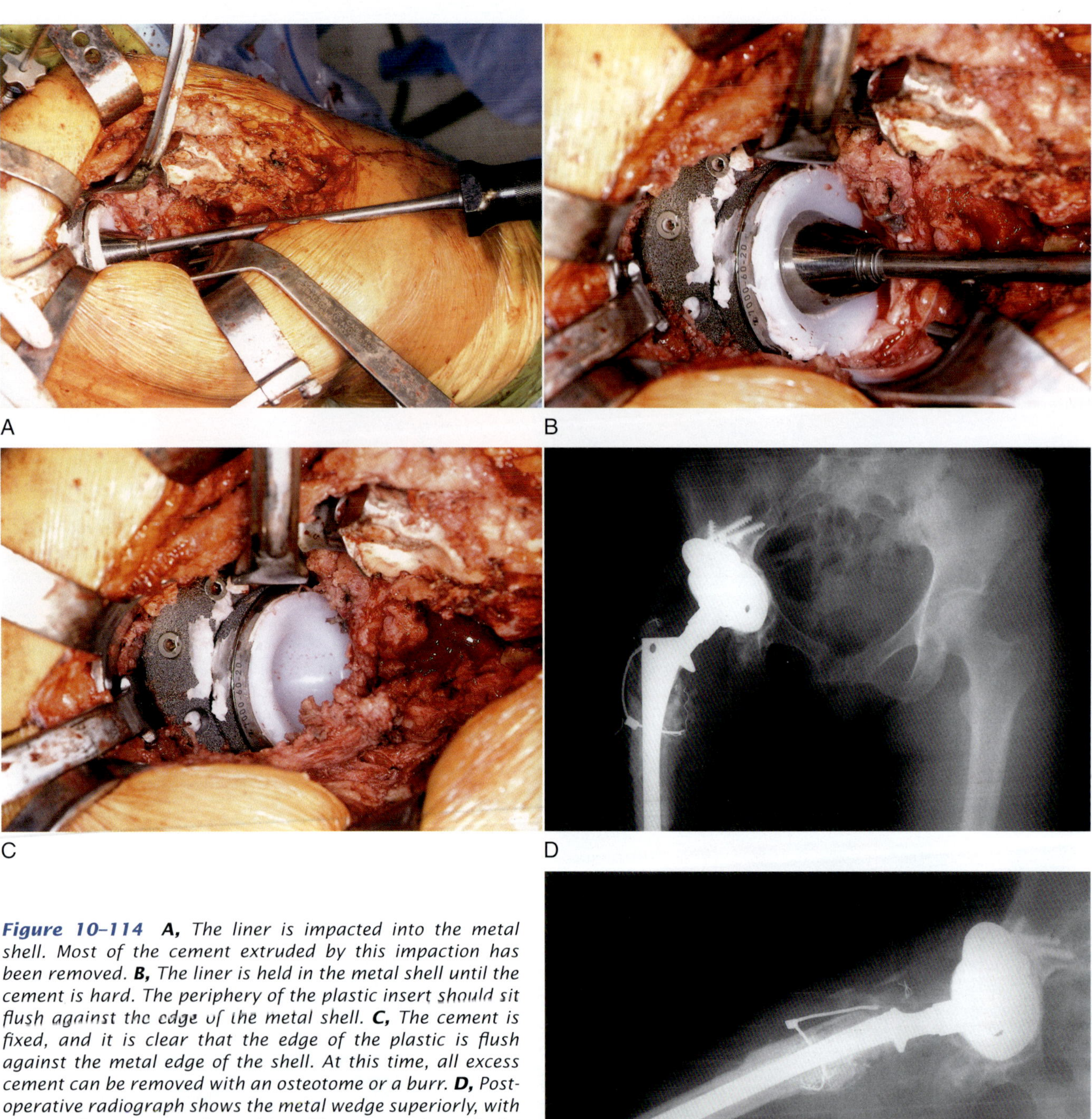

Figure 10–114 ***A,*** *The liner is impacted into the metal shell. Most of the cement extruded by this impaction has been removed.* ***B,*** *The liner is held in the metal shell until the cement is hard. The periphery of the plastic insert should sit flush against the edge of the metal shell.* ***C,*** *The cement is fixed, and it is clear that the edge of the plastic is flush against the metal edge of the shell. At this time, all excess cement can be removed with an osteotome or a burr.* ***D,*** *Postoperative radiograph shows the metal wedge superiorly, with the cup in an anatomic position. The screws through the wedge can be seen. There are also broken fragments of screws from the previous operation.* ***E,*** *Lateral radiograph shows the acetabular reconstruction, with excellent fit of the cup against the host acetabular bone and the wedge superiorly.*

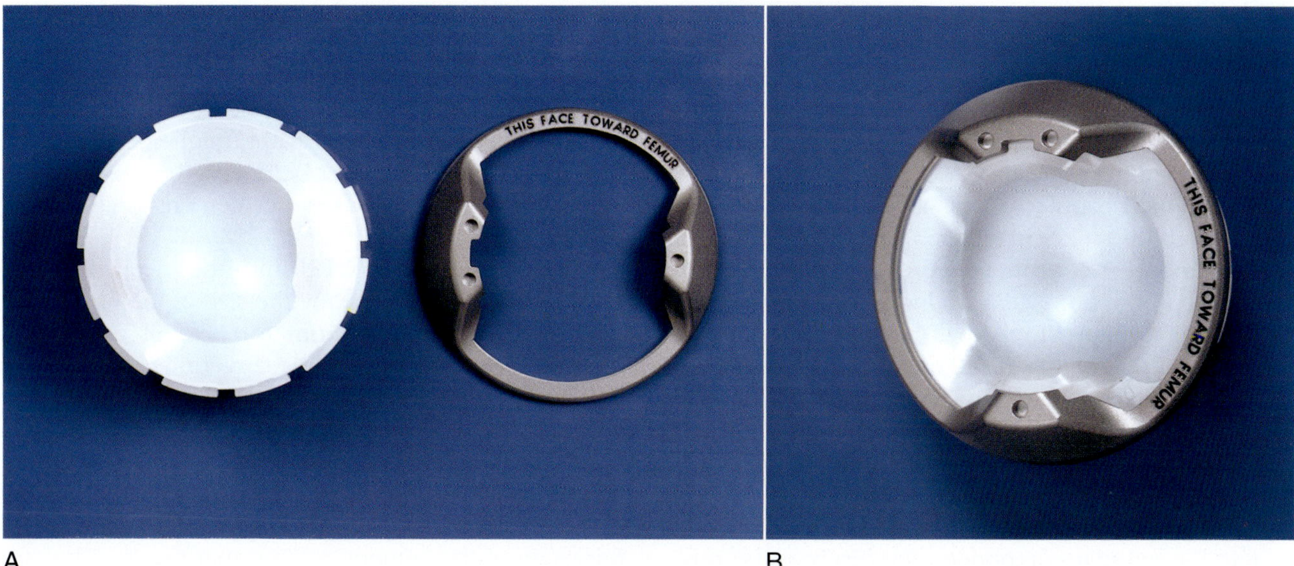

A B

Figure 10–115 **A,** *The two parts of the constrained liner: the plastic with cutouts, and the metal ring that augments the locking constraint.* **B,** *The assembled constrained liner shows the position of the ring on the prominent plastic and the cutouts available for promoting range of motion without impingement.*

The cup plane measurement will provide information about the inclination and anteversion of the cup (see Chapter 7). The computer can be used to ensure the position of the acetabular cup. Verifying the position of the acetabulum enables the surgeon to select the correct liner to protect against impingement. Choosing the largest femoral head possible is also the wisest decision.

Addition of a Constrained Liner

One of the best implant additions for revision surgery is the constrained liner. It has significantly reduced the dislocation rate after revision because it allows mechanical protection against dislocation in patients who have severely compromised soft tissue.

There are only two constraints against dislocation for patients who have severe compromise of the static (capsular) and dynamic (muscular) soft tissues of the hip. The first is biologic constraint, but this cannot be expected to occur in patients who do not have functioning muscles and who have had multiple hip operations. With multiple hip operations, the capsule simply does not form a strong structure (which is one good reason to do an extended slide in patients with multiple revisions). The second means of stability is mechanical, which is what the constrained liner provides. I have had good success with the Osteonics constrained liner (Osteonics, Rutherford, N.J.); however, one disadvantage is that it has an elevated lip that promotes impingement. Currently, I use the Epsilon constrained liner (Zimmer) because it has cutouts of the polyethylene

wall that allow range of motion of the hip and reduce the risk of impingement (Fig. 10–115).

When the acetabular metal shell (either a retained metal shell or a newly implanted metal shell) is fixed to bone, the trial constrained liner is placed into this metal shell (Fig. 10–116). If the constrained liner is going to be cemented into the metal shell, the size selected should allow the periphery of the plastic to fit flush against the edge of the metal shell. The liner should not be so small that it falls into the metal shell or that it toggles when seated against the metal rim. It

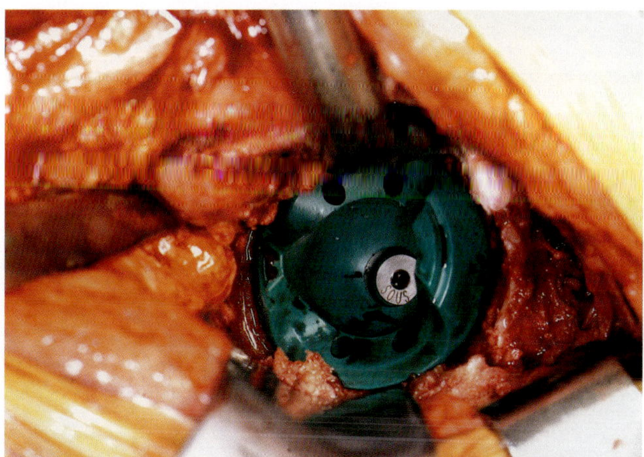

Figure 10–116 *The trial-constrained liner is in place, with the cutouts in the appropriate position to minimize the risk of impingement. The correct position of the trial liner in the metal shell should be marked with methylene blue or a Bovie electrocautery to ensure that when it is locked or cemented in place, the same position is obtained.*

should not be so large that the plastic protrudes from the metal, and the polyethylene liner should not be angulated inside the metal to increase or decrease anteversion. The sizing of the trial liner cannot be done correctly until all the soft tissue has been removed from the periphery and inside the shell.

When an insert of the correct size has been selected, the hip should be taken through a range of motion so that the cutout areas can be correctly positioned to provide maximum protection against impingement (Fig. 10–117). This usually means that the superior flange of plastic is placed between the 12 and 2 o'clock positions on the metal shell. A mark should be made on the iliac bone with methylene blue or Bovie electrocautery so that the location of the apex of the flange can be easily identified during cementation.

When a constrained liner is used in a freshly implanted acetabular component, the hip must be protected for at least 3 months. There is so much more torsional force at the interface with constrained versus nonconstrained liners that there is a history of constrained liners becoming loose quickly. I favor a cast for these patients for at least 6 weeks and two crutches with almost no weight bearing for a total of 3 months. If the patient can be trusted to be totally compliant and clearly understands the consequences, two crutches with almost no weight bearing can be used for 3 months without a cast. The surgeon must make this choice, but it is better to err on the conservative side to protect the operation and the patient.

Cementation of the Liner into the Metal Shell

Preparation for cementation of the liner into the shell is done while the cement is being mixed. A 4.5-mm drill bit is used to remove the soft tissue from inside the screw holes so that they can be used for interdigitation of the cement between the plastic and the metal (Fig. 10–118). Additionally, the back side of the polyethylene liner should be roughened with a high-speed burr (Fig. 10–119). These should not be deep grooves, but roughening the surface allows better cement fixation to the surface of the plastic.

Cement should be placed into the metal shell when it is still fairly liquid. Usually the size of the plastic insert does not leave much room for cement between the plastic and the cup. The surgeon cannot control whether there is a 1-mm, 2-mm, or 4-mm cement column between the plastic and the bone. Because the constrained liner and the cup are often from different manufacturers, the size is selected based on the fit of the plastic into the metal, with no regard for the thickness of the cement column that results. Therefore, if the cement is too viscous, the plastic insert will not fully seat against the metal shell, and the construct will not be perfect. A bulb syringe can be used to pressurize the cement into the screw holes (Fig. 10–120). The bulb must be very wet so that it does not stick to the cement. The liner is then impacted into the metal shell. Cement will extrude from the interface between the plastic and the metal. Again, it is absolutely critical that the plastic rim of the insert be flush against the metal rim of the shell. With a constrained insert, the inserter tool must be smaller than the head size of the insert so that the tool is not locked into the insert. For instance, if the femoral head is 32 mm, a 28-mm impactor should be used (Fig. 10–121). The cement is cleaned from the edges of the metal-plastic interface. The impactor holds the plastic in place while the cement is polymerizing and until the cement is hard (Fig. 10–122).

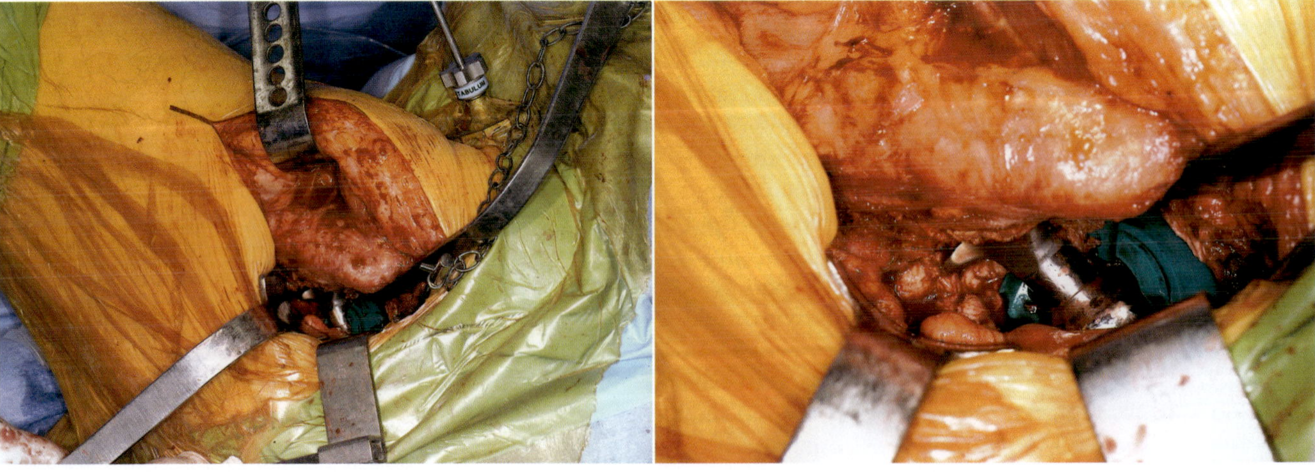

A   B

Figure 10–117 ***A,*** *The leg is moved into flexion and internal rotation and extension and external rotation. The photograph show the leg in flexion and internal fixation and the metal neck in the cutout area, indicating that the position of the constrained liner is good for this hip.* ***B,*** *Close-up view of the metal neck in the cutout with the hip in flexion and internal rotation.*

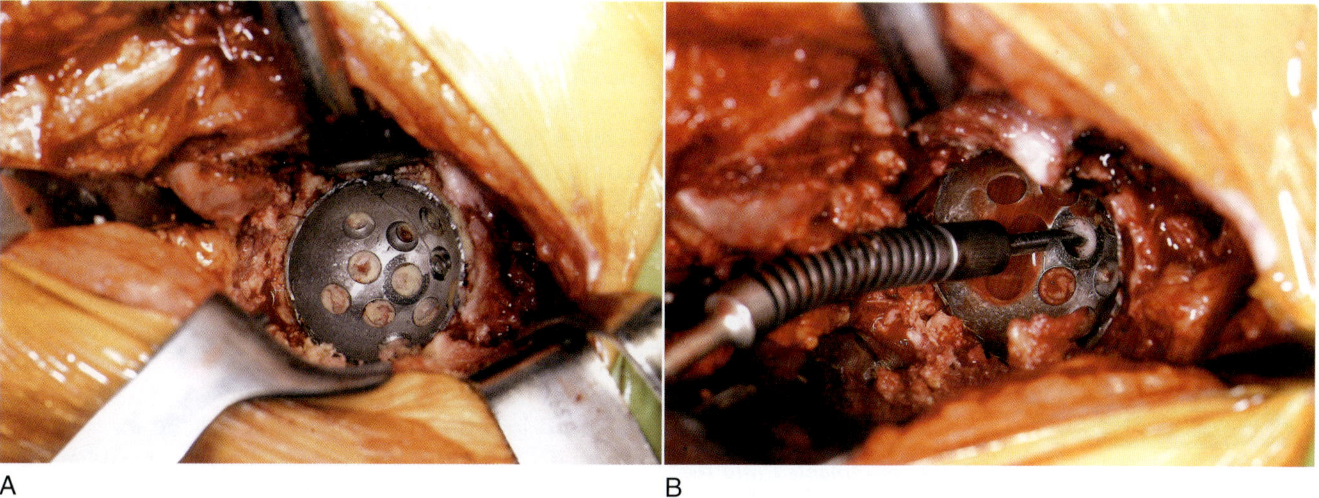

A   B

Figure 10–118   **A,** *The periphery and the internal surface of the acetabular cup have been cleared of all scar tissue. The screw holes still have tissue occluding them, which must be removed for cement fixation of a liner.* **B,** *A 4.5-mm drill bit is used to clear the tissue out of these holes in the acetabular shell.*

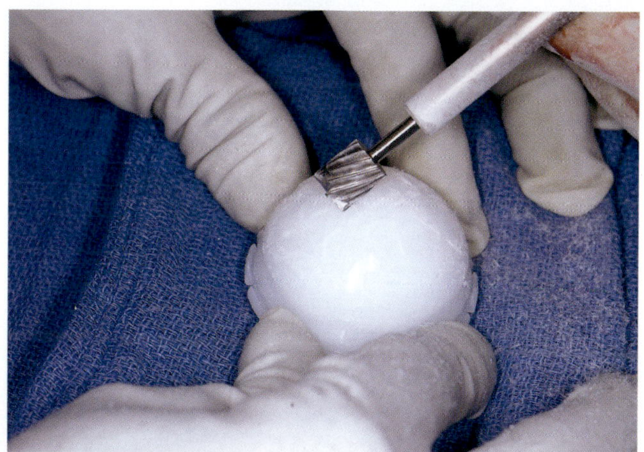

Figure 10–119   *The power burr is used to scratch and roughen the polyethylene liner to allow mechanical interdigitation of the cement and the plastic when it is cemented into the shell.*

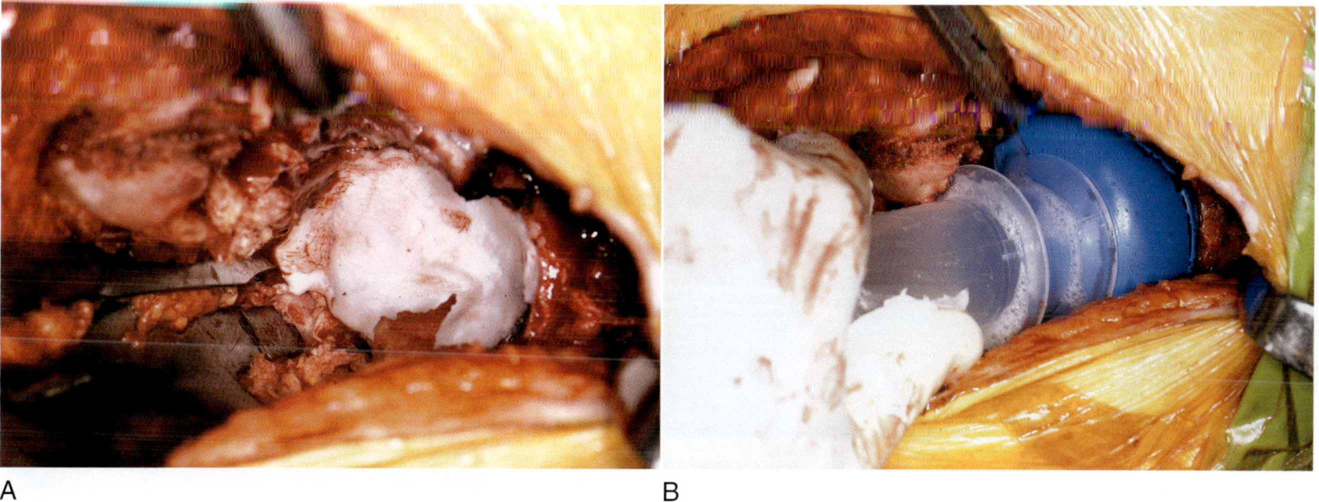

A   B

Figure 10–120   **A,** *Cement has filled the metal shell. It should not be inserted in a thickened, viscous state, or it will be difficult to completely seat the plastic rim against the metal rim.* **B,** *The cement can be pressurized into the screw holes with a bulb syringe. This technique is not necessary when cementing a plastic insert into a cup, but it is useful when cementing an acetabular component into acetabular host bone.*

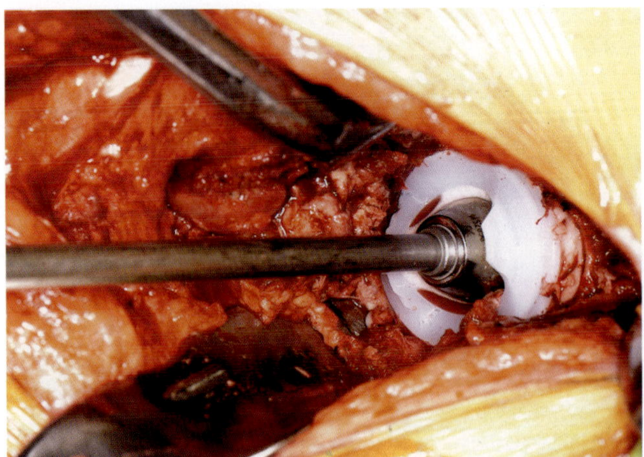

Figure 10–121 *The constrained liner is cemented into the metal shell, with the prominent plastic positioned just as it was during the trial to allow the same range of motion. An impactor smaller than the inner diameter of the liner should be used (e.g., a 28-mm impactor for a 32-mm liner). If an impactor of the same size is used, it could become locked in the plastic.*

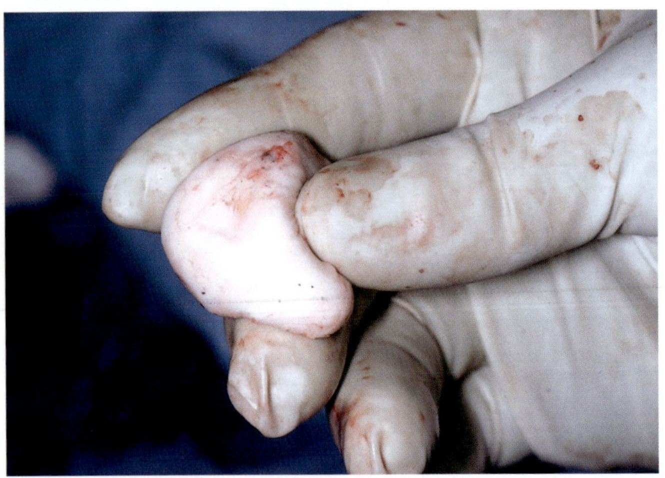

A

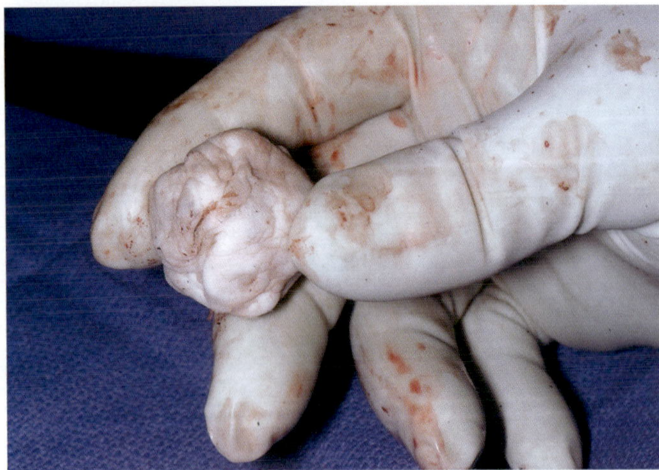

B

Figure 10–122 ***A,*** *The liner is held in place until the cement is hard. This can be judged by periodically pinching the cement; if it indents, it is not yet polymerized.* ***B,*** *When the cement can no longer be indented, the fixation is complete.*

One of the most difficult aspects of cementing the constrained liner into the shell is cleaning the locking mechanism of the metal ring sufficiently. A tool simplifies the insertion of the ring by seating it against the flanges so that it can be malleted into position (Fig. 10–123), but it will not lock if there is cement in the locking mechanism. Therefore, the surgeon has to be meticulous about cleaning the locking mechanism rim while the cement is setting. It is usually necessary to remove the impactor to gain access to the entire locking rim. Even with compulsive cleaning, however, sometimes the ring will not lock into place. If this is the case, I cut the ring and remove it, because the hip is already reduced into the constrained liner. If the hip were dislocated out of the constrained liner, it would weaken the plastic locking mechanism, which is now the only true constraint. Therefore, by cutting the metal ring with a carbide burr and removing it, the plastic locking mechanism is as secure as it can be without the addition of the ring (Fig. 10–124). I have had good success with the constrained liner, even in those few cases when I could not use the metal ring.

In my opinion, the greatest technical innovation for revision of the liner in the last decade has been the cementing of inserts into cups. I have used this technique many times to avoid having to remove a metal shell (which would require that the patient undergo complete revision of the acetabulum). With this technique in a retained cup, the patient can walk immediately, with full weight bearing, and the patient's function is much better, much more quickly. Even if the femoral component has been revised, weight bearing can usually progress much more rapidly, because limited weight bearing is generally used after revision operations to protect the acetabulum.

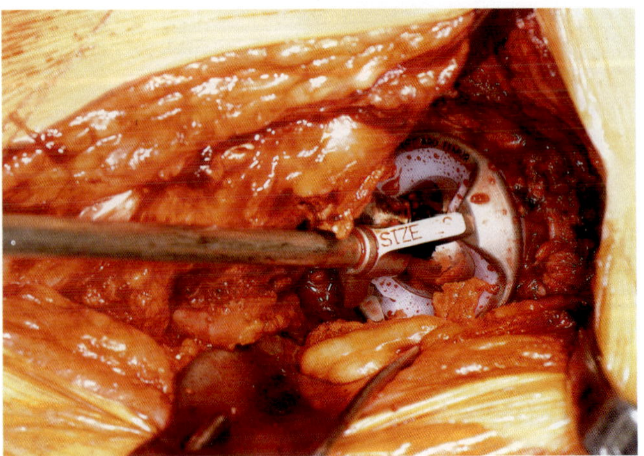

Figure 10–123 *A tool aids in inserting the metal ring onto the plastic. The locking groove for the liner must be entirely cleared of cement for this locking mechanism to be secured.*

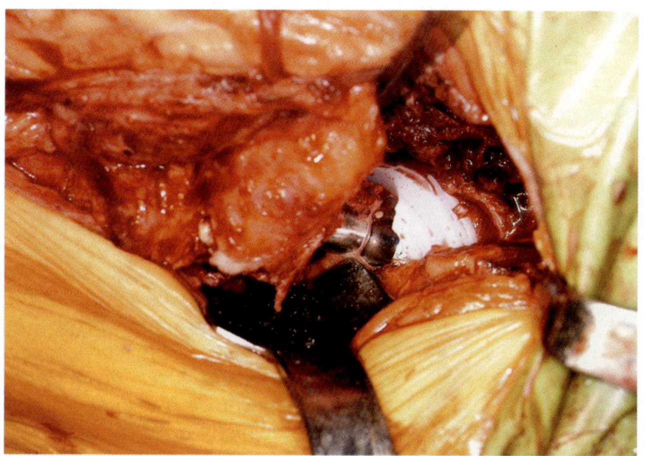

Figure 10–124 *If the locking ring cannot be secured, it should be cut with a carbide bit and removed. The hip has already been reduced, and taking the femoral head back out of the polyethylene would disrupt the augmented constraint. Even without the ring, there is some constraint of the femoral head within the plastic; this should provide adequate protection, particularly if the plastic is positioned so that there is no impingement during range of motion.*

I have had only one failure of a cemented liner since I began using this technique in the early 1990s. This failure occurred with the first insert I cemented, which became loose. It was from this case that I learned that the rim of the plastic must be flush against the rim of the metal. When the principles of cementing an insert into a metal shell are rigidly adhered to, the durability of this construct is clearly better than the mechanical locking mechanism that was previously used. Confidence in the cementation of polyethylene liners in metal shells is expressed by the designers of trabecular metal cups, who use this as one fixation method.

REHABILITATION TECHNIQUES

Rehabilitation after revision surgery requires protection of the bone and soft tissues of the hip and thigh. After primary surgery, the patient can bear full weight immediately because the bone is strong and the injury to soft tissues and bone has been very controlled. After revision surgery, the bone is weak in the acetabulum, the femur, or both, and the injury to the soft tissues is much greater than with a primary operation. It is important for the surgeon to inform the patient that expectations after a revision operation are much different from those after a primary operation. After a primary operation, many patients are able to be fully functional within 1 month. After a revision operation, they may not be fully functional for 6 months.

Weight Bearing

Almost every revision requires limited weight bearing for a minimum of 6 weeks, which means the use of two crutches or a walker. For older patients or those with poor balance, the walker is the preferred assistive device, providing better protection from falls and further injury. Younger, stronger, more active patients need crutches to satisfy their functional needs. Regardless of the assistive device, the maximum amount of weight bearing allowed in the first 6 weeks is 50%— less if there is concern about the strength of the bone or fixation. However, the need for less than 50% weight bearing is usually an indication for a cast.

Whether limited weight bearing is carried beyond 6 weeks, to 3 or 6 months, is dependent on the presence of a supporting bone graft. If I use a bone graft that will have to carry weight, such as a superior acetabular bone graft, I do not permit full weight bearing for 3 to 6 months, depending on the weight and activity of the patient. The heavier or more active the patient, the longer the duration of limited weight bearing.

Despite the limitation on weight bearing, patients can and should be community ambulators. I encourage young, strong patients to use their crutches and take a daily walk for exercise and therapy. This is good for the cardiovascular system, the spirit, and muscular reconditioning. Older patients may need a wheelchair to go to restaurants, attend church, and visit friends. It is critical, however, that all patients be allowed community ambulation with whatever type of assistance they need to prevent severe postoperative depression.

Cast or Brace

The use of an external support device following a revision operation is not uncommon, and it is essential that the surgeon be willing to discharge a patient with an external device, if necessary. These are complex operations with complex bony and soft tissue injuries. An orthopedic surgeon does not hesitate to use a cast when appropriate with a traumatic bony or soft tissue injury, and he or she should not hesitate to use a cast or brace following a total joint replacement operation.

Some surgeons brace every patient after revision to protect against dislocation (Fig. 10–125). The risk of dislocation after a revision operation is as much as ten times higher than that after a primary operation. The rate of dislocation after revision varies from 3% to 30% in the experience of surgeons, but with the options of large femoral heads and constrained liners, this rate should be no more than 5% in the future. In addition, use of the computer allows the mating of the acetabu-

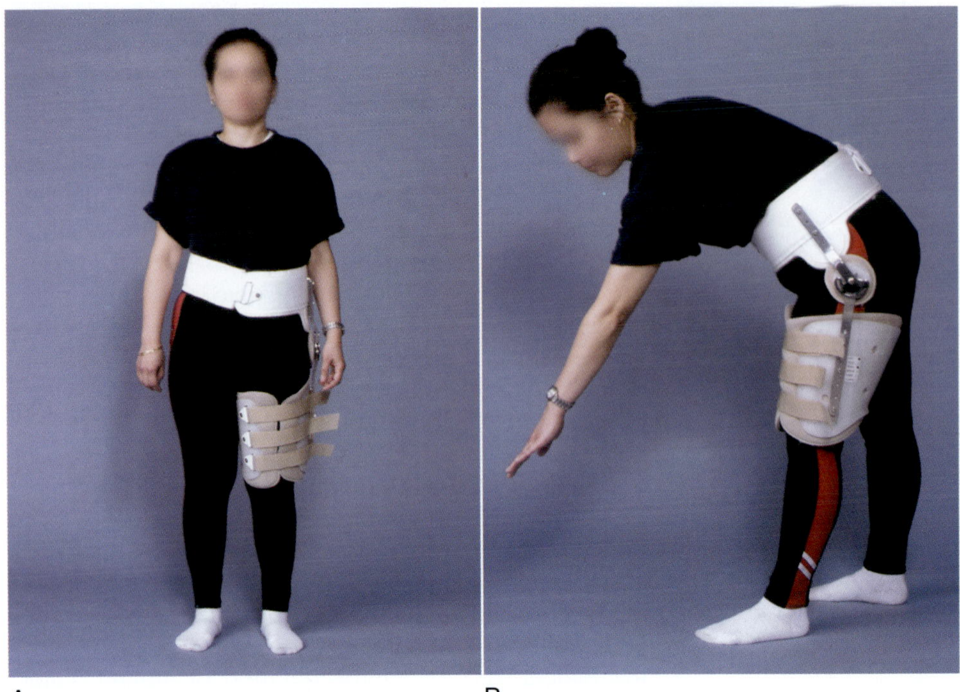

A   B

Figure 10–125 **A,** *A hip brace is commonly used to reduce range of motion after hip replacement. This brace can also be used after dislocations. Another choice is a knee immobilizer, which also reduces hip range of motion; however, with prolonged use, the knee immobilizer can cause residual stiffness and discomfort in the knee.* **B,** *The brace limits the amount of bend available at the hip, which provides protection against dislocation and impingement of the hip replacement.*

lum and femoral component in a revision to be more accurate, even when the usual acetabular bony landmarks are absent.

Bracing has a positive effect on preventing dislocation. However, the surgeon cannot be sure that the patient will leave the brace on, and most patients do not leave the brace on for 24 hours a day. There are also some patients who suffer a dislocation with the brace in place. Therefore, in my experience, the use of a brace to avoid dislocation should be limited to those patients who are trustworthy, who have soft tissue imbalance that can be protected with a brace, and who can be well fitted with a brace (for some body sizes, a brace is simply not practical). The longest time that a patient can be expected to tolerate a brace is 3 months. A brace will never compensate for poor component position, however.

If I believe that external protection is needed, I prefer protection that does not allow motion of the joint and that is not removable by the patient. I commonly use the pantaloon cast after revision operations and have great confidence in it (Fig. 10–126). It is almost always the acetabular bone that causes concern, and the pantaloon cast, which prevents motion of the joint, provides good protection of that bone. Patients with severely complex acetabular bone discontinuity or bone grafts can achieve healing with this cast and toe-touch weight bearing for 3 months, followed by 50% weight bearing for an additional 3 months. I recommend the pantaloon cast whenever there is a question about

acetabular fixation or hip stability because of soft tissue imbalance in a patient in whom a constrained liner is not recommended. Use of a constrained liner in a patient with very poor acetabular bone also requires a cast; otherwise, fixation of the acetabular component to poor bone may not occur because of the stresses present with a constrained liner.

A pantaloon cast extended into a spica cast is required to protect the femoral bone. If there is poor femoral fixation because of femoral fracture or after repair of some periprosthetic fractures, a spica cast is needed. When I use the spica cast, I incorporate knee hinges to allow knee motion and usually an ankle hinge for ankle motion. The spica cast is usually required for 2 to 3 months, and it is preferable not to keep the knee and ankle stiff for this amount of time. The hip joint is immobile with this cast. The need for a spica cast has been rare in my experience, but there are some cases when it is necessary.

Physical Therapy

Physical therapy after revision surgery is more common than after a primary operation. Patients usually do well on their own after primary operations, and simple daily walking provides them with the necessary confidence and improvement in leg strength. Patients are rarely as functional after revision surgery. There is more nagging discomfort, less endurance capability, and less physical capability, often with some impaired balance, after a

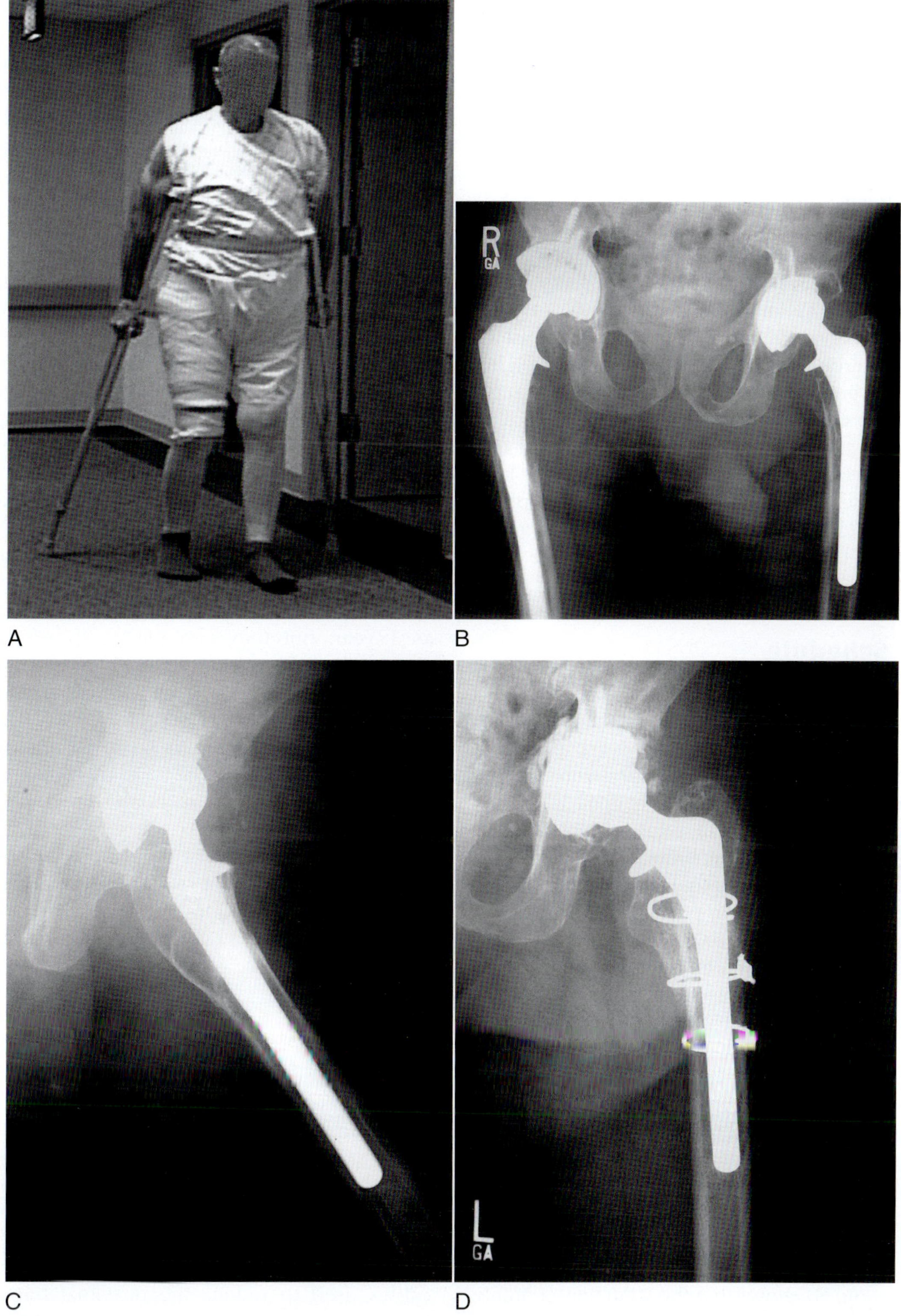

Figure 10–126 *A, The pantaloon cast is used for immobilization of the hip after revision operations. B, Preoperative x-ray of a patient who has severe wear of the acetabulum and osteolysis of the acetabulum and femur, trochanter, proximal femur, and pelvis in zone 1. C, Lateral x-ray shows severe osteopenia of the greater trochanter and proximal femur below the spot weld at the end of the coating. D, The operation for this patient consisted of an exchange of the plastic insert, with a Durasul liner cemented into the fixed cup. Cement can be seen around the metal shell from fixation of the liner. During the operation, however, with the femur retracted anteriorly, the osteolytic femur fractured and had to be repaired with three cables. The patient was then placed in a pantaloon cast for 3 months to allow the bone to heal. The presence of the fiberglass cast is evident by the fuzziness of the x-ray and the stippling between the pelvis and the femur. The femur healed, and the patient functions satisfactorily, but with a limp.*

revision operation. In spite of preoperative counseling, many patients still expect to have results consistent with their primary operations. Therefore, the use of physical therapy is good for patients both mentally and physically. Physical therapy allows them to believe that they have done everything possible to restore their leg strength and coordination. A good physical therapist can teach patients their limitations, help them curtail their expectations, and get them to accept their physical disabilities and adapt to them.

The timing of physical therapy is dependent on the complexity of the operation. For many patients, it is best to heal for 6 weeks before the therapist begins muscle-strengthening exercises. I prohibit the use of leg weights on all hip replacement patients, either primary or revision, for at least 6 weeks and usually 3 months. The extremity simply cannot tolerate this level of load, and it increases the patient's pain. If the surgeon has any concern about the quality of fixation, the use of physical therapy should reflect it. Clearly, if a brace or a cast is used, physical therapy cannot fully commence until after its removal.

Recovery Schedule

It is important for revision patients, and surgeons who perform revisions, to understand that complete healing is a 1-year process. There is usually very poor leg strength for 3 months after revision. Patients are on crutches during this time, and the magnitude of the operation has caused significant weakness of the hip musculature. There is also more stress on the back, and it is common for patients to have low back pain for months after a revision. The opposite leg can become sore because of overload due to protection of the operative hip. All these are common complaints, and patients should be reassured that this is a normal healing pattern.

The healing pattern after revision surgery should be outlined for patients in 3-month segments. For the first 3 months, patients will be using an assistive device, will have limited physical capability, and will have pain and weakness in the leg.

During the second 3 months, the strength of the leg will begin to improve, and patients will be able to function without an assistive device, depending on the complexity of the revision. At this time, patients can begin physical therapy and start a simple exercise routine, such as riding an exercise bike. For someone with a very simple revision, certain activities, such as golf, can be resumed if the leg will tolerate it. Many of the decisions regarding the patient's progress during this period have to be individualized according to the patient and the operation performed.

The third 3-month period brings more comfort, more endurance, and more physical capability. Patients will be free of assistive devices and will be able to begin engaging in activities they enjoy. They need to be warned not to expect to walk a golf course for as long as 1 year, but they can play golf using a cart. The resumption of sporting activities must be an individualized decision based on leg strength and healing of the operation.

By the fourth 3-month segment, patients begin to gain confidence that the operation has worked, and they also become aware of the level at which it has worked. Patients start to understand what their limitations are and what their expectations should be. They begin to adapt to the permanent limitations caused by the revision operation. The healing curve shown in Chapter 11 is simply prolonged for revision patients.

X-ray Example 1: The preoperative x-ray is shown in Figure A. This patient has varus femoral necks, which can result in a higher risk of fracture with impaction of the stem. A second fracture risk is a large anterior bow of the femur, as seen on the lateral x-ray (see Fig. A). The postoperative anteroposterior pelvis x-ray (Fig. B) shows that the stem was certainly not too big for this canal. At surgery, because of the varus neck, the femoral implant had to be malleted deeper into the bone to equalize the leg lengths. Still, as seen in the postoperative lateral x-ray (Fig. C), there is no indication that the stem was wedged into the femur, causing a fracture. The patient returned to the office at 6 weeks for follow-up, and the x-ray shown in Figure D was taken. Clearly, the stem has sunk, and the femur has fractured. It was assumed that an intraoperative fracture was not recognized. The femur below the fracture remained intact (Fig. E), which means that good fixation with a revision stem can be obtained. The revision was completed with cables used to reduce the proximal fracture, and a long revision stem was inserted (Fig. F). The lateral x-ray of the revision operation is shown in Figure G. The postoperative x-rays were obtained 4 months after revision and show good healing at the fracture site. The patient was free of pain and ambulating with full weight bearing at that time.

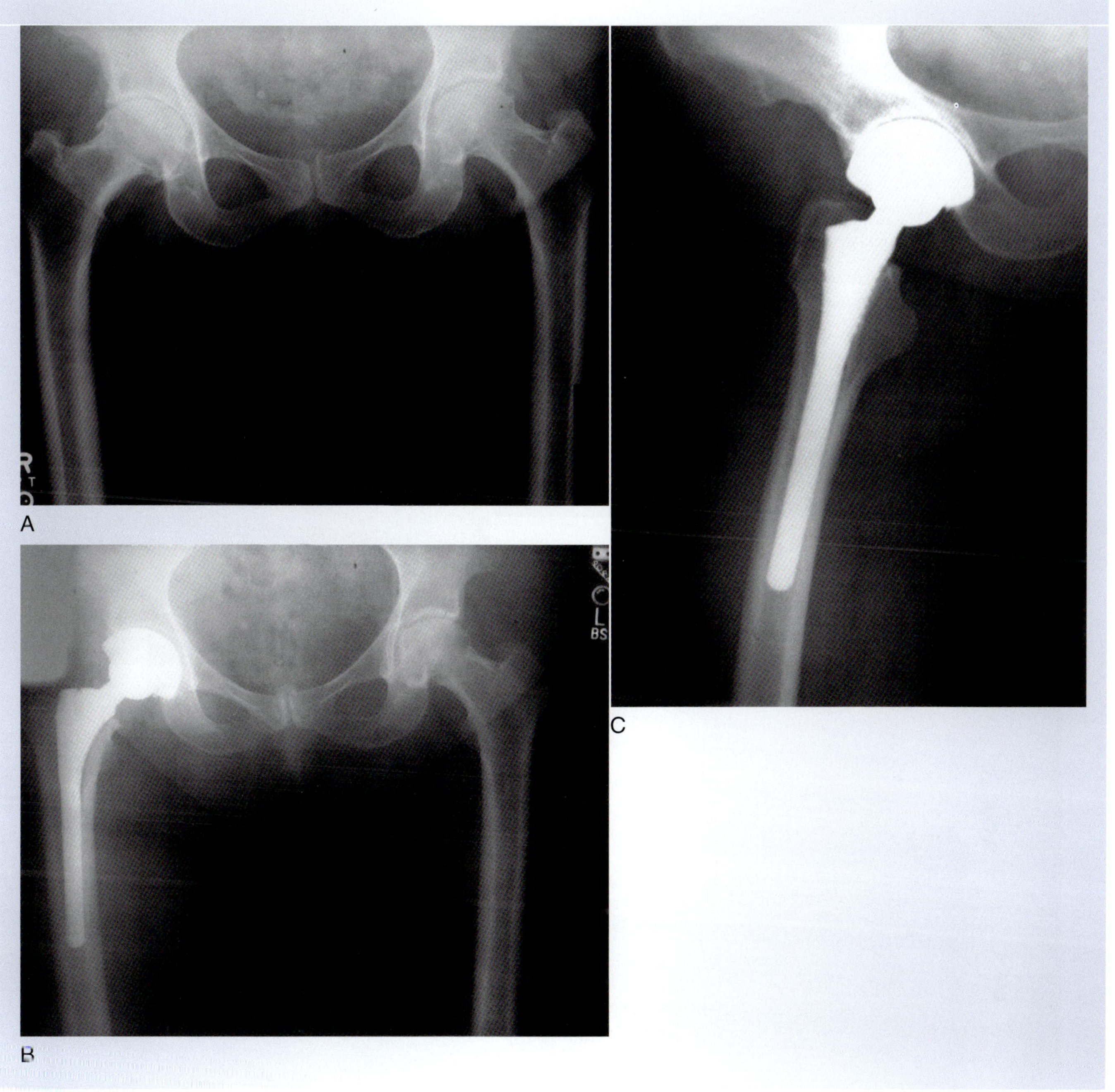

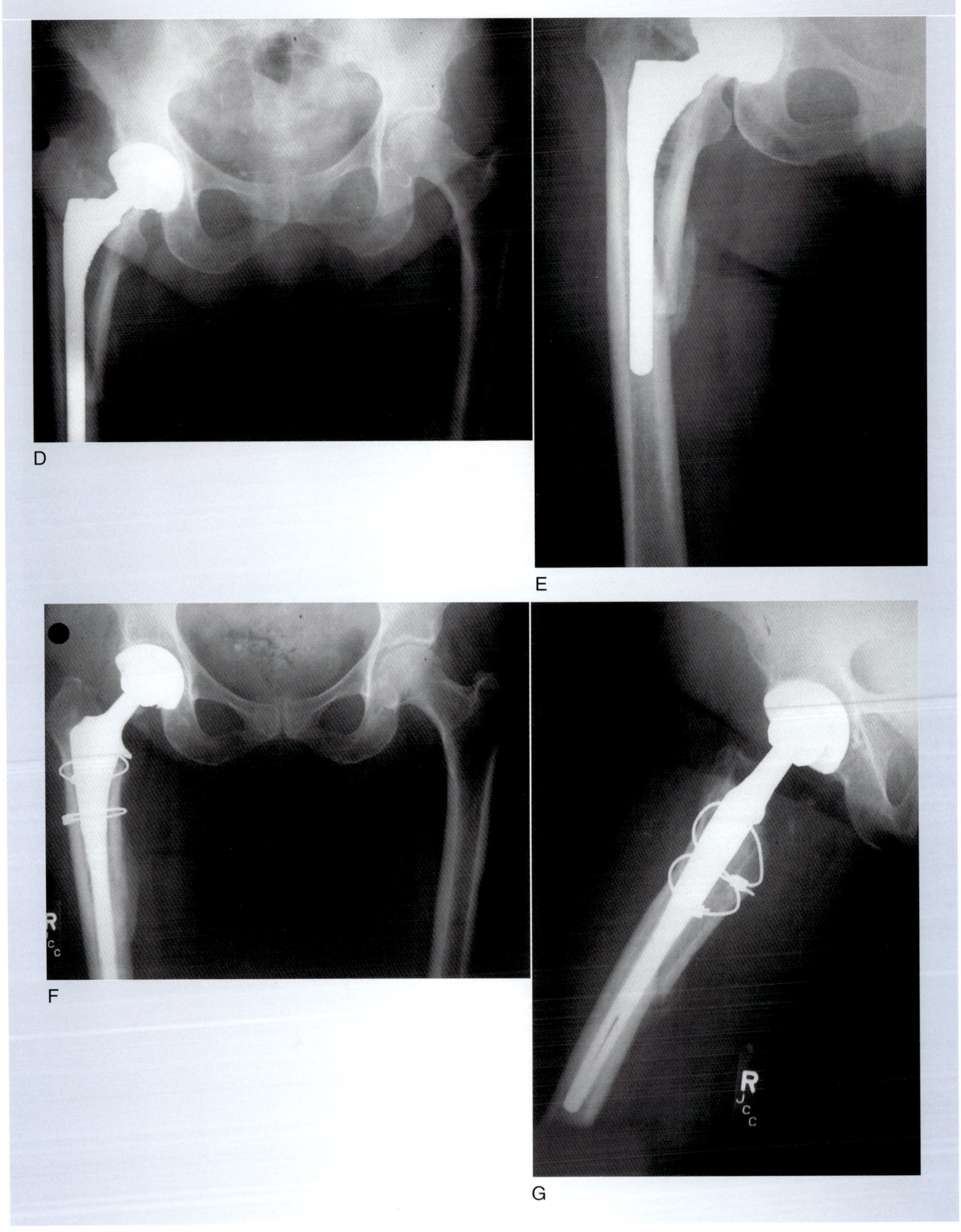

D

E

F

G

X-ray Example 2: The preoperative x-ray is shown in Figure A. The operation was performed without complication, and the postoperative x-ray is shown in Figure B. Four weeks after the operation, the patient caught her leg between two pieces of furniture at home and had a twisting fall. She suffered a fracture of the proximal metaphysis, with sinking of the stem (Fig. C). Interestingly, the patient had a fracture rather than a dislocation, confirming the stability of the reconstruction. The revision of this operation was straightforward, with removal of the sunken and loose implant and reduction and fixation of the fracture with cables. A stem one size larger was inserted to compensate for the enlargement of the metaphysis by the fracture (Fig. D). This patient's revision healed and functioned like a primary hip replacement. It should be observed that if the collar is left proud, as was done in this patient, the iliopsoas tendon must be recessed so that it does not impinge on the collar and cause groin pain.

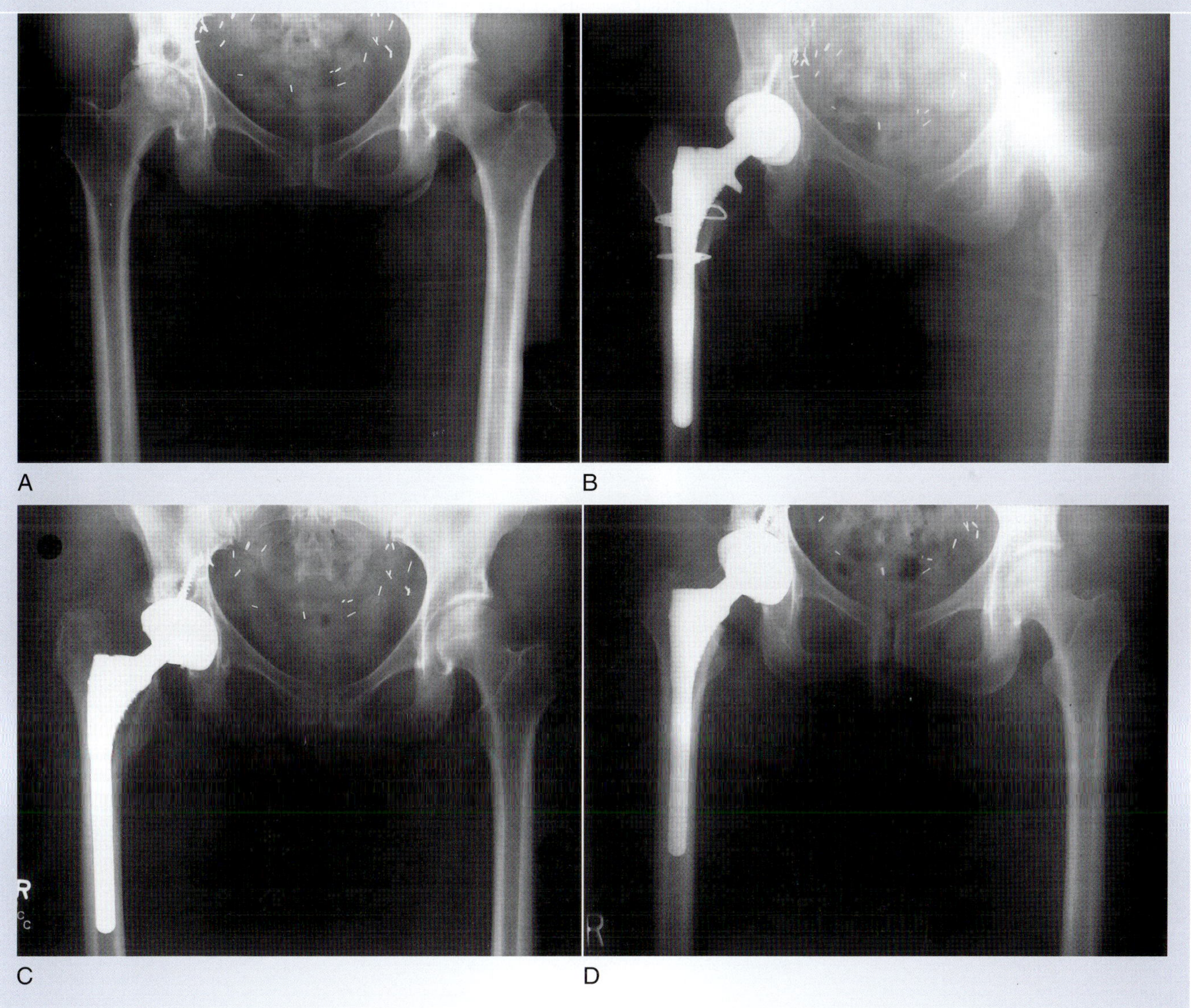

X-ray Example 3: This patient had a right total hip replacement performed 5 years before the left total hip replacement. The left hip replacement had no difficulties at surgery, but the patient returned 1 month later with a left hip infection caused by an enterococcus (Fig. A). At the time of open debridement, the loose cup was removed, and an attempt was made to save the cemented stem. Antibiotic-impregnated cement was used to loosely cement a constrained liner as a spacer (Fig. B). Trying to "cut corners" and save an implant is rarely successful, and this case was no exception. In a third operation, the cemented stem had to be removed, and a new spacer was placed for the cup and the stem (Fig. C). Because the infection was caused by a vancomycin-resistant enterococcus, in the third procedure the cement was mixed with seven doses of vancomycin for every bag of cement (Arlen Hanssen of the Mayo Clinic taught me that vancomycin-resistant enterococcal infections can be treated successfully with very high doses of vancomycin in the cement spacer). The infection was controlled, and 2 months after the placement of the spacer, the stem was reimplanted in a fourth operation (Fig. D). Again, the cement was mixed with high doses of vancomycin. Three years later, the patient functions well with little discomfort. The lateral x-ray is shown in Figure E.

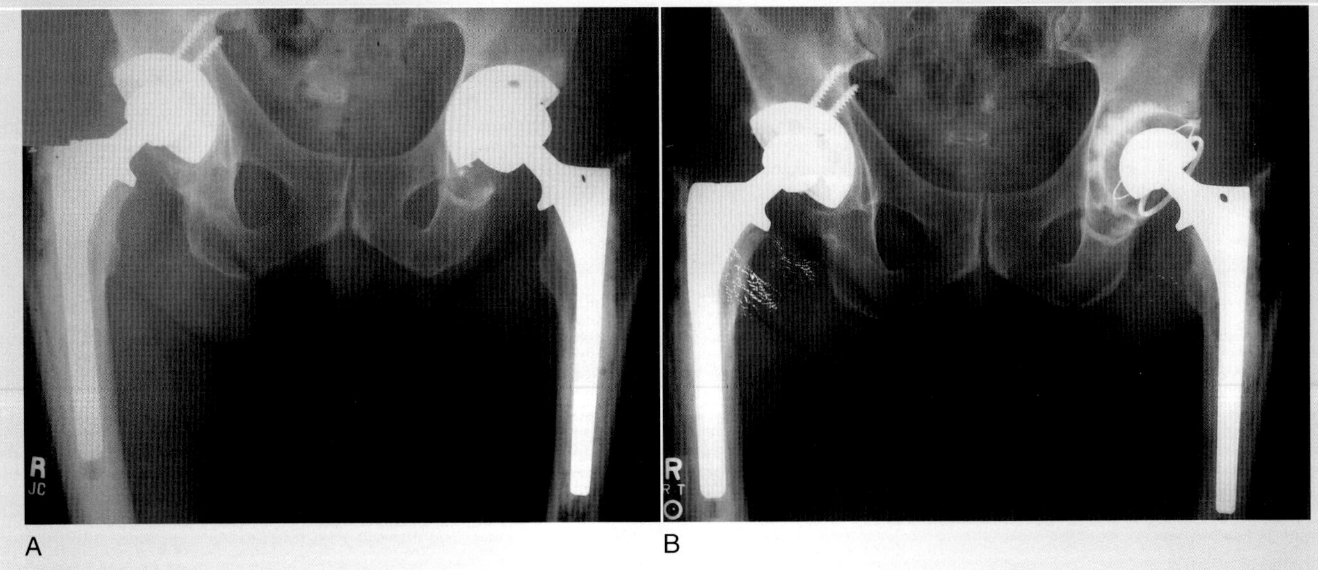

A   B

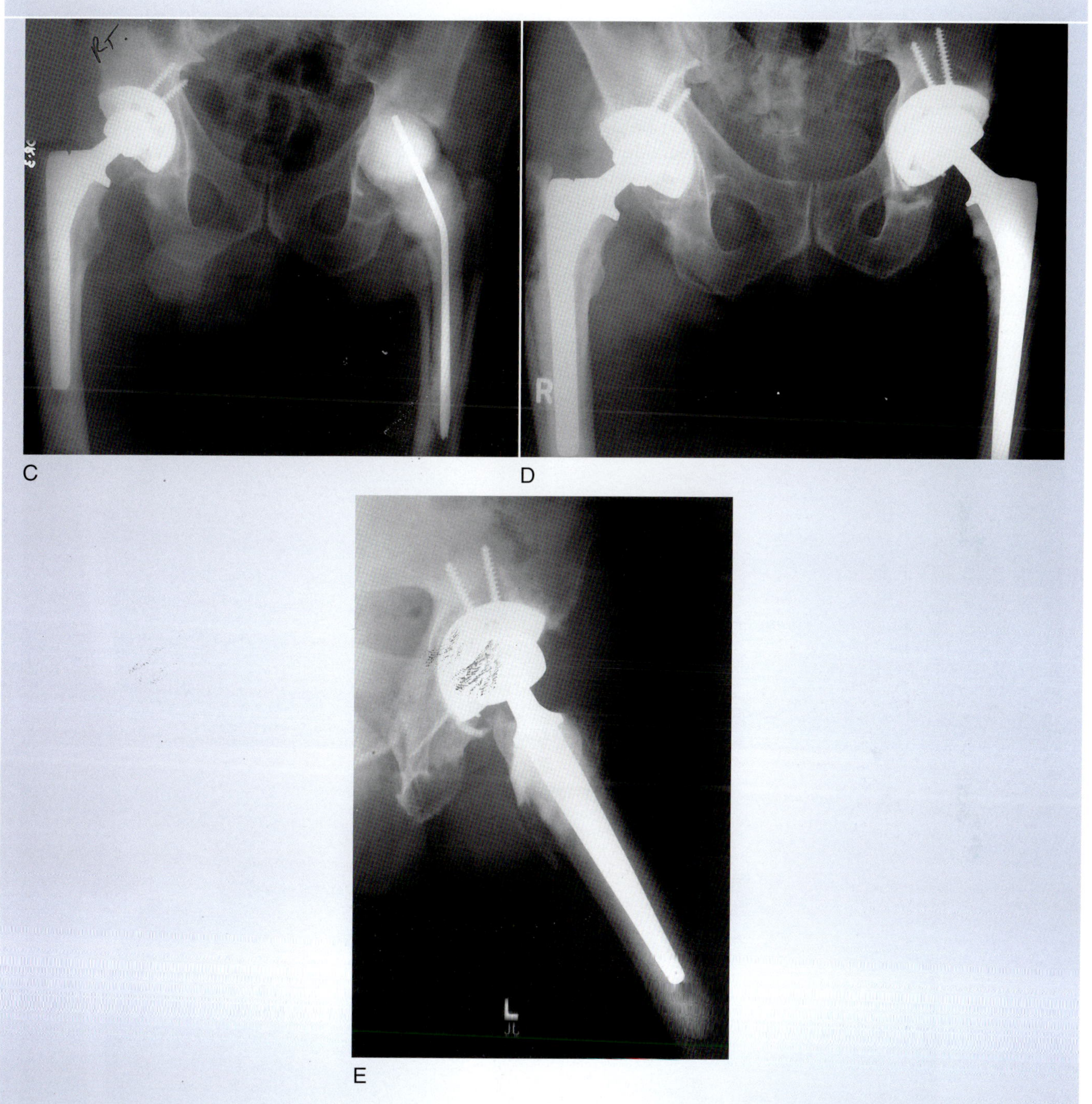
R.T.
R
L

X-ray Example 4: This patient required bilateral total hip replacement for severe osteoarthritis (Fig. A). Postoperatively, the acetabulum for the left hip had essentially no anteversion, as observed by no apparent opening of the acetabular mouth. Even though a 38-mm head was used, the poor mating of the femoral head and cup and an obviously poor anteversion resulted in a high risk for dislocation (Fig. B), which did occur. At the time of revision, the anteversion of the cup was measured by computer as 5 degrees (Fig. C). Revision was accomplished with 20 degrees of anteversion of the cup, as seen by the opening of the acetabulum in Figure D. I normally prescribe aspirin for deep venous thrombosis prophylaxis. This patient, however, required chemical anticoagulant treatment for prophylaxis of venous thrombosis, and the occurrence of heterotopic bone can be seen in this hip. Heterotopic bone does not occur when aspirin is used.

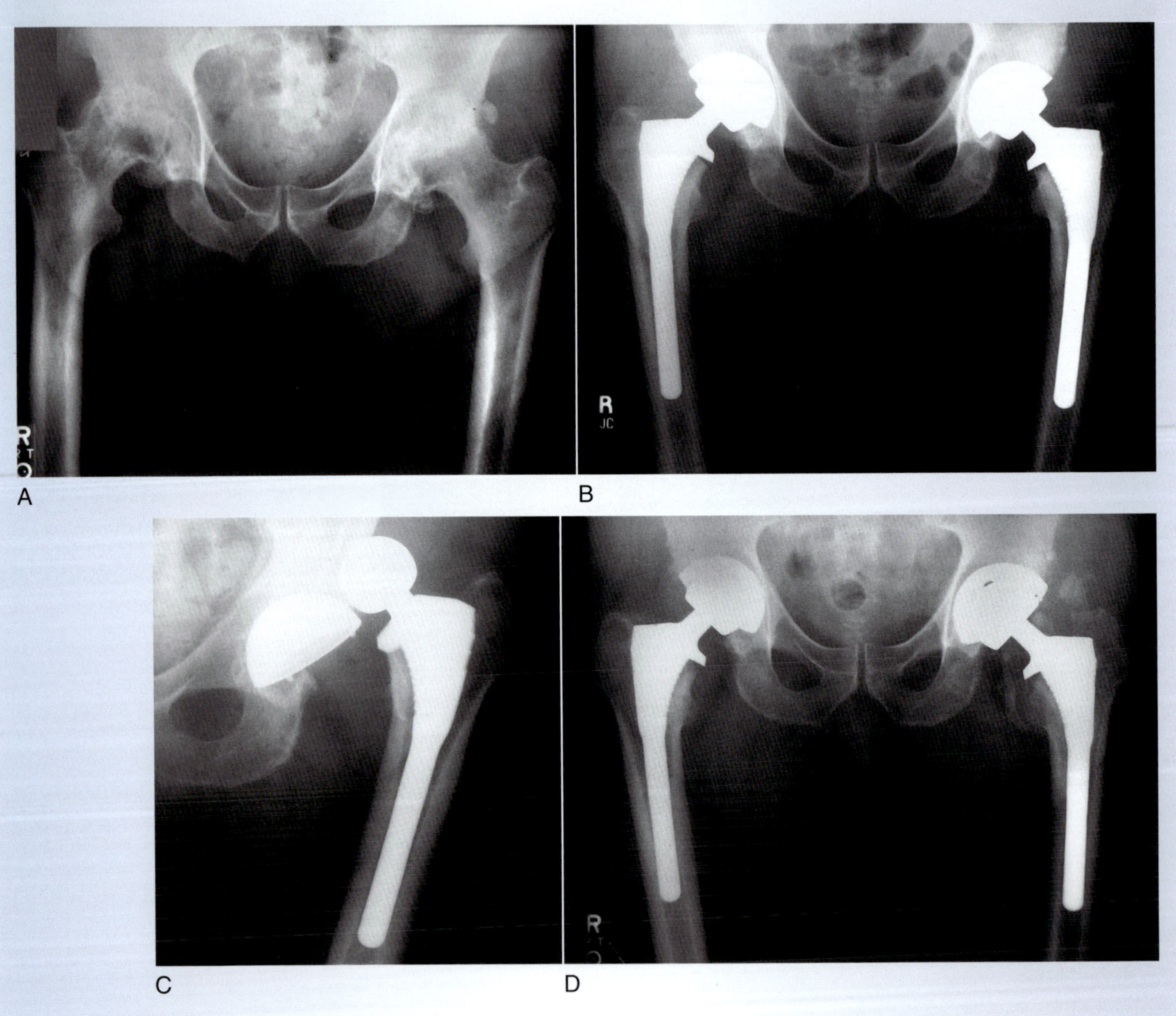

A

B

C

D

References

1. Paprosky WG, Lawrence J, Cameron H: Femoral defect classification: Clinical application. Orthop Rev 19(Suppl):9, 1990.
2. Udomkiat P, Dorr LD, Won YY, et al: Technical factors for success with metal ring acetabular reconstruction. J Arthroplasty 16:961-969, 2001.
3. Glassman AH, Engh CA, Bobyn JD: A technique of extensile exposure for total hip arthroplasty. J Arthroplasty 2:11-21, 1987.
4. Aribindi R, Paprosky WG, Nourbash P, et al: Extended proximal femoral osteotomy. Instr Course Lect 48:19-26, 1999.
5. Dorr LD, Wan Z: Ten years of experience with porous acetabular components for revision surgery. Clin Orthop 319:191-200, 1995.

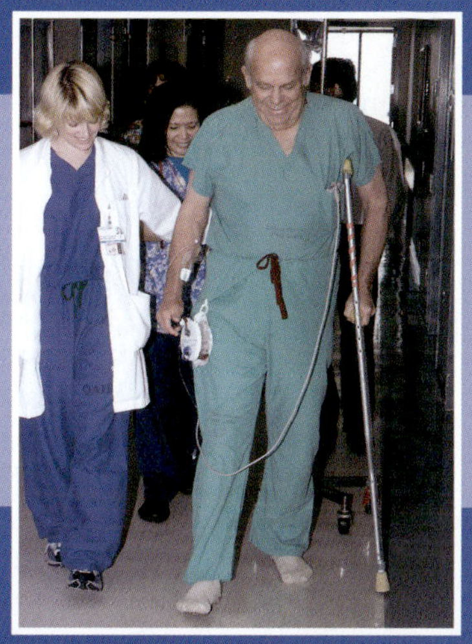

Rehabilitation after Primary Total Hip Replacement

This chapter summarizes my personal experience with the process of rehabilitation after primary total hip replacement. I had right total hip replacement with a traditional-length incision. I kept a diary for the first 6 months after my operation, and my experience has significantly changed my postoperative treatment of patients. I now allow patients to be much more liberal in their activities, and I changed my mind about the necessity for dislocation precautions, even after a posterior approach. I realized that the dislocation classification I had previously published as being "positional" is actually caused by impingement in most patients.[1] If the components are well mated and impingement is avoided at surgery, and if simple positional maneuvers are used by the patient, the risk is essentially zero.

PATTERN OF HEALING

The pattern of healing was clarified by my own experience. There is an initial healing-in period that lasts for 1 to 3 weeks, depending on the patient's age. For some patients with other mental or physical limitations, the healing-in period may extend as long as 6 weeks, but this is rare. The healing-in period is comparable to the running-in period of implants. The latter is a period usually lasting from 6 weeks to 3 months during which there is settling between the femoral head and the plastic articulation surface. This is a time of rapid adjustment to a change in the environment. The healing-in period is the body's adjustment to a change in the hip environment and to the metabolic changes caused by anesthesia, surgical trauma, and medication. I consider the healing-in phase complete when the patient can go the entire day without taking a nap, can do 4 to 6 hours of productive work during the day, can walk 1 mile outdoors (provided there is no medical or physical impediment), and can participate in social activities.

After the healing-in period, the rehabilitation process consists of three phases that together last about 1 year. During phase 1 (postoperative weeks 3 to 12), the patient regains energy and stamina. By the end of this phase, almost all patients have returned to a nearly normal daily routine, even though they still have some symptoms. In phase 2 (months 4 to 6), the strength of the leg significantly improves; the patient has increased endurance for all activities, including activities of daily living, and can increase sporting activities. Phase 3 (months 7 to 12) brings continual improvement in the patient's metabolism and all other aspects of the hip replacement. At 1 year, the patient realizes that he or she is significantly better than at 6 months.

Healing-in Period

The healing-in period is the body's immediate adaptation to the surgical trauma. Almost all total hip replacement patients are admitted to the hospital on the morning of the operation, and the healing-in period actually begins on the day of surgery.

Day of Surgery. I woke up at 3:30 AM and showered. Patients are not allowed to have anything to eat or drink after midnight the day before surgery, so I watched as my wife, Marilyn, had her morning coffee. My situation was unique, in that Dr. Chit Ranawat, who performed my surgery, stayed at my home the night before and rode to the hospital with me. He and I had operated at a conference in Las Vegas on Tuesday and then returned to my home Wednesday. My 90-minute surgery was scheduled for 6:00 AM Thursday so that it would be over before the normal surgical day began.

When we arrived at the hospital, I went directly to the preoperative preparation area, where I was given preoperative oral medications and the epidural was inserted. I was also given enough intravenous medication so that I have some memory of being moved from the transportation gurney to the operating table but no other memory of the operating room. I believe that most patients would prefer to be oblivious to their surroundings while they are being brought to the operating room and anesthesia is induced, and I learned that they are indeed unaware of what is going on.

My next memory was noting that the axillary roll was uncomfortable in my armpit. I mentioned to the anesthesiologist that I probably would not be able to tolerate that position for the entire operation, and he told me that the operation was over. I was amazed that I had absolutely no memory of the event.

I was taken to the recovery room, where the sedative used during the operation (propofol) was withdrawn, and I woke up completely. I knew that Dr. Ranawat had done a good job because he was very happy in the recovery room. Everyone was in a good mood, which included Dr. Chorn, the anesthesiologist; Dr. William Long, who had assisted Dr. Ranawat; and my wife. I was happy because I could move my foot. My friend Rich Cadarette, who is the Zimmer representative in Los Angeles, was also there; another one of my surgeon friends, Ben Bierbaum, phoned from Boston to check on my outcome. I found it very comforting to have support people around to reassure me that the operation was successful. Therefore, I now allow family members into the recovery room so that they can see for themselves that the patient is doing well and so that the patient has the comfort of their presence. Another surgeon, Richard Rothman from Philadelphia, even allows patients to talk to their family members on the telephone from the operating room at the completion of the operation.

Within an hour of my arrival in the recovery room, I was moved to my room (about 8:30 AM). There, my total joint nurse, Vi Gabule, RN, took over. For the next

48 hours, she was my boss. Confidence in the nursing staff is clearly important in this early postoperative period, when the patient is somewhat helpless. Most patients hate giving up control to people they have never met (the nurses), so it is important for the nurses to be as human and as professional as possible, so that the patient believes that he or she is receiving the best treatment.

I felt no pain as I lay in bed. However, my leg hurt with movement, and it felt too heavy to move. I was much more comfortable with my leg on pillows than having it in a slings-and-springs support device. Since my experience, I now place the patient's leg on pillows and forgo the use of any abduction pillow or slings-and-springs device. In the late morning, my Foley catheter was removed, and I learned that urinating afterward is painful (at least for a man). The first two times, I had the sensation of urinating through razor blades. As a result, I no longer routinely use a Foley catheter, except in those patients who need it for medical reasons, such as incontinence or severe strictures of the urethra. Because the epidural is pulled immediately after the operation, a Foley is not needed for reasons of anesthesia. The Foley is just one more source of pain that can be eliminated.

At 11:30 AM (4 hours after completion of the operation), the physical therapist got me up and we walked one loop around the hall. I started the walk with a walker and then converted to one crutch (Fig. 11–1). It is a real feeling of accomplishment to be able to put

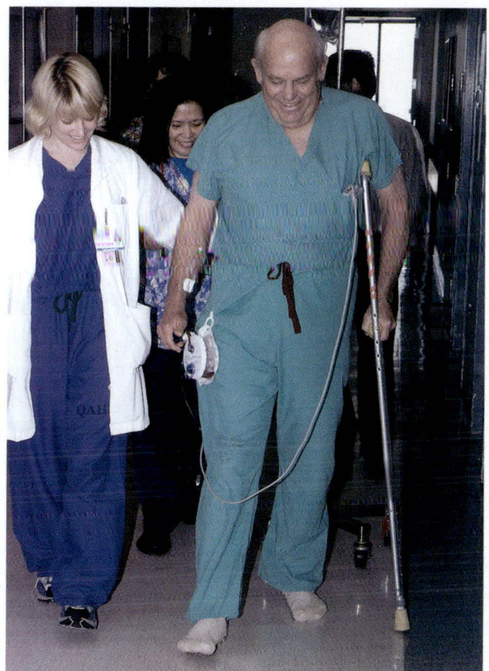

Figure 11–1 *Dr. Dorr walking with a single crutch 4 hours after his surgery with physical therapist Lynn Loxterman. In the background is Vi Gabule, Dr. Dorr's total joint nurse.*

weight on the leg and walk without the aid of a walker as quickly as possible. One of the most valuable lessons I learned from my experience is the importance of the patient's confidence in the recovery process. I had a real "high" when I returned to the room because my leg was strong enough to bear my full weight with the support of only one crutch.

Most of the afternoon was spent taking phone calls from local friends and surgeon friends such as Cecil Rorabeck, Charles Engh, and George Etheridge in Florida. I took a second walk with crutches in the afternoon. In the evening, I had little appetite, so I ate some soup and drank water.

I used ice on my hip almost constantly during the first 48 hours. For obvious reasons, the ice needs to be changed every 3 to 4 hours, and the plastic bag containing it needs to be intact. This is an inexpensive and effective means of controlling discomfort, and I use it on all patients now.

That first night I took a hydrocodone-acetaminophen pill every 3 hours. This medication was welcomed, because it seemed that just as my leg started to ache, the nurse would come with the pill. Moving the leg produced the most pain, and the leg was so heavy that I had to use to my hands to help move it. Being packed with a pillow on the lateral side of my buttock (which elevated the wound slightly) and having a pillow along the lateral side of my leg so that it could fall into an externally rotated position in the pillow allowed me to rest comfortably (Fig. 11–2). I was urinating frequently at night because of the intravenous fluids and the medication. However, I had no nausea, no vomiting, and no feeling of discomfort as long as I lay still. I was able to sleep fitfully because of the preemptive pain medication I received; without it, I would not have slept. I already knew the importance of preemptive pain medication, which had been taught to me by Dr. Tom Mallory, but my experience accentuated this lesson. I am now compulsive about the use of preemptive pain medication for the first 2 nights.

Day 1. I was awake by 6:00 AM, and Jeri Ward, RN, brought me a muffin and coffee. I learned that coffee is not necessarily a good idea in these first few days because it can cause stomach upset, and the caffeine, on top of all the other medications, can make one feel a bit "antsy." I was given 20 mg of oxycodone in the morning. I appreciated this medication because the leg ached. It hurt to put any pressure on the leg, but I was able to walk with a walker around the room and do my morning hygiene at the sink. After walking, I sat in a high chair for 1 hour. The leg had to be supported when sitting; it should not be allowed to hang free. Afterward, I was fatigued and slept.

I continued to have little interest in eating, although that evening Marilyn and my son Michael brought some

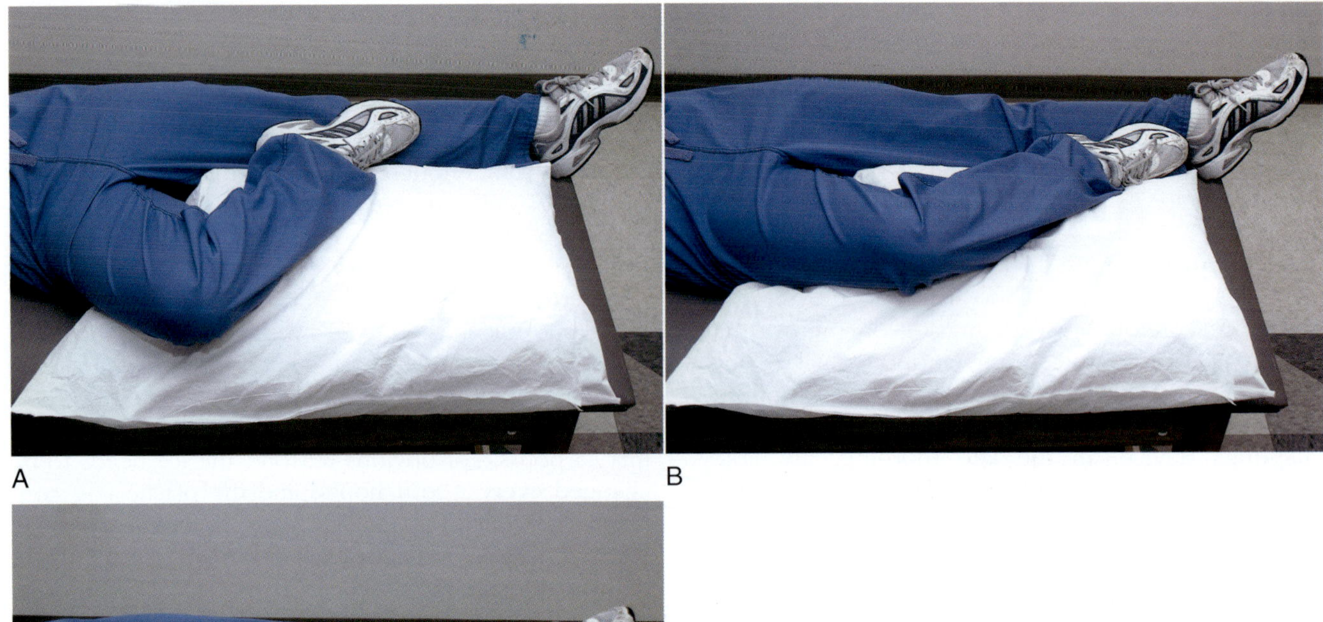

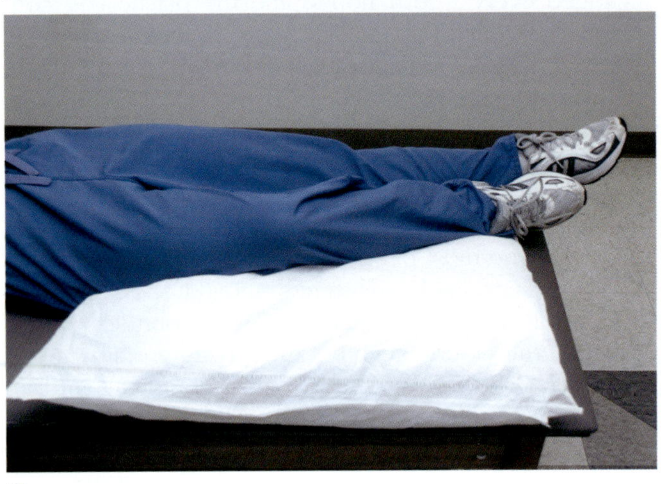

Figure 11-2 **A,** *Comfortable positions for the leg when lying down. A pillow is used to support the leg in external rotation and flexion.* **B,** *The pillow can be brought up under the buttock, and the leg can be moved in various positions of external rotation.* **C,** *Even when the leg is in extension, it is more comfortable lying on a pillow with external rotation.*

food from one of our favorite restaurants that I found appetizing. I was certainly drinking a lot of water. My hematocrit was 33 (my preoperative hematocrit had been 44). However, I had no dizziness, no lightheadedness, and no nausea or vomiting. I had been given an autologous unit of blood during the operation, and I am certain that this "blood doping" contributed to my ability to ambulate with such strength and confidence.

That night, I continued to receive hydrocodone-acetaminophen every 3 hours until 1:00 AM; then I was able to sleep until 6:00 AM without medication.

Day 2. Jeri Ward again brought me coffee and a muffin at 6:00 AM. The muffin tasted great, but I avoided the coffee this time. I was given 10 mg of oxycodone, which relieved the heavy ache in my leg. I read the newspaper and tried to have a bowel movement, without success. At 9:30 AM, I walked using the walker because my leg felt sore; I tried sitting up after walking, but I felt lousy, so at 10:15 I took a nap. During the nap, I sweated so heavily that I soaked all the bedclothes. I had slept for $1\frac{1}{2}$ hours, and when I awoke, I felt very

good. My son Randy was there, and we visited a while. When Marilyn arrived, I announced that I was going home that day. I looped around the hall with a cane, did stairs easily, and left the hospital at 2:30 PM.

When I arrived home at 3:30, I was very hungry. Mike went to a local Mexican restaurant because I was starving for carbohydrates and wanted nachos and jalapeño peppers. After eating, I went straight to bed at 4:30 in the afternoon. I packed my leg with pillows and had to lie on my back because I was too sore to be on my side. I had another episode of heavy sweating. I took two hydrocodone-acetaminophen pills that night—one early in the evening and another at 1:00 AM. Having a urinal at home was a great help, because it meant that I could empty my bladder without having to get up and walk to the bathroom. When I did get up, I was using two crutches, so it would have been a real chore to get to the bathroom. All male patients should be sent home with a urinal, and female patients can try a female urinal or a bedside commode. I slept very well that night and awoke at 7:30 the next morning.

Day 3. It was nice to be home, and I became an advocate of discharging patients as early as possible. The comforts of home and the feeling of independence were great. However, patients will require some help at home for at least a week, so the family must be willing and able to provide the necessary care. For patients without such family support, a longer hospitalization is preferable. It is not necessary for these patients to go to a rehabilitation unit, but a 4- to 5-day hospital stay will facilitate their independence at home.

On this day, I learned a lot about comfortable sitting positions. I sat in a high chair to read the newspaper, but this became uncomfortable after about an hour. I tried a regular chair with the blue hip cushion, but that was terrible. I then rigged the couch with firm supports under the cushions. This made the couch comfortable to lie on, and my leg felt good with a pillow under the knee and the leg leaning against the side of the couch for support. I was able to sleep on the couch and took a 2-hour nap after reading the newspaper. However, it was hard to get up from the couch. The first time I tried, my knee rolled in and I got a shot of pain through the repaired tissues. There was nowhere to support my hands to push myself up out of the couch.

I was now walking in the house with a cane. I had abandoned the single crutch after less than 24 hours because I found the cane much easier to use.

In the afternoon, I tried changing from the chair with a cushion to the chair with regular pillows. This was still somewhat uncomfortable because my right buttock was still sore. However, the day went quickly. I had another nap in the afternoon. I also went outdoors with Marilyn and took a half-mile walk with my cane, which boosted my confidence. That night I took one pain pill at 1:00 AM.

Day 4. When I woke up this morning, I decided to tackle the problem of sitting. I found that the recliner chair was a big improvement and quite comfortable, I simply had to remember to bring the chair to an upright position, slide to the front of the chair, and get up with my leg under me.

I was becoming more independent. I could dress myself, using the dressing stick to ease the process of putting on my pants. I could easily bend to touch my knees, and I could pick something up off the floor by lifting and extending my right leg and leaning over my left leg. I could not get my sock and shoe on my right foot, however, so Marilyn did this for me.

I was now having regular daily bowel movements. For the first 3 weeks, having an elevated toilet seat made it much more comfortable to sit with my sore buttock. I could actually go downstairs normally, although I continued to go one step at a time. I now had enough leg strength to lift my leg in and out of bed, and I was walking in the house without a cane and using the cane only outdoors.

My anterior wound was swollen, and the posterior wound was soft. I was still using povidone-iodine (Betadine) on the wound and a new dressing after I showered, but I had no drainage, so this was really not necessary. I took a 2-hour nap on the couch late in the morning, and I worked in the afternoon writing thank-you letters and answering mail that had been brought from the office. I walked two thirds of a mile twice that day, and I was proud of myself for increasing my distance each time. That night I took two pain pills—one early and one around 1:00 AM.

Day 5. By now I was able to accomplish quite a bit of work during the day. The recliner became my office (Fig. 11–3). I read the newspaper and watched the French Open tennis tournament on TV for entertainment. I was hobbling around without the cane indoors. My leg was definitely getting stronger. The sweats, which I continued to have when I slept, finally stopped by the fifth day. I am not certain if the sweats were caused by the pain medication I took at night or were a function of my body's elimination of the drugs and anesthesia given me in the hospital. In any case, it was good to stop having them, because they were uncomfortable. I can understand why some patients think that this means they are sick or having a complication.

My attention span was still short, but I could do simple work such as dictation and answering mail. I was taking longer and longer walks. Interestingly, I still had no appetite for anything other than light food.

While lying in bed that evening, I had an episode in which my right hip and knee flexed. I turned to my left and allowed my right leg to internally rotate and fall to the left and felt a sharp pain posteriorly. I realized that keeping a pillow between my legs was far more comfortable than going through these painful episodes, so I continued to do it. In fact, I had used a pillow before my surgery for comfort, and it has become such a habit that I still use it today.

Day 6. My metabolism was returning to normal. Food was more appetizing, and I actually ate a small amount of steak. I walked 1 mile with a cane, and I could go down stairs normally. I went the entire day without taking a nap. Showering was easy. I went to my golf club in the afternoon and had a gin and tonic, but based on my experience, I would not recommend drinking alcohol during the healing-in period. It depresses the metabolism and definitely decreases the attention span. That night (and during my entire 2-week healing-in period), I took a hydrocodone-acetaminophen at 1:00 AM, which allowed me to sleep comfortably the second half of the night.

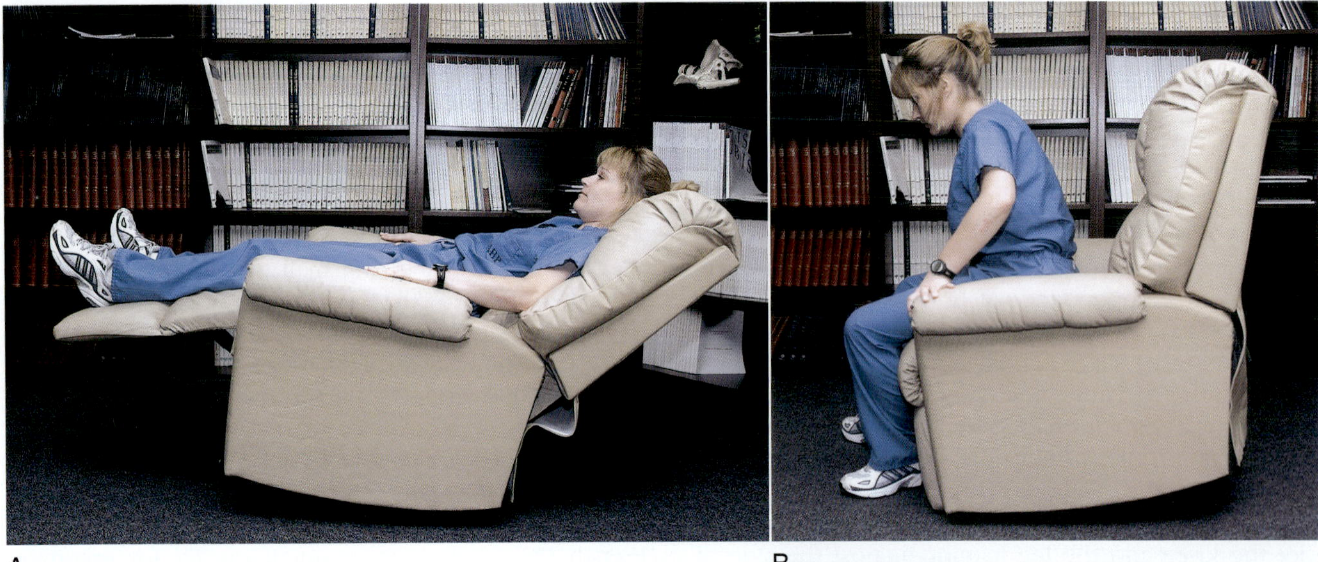

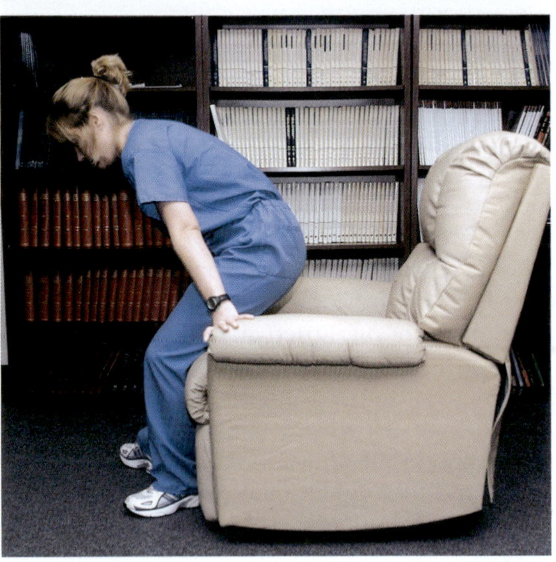

*Figure 11–3 **A,** A recliner chair can be used safely. In the past, there was concern about dislocation with the use of recliners. However, a recliner is dangerous only if someone tries to stand up without first collapsing the chair from the reclined position to the normal sitting position. **B,** The recliner has been collapsed into the regular upright position. By sliding to the front of the chair and using the arms, it is easy to rise from the recliner. Observe that the right foot (operative leg) is in external rotation. **C,** The right foot remains in external rotation until the patient is fully standing. Early after surgery, the leg will be sore and weaker than usual, so it is necessary to push up with the arms.*

Day 7. I had the surgery 1 week ago today. In the morning I went to the hospital and had a duplex scan, which was normal (thank goodness). Jim Morris and Mike Smith filmed me walking in the hall with a cane and doing stairs to show what a patient is capable of 1 week postoperatively. I went to my office for the first time and spent about an hour doing paperwork and then went home. I rested in the afternoon and did not take a walk because I was fatigued. I went to bed early. I still had aching at night and took my usual 1:00 AM pain pill.

By the end of my first week of healing in, I had learned the tricks of using pillows in bed and a recliner chair to achieve comfort. I learned that the patient can do little to accelerate the process and must simply adapt to the new circumstances and the reduced energy level.

Day 8. The days were less exciting after the first week, and the lessons were fewer. My daily routine was becoming repetitive. I was now carrying the cane for some of my 1-mile walk. I continued to work mostly in the recliner. I was eating regularly and still used a pain pill at 1:00 AM.

Day 9. I increased my walking distance to nearly 2 miles and accompanied my wife to a party at night. I drank three gin and tonics at the party, and on my return home, I fell into a very deep sleep that lasted 5 hours. This reinforced my conviction that it is not a good idea to add alcohol to the medications being taken and the altered metabolism during the healing-in phase.

Day 10. Again, I walked nearly 2 miles and went to a movie and a Mexican restaurant, without a cane, in the afternoon.

Day 11. I went to the golf club to putt and chip, which I did for 30 to 40 minutes. After this, plus a 2-mile walk, my leg was sore. However, the return to normal activities was important for my confidence. I was now eating regular food, although my appetite was still not entirely normal. I no longer needed the pain medication at night, but I continued to have trouble finding a comfortable position. My right leg was still heavy and weak, so it was difficult to turn to my left side. I would use the headboard of the bed to leverage myself onto my left side, and once I was there, I was comfortable.

Day 12. I awoke at 5:30 AM, most likely because I did not take a pain pill during the night and this is my usual time to arise. I perused the newspaper, finished a book I was reading, and then took a nap. At 10:15 I went out and got a haircut (this is not really a necessity for me, but it was something to do). I then went to my office and fiddled around for about 2 hours. I did all this without the cane. In the afternoon, I stopped at the golf club and chipped and putted for about an hour and a half. My leg felt sore after this, so I did not take a walk. I returned home and did two journal manuscript reviews and took another nap. That evening, I attended a 90-minute research meeting at a local restaurant, where I had one alcoholic drink. Clearly, I was still not tolerating alcohol well. My activity was now nearly normal for a low-energy day. That night, I had trouble sleeping because of the inability to make the leg comfortable and turn over easily. I took a pain pill at 3:00 AM.

All the Steri-Strips were now off my wound, and the subcuticular tags at the proximal and distal ends of the wound had been removed.

Day 13. After the 3:00 AM pain pill, I slept until 10:30. However, I awoke with great energy and had a productive day. I dictated notes and letters from the previous night's meeting, dictated manuscript reviews, and made some phone calls. In the afternoon, I took a 2-mile walk, my leg felt strong, and I walked 1 of those miles without the cane. I worked all afternoon on paperwork and at 4:30 went on a social outing.

Healing-in Summary. The key to success in these first 2 weeks is rest. It is critical to take naps as needed. Some patients are resistant, but I tell them that rest means:

R—Remember

E—Everything

S—Stabilizes in

T—Time

I also believe that no physical therapy is best. The hip heals itself easily because it is a ball-and-socket joint, which means that the phasic firing of the surrounding muscles occurs much more easily than with a knee joint, for instance, which requires complex interaction of the opposing muscle groups. If the patient is simply willing to walk, the leg will recover. Physical therapy may actually deter the healing process by making the leg sore. During the healing-in period, my leg became sore a number of times, and it was necessary for me to modify my activities accordingly. A well-meaning physical therapist pushing hard on the leg to try to accelerate the regaining of strength can do more harm than good.

Social activities are important during this time to keep up the patient's spirits. The realization that normal activities can be performed, and normal social events can be attended, is a great boost to the patient's morale. Another important confidence-building activity is to do "head work" while resting the leg. The feeling of being productive gives the patient absolute confidence that the operation was a success.

Looking back at my record, I believe that I completed the healing-in phase by 2 weeks. I have seen this phase completed in 1 week in patients younger than 50 years, and I have seen it last for 6 weeks in patients older than 80. Regardless of age, this phase is definitely shorter than it was when intravenous narcotics were used for pain control. The use of intravenous narcotics, and the accompanying lethargy, slows every step of the healing-in phase. Modern pain management techniques are a wonderful advance for hip replacement patients.

Rehabilitation Process

In the first phase of rehabilitation, there is a steady increase in energy and stamina, and patients see weekly improvement. The pace of recovery slows during phase 2 and slows even more in phase 3.

Phase 1: Weeks 3 to 12

In this first phase, patients progressively increase their productivity by returning to work and gradually increasing the number of hours worked each day. They can also participate in social events and exercise. Patients still experience greater than normal fatigue during this period, however, and require more sleep. The time to achieve full productivity varies with the patient, just as the healing-in phase can vary. I was near full productivity by the sixth week, which means that I was able to operate and see patients on a normal schedule and work a normal week. I still had much more fatigue and slept more hours and certainly did not accomplish as much research, writing, and review work as I normally would. By 12 weeks, nearly everyone is back to a normal level of productivity, can play sports such as golf, and has resumed a regular exercise routine. I consider this phase to be the one in which the patient regains stamina.

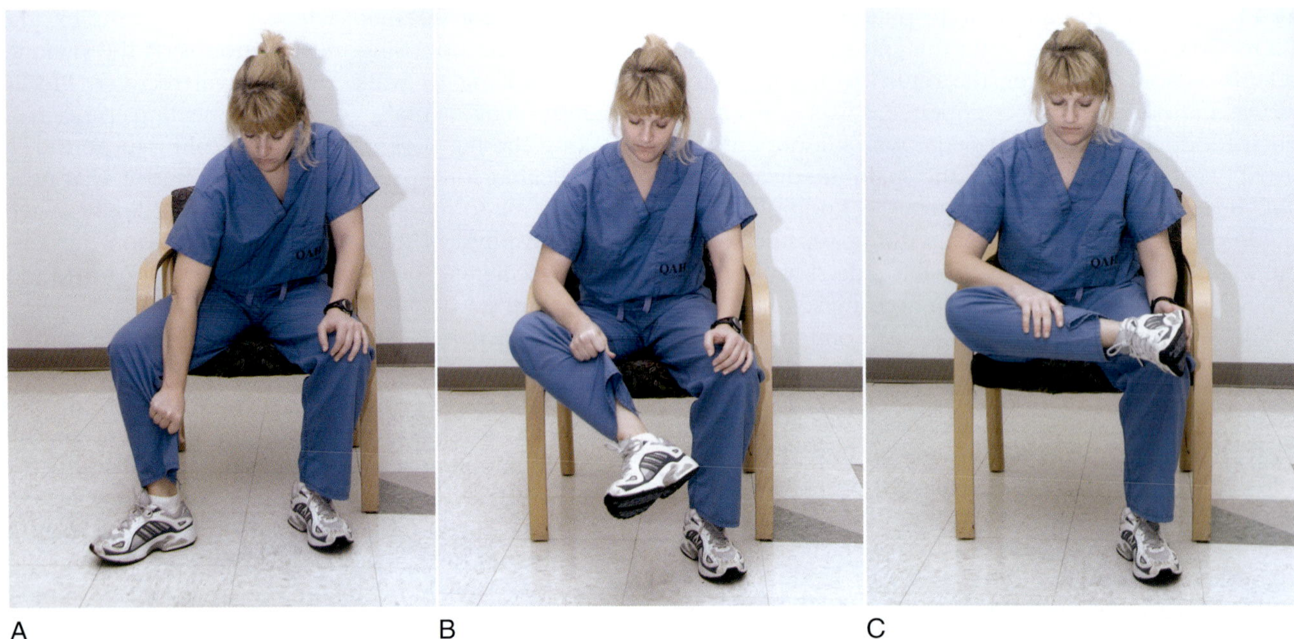

Figure 11–4   *A, In the early postoperative period, the leg will be weak and the area of the incision will be sore. Therefore, it is helpful to grab a pant leg to bring the foot across to the opposite knee. B, The leg can also be lifted. It may be a few days or weeks until the leg is flexible enough to get the foot all the way to the opposite knee and until the posterior hip soreness allows this to be done without lifting the leg. C, It is safe to cross the leg to the opposite knee, which is a good position for putting on socks and shoes.*

Week 3. My third postoperative week began with a trip from Los Angeles to Minnesota, where we have a home on Lake Minnetonka, near Wayzata. I intended to continue my recovery there, in a less stressful environment. I could easily ambulate through the airport using a cane. I slept for 2 hours during the 3-hour flight to Minneapolis. I was also sleeping more easily at night because I was much more comfortable in the side-lying position, particularly the left side. During this week, I walked daily, and my wife and I went on daily excursions to the bookstore, out for lunch, or out to eat in the evening. I still could not tolerate alcohol well, as demonstrated by the night I had two drinks that wiped me out.

I noticed during my walks that I was usually sore for the first part of the walk, but then my walk became stronger and I felt comfortable after the walk. The soreness I had with weight bearing was mostly with heel-strike, with none occurring on toe-off. Therefore, extension of the hip was not painful; my pain was primarily with flexion and loading of the hip. The pain with loading was primarily in the acetabulum (pelvic bone); I had no thigh pain. I had capsular pain that would pull in the back of the hip if I leaned forward beyond its limit or when I tried to lift my foot onto the opposite knee to put on my sock and shoe (Fig. 11–4). I was working on externally rotating my hip and knee and lifting my foot onto the opposite knee as a stretching exercise. Because of this painful pulling on the pos-

terior capsule, it was easier to put on my sock and shoe by going down between my legs, keeping my right knee and foot pointed out, and sliding them on (Fig. 11–5). (Thank goodness for slip-on shoes.) For medication, I was still taking 10 mg of valdecoxib (Bextra*) every morning, but no pain pills at night.

I was able to play golf, which consisted mostly of chipping and putting, for about an hour. I stopped using the TED hose (thigh-high compression stockings) during this week. I was clearly so active that they were of no benefit. Patients who are fully ambulatory the day of surgery and remain so when they go home do not need to use TED hose after 1 to 2 weeks. TED hose can be reserved for low-activity patients or those who have swelling in the leg.

During this week we traveled by car to Rochester, Minnesota, to visit Arlen and Mary Hanssen and their girls. This was a fun day and emphasizes the benefit of social activities.

My productivity this week consisted of mostly head work. I worked on letters and mail and writing. I also did a good deal of reading.

Week 4. By the fourth week, I was able to play golf for 2 hours and began to hit the ball from 150 yards into the green and then play the green side shots. I was

---

*This drug was taken off the market in April 2005.

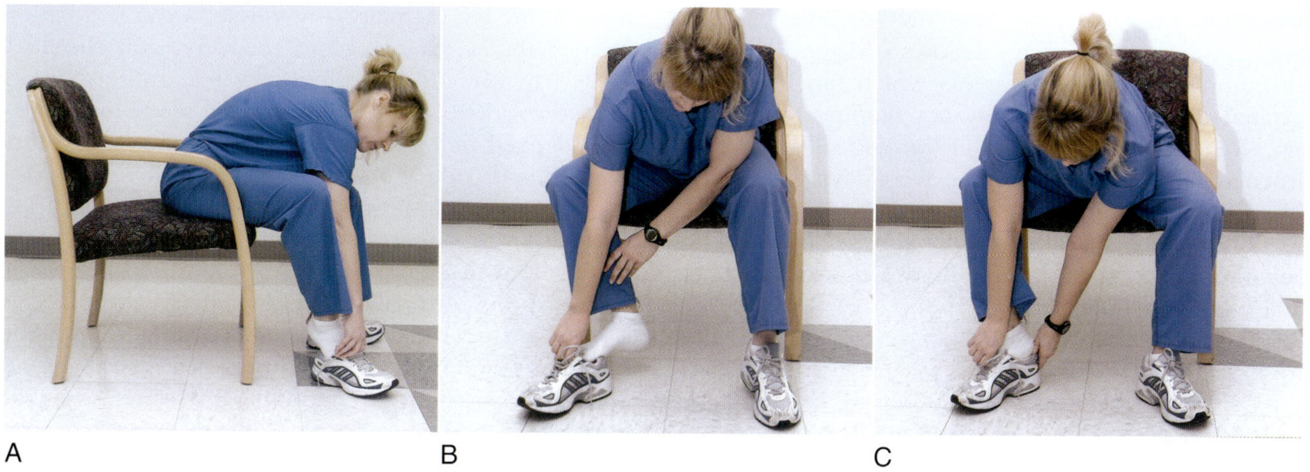

A   B   C

Figure 11–5 **A,** *Socks and shoes can be put on by leaning forward with the body inside the knee of the operative leg. The operative leg should be abducted and externally rotated for this technique.* **B,** *It is fine for the body to be fully flexed forward when the right (operative) leg is in this position. There may be soreness initially, but this will gradually resolve over time.* **C,** *As the soreness disappears from the hip, both hands can be used to dress and to tie shoes.*

riding my exercise bike for 50 minutes, in addition to walking 2½ miles. I did not take Bextra this week, but I took two ibuprofen (Advil) tablets before playing golf. My routine was becoming quite normal for our Minnesota lifestyle. I could sleep on either side, and my leg felt strong. In the second half of the week, I began playing golf with the long clubs and started hitting with Marilyn from the women's tee, first using a five wood and then a three wood. When I had no difficulty with this and no soreness afterward, I proceeded to the men's tee using a driver. I was playing up to nine holes by the end of month 1. I observed that overloading my leg still produced weakness and soreness.

One interesting thing I noted was that during my walks that first month, my hip almost always had a click toward the end of the walk. The more fatigued my leg was, the more frequent the click. Clearly, the capsule of the hip had not healed yet and had not sealed or tightened around the femoral head and neck. There was some distraction of the femoral head from the cup, and I could feel it as it would piston. I did not experience this feeling while doing activities around the house (except on a few occasions), but it was very common at the ends of my walks during the first month. The clicking began to diminish week by week during the second month. By 3 months postoperatively, it was uncommon but still occurred whenever my leg was fatigued; it did not disappear entirely until about 6 months postoperatively

Weeks 5 and 6. I returned to Los Angeles and began to see patients as usual, with no problem with my leg. I was riding my exercise bike and gradually increasing the resistance. By the end of 3 months, I had tripled the resistance from the amount I had started with postoperatively.

At 5 weeks after the operation, I performed a live demonstration surgery for an orthopedics meeting, then traveled about an hour to join the meeting and participate in an afternoon seminar. I have to admit that I had some anxiety about doing a live operation after not operating for 5 weeks, but both the patient and I had a good result. I was definitely getting back into my usual routine and was able to increase my productivity.

Weeks 7 and 8. By now, I was back to my normal routine. I saw patients on Monday, operated on Tuesday and Wednesday, and saw patients again on Thursday. On Friday, I did research work or traveled to teach at a medical meeting. Although I was able to keep up this routine, I was quite stiff, particularly in the lower back, on Tuesdays and Wednesdays after standing and operating for 6 to 7 hours, with some breaks.

I experienced some start-up pain and limping, particularly after putting on my sock and shoe (by bringing my leg across and placing my foot on the opposite knee) but also after riding in a car for a while or even sitting for long periods (such as at a dinner). The capsule was still sore, and the leg position while putting on my sock and shoe stretched that posterior capsule and caused some pain when I first got up. I would have start-up pain and stiffness and limp for 1 to 2 minutes. By 3 months, the start-up stiffness usually lasted for only two or three steps. It did not completely resolve for 6 months. This was clearly capsular discomfort, because there was no thigh pain and no acetabular bone pain.

During this 2-week period, I began to play a full 18 holes of golf. I rode in a cart for most of the holes, but I was still stiff at night. I continued to take two Advil when I played golf.

Weeks 9 to 12. During this time, my schedule was full. I attended a meeting of my fellows (doctors I helped train), and they could not guess which hip had been operated on, so clearly I was not limping much. My limp would generally appear at the end of a full day, particularly if I played golf. The weekdays were filled with my normal routine of seeing patients, operating, and doing research. By this time, almost anyone who does not have to stand or lift all day long can return to a full work schedule.

For medication, I took Advil before playing golf, and I took 20 mg of Bextra in the morning before I operated, because I knew that I would be standing for most of the day. I did not need any pain medication at night. My appetite had returned to normal, and I was eating my usual type and volume of food.

Phase 2: Months 4 to 6

In the second phase of recovery, there is a noticeable increase in the strength of the leg, and activities that require endurance are easier to perform. Sporting activities can be resumed. However, I learned that playing vigorous sports such as racquetball should be postponed a bit longer. When I played racquetball during this period, I observed that I was playing mostly with my left leg and favoring my right leg. I noticed the same pattern when I walked the golf course. Because I tried to be too athletic too soon, I overloaded my left leg and, toward the end of this period, tore the meniscus of my left knee, causing additional discomfort and disability. I did not have any locking or effusion, so I let the tear grind itself away rather than having arthroscopy. My knee healed after several weeks, and I resumed playing racquetball and golf, but it was almost as if nature had forced me to take it easy so my hip could heal. When I returned to sports after my knee healed, my hip had had sufficient time to gain strength (I continued to ride the exercise bike regularly), so I was no longer a left-legged sportsman. I could move laterally quite well when playing racquetball and could walk inclines, up and down, equilibrating the weight on my legs. This experience should teach both doctors and patients that vigorous sports are not advisable for at least 6 months after the operation.

Month 4. During this month, the capsule soreness was significantly reduced, although I still had both mild thigh pain and mild acetabular bone pain. This was certainly not uncommon after standing and performing surgery all day. I also felt mild thigh pain from walking the entire golf course; it did not require any medication, but it was present. I used anti-inflammatory medications before surgery (Bextra) and before golf (Advil). Riding an exercise bike did not bother me, and in fact,

it made my leg (actually, my whole body) feel better. I learned that at this stage of recovery, golf should be limited to one or two times a week; more than that caused overload of the right leg and made me more of a left-legged person. If I played golf one or two times a week and rode the exercise bike on the other days, my leg strength improved almost weekly. It was apparent that I was still arm swinging, mostly when I played golf, so my legs were not really participating in the swing as they normally should.

I must stress the importance of keeping up a walking program (preferably daily) during the first 3 months and, if possible, for 6 months. I became somewhat bored with walking and rode my exercise bike more often than I walked (although I did walk the golf course) in the second 3 months. I rode the exercise bike between 40 and 60 minutes and at the highest resistance I could tolerate so that I got good exercise, both cardiovascular and for my legs.

Month 5. Marilyn and I returned to Minnesota, and I maintained my regular schedule. I would ride the exercise bike daily and go to the golf course and practice for up to 2 hours. Golf relaxed me and filled my day. I still took Advil before playing golf. I was beginning to be able to walk even the hilly parts of the golf course, but I did not walk a full 18 holes during most of this month.

I walked without a limp during most of the day, but I sometimes limped if I had some start-up fatigue after sitting for a long time, in the morning when I first got up, and particularly after I exercised for a while, sat down, and then got up. This is a normal level of disability at this time.

I could lean down to pick something up off the floor or to get my golf ball out of the hole, but I always leaned down inside my right leg and with my right knee pointing out (Fig. 11–6). Whenever I got out of the car on the driver's side, I had to drag my right foot across the floor to the edge of the door and then lift the leg out of the car; then I could load it and walk normally. This weakness has persisted; I still have to slide the foot across the floor of the car a little bit, but the muscle is now strong enough to lift the leg out of the car. Perhaps this is the cost of cutting the external rotators with a posterior approach. I still get into a car sideways and then swing my legs around (Fig. 11–7); this way just seems more comfortable. To put on socks and shoes, I could easily lean down between my knees or put my leg up on a stool and lean down inside my knee to tie the shoe (see Fig. 11–5). I could cross my leg fairly easily and pull the foot up far enough to put on a sock and tie the shoe (see Fig 11–4). There is some persistent stiffness and weakness with this maneuver, which may be another consequence of cutting the external rotators.

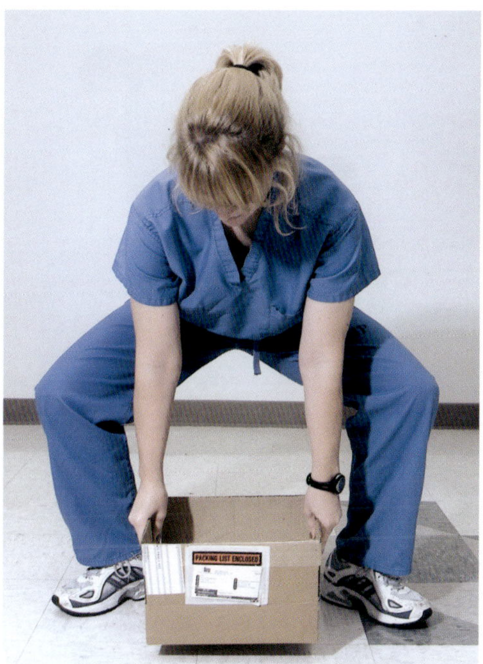

Figure 11–6 *The best technique for picking up items from the floor is to lean down between the knees in a squat-type position. Leaning straight forward is harder on the back, and if the hamstrings are tight, it is difficult to get all the way to the floor. This position is safest for the back and is safe for the hip.*

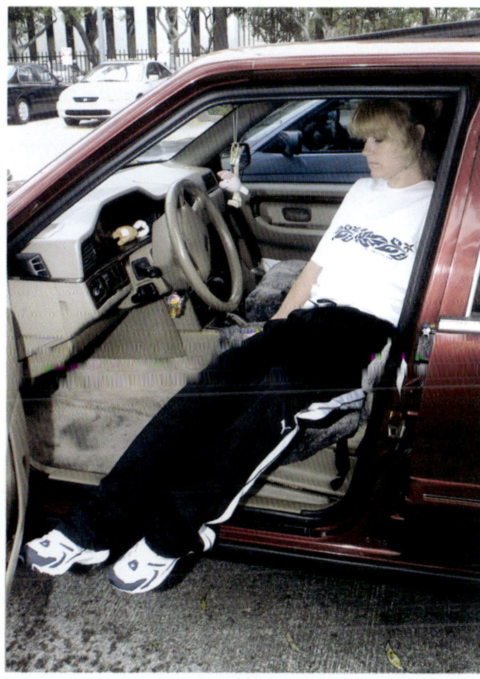

Figure 11–7 *Getting into and out of a car is best done by swinging the legs in from a sideways position.*

I could now get up from chairs without arms. Previously, I needed to use the chair arms to help me get out of the chair. I rose from chairs by pointing my right knee outward and keeping that leg a bit more extended than my left leg; as I stood up, I drew my right leg under my body (Fig. 11–8). This is the way I began getting into and out of chairs immediately after surgery, and the habit became ingrained. Even when I do not use the arms of a chair, I start with my right knee pointing out and bring the right leg under me as I get up.

I began playing racquetball during the fifth month. I could run after the ball and had no abnormal sensation. I had no residual discomfort or pain in the hip after playing racquetball, but as I mentioned previously, I was playing left-legged and favoring the right leg to protect it. By 6 months postoperatively, I had injured my left knee because of this compensation. During the fifth month, I could ride the exercise bike almost normally for 45 minutes with a high resistance (10 to 12 out of 20). I still fatigued more easily, and I needed 8 to 10 hours of sleep to recover from a full day of work and other activities.

I still felt stiff after performing surgery all day and usually took Advil in the morning before surgery or in the evening after surgery. I no longer took Bextra. It is interesting that this stiffness persisted for nearly 15 months, predominantly in my lower back. This is a good example of the deconditioning of muscles that occurs from arthritis and then during recovery after hip replacement. The muscles require a long period of conditioning to regain their normal tone, and this is not something that can be accelerated in any way. Muscle endurance can be increased, but it can be maximized only with time. Bone is known to have a standard osteon remodeling time, and I believe that the final endurance conditioning of muscles is similar to the osteon remodeling time for bone.

I still had episodic pain in the capsule and start-up pain that was fairly intense after certain activities and was present after crossing the leg. I wonder whether the capsular pain persists not only because of healing but also because of the run-in wear of the hip and the debris that is created, which causes inflammation in the capsule. No matter what type of articulation surface is used, there is run-in wear that creates debris, which is a foreign material to the capsule. The capsule clearly adapts to the debris over time, but at this early stage, I think the debris causes an inflammatory response in the capsule.

Another interesting observation was that I definitely had greater stiffness after drinking alcohol, and the more alcohol I had, the stiffer the leg was.

During the fifth month, I became aware of a neurologic pattern I had adopted to protect my right hip and leg. I stood on my left leg in surgery, pushed harder with my left leg on the exercise bike, and played

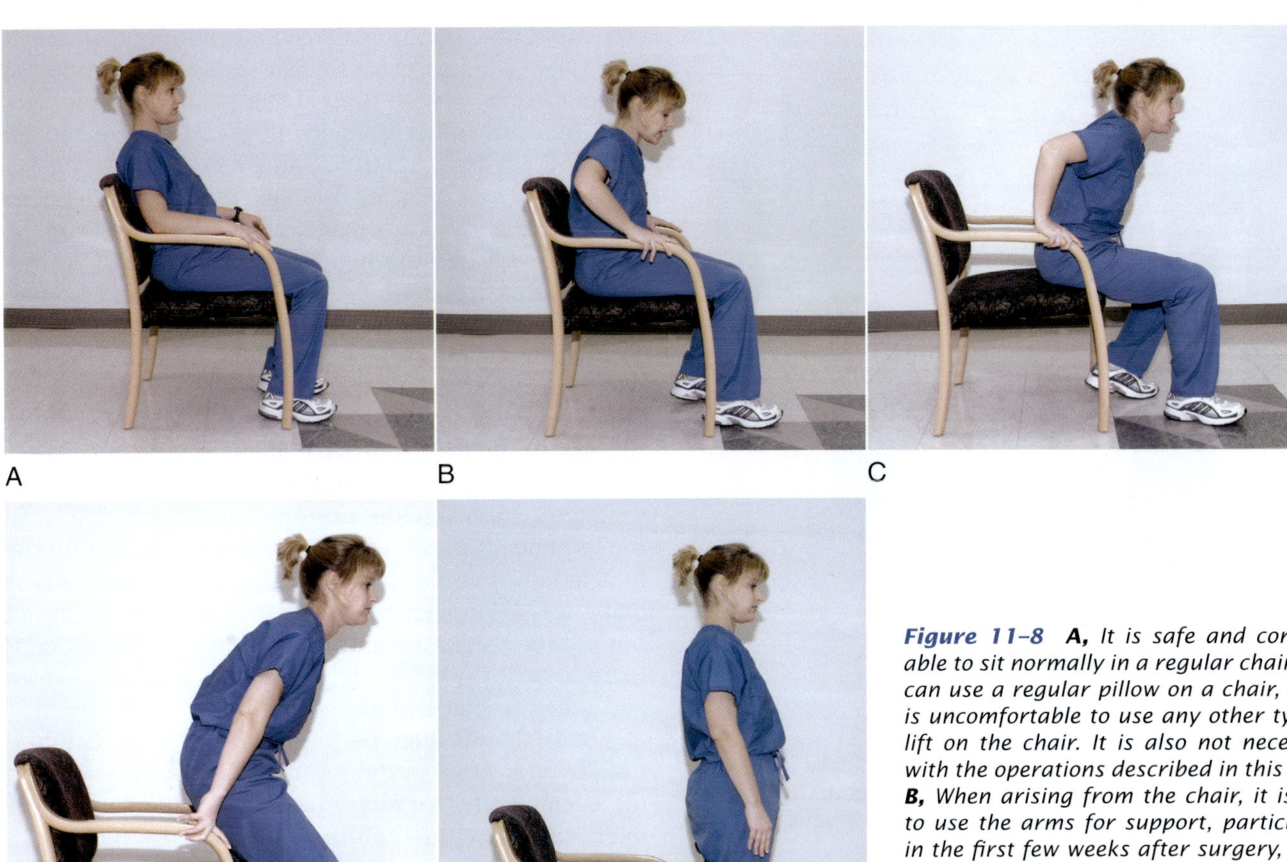

Figure 11–8 *A, It is safe and comfortable to sit normally in a regular chair. One can use a regular pillow on a chair, but it is uncomfortable to use any other type of lift on the chair. It is also not necessary with the operations described in this book. B, When arising from the chair, it is best to use the arms for support, particularly in the first few weeks after surgery, when the leg is still weak and sore. C, By sliding to the front of the chair, it is easy to push up out of the chair without struggling. D, Keeping the right foot turned outward and the right (operative) leg in front of the left leg provides both safety and comfort for the hip. E, After rising from the chair, simply pull the right leg back under the body, and proceed with a normal gait.*

racquetball more off my left leg and had difficulty going to my right. Once I became aware of this pattern, I made a conscious effort to reverse it. I believe that this is advisable for all patients, particularly those who want to participate in athletics. It is necessary to understand this neurologic pattern of protecting the operative extremity and overloading the nonoperative extremity. When I consciously tried to reverse this pattern, I was able to break it, but it took some time. In my case, I think the downtime from my knee injury helped break the pattern. Clearly, overloading my left leg caused the injury to my knee, and I would be unable to participate in vigorous sports until I was equilibrating my weight between my right and left legs.

During this month, my wife also made the comment that I was getting my fast walk back. I have always been in a hurry, but this observation by my wife indicated that my leg was getting stronger.

Month 6. My sixth month was compromised by my knee injury. However, I was certainly able to perform all my medical responsibilities. I traveled to Turkey for a conference, and no one there knew that I had had a total hip replacement. When I mentioned my recent operation, none of the doctors could tell which side it was. The hotel in Turkey did not have an exercise bike, so I tried to use the elliptical machine, but it made my knees sore; they were clearly suffering from my overload neurologic pattern. However, I walked all over Istanbul without any symptoms, and I noticed that I was getting into and out of cars better. I still had some tightness in the back of my hip.

By this time, my hip felt like it was in a steady state. I occasionally felt some aching in the capsule or acetabular bone if my hip was cramped or twisted. This was a transitory ache that seemed to be a consequence of some impingement of the capsule. I still had some start-up stiffness, but the start-up pain was gone. This stiffness occurred only after sitting for quite some time (such as a movie). I had absolutely no standing or walking pain.

An x-ray showed good fixation and wear. The amount of run-in wear measured by Dr. Zhinian Wan was 0.03 mm.

By the end of 6 months, it was obvious that the increased strength of my hip was the greatest improvement during phase 2. I could move laterally in racquetball. I could run more easily and without hesitation. I could stand on either leg to put on my pants, and my balance was good enough to do this. I was getting into and out of the car without any discomfort, but I still had to drag my foot somewhat on the driver's side. I still got posterior capsule pain with my leg crossed, and I still had lower back stiffness after standing all day.

One other observation is that I did not have the same balance I had before I got arthritis, and this is still true today. I do not have grossly abnormal balance or any trouble with balance. However, my righting mechanism is not quite as quick, and I am more likely to lose my balance when I make a quick twisting move or have a slight stumble. I cannot say whether this is a consequence of reduced muscle strength, reduced proprioception, or a central neurologic change. However, there is clearly a difference in balance, and I have heard this same complaint from many patients, so I know that it is real. This slight change in balance seems to be permanent.

Phase 3: Months 7 to 12

During this 6-month period, there is subtle improvement in all areas after the hip replacement. The body metabolism becomes more stable, the sleep requirement is not as great, the tolerance of stress is better, and the workday is easier.

At 8 months, I still had some start-up stiffness, but this was gone by 1 year. I still needed to slide my foot to get out of the car on the driver's side, but this had improved. I occasionally had some thigh pain that persisted for 48 hours after a hard racquetball game, but it did not require any medication. I still had some reduced range of motion for external rotation of the right leg onto the left knee, although I could put on my socks and shoes, and I could cut my toenails with difficulty. By the eighth month, I could play racquetball well and even won a game every once in a while. I could walk the golf course without any difficulty. I could operate 8 hours with some back soreness, and I could tolerate seeing patients all day.

By the middle of this third phase, I had recovered well from the operation, and I realized that it had been extremely successful. My gratitude to Dr. Ranawat for

doing such a wonderful job deepened with each improvement. I now understand why patients are so grateful to those of us who accomplish a successful total hip replacement. It is life changing, taking one from a disabled, painful state to a normal life. Clearly, my leg was not the same as before I had arthritis; I still had some discomfort with certain activities. However, the result was certainly acceptable, and I was continuing to improve with time.

By the end of the first year, I was participating in all the activities I wanted to, including playing racquetball and golf, operating, traveling, and attending social activities. At 1 year, I continued to have some stiffness in my back after performing surgery. I still had to be careful about scheduling too much activity on a given day, such as playing racquetball in the morning and then standing to operate for 8 hours, which would significantly increase my back stiffness. And if I played golf, that would be my only physical activity for that day. By adapting my schedule to what my leg could tolerate, I was able to do everything I wanted to do.

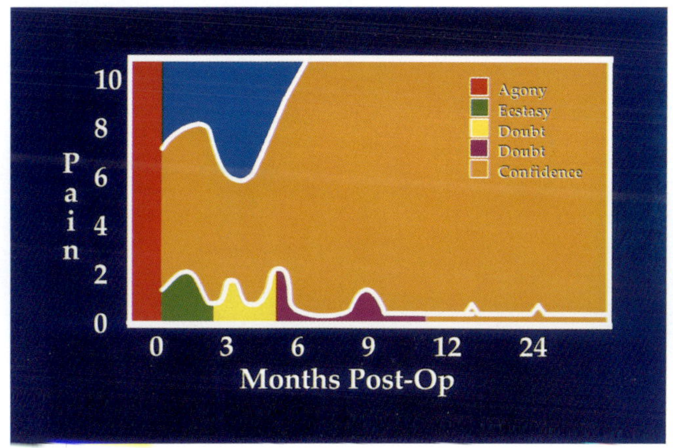

Figure 11-9 *The healing curve. The pain scale is shown along the vertical axis, with a range from 0 to 10, and the postoperative months are shown on the horizontal axis. The period just before surgery is one of agony for patients; in addition to pain, there is functional disability that severely limits their activities. In the first few weeks after surgery, the pain is significantly diminished, and patients are ecstatic about being rid of the pain and the realization that this operation is going to make them better. Between 2 and 6 months, some patients experience a period of doubt because they have episodes of discomfort. These episodes of pain and limping, which are usually caused by a gradual or significant increase in activity, make them wonder whether something has gone wrong with the operation. This period of doubt can extend beyond 6 months for patients who are anxiety prone and for those who did not receive good preoperative and postoperative education and counseling. After 3 to 4 months, almost all patients experience a surge in their confidence, which continues to grow. All patients who have not had a complication have supreme confidence in the success of their operation by 1 year, which is sustained thereafter.*

Continuation of Recovery: Months 12 to 18

Although the majority of recovery has been accomplished by 1 year, it is not over. Healing reaches a steady state by 1 year, with the majority of the healing being stabilized. However, changes continue to occur between 12 and 18 months after surgery. In that period, the stiffness in my back disappeared, and I no longer had to take Advil before I operated. My leg functioned very well for all activities. I traveled quite extensively for medical purposes between 15 and 18 months after surgery and had absolutely no difficulty with the leg. I continued a regular exercise program using the exercise bike. This regular routine was important, because if I missed a few sessions of working out, my leg would ache more. I believe that maintaining the conditioning of the hip muscles adds to the comfort and endurance of the leg.

I have developed a healing curve for total hip replacement (Fig. 11–9). This must clearly be a bell curve. Some patients will have acceleration in some phases of recovery, and some will have retardation. However, this curve is applicable to most patients, and if doctors and patients understand the healing curve, they will keep their expectations in line, will not panic at the occurrence of episodic pain, and will know that recovery and improvement will continue—for as long as 2 years. One of the reasons that follow-up studies of hip replacement are so difficult to perform is that after 2 years, patients are in such good shape that they cannot be bothered going back to the doctor. This confirms the time frame of the healing curve.

Reference

1. Dorr LD, Wan Z: Causes of and treatment protocol for instability of total hip replacement. Clin Orthop 355:144-151, 1998.

Note: Page numbers followed by f refer to figures; those followed by t refer to tables.

B

Contractures, hip, bilateral hip replacement
and, 12-13
causes of, 17
release of, 17-19, 18f, 19f
Converge (APR) cup, 25, 96, 247
Converge shell, 156
Corkscrew, for removal of femoral head
from wound, 187, 188f
Cortical bone, of cotyloid notch, 68, 69f
acetabular reaming and, 145, 145f
impingement and, 133, 133f
in acetabular exposure, 81, 83, 83f
in anterolateral approach, 206, 206f
in posterior approach in revision
surgery, 216, 217f
in standard posterior exposure, 38,
39f, 40f
of femoral neck, removal of, 233
Cosmesis, in posterior mini-incision vs.
standard technique, 56
Cotyloid notch, 19
cortical bone of, 68, 69f
acetabular reaming and, 145, 145f
impingement and, 133, 133f
in acetabular exposure, 81, 83, 83f
in anterolateral approach, 206, 206f
in posterior approach in revision
surgery, 216, 217f
in standard posterior exposure, 35,
38f, 39f
in dysplastic acetabulum, 96, 96f
in leg length assessment, 196
medial wall in, 144f
COX-2 inhibitors, for pain, 4, 5
Crowe dysplastic acetabula, fixation of,
type I, 92, 92f, 167, 168f
type II, 92, 93f, 167, 169f
type III, 92, 93f, 167, 170f
type IV, 92, 92f, 94f, 167, 171f, 172f
in acetabular preparation, 93, 94f, 95-97,
95f-98f
Crutches, postoperative use of, 7t, 8, 265,
279, 279f
with constrained liner, 262
Cup holder, insertion of acetabular
component with, 147f
Cup Out, for removal of acetabular cup,
248, 249f

D

Darvocet (propoxyphene and
acetaminophen), 4, 5
Darvon (propoxyphene and
acetaminophen), 4, 5
Dead space, elimination of, in anterior
mini-incision, 199f
in closure of posterior flap, 51, 53f
in posterior mini-incision, 75f
vs. standard posterior technique, 56
in revision for trochanteric nonunion,
227, 227f
femoral head size and, 51, 117, 118
Deep venous thrombosis, prophylaxis for,
in anterior approach, 181, 182f
Depo-Medrol (methylprednisolone), for
intra-articular injection, 4, 5

Diaphyseal fixation, of femoral revision
stem, 237, 237f
Diaphyseal fracture, in revision surgery,
237-238, 239f, 240
risk of, in removal of cementless stem,
220, 223
Diaphyseal stem, grit-blasted surface vs.
porous coating of, 25
Diary, of rehabilitation period, 278-290
Diprivan (propofol), 3
Discharge, hospital, safety precautions and,
8
use of assistive devices and, 7t, 8
rapid, physical therapy technique for, 6-
12
Dislocation, congenital, acetabular position
in, 98f
constrained liner and, 261
controlled, in posterior mini-incision, 64,
65f, 78
in revision surgery, 214-215, 215f
in standard posterior approach, 32, 34f
of femoral head, in anterior mini-
incision, 186, 186f
in posterior mini-incision, 64, 78
in standard posterior exposure, 32,
34f
with PROfx table, 181
precautions against, 11-12, 11f, 12f, 13f,
261
revision surgery for, 274f
risk of, after revision surgery, 265-266
anterior approach and, 180
Distal window of the iliofemoral approach,
180
Divot, for determining leg length and
offset, 149
for removal of cementless stem, 219, 220f
for removal of femoral implant in
revision surgery, 220f, 232
Dolasetron (Anzemet), for postoperative
nausea and vomiting, 3
Dorsal horn neurons, neurotransmitters
from, 4
Draping, 138, 138f
Drill and screw technique, for removing
acetabular insert, 247-248, 247f, 248f
Driving, after surgery, 17
Dynasil liner, articulation surface of, 28
cementing of, 246, 246f, 247f
placement of, 91f
removal of, 247, 247f, 248f
Dysplasia, acetabular. *See* Acetabulum,
dysplastic.

E

Electrocautery, Bovie, for gluteus maximus
splitting, 230, 231f
for marking femoral neck cut, 32, 35f
in acetabular exposure, 60, 62, 63f, 78
in anterolateral exposure, 205f
in revision surgery, 215, 230, 231f
in standard posterior exposure, 30, 32,
35f
Enterococcal infection, revision surgery for,
272f, 273f

Epicondyle(s), in registration of plane of
leg, 140, 142f
Epidural anesthesia/analgesia, postoperative
physical therapy and, 8
vs. general anesthesia, 3
Epidural catheter, in bilateral hip
replacement, 14
starting infusion in, 3-4
Epsilon constrained liner, 261, 261f
Exercise(s), postoperative, muscle
strengthening, 268
routine, 268
Exercise bike, postoperative use of, 285,
286, 287
Expense, computer navigation and, 132
Extended anterior slide, closure of, 223,
223f, 224f
for cement removal, 233, 234f
for controlled removal of greater
trochanter, 219, 220
for removal of femoral implant, 222-223,
222f-224f, 232, 232f
vs. femoral window, 219, 220
in revision surgery, 212, 222-223, 222f-
224f
muscle preservation and, 230
External oblique muscle, 67, 68f
External rotators, in anterior mini-incision,
192, 193f, 194f
in posterior mini-incision, 62, 63f, 64,
65f, 78, 79f
in revision surgery, 212
in standard posterior exposure, 30, 32,
32f, 33f, 34f
suture closure of, 51, 53f
Extraction device, for removal of femoral
implant, 219, 232

F

Fascia, between gluteus medius and
gluteus minimus, 62, 63f
of gluteus maximus, incision of, 30, 60,
62, 62f
splitting of, in standard posterior
exposure, 30, 32f
Fat, over external rotators, 30, 32, 32f, 33f
pericapsular, overlying hip capsule, 184,
184f
subcutaneous, 184, 184f, 203f
Fat embolism, in bilateral hip replacement,
13-14
Femoral base plate, for computer guidance
system, 73f
removal of, 97, 99f
Femoral canal. *See also* Intramedullary
canal.
in cemented fixation, 123
opening of, 123, 124f
preparation of, 123, 125f, 126, 126f
opening of, 97
with broach, 192, 194f, 195f
with burr, 48, 49f, 72f
with cemented fixation, 123, 124f,
125f, 126, 126f
reaming of, in revision surgery, 235,
236f, 237, 237f, 238f